THIRD EDITION

CLINICAL HANDBOOK
of PEXDIATRICS

D0169978

EDITOR
M. William Schwartz

Associate Editors

Lawrence Brown

Bernard J. Clark III

Catherine S. Manno

Seth L. Schulman

Joseph Zorc

LIPPINCOTT WILLIAMS & WILKINS
A Wolters Kluwer Company

Philadelphia • Baltimore • New York • London
Buenos Aires • Hong Kong • Sydney • Tokyo

Executive Editor: Neil Marquardt
Managing Editor: Daniel Pepper
Marketing Manager: Scott Lavine
Senior Production Editor: Karen Ruppert
Compositor: TechBooks
Printer: Malloy

Library of Congress Cataloging-in-Publication Data

Clinical handbook of pediatrics / editor, M. William Schwartz ; associate editors,
   Lawrence Brown, Bernard J. Clark III, Catherine S. Manno. — 3rd ed.
      p. ; cm.
   Includes index.
   ISBN 0-7817-3649-8
   1. Pediatrics—Handbooks, manuals, etc.   I. Schwartz, M. William, 1935–
   [DNLM: 1. Pediatrics—Handbooks.   WS 39 C6405 2003]
   RJ48.C55   2003
   618.92—dc21

                                                                    2002043420

                                          03   04   05   06   07
                             1   2   3   4   5   6   7   8   9   10

CONTENTS

ELIZABETH R. ALPERN, MD, MSCE
Assistant Professor of Pediatrics
University of Pennsylvania School of
Medicine
Attending Physician, Emergency
Department
The Children's Hospital of Philadelphia
Philadelphia, Pennsylvania

CRAIG A. ALTER, MD
Associate Professor of Pediatric
Endocrinology
University of Pennsylvania School of
Medicine
Pediatric Endocrinologist
The Children's Hospital of Philadelphia
Philadelphia, Pennsylvania

ROBERT N. BALDASSANO, MD
Assistant Professor of Pediatrics
University of Pennsylvania School of
Medicine
Director, Center for Pediatric
Inflammatory Bowel Disease
The Children's Hospital of Philadelphia
Philadelphia, Pennsylvania

JILL M. BAREN, MD, FACEP, FAAP
Assistant Professor of Emergency Medicine
and Pediatrics
University of Pennsylvania School of
Medicine
Hospital of the University of Pennsylvania
The Children's Hospital of Philadelphia
Philadelphia, Pennsylvania

ANDRIA BARNES RUTH
Associate Professor of Pediatrics
Gastroenterology Division
The Children's Hospital of Philadelphia
Philadelphia, Pennsylvania

LOUIS M. BELL
Chief of General Pediatrics
Professor of Pediatrics
The Children's Hospital of Philadelphia
Philadelphia, Pennsylvania

NATHAN BLUM, MD
Attending Physician
Child Development and Rehabilitation
Medicine
The Children's Hospital of Philadelphia
Philadelphia, Pennsylvania

STEVEN M. BOROWITZ, MD
Pediatric Physician
University of Virginia
Charlottesville, Virginia

MICHAEL C. BRAUN, MD
Assistant Professor of Pediatrics
Institute of Molecular Medicine
The University of Texas Medical School
at Houston
Houston, Texas

AMY R. BROOKS-KAYAL, MD
Assistant Professor of Pediatrics and
Neurology
University of Pennsylvania School of
Medicine
Attending Physician, Neurology and
Pediatrics
The Children's Hospital of Philadelphia
Philadelphia, Pennsylvania

JAMES M. CALLAHAN, MD
Associate Professor of Emergency Medicine
SUNY Upstate Medical University
Attending Physician, Pediatric Emergency
Department
University Hospital
Syracuse, New York

AARON E. CARROLL, MD
Clinical Scholar
Robert Wood Johnson Scholars Program
University of Washington
Seattle, Washington

MARINA CATALLOZZI, MD
Fellow, Craig-Dalsimer
Division of Adolescent Medicine
The Children's Hospital of Philadelphia
Philadelphia, Pennsylvania

CINDY W. CHRISTIAN, MD
Assistant Professor of Pediatrics
University of Pennsylvania School of
Medicine
Director, Child Abuse Services
The Children's Hospital of Philadelphia
Philadelphia, Pennsylvania

ESTHER K. CHUNG, MD, MPH
Assistant Professor of Pediatrics
Thomas Jefferson University
Medical Staff
Alfred I. duPont Hospital for Children
Wilmington, Delaware

BERNARD J. CLARK, III, MD
Associate Professor of Pediatrics
University of Pennsylvania School of
Medicine
Senior Cardiologist
The Children's Hospital of Philadelphia
Philadelphia, Pennsylvania

MITCHELL I. COHEN, MD
Pediatric Cardiologist
Phoenix, Arizona

MONICA H. DARBY, BS
Staff Pharmacist
The Children's Hospital of Philadelphia
Philadelphia, Pennsylvania

HENRY R. DROTT, PhD
Director, Clinical Chemistry Laboratory
The Children's Hospital of Philadelphia
Philadelphia, Pennsylvania

JOEL FEIN, MD
Associate Professor of Pediatrics and
    Emergency Medicine
University of Pennsylvania School of
    Medicine
Attending Physician
Emergency Department
The Children's Hospital of
    Philadelphia
Philadelphia, Pennsylvania

JANET H. FRIDAY
Assistant Professor of Pediatrics
Connecticut Medical Center
Hartford, Connecticut

SUSAN A. FRIEDMAN, MD
Assistant Professor of Pediatrics
University of Pennsylvania School of
    Medicine
Associate Physician, Neonatal Follow-up
    Program
Director of Well Newborn Nursery
The Children's Hospital of Philadelphia
Philadelphia, Pennsylvania

ANGELO P. GIARDINO
Medical Director
St. Christopher's Hospital
Department of Pediatrics
Philadelphia, Pennsylvania

MARC H. GORELICK, MD
Associate Professor of Pediatrics and Chief,
    Pediatric Emergency Medicine
Medical College of Wisconsin
Medical Director, Emergency Department
The Children's Hospital of Wisconsin
Milwaukee, Wisconsin

AMY B. HIRSHFELD, MD
Instructor, Pediatrics
University of Pennsylvania School of
    Medicine
Cardiology Fellow
The Children's Hospital of
    Philadelphia
Philadelphia, Pennsylvania

DOUGLAS M. HOFFMAN, MD
Assistant Professor of Pediatrics
Boston University School of Medicine
Associate Director, Adolescent Center
Boston Medical Center
Boston, Massachusetts

TIMOTHY M. HOFFMAN, MD
Assistant Professor of Pediatrics, Division
    of Cardiology
The Ohio State University College of
    Medicine
Columbus Children's Hospital
Columbus, Ohio

MICHAEL D. HOGARTY, MD
Assistant Professor of Pediatrics
University of Pennsylvania School of
    Medicine
The Children's Hospital of Philadelphia
Philadelphia, Pennsylvania

DOUGLAS HYDER, MD
The Children's Hospital of Philadelphia
Philadelphia, Pennsylvania

PAUL ISHIMINE
Division of Emergency Medicine
Children's Hospital Health
    Center of San Diego
UCSD School of Medicine
San Diego, California

THOMAS L. KENNEDY III, MD
Professor of Clinical Pediatrics
Yale University School of Medicine
Chairman, Pediatrics
Bridgeport Hospital
Bridgeport, Connecticut

RICHARD M. KRAVITZ, MD
Assistant Professor of Pediatrics
Division of Pediatric Pulmonary Diseases
Duke University Medical Center
Durham, North Carolina

ANN-MARIE LEAHY, MD
The Children's Hospital of Philadelphia
Philadelphia, Pennsylvania

MARY B. LEONARD
Assistant Professor of Pediatrics
Pediatric Neurology
The Children's Hospital of Philadelphia
Philadelphia, Pennsylvania

LORRAINE LEVITT KATZ, MD
Assistant Professor of Pediatrics
University of Pennsylvania School
    of Medicine
Attending Physician
Division of Endocrinology
The Children's Hospital of Philadelphia
Philadelphia, Pennsylvania

CHRIS ALEXANDER LIACOURAS, MD
Associate Professor of Gastroenterology
and Nutrition
University of Pennsylvania School
of Medicine
Pediatric Gastroenterologist
The Children's Hospital of Philadelphia
Philadelphia, Pennsylvania

DANIEL J. LICHT, MD
Instructor, Department of Neurology
University of Pennsylvania Medical School
Instructor, Child Neurology Division
The Children's Hospital of Philadelphia
Philadelphia, Pennsylvania

KATHERINE MACRAE DELL, MD
Assistant Professor of Pediatrics
Case Western Reserve University
Attending Pediatric Nephrologist
Rainbow Babies and Children's Hospital
Cleveland, Ohio

RANDOLPH P. MATTHEWS, MD
Clinical Instructor, Pediatrics
University of Pennsylvania School of
Medicine
Senior Fellow, Division of Gastroenterology
and Nutrition
The Children's Hospital of Philadelphia
Philadelphia, Pennsylvania

SHOSHANA T. MELMAN, MD
Associate Professor of Pediatrics
Drexel University College of Medicine
Division of General Pediatrics
St. Christopher's Hospital for Children
Philadelphia, Pennsylvania

KEVIN MEYERS, MD
Assistant Professor of Pediatrics
University of Pennsylvania School of
Medicine
Pediatric Nephrologist
The Children's Hospital of Philadelphia
Philadelphia, Pennsylvania

NAHUSH A. MOKADAM

THOMAS J. MOLLEN, MD
Clinical Associate, Neonatology
The Children's Hospital of Philadelphia
Philadelphia, Pennsylvania

LAURA MULREANY, MD
Pulmonary Medicine Fellow
The Children's Hospital of Philadelphia
Philadelphia, Pennsylvania

MICHAEL MULREANY, MD
The Children's Hospital of Philadelphia
Philadelphia, Pennsylvania

FRANCES M. NADEL, MD
Assistant Professor of Pediatrics
University of Pennsylvania School of
Medicine
Attending Physician, Emergency
Department
The Children's Hospital of Philadelphia
Philadelphia, Pennsylvania

MICHAEL NORMAN, MD
Consultant
Charlotte, North Carolina

CYNTHIA NORRIS, MD
Associate Professor of Pediatrics
Hematology Division
Medical Director, Hematology Acute Care
Unit
The Children's Hospital of Philadelphia
Philadelphia, Pennsylvania

GILBERTO R. PEREIRA
Professor of Pediatrics
Senior Neonatologist
The Children's Hospital of Philadelphia
Philadelphia, Pennsylvania

NATASHA S. R. PEREIRA, MD
Attending Physician
Emergency Medicine, Urgent Care
The Children's Hospital of Philadelphia
Philadelphia, Pennsylvania

JONATHAN PLECHTER
Assistant Professor of Pediatrics
Division of Adolescent Medicine
The Children's Hospital of Philadelphia
Philadelphia, Pennsylvania

JILL C. POSNER, MD
Assistant Professor of Pediatrics
University of Pennsylvania School of
Medicine
Attending Physician
Emergency Department
The Children's Hospital of Philadelphia
Philadelphia, Pennsylvania

MADHURA PRADHAN, MD
Instructor, Department of Pediatrics
University of Pennsylvania School of
Medicine
Attending Physician
Nephrology Department
The Children's Hospital of Philadelphia
Philadelphia, Pennsylvania

CLAUDIO RAMACIOTTI, MD
Pediatric Cardiologist
Children's Medical Center of Dallas
Dallas, Texas

MITCHELL ROBERTS, MD

JACK RYCHIK, MD
Medical Director, The Fetal Heart Program
Director, Echocardiography Laboratory
Attending Cardiologist
The Children's Hospital of Philadelphia
Philadelphia, Pennsylvania

MARTA SATIN-SMITH
Children's Hospital of the King's Daughters
Department of Endocrinology
East Virginia School of Medicine
Norfolk, Virginia

COURTNEY SCHREIBER, MD
Hospital of the University of Pennsylvania
Philadelphia, Pennsylvania

SETH L. SCHULMAN, MD
Associate Professor of Pediatrics
University of Pennsylvania School of
  Medicine
Attending Physician
Nephrology Department
The Children's Hospital of Philadelphia
Philadelphia, Pennsylvania

CHARLES I. SCHWARTZ, MD, FAAP
Assistant Clinical Professor of Pediatrics
University of Pennsylvania School of
  Medicine
General Pediatrician
Phoenixville Hospital
Phoenixville, Pennsylvania

MITCHELL SCHWARTZ
General Pediatrician
Philadelphia, Pennsylvania

SAMIR S. SHAH, MD
Clinical Instructor, Pediatrics
University of Pennsylvania School
  of Medicine
Fellow, Divisions of General Pediatrics and
  Infectious Diseases
The Children's Hospital of
  Philadelphia
Philadelphia, Pennsylvania

KATHY N. SHAW, MD, MSCE
Professor of Pediatrics
University of Pennsylvania School of
  Medicine
Chief, Division of Emergency Medicine
The Children's Hospital of Philadelphia
Philadelphia, Pennsylvania

LAURA N. SINAI, MD, MSE
Lockman-Lubell Pediatrics Associates
Fort Washington, Pennsylvania

KIM SMITH-WHITLEY, MD
Associate Director, Sickle Cell Program
Attending Physician
Hospital of the University of Pennsylvania
Philadelphia, Pennsylvania

**PAUL S. THORNTON, MB, BCh,
MRCPI**
Assistant Professor of Pediatrics
University of Pennsylvania School
  of Medicine
Clinical Director, Hyperinsulinism Center
Division of Endocrinology
The Children's Hospital of Philadelphia
Philadelphia, Pennsylvania

NICHOLAS TSAROUHAS, MD
Assistant Professor of Pediatrics
University of Pennsylvania School
  of Medicine
Attending Physician, Emergency Medicine
The Children's Hospital of Philadelphia
Philadelphia, Pennsylvania

STUART WEINZIMER, MD
Assistant Professor of Pediatrics
Yale University School of Medicine
New Haven, Connecticut

CATHERINE C. WILEY
General Pediatrics
Connecticut Medical Center
Hartford, Connecticut

JAMES F. WILEY III
Chief of Emergency Medicine
Department of Pediatrics
Connecticut Medical Center
Hartford, Connecticut

ALBERT C. YAN, MD
Assistant Professor of Pediatrics and
  Dermatology
University of Pennsylvania School
  of Medicine
Attending Physician, Pediatric
  Dermatology
The Children's Hospital of Philadelphia
Philadelphia, Pennsylvania

JOSEPH ZORC
Assistant Professor of Pediatrics
Department of Emergency Medicine
The Children's Hospital of Philadelphia
Philadelphia, Pennsylvania

KATHERINE ZSOLWAY, DO
The Children's Hospital of Philadelphia
Philadelphia, Pennsylvania

Preparing this third edition of the *Clinical Handbook of Pediatrics* and reviewing the past two editions gives an interesting perspective to the state of pediatrics. For many topics, such as abdominal masses and proteinuria, little has changed. For others, such as ear pain, (otitis media), the debate continues on when and if to treat with antibiotics. Unfortunately, child abuse continues to be a problem with no real breakthroughs in prevention or treatment. On the other hand, control of HIV transmission to newborns has been reduced dramatically with treatment of the mothers prior to delivery. Survival of patients with hypoplastic left heart syndrome exceeds 90% at major cardiac surgical centers. New treatment of diabetes has improved the lifestyles of many patients. Immunizations continue to reduce childhood infections and meningitis. New viruses continue to threaten our health and keep cable news shows discussing them with resultant increased fear from viewers.

The challenge in organizing this edition was to make sure that these improvements were integrated into the text, keeping to the philosophy of describing practical approaches to the common problems of children. The authors of the chapters succeeded in reaching this objective. Many new authors replaced writers from the first two editions; they took over editing or rewriting the chapters with great skill and enthusiasm. The various editors fulfilled their mission of conciseness so that the book did not exceed the allotted space. I appreciate their efforts.

Special thanks to the associate editors Larry Brown, BJ Clark, Catherine Manno, Seth Schulman, and Joe Zorc, who, despite many demands on their time, worked with the authors to complete this revision on time. The staff at Lippincott Williams & Wilkins changed from the last edition but the new personnel, especially Dan Pepper and Karen Ruppert, kept the project on schedule. My special thanks to Cheryl Kosmowski who coordinated the project and handled communications between the authors, editors, and publisher.

M. William Schwartz
Philadelphia

1

Patient History and Physical Examination Write-Up

M. William Schwartz

This chapter presents a guide to a full patient write-up. Not every item described in this chapter is necessary in every write-up. The write-up is a document that records only the most pertinent information; the reader should not be overwhelmed with details that do not tell the patient's story.

▼ HISTORY

Chief Complaint

The chief complaint should be recorded in the patient's or parent's own words. The age and sex of the patient, as well as the duration of the problem, should also be noted.

History of Present Illness

A clear, concise chronology of important events surrounding the problem should be obtained. When did the problem start? How has it changed over time? What tests and treatments were performed? Include only important negatives. This is not the place to show that you asked all the questions.

Medical History

▼ **Prenatal history**—mother's weight gain; number of pregnancies; length of pregnancy; presence of complications, abnormal bleeding, illness, or exposure to illness; medications taken during pregnancy

▼ **Birth history**—parity of mother; birth weight; duration of labor; use of induction, anesthesia, or forceps

▼ **Neonatal history**—jaundice, cyanosis, respiratory problems, or other conditions present at birth; positive physical findings that relate to the current problem; feeding method; time spent in the hospital; discharge (with mother, or later?)

▼ **Developmental history**—milestones for smiling, rolling over, sitting, standing, speaking, and toilet training; growth landmarks for weight gain and length

▼ **Behavioral history**—personality, friends, play activities, interests, favorite television programs, sleeping and eating habits, sexual activity

▼ **Immunization history**—immunizations by type and date, dates of recent boosters, recent tuberculosis testing results

---

✄ HINT A statement in the patient's write-up that the patient's immunizations are "up to date" does not indicate whether recent changes in the recommendations were followed. Specific dates should be provided whenever possible.

▼ **Past medical history**—childhood illnesses, estimated frequency of infections

▼ **Surgical history**—procedures, complications, dates of each

Review of Systems

Do not duplicate the history of the present illness in this section of the write-up.

- ▼ **Head**—injuries, headaches, hair loss, scalp infections
- ▼ **Eyes**—acuity of vision; use of glasses; history of discharges, abnormal tearing, or injuries; prior surgery
- ▼ **Ears**—acuity of hearing; history of otitis, discharges, or foreign bodies
- ▼ **Nose**—breathing difficulties, discharges, bleeding, sinus infections
- ▼ **Oral cavity and throat**—frequency of sore throats, dental problems, bleeding gums, herpes infections, ulcers
- ▼ **Lungs**—exercise tolerance (ability to keep up with peers during exercise), breathing difficulties, cough, history of pneumonia, wheezing, pains, hemoptysis, exposure to tuberculosis, previous chest radiographs
- ▼ **Heart**—exercise tolerance; history of murmurs; history of rheumatic fever in patient or family; history of Lyme disease or other infections that may affect the heart; feeling of heart racing, dyspnea, orthopnea, or chest pain; cyanosis; edema
- ▼ **Gastrointestinal system**—appetite, weight changes, problems with food (e.g., allergy, intolerance), abdominal pain (location, intensity, precipitating events), bowel movements (number and character), jaundice, rectal bleeding
- ▼ **Genitourinary system**—history of infection, frequency of urination, dysuria, hematuria, character of the urine stream, bed wetting, urethral or vaginal discharge, age of menarche
- ▼ **Extremities**—joint or muscle pain, muscle strength, swelling, limitation of movement
- ▼ **Neurologic system**—seizures, weakness, headaches, tremors, abnormal movements, development, school achievement, hyperactivity
- ▼ **Skin**—rashes, type of soap and detergent used

Family History

Ages of Parents and Siblings

- ▼ **Family history of illness**—seizures, asthma, cancer, behavior problems, allergies, cardiac disease, unexplained deaths, lipid disorders
- ▼ **Deaths in family**—causes of, age of family member at the time
- ▼ **Social history**—other household members, sleeping arrangements, marital status of the parents, parents' employment status, health insurance status

---

⚨ HINT   In a patient with a suspected metabolic disorder, the most important question concerns early deaths of the patient's siblings or cousins. In a patient with a suspected infectious disease problem, the most important question concerns the patient's contact with others who are ill.

▼ PHYSICAL EXAMINATION

- ▼ **General appearance**—cooperation, evidence of acute or chronic illness, evidence of disproportion of height and weight, deformities
- ▼ **Measurements**—height (length) and weight compared with average percentiles for the patient's age
- ▼ **Skin**—rashes, distinguishing marks (e.g., nevi, hemangioma)

▼ **Lymph nodes**—size, location, tenderness, or warmth
▼ **Head**—contour, abnormal appearance, size and shape of the fontanelles, bruits
▼ **Eyes**—color of sclerae and conjunctivae, nystagmus, photophobia, estimate of vision, pupil size and reaction to light, appearance of fundus (i.e., color and sharpness of the disc, arteries, and veins; presence of hemorrhages or exudates)
▼ **Ears**—gross deformities of the pinna or abnormal openings (e.g., branchial cleft sinus), tenderness caused by traction on external ear, exudate in the ear canal, appearance of the tympanic membrane, ability to see ossicles, movement of tympanic membrane following air insufflation
▼ **Nose**—patency, flaring, color of the mucous membranes, presence of polyps, color and amount of any exudates
▼ **Oral cavity and throat**—color of the mucous membranes, number and condition of teeth, evidence of exudate, condition of the tongue, tonsil size, movement of the tongue and posterior pharynx, presence of ulcers
▼ **Neck**—range of motion, palpable lymph nodes or thyroid, position of trachea, symmetry, tenderness, carotid pulsations
▼ **Chest**—contour, equal excursion with respirations
▼ **Lungs**—retraction; percussion symmetry; air entry; breath sounds heard equally well in all segments; evidence of rales, wheezing, or rhonchi (transmitted sounds from the upper airway); friction rub
▼ **Heart**—visible pulsations, thrills, heart sounds (ease of hearing, quality, description of second heart sound at the base), rate, rhythm, murmurs [location, diastolic or systolic], grade (I–VI), quality (blowing, coarse, vibratory), transmission]
▼ **Abdomen**—shape (distended or flat), visible veins, peristalsis, quality of bowel sounds, tenderness, palpable organs
▼ **Back**—range of motion; evidence of kyphosis, lordosis, or scoliosis (determined by examining the spine with the patient bent forward); dimples or cysts in the sacral area
▼ **Genitalia**
  ▼ **Girls**—evidence of fused labia, imperforate hymen, or enlarged clitoris; color of mucosa; evidence of infection (e.g., discharge, foul odor); pubic hair
  ▼ **Boys**—palpable testes; condition and ease of retraction of foreskin; evidence of infection (e.g., discharge); location and size of meatus; pubic hair
▼ **Anus**—evidence of hemorrhoids, fissures, sphincter tone, presence of stool in the vault, masses
▼ **Extremities**—range of motion; presence of deformities, a limp, or dislocated hips
▼ **Muscles**—size, tone, strength
▼ **Neurologic system**
  ▼ **Abnormal movement**—tremors, twitches, athetosis
  ▼ **Coordination**—rapid alternating movements, finger-to-nose, heel/toe gait, past pointing, ability to perform rapid alternating movements of the hands, ability to stand with eyes closed and move the heel down the opposite shin
  ▼ **Cranial nerve function**—see Chapter 2, "The Physical Examination," Table 2.3

▼ **Reflexes**—symmetry of deep tendon reflexes; biceps, triceps, patellar, and Achilles reflexes; plantar, cremasteric, and anal wink reflexes; sucking, rooting, and Moro reflexes (in infants)
▼ **Sensory examination**—touch, pain, temperature, position, vibration

▼ HINTS FOR PATIENT PRESENTATIONS

One of my images of hell is to be forced to spend a day listening to medical students' case presentations on rounds—both of them. —Burt Sloane

Consider the Audience and Setting

The group members often have short attention spans, are usually standing, and often have other obligations. Make a **brief presentation,** no longer than 2 minutes, that offers highlights of the problem and leads the audience to the diagnosis. This is not the time to demonstrate your thoroughness or compulsive nature.

Also **consider the style** of the preceptor and those attending. Some may prefer a Socratic dialogue while others want a more detailed presentation. Keep in mind that the Socratic style leads to interactive questions and answers. It is important, however, to appreciate the time pressures of audiences in inpatient rounds or clinics.

In contrast, **grand rounds** or formal case presentations may last as long as 10 minutes. These presentations focus on a diagnostic dilemma with many differential diagnoses, provide data for someone else to discuss with regard to findings and reaching a diagnosis or treatment, and include detailed histories, many negative findings, and most laboratory test results.

Decide What Information Is Important to Include

It is important to **decide what negative information to include** in the presentation and what to rule out. The negative information should help to exclude one or two of the major differential diagnoses. For example, you should mention respiratory distress in a case of cardiac failure but not in a case of urinary tract infection. Likewise, you should mention family history in a case of asthma or mental retardation but not in leg trauma.

After gathering information about the patient's problem, **select the highlights,** arranging them in an interesting and logical manner to lead to the diagnosis.

Organize the Presentation

The following format is suggested.

Chief Complaint

State in the patient's or parent's words the reason for referral or admission. Mention the patient's age and the source of the referral. Avoid starting with a list of descriptors (e.g., "product of a gravida 1, para 1 full-term pregnancy" or "was well until 2 days before admission, when the following events occurred").

History of Present Illness

Give a summary of the pertinent events preceding admission and the changes in the patient's condition that precipitated the visit.

Review of the Patient History

Include only information that suggests the diagnosis or rules out major differential diagnoses. Consider the patient's developmental history, immunization history, past medical history, and family and social history.

Physical Examination Findings

Discuss how the child looked, but include only pertinent positive findings and the few negative findings that help to eliminate major differential diagnoses or lead to the diagnosis. If applicable, include other information such as the parents' expectations for the visit. Finally, summarize the facts that lead to the diagnosis.

Audience Questions

Be prepared for questions. They are compliments and mean that the audience was listening and thinking about the problem and the information you discussed. Questions are not criticisms of an incomplete presentation. Therefore, do not respond by adding more detail to your next presentation.

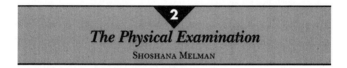

2

The Physical Examination

SHOSHANA MELMAN

▼ GENERAL CONSIDERATIONS
Performing the Physical Examination

The physical examination of a child is as much an art as a scientific procedure. The goal is to make the examination as productive and nontraumatic as possible for both the child and yourself.

To **minimize fear** in young children, conduct most of the physical examination with the child sitting on the parent's lap or nestled against his or her shoulder. Talk with the parent first, while seeming to ignore the child, so that the child has a chance to study you. Speak quietly, using a friendly tone of voice. Move gently and slowly, avoiding loud, sudden movements.

The physical examination is routinely presented and written in standard (adult) order, although it may not be carried out in that sequence. Children about 8 years and older can usually be examined easily in standard adult order, but with younger patients it is important to **examine the most critical areas first,** before the child cries. Always start with observation. Next, in a young child with a specific presenting complaint, it is often helpful to examine the corresponding organ system. In a young child with no specific complaints, palpate the fontanelles, then auscultate the heart and lungs. Wait until the end of the examination to check the most threatening areas (e.g., the ears and oral cavity).

Special Concerns
Mental Status

Because children often cannot vocalize their symptoms, their overall mental status is an essential clue to their degree of illness. Will the child smile or play? Observe interactions with parents or siblings. Be careful to differentiate a child who is simply tired from one who is lethargic (difficult to arouse). Similarly, distinguish the cranky child who comforts easily from one who is truly irritable and inconsolable.

> **HINT** Cranky, febrile young children are often much more pleasant after their fevers are brought down. Children with meningitis are not easily comforted by being held; in fact, when picked up they may cry more.

Hydration Status

Physical findings consistent with dehydration include an increased pulse, decreased blood pressure, sunken fontanelles, dry mucous membranes, decreased skin turgor, and increased capillary refill time (more than 2 seconds).

▼ VITAL SIGNS AND STATISTICS

Temperature

Body temperatures are more labile in children than in adults and can be raised depending on the time of day (i.e., in the late afternoon) or following vigorous activity, excitement, or even eating.

A child's **normal oral temperature** is similar to an adult's, typically about **98.6°F.** The rectal temperature is typically approximately 1° higher than the oral equivalent, and an axillary temperature (the least accurate method) is typically about 1° lower. Study results regarding the reliability of tympanic thermometers have been mixed; they are often used in low-risk older children in busy office settings.

> **HINT** An infant or young child can have a temperature of 103°F–105°F, even with a minor infection. In contrast, a sick newborn may have a lower than normal temperature.

Pulse Rate

In an infant, palpate for pulse rate over the brachial artery. In an older child or adult, the wrist is generally the optimal location. Pulse rate is usually **120–160 beats/min in the newborn** and steadily **declines as the child grows.** A typical teenager's pulse rate would be 70–80 beats/min.

> **HINT** In infants and children, the pulse rate responds much more distinctly to disease, exercise, or stress than it does in adults.

Respiration Rate

The most accurate measurements are obtained while the patient is asleep. In infants and young children, breathing is mostly diaphragmatic; the respiratory rate can be determined by **counting movements** of the abdomen. In older children and adolescents, chest movement should be **directly observed.** Normal pediatric respiratory rates are summarized in Table 2.1.

> **HINT** Infants typically exhibit "periodic breathing," short periods of rapid breathing followed by several seconds without a breath. Pauses of 10 seconds or more are abnormal.

TABLE 2.1. Normal Pediatric Respiratory Rates (Respirations/Min)			
Newborns	Toddlers	School-age Children	Adolescents
30–50	20–40	15–25	12

Blood Pressure

To obtain an accurate blood pressure measurement, **patient relaxation** is especially critical. Explain to a young child that the "balloon" will squeeze his arm, and encourage him to watch the display.

Cuff width is also important. Choose a cuff width that covers 50%–75% of the upper arm length. A too-narrow cuff may artificially increase the blood pressure reading.

If you are concerned about the possibility of heart disease, check blood pressure in **all four extremities.** Compare blood pressure measurements with standard norms for age and sex.

Length (Height)

To obtain a length measurement, place the infant on a firm table. Hold the baby's feet against a stationary board, keeping the knees straight, and bring a movable upright firmly against the baby's head to measure the infant's recumbent length.

Children older than 2 years can be measured with the child standing erect. The child should be positioned with feet flat, eyes looking straight ahead, and occiput, shoulders, buttocks, and heels against a vertical measuring board.

Figure 2.1 shows the National Center for Health Statistics percentiles for physical growth in girls and boys from birth through the age of 20 years.

Weight

Routinely **weigh infants unclothed.** For patients in whom small variations in weight are important, it is helpful to consistently use a single scale, preferably at the same time of day.

The growth charts in Figure 2.1 include **body mass index, or BMI** (wt/ht^2). This number is used in patients ≥ 2 years of age to determine if weight is appropriate for height. By plotting BMI for age, health care providers can achieve early identification of patients at risk for being overweight/obese.

▼ HEAD
Head Circumference

Start your examination of the head by measuring the head circumference at the maximum point of the occipital protuberance posteriorly and at the mid-forehead anteriorly. **Microcephaly** (small head size) could result from abnormalities such as craniosynostosis (premature fusion of the sutures) or congenital "TORCH" infection. **Macrocephaly** (large head size) could be caused by problems such as hydrocephalus or an intracranial mass. Normal head circumferences are presented in Figure 2.2.

A. GIRLS: BIRTH TO 36 MONTHS

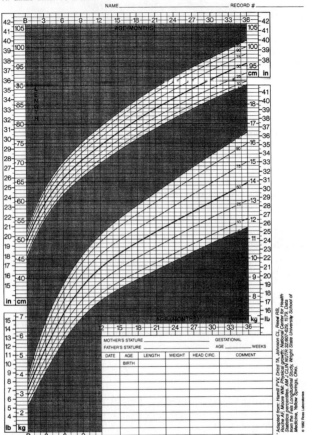

FIGURE 2.1. National Center for Health Statistics (NCHS) percentiles for physical growth in girls.
(A) Girls, age 0–36 months. (B) Girls, age 2–18 years. (C) Boys, age 0–36 months. (D) Boys, age 2–18 years. (Used with permission of Ross Products Division, Abbott Laboratories, Columbus, OH 43216; from NCHS Growth Charts, ©1982 Ross Products Division, Abbott Laboratories.)

Skull Depressions

Depressions of the skull may represent fractures but are most commonly **sutures** (i.e., membranous tissue spaces that separate the skull bones) and **fontanelles** (i.e., areas where the major sutures intersect, also known as "soft spots"). The cranial sutures usually overlap in the newborn because

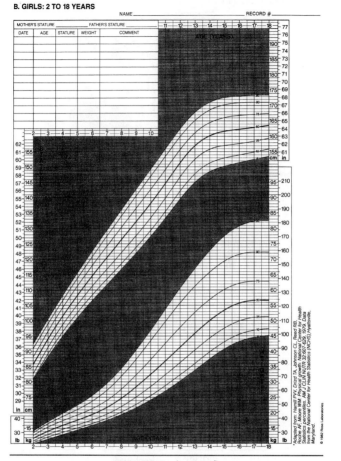

FIGURE 2.1. (continued)

of intrauterine pressure. Sutures that are widely palpable after 5–6 months of age may indicate hydrocephalus.

The anterior fontanelle is 4–6 centimeters in diameter at birth and usually closes between the ages of 4 and 26 months. The posterior fontanelle is usually 0–2 centimeters at birth and generally closes by age 2 months. When describing fontanelles, mention their status (open or closed), size, and fullness. If palpated while the baby is sitting, a tense or elevated fontanelle may reflect increased intracranial pressure. A depressed fontanelle can be a sign of dehydration.

C. BOYS: BIRTH TO 36 MONTHS

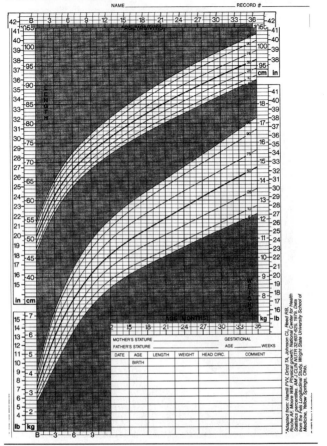

FIGURE 2.1. (continued)

▟ **HINT** At birth, the anterior fontanelle may appear closed as a result of overriding sutures from molding of the head during parturition.

▟ **HINT** Try to examine the anterior fontanelle with the child calm and sitting upright.

Head Shape

Observe the shape of the child's head. Areas of **flatness,** especially in the occipital or parietal regions, may be caused by lying too long in one position

D. BOYS: 2 TO 18 YEARS

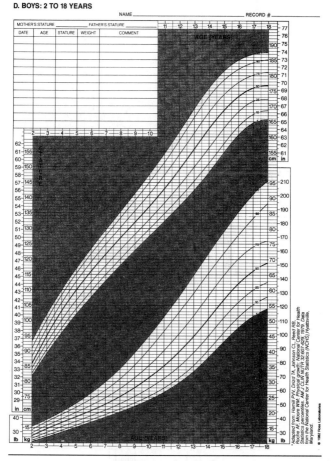

FIGURE 2.1. (continued)

and may occur in an infant suffering from neglect, prematurity, or mental retardation. **Frontal bossing** may be a sign of rickets. Areas of **localized head swelling** could be caused by neoplastic, infectious, or traumatic processes.

Newborns often have **caput succedaneum** (a soft swelling of the occipitoparietal scalp) caused by injury during birth. **Cephalohematoma,** another birth injury, is a swelling caused by subperiosteal hemorrhage involving one of the cranial bones. In cephalohematoma, the swelling does not cross the suture lines as it does in caput succedaneum.

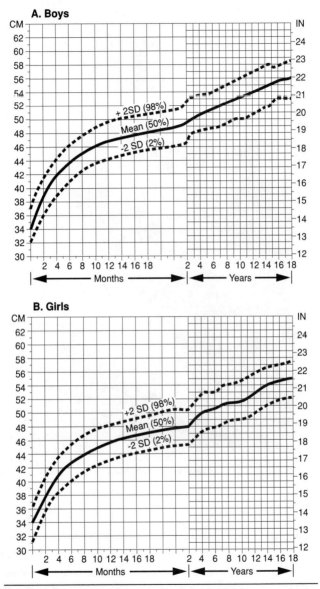

A. Boys

B. Girls

FIGURE 2.2. Head circumferences in boys *(A)* and girls *(B)*. *CM* = centimeters; *IN* = inches; *SD* = standard deviations. (Redrawn with permission from Horan MJ, Nelhaus G: Head circumference from birth to eighteen years. *Pediatrics* 79:1–25, 1987.)

Percussion and Auscultation of the Head

Percussion of the head may reveal **Macewen sign** [a resonant sound in children with closed fontanelles that indicates increased intracranial pressure (ICP)] or **Chvostek sign** [contraction of the facial muscles in response to percussion just below the zygomatic (cheek) bone]. Chvostek sign can be found in normal newborns as well as in children with hypocalcemic tetany. Percussion over the parietal bone may produce a **"cracked-pot sound,"** a normal finding prior to suture closure.

Auscultation of the head for **bruits** is not particularly useful until late childhood. Systolic or continuous bruits may be heard in the temporal area until age 5. Abnormal conditions that may be associated with bruits include arteriovenous malformation (AVM), cerebral vessel aneurysms, brain tumors, and coarctation of the aorta.

Inspection of the Hair and Scalp

The child's hair should be assessed for quantity, color, texture, and infestations. **Alopecia** can be congenital, caused by a fungal infection (tinea capitis), or the result of excessive hair pulling (trichotillomania). **Dry, coarse hair** may be a sign of hypothyroidism, and **fine, thin hair** may be seen in children with homocystinuria. In children with **pediculosis capitis** (head lice), close inspection reveals small, adherent, white nits.

▼ EYES

The eye examination is very important, providing information about the eyes and, in many cases, systemic problems. It is usually counterproductive (not to mention unkind) to try to pry a child's eye open. Instead, **distract the patient** with a toy or other object whenever possible to gain cooperation. A recalcitrant newborn can be encouraged to open his eyes by having an assistant gently rotate the baby from side to side while supporting him vertically (i.e., under the arms).

Assessment of the Eyes

Range of Motion and Orientation

Check for full range of motion by attracting the child's attention with a toy or piece of equipment. **Strabismus** (a condition in which the eyes do not move in a parallel manner) can manifest as **esotropia** (turning in of an eye) or **exotropia** (turning out of an eye). The following tests can be used to test for strabismus:

▼ **Corneal light reflection**. Have the baby focus on a small light. When the child is looking at the light, the reflection of the light from each cornea should be symmetrically placed. Asymmetries suggest the presence of strabismus.

▼ **Cover–uncover test.** The child focuses on a light, and one eye is covered and then uncovered. If either eye moves, strabismus may be present.

HINT   Intermittent esotropia or exotropia in a young infant may be normal, but deviations beyond 6 months of age can cause permanent vision loss.

Distance Between the Eyes

Observe the distance between the eyes, which can be documented as either the inner canthal distance (Fig. 2.3) or the interpupillary distance. **Hypotelorism** (abnormal closeness of eyes) is frequently found with holoprosencephaly sequence, maternal phenylketonuria, trisomy 13, and trisomy 20p. **Hypertelorism** (increased distance between the eyes) is frequently associated with a wide number of syndromes, including Apert syndrome, DiGeorge sequence, fetal hydantoin effects, Noonan syndrome, trisomies 8 and 9p, and absence of corpus callosum.

Nystagmus and "Setting Sun" Sign

Observe for nystagmus (rhythmical movements of the eyeballs) and "setting sun" sign (in which the eyes constantly appear to be looking downward).

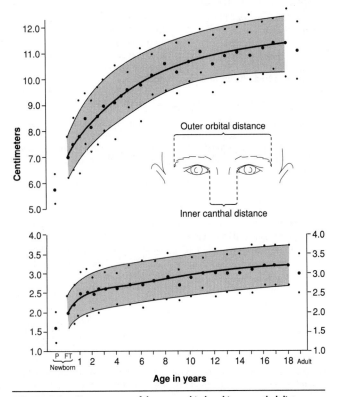

FIGURE 2.3.   Measurements of the outer orbital and inner canthal distance.
FT = full-term infant; *P* = premature infant. (Redrawn with permission from Laestadius ND, Aase JM, Smith DW: Normal inner canthal and outer orbital dimensions. *J Pediatr* 74(3):465–468, 1969.)

Nystagmus may be physiologic or it may be found with early loss of central vision, labyrinthitis, multiple sclerosis (MS), intracranial tumors, or drug toxicity. "Setting sun" sign may be seen with hydrocephalus or intracranial tumor, but also may be transiently noted in some healthy infants.

General Appearance

Check for an abnormal upward, outward **eye slant** and for **epicanthal folds** (vertical folds of skin over the medial portions of the eyes). Both can be associated with Down syndrome.

Assessment of the Individual Eyes

Visual Inspection

The following should be noted:

▼ **Pupil size and reaction to light**—both direct and consensual
▼ **Condition of the eyelids**—potential abnormalities include edema (swelling), erythema (redness), drooping, or the presence of masses
▼ **Hazy corneas**—caused by congenital glaucoma or inborn errors of metabolism
▼ **Injected or inflamed conjunctivae**
▼ **Icteric sclerae**

⚕ HINT A jaundiced child will have icteric sclerae, but a child with carotenemia (e.g., from too much enthusiasm for carrots) will have clear sclerae.

▼ **Brushfield spots on the irises**—small white spots frequently associated with Down syndrome
▼ **Excess tearing**—caused by congenital obstruction of the nasolacrimal duct

Funduscopic Examination

In infants, a minimal funduscopic evaluation consists of evaluation of the **red reflex:** the ophthalmoscope is set at 0 diopters; at a distance of approximately 1 foot away from the infant, a reddish orange color should be visible through the pupil. Leukocoria, a **white pupillary reflex,** can indicate serious disease, including cataracts, retinal detachment, or retinoblastoma. Inflammation or opacity of the **cornea** should be noted. Finally, if possible, the **optic disc and vessels** should be examined, ruling out fundal lesions and papilledema.

Vision Screening

The infant's vision and visual fields should be screened, using a brightly colored object. Note the infant's response to an object brought from behind her **(peripheral vision)** and her ability to track an object in front of her **(central vision).** Formal vision testing (often using the Snellen E Chart) can usually start at about age 4 years (see Chapter 3, "Developmental Surveillance").

⚕ HINT Normal newborns typically have about 20/400 vision, improving to about 20/100 by 6 months of age.

⚕ HINT Newborns often do not produce visible tears in the first few days of life.

▼ EARS

External Examination

Rashes that favor the postauricular area include seborrheic dermatitis, measles, and rubella. **Pain** on gentle traction of the pinna or tragus can signal external otitis.

Otoscopic Examination

Before examining the tympanic membrane, ensure that any uncooperative child is **well restrained.** One simple method is to have the parent firmly hold the supine child's raised arms against either side of the head. This also allows easy access for the oral examination that follows.

✂ HINT In an uncooperative child, press your otoscope hand against the patient's face. If the child suddenly moves despite proper restraint, the otoscope will move in tandem, decreasing the likelihood of injury.

It is also critical to **properly position the child's ear.** For an infant, pull the pinna down and back. For a school-aged child, pull straight back. For an adolescent, pull up and back.

▼ Check the tympanic membrane for **continuity.** Is it intact or perforated? Are there myringotomy tubes in place?
▼ Note the **color** and **degree of lucency.** Redness can indicate inflammation or merely be caused by a child's crying. A dull, purulent appearance indicates infection.
▼ Observe for **bulging** of the tympanic membrane, which suggests the presence of pus and fluid in the middle ear.
▼ Check for **visibility** of the bony landmarks and the cone of light reflex (which is absent with inflammation).
▼ Assess **mobility,** using a squeeze bulb. Poor movement can indicate the presence of fluid or purulent material in the middle ear.

Determining Hearing Acuity

Determining hearing acuity clinically is difficult in babies and young children. Watch the child's face as you make noise with a rattle or rustle paper behind each ear. Check to see if the child is **startled** by the sound (usually by age 1 month) or **looks toward the source** of the sound (by about age 5 months).

✂ HINT One helpful approach to determining hearing acuity in infants and young children is simply to ask the parents.

▼ NOSE

Check the **nasal mucosae.** Pale, boggy mucosae with a watery discharge suggest allergy, whereas hyperemic mucosae with a mucopurulent discharge suggest infection. Be alert for the possibility of nasal **foreign bodies,** which often present with a unilateral, malodorous rhinorrhea. Examine the **nasal septum** for deviation, ulcerations, perforation, or bleeding. Check the **nasal turbinates** for bogginess or polyps.

ﾂ HINT A newborn who is cyanotic when calm but pink when crying may have pulmonary disease with collapsed alveoli. Another possible diagnosis is choanal atresia (a congenital failure to develop openings between the nose and the nasopharynx).

▼ ORAL CAVITY
Lips and Buccal Mucosa

Examine the lips for **asymmetry, fissures, clefts, lesions,** and **color.** Gray or purple lips may reflect cyanosis. Vigorous sucking can produce a callus on the lips. Small vesicles on an erythematous base can indicate herpes simplex infection.

Assess the buccal mucosae for **moistness,** and check for **lesions.** For example, tiny white dots on an erythematous base may be Koplik spots–an early sign of measles. Small, white adherent patches may be oral thrush (*Candida* infection). Note any **strange odors** to the breath [e.g., sweet (acetone), ammoniac (uremia)].

Tongue

Examine the tongue, checking for color, size, coating, and dryness. A bluish color to the tongue indicates central cyanosis, which reflects the presence of unsaturated hemoglobin (methemoglobinemia). A **"strawberry" tongue** (characterized by large red papillae) may be seen with scarlet fever.

Teeth and Oropharynx

Examine the **teeth** for number and condition. Observe the **tonsils** for color or exudate. Check the **palate** for a high arch, cleft, or mucosal lesions. The palates of newborns often have small, whitish epithelial masses known as Epstein pearls. Examine the **posterior pharynx** for exudate, vesicles, or bifid uvula.

▼ NECK
Torticollis

Check for torticollis (fixed position of the head to one side), which may be **congenital** or **acquired.** Congenital torticollis may be caused by injury to the sternomastoid muscle. Acquired torticollis has many causes, including cervical spine disease, gastroesophageal reflux disease (GRD), posterior fossa or brain stem tumors, and infections within the head or neck.

Range of Motion

Have the child touch the chin to the chest (to test the inferior cervical spine), look up and move the head side to side (to test the atlantoaxial joint), and bend the neck laterally ear to shoulder (to test the lower cervical spine). Always examine ill children for the presence of nuchal rigidity, which can signal the possibility of meningitis. To help rule out **nuchal rigidity** in a young child, encourage him to look up and down by shining a bright light or shaking noisy objects (e.g., keys).

ﾂ HINT Children younger than 2 years do not consistently develop nuchal rigidity with meningitis.

Palpation, Auscultation, and Visual Inspection of the Neck

Palpate the **thyroid gland,** evaluating both lobes for swelling, symmetry, consistency, and surface characteristics (e.g., smooth versus nodular).

✄ HINT Lymph nodes are relatively more prominent in children than in adults. Shotty cervical (as well as axillary and femoral) lymph nodes (up to 1 cm in diameter) are normal in children younger than 10 years of age.

Auscultation may reveal a bruit, suggestive of thyrotoxicosis.

Examine the **neck** for other swellings or defects, including dermoid cysts, branchial cysts, and thyroglossal duct cysts. A thyroglossal duct cyst arises from a remnant of the embryonic thyroglossal duct. It is usually located in the midline, anywhere between the tongue and hyoid bone. It should move up when the patient sticks out her tongue or swallows.

▼ NEUROLOGIC SYSTEM

Assessment of Developmental Milestones

Assessment of a young child's developmental milestones is critical to the overall neurologic examination. Therefore, a **screening developmental examination,** such as the Denver II (see Chapter 3, "Developmental Surveillance," Figure 3.1), should be a part of every well-child neurologic assessment.

Assessment of Reflexes

Examination of the infantile reflexes is described in Table 2.2.

Test **deep tendon reflexes** using your finger, a reflex hammer, or the side of a stethoscope bell. Check for ankle or knee clonus (quick, repetitive muscle contractions). Bilateral clonus may be normal in an infant but can also reflect exaggerated muscle tone and deep tendon reflexes.

Assessment of Cranial Nerve Function

Examination of the cranial nerves is described in Table 2.3.

Sensory Examination

Assess an infant's general sensation by checking for a response to light touch.

Assessment of Coordination

Assess the child's coordination as he reaches for a toy, crawls, or walks. Check for unusual muscle movements:

▼ **Fasciculations**—twitchings of groups of muscle fibers
▼ **Tremors**—trembling movements of the extremities
▼ **Chorea**—irregular, spastic, involuntary movements
▼ **Athetosis**—constant, slow, writhing movements, sometimes found in normal infants and in children with cerebral palsy (CP) and tuberous sclerosis
▼ **Spasmus nutans**—periodic head nodding, sometimes associated with GRD, decreased intelligence quotient (IQ), or neuroblastoma and often combined with nystagmus and head tilt

TABLE 2.2.   Infantile Reflexes

Reflex	Usual Infant Age	Method of Elicitation	Description of Reflex
Moro (startle) reflex	Birth to 4–6 months	Lift the baby's head 15°, and then let it fall gently into your hands	Arms suddenly extend then flex, various movements of legs
Asymmetric tonic neck reflex	Birth to 4 months	Place the baby supine, head turned to one side	Isolateral arm and leg extend, contralateral arm contracts, like a fencer
Babinski reflex	Birth to 18 months	Stroke the dorsum of the baby's foot	Toe dorsiflexion, fanning
Palmar grasp reflex	Birth to 4 months	Place finger on the baby's palm	Involuntary grasping motion
Rooting reflex	Birth to 4 months	Touch corner of the baby's mouth	Head turns to side, baby opens mouth
Parachute reflex	6–7 months	Hold baby prone, move carefully downward	Extension of arms (to break fall)

HINT   The most critical part of the routine neurologic examination is your impression of the child's developmental abilities and general responsiveness. A reluctant toddler will often walk if her parent moves several steps away from her and offers encouragement. Entice the child to play with an interesting toy or object.

▼ CHEST AND LUNGS
Shape of the Chest

A **barrel-shaped chest** in a child older than 6 years can be associated with acute asthma or a chronic pulmonary disease such as cystic fibrosis. **Pectus excavatum** (a funnel-shaped chest) is caused by a congenitally depressed sternum and costal cartilages. **Pectus carinatum** ("pigeon chest") is characterized by protrusion of the sternum and costal cartilages. Although this is often an idiopathic problem that is not associated with actual medical difficulties, pectus carinatum is sometimes caused by rickets or osteoporosis.

Assessment of Breathing

Check carefully for signs of **respiratory distress,** including nasal flaring, retractions, or grunting. Nasal flaring refers to a widening of the nostrils, which often occurs with each inspiration in respiratory distress. Retractions are movements of the spaces between the ribs, occurring with each breath in a child with respiratory distress. Grunting is an end-expiratory sound, most often heard in the newborn or infant with respiratory distress.

TABLE 2.3.   Examination of the Cranial Nerves

Cranial Nerve	Function	Elicitation Technique	Potential Abnormalities
I: Olfactory nerve	Smell	Cannot assess until child can speak	...
II: Optic nerve	Vision	In newborns, note response to objects brought from behind (peripheral vision) and ability to track objects in front (central vision)	Deviation from typical visual acuity (newborn = 20/400; improving to about 20/100 by age 6 months)
		Children 4 years and older can undergo formal vision testing	
III: Oculomotor nerve	Elevation of upper eyelid, upward and downward gaze	Observe ocular movements and pupillary reflexes	Ptosis, pupil dilatation, nystagmus
IV: Trochlear nerve	Upward gaze		
V: Trigeminal nerve	Chewing, sensation on face, forehead, lips, and tongue	Evaluate corneal reflexes, check facial sensation with a piece of gauze	Absent responses
VI: Abducens nerve	Lateral gaze		
VII: Facial nerve	Facial muscle control (eyelid closure, forehead wrinkling, asymmetry of face), taste (anterior two-thirds of tongue)	Check for facial symmetry at rest and when the child is smiling or crying	Asymmetry
VIII: Vestibulocochlear nerve	Hearing	In newborns, check for acoustic blink (in response to a loud noise); by age 4 months, baby should turn to sound	Absent responses
IX: Glossopharyngeal nerve	Taste (posterior two-thirds of tongue), elevation of palate, sensory gag reflex	Observe ability to handle secretions or beverages	Difficulty swallowing
X: Vagus nerve	Swallowing, movement of pharynx		
XI: Accessory nerve	Turning head, shrugging shoulders	Assess the child's posture	Head tilt or shoulder drop
XII: Hypoglossal nerve	Protrusion of tongue	Ask cooperative child to stick out her tongue	Fasciculations or deviations from midline (tongue moves to side of lesion)

Percussion of the Lungs

Hyperresonance is usually caused by an increased amount of air in the chest (e.g., as in patients with asthma). **Dullness** is normally heard over the scapulae, liver, heart, and diaphragm.

Auscultation of the Lungs

In an infant, press the diaphragm of a small stethoscope firmly to the chest wall. Position the head in the midline, facing forward. Do not be reluctant to examine the lungs of a crying baby. Inspiratory sounds are actually enhanced by the deep inspiration.

⚤ HINT Warm your stethoscope before auscultation.

Breath Sounds and Air Movement

Listen carefully for breath sounds, **comparing air movement** in the two lungs. Decreased breath sounds suggest decreased air exchange. It is important to evaluate air movement because a patient with severe asthma can have such overwhelming obstruction that no wheezing is heard. **The patient with severe asthma but no wheezing may be in impending respiratory failure!**

⚤ HINT Breath sounds tend to be harsher sounding (more bronchial) in children (as compared with adults) because the thinner chest wall of the child does not muffle the breath sounds as much.

Chest Sounds

Identify adventitious chest sounds:

▼ **Rales** are fine crackles, usually heard best at the end of inspiration, that generally reflect the presence of fluid or exudate in the alveoli. In patients with rales, consider bronchopneumonia, atelectasis, and congestive heart failure.

▼ **Rhonchi** are coarse inspiratory and expiratory sounds, caused by secretions in the upper airway. They are often caused by crying or upper respiratory infection.

▼ **Wheezes** are palpable and audible vibrations, often musical in character, produced when air flow is restricted. Expiratory wheezes are most common and typically reflect lower airway obstruction. Wheezes are most commonly found with asthma and bronchiolitis. Other causes include congestive heart failure and foreign body aspiration.

Extraneous Sounds

▼ **Peristalsis,** if heard in the pulmonary examination, can suggest a diagnosis of diaphragmatic hernia (an abnormal opening of the diaphragm that allows the protrusion of abdominal contents into the chest).

▼ **A pleural friction rub** (a coarse grating sound with each breath) is occasionally present with pneumonia, lung abscess, or tuberculosis.

⚤ HINT Young children cannot cooperate as well as older children with a lung examination. Therefore, auscultation is not as reliable as in an older child, and a chest radiograph should be ordered more readily.

▼ CIRCULATORY SYSTEM

Many general physical examination clues can signal a child with cardiac disease. Typical observations include poor growth (weight affected more than length), developmental delay, cyanosis, clubbing of the fingers or toes, tachypnea, tachycardia, and peripheral edema. Routinely compare femoral pulse strength with right-arm pulse strength, which can be decreased in patients with coarctation of the aorta.

When examining the heart, first observe for **chest deformities** and **cardiac pulsations.** Palpate for the **point of maximum impulse (PMI).** In children younger than 7 years, the heart's general horizontal position usually results in a PMI in the fourth intercostal space, to the left of the midclavicular line. In children older than 7 years, the PMI is usually in the fifth to sixth intercostal space within the midclavicular line. A PMI displaced down or lateral to these sites can indicate congestive heart failure.

The PMI may feel prominent in a thin child, in a child who has just finished exercising, or in a child who is anxious, febrile, in impending heart failure, or hyperthyroid. It is decreased in patients with pericardial or pleural effusions or pneumomediastinum (presence of gas or air in the mediastinal tissues). Thrills and pericardial friction rubs manifest as fine or coarse vibrations.

Listen with the child in both the **supine** and **sitting positions.** Listen over the whole precordium, especially at the apex, the pulmonic area (second interspace, left of the sternum), the aortic area (second interspace, right of the sternum), and the tricuspid valve (fourth interspace over the sternum). Listen for a split second heart sound (S_2), heard best over the pulmonic area during inspiration. [This finding is more obvious in school-aged children than in adults. It is usually only a potential problem if there is a large, fixed split, such as that found with atrial septal defect (ASD)].

▼ **Are the heart sounds clear?** Distant sounds can suggest pericardial fluid.
▼ **Is there a third heart sound (S_3)?** (Usually heard at the apex, an S_3 may indicate mitral valve prolapse or ASD.)
▼ **Is there a gallop rhythm and other physical signs consistent with congestive heart failure?**

Rhythms

Sinus arrhythmia refers to the normal variation in pulse rate found with respiration. It is particularly prominent in young teenagers. Pulse rate increases with inspiration and decreases with expiration. **Premature ventricular contractions** are fairly common in the pediatric population. Generally, they should number less than 6 per minute at rest and decrease with exertion.

Murmurs

Description

Murmurs are described as follows:

▼ **Loudness**—reported as grade I to grade VI
▼ **Timing in the cardiac cycle**—described as diastolic or systolic, early or late
▼ **Pitch**—high or low
▼ **Quality**—blowing, musical, or rough
▼ **Location**—e.g., apex, left lower sternal border
▼ **Transmission across the chest**—e.g., radiating to the right lower sternal border

Innocent Murmurs

Nonpathologic murmurs typically heard in childhood include Still murmur and venous hum. **Still murmur** is the most common murmur in children between the ages of 2 years and adolescence. It is typically described as musical or vibratory, short, high-pitched, early systolic, and grade I to III. It is usually heard best in the apical region. A **venous hum** is a continuous, low-pitched murmur heard under the clavicle and in the neck. It is caused by blood draining down the jugular vein. See Chapter 56, "Murmurs."

▓ HINT The most important first step in assessing a murmur is to distinguish innocent from pathologic. Innocent murmurs are typically grade III or less, systolic in timing, and with no accompanying signs of cardiovascular disease.

▼ ABDOMEN

A successful abdominal examination is especially reliant on having the **patient relaxed.** Position the patient in a supine position, with her knees bent and her arms at her sides. Warm your stethoscope and hands and then allow your hand to rest quietly for a moment on the patient's abdomen before making initial probing movements. To reduce ticklishness, place the child's hand on yours. Talking with the child about her siblings, friends, or school can be a useful distraction. It can also be helpful to allow children to examine your stethoscope while you examine them.

Abdominal Contour

Examine the abdominal contour. Is the abdomen flat, protuberant (common in toddlers), scaphoid (depressed, sometimes found with diaphragmatic hernia), or distended? Check for diastasis recti (vertical separation of the rectus abdominis muscles).

Abdominal Wall Motion

Respirations are generally abdominal in children younger than 6–7 years. In young children, absence of abdominal wall motion may be caused by peritonitis, diaphragmatic paralysis, or large amounts of fluid or air in the abdomen. In older children, respirations that are mostly abdominal can indicate pneumonia or other pulmonary disorders.

Auscultation

Auscultation of the abdomen should be done **before palpation** to avoid altering the sounds of peristalsis. **Normal sounds** are short and metallic, occurring every 10–30 seconds. **Excessively frequent and high-pitched sounds** can indicate early peritonitis, gastroenteritis, or intestinal obstruction. **Absence of sounds** for more than 3 minutes can occur with paralytic ileus or peritonitis. Vascular obstruction may be indicated by a murmur over the aorta or renal arteries. It is especially important to check for vascular obstructions in any child with hypertension.

Percussion

Percussion can be useful to assess the liver (and occasionally the spleen) and to identify ascites, abdominal masses, or air in the gastrointestinal tract. Babies often have more swallowed air in their gastrointestinal tracts than do adults.

Percuss lightly in all **four quadrants** to assess general distribution of tympany and dullness. Tympany is generally the predominant sound. A distended abdomen with little tympany may contain fluid or solid masses. Dullness is typically found over the liver, over a full urinary bladder, or over masses.

To determine **liver span,** percuss the upper and lower borders in the right midclavicular line, and measure the vertical distance. Normal spans are approximately 2 centimeters at 6 months, 4 centimeters at 3 years, 6 centimeters at 10 years, and 8 centimeters in adults. Causes of hepatomegaly include passive congestion, hepatitis, and tumor.

Palpation

💾 HINT For crying children, palpate immediately on inspiration. The child often will relax his abdominal musculature for a moment.

Abdomen

Palpation of the abdomen is best done **on inspiration and on deep expiration.** Place one hand on the patient's back and the other on the abdomen. First palpate lightly, then deeply. Start in the left lower quadrant and continue in a clockwise manner. If any area seems tender, palpate that area last.

Rigidity (a tense abdomen) can indicate a surgical condition but is sometimes caused by voluntary muscle tightening in a frightened child.

Check for **tenderness,** trying to localize the point of maximum pain. The location of the tenderness can offer clues regarding the cause (Table 2.4). Rebound tenderness is associated with peritoneal inflammation.

💾 HINT When checking for abdominal tenderness, ask a young child, "Does this feel OK?" Toddlers and preschoolers will often nod yes indiscriminately when asked if something hurts. Facial expression is the most reliable sign of true tenderness.

TABLE 2.4. Suggested Causes of Abdominal Tenderness According to Location

Location of Abdominal Tenderness	Possible Causes
Right upper quadrant	Acute hepatomegaly, hepatitis, intussusception
Left upper quadrant	Intussusception, splenic enlargement or rupture
Midline upper abdomen	Gastroenteritis, gastric or duodenal ulcer
Right lower quadrant	Appendicitis, abscess
Left lower quadrant	Constipation
Midline suprapubic area	Cystitis
Lower abdomen in general	Gastroenteritis, tumor, Meckel diverticulum, ovarian or testicular torsion
Poorly localized	Pneumonia, mesenteric adenitis, peritonitis, sickle cell crisis

Spleen

The spleen is often normally palpated in the first few years of life. It can be enlarged with infection (especially infectious mononucleosis), sickle cell or other hemolytic anemias, or leukemia. See Chapter 76, "Splenomegaly."

Liver

The liver generally can be palpated 1–2 centimeters below the right costal margin. Its edge is usually sharp and soft. A pathologically enlarged liver usually extends more than 2 centimeters below the right costal margin and has a rounded, firm edge. See Chapter 42, "Hepatomegaly."

Kidneys

In newborns, the kidneys can be gently trapped between the examiner's hands, allowing examination for masses. In all children, percussing gently over the costovertebral angles bilaterally can reveal tenderness over the kidneys.

▼ GENITALIA

In infants, first assess the genitals for **ambiguity.** Is the baby "boy" really a virilized female with clitoromegaly and fused labial folds? Is the baby "girl" a male with a micropenis?

When examining children and teenagers, always respect the **patient's modesty.** Provide a gown and be sure to have a chaperone present.

Boys

▼ **Examine the glans penis and locate the meatus.** Is it ventrally displaced (hypospadias) or dorsally displaced (epispadias)? Observe for inflammation of the glans penis (balanitis) or of the prepuce (posthitis). Is there a penile discharge?

▼ **Note whether the child has been circumcised.** In an uncircumcised boy, is there phimosis (i.e., an inability to retract the foreskin)? Normally the foreskin is not retractable until age 2 years.

▼ **Observe for scrotal masses.** Hydrocele is caused by an accumulation of fluid in the tunica vaginalis. You may demonstrate the fluid by shining a light to the scrotum. (Unlike inguinal hernias, hydroceles do not reduce.) Palpate for the testicles and note their location. In determining the presence of a retractile testis, it is helpful to have the boy sit cross-legged; the testes can then be "milked down" from the inguinal canal. Check for testicular masses.

Tanner staging of penis, testes, scrotum, and pubic hair development is described in Table 2.5.

Girls

▼ **Observe the labia majora and minora.** Are the labia minora fused? Is the fusion complete? (Sometimes a thin membrane can be gently opened with a cotton swab.)

▼ **Check for enlargement of the clitoris.** Examine the introitus (vaginal opening) for size, discharge, excoriation, or scarring. Pseudomenstruation (i.e., a usually minimal, bloody vaginal discharge caused by placental transfer of maternal hormones) may be noted in newborn girls. Infections, bleeding, or bruising may be an indication of sexual abuse. Is the hymen intact?

TABLE 2.5. Tanner Staging of the Penis, Testes, Scrotum, and Pubic Hair

Tanner Stage	Penis	Testes	Scrotum	Pubic Hair
1	Immature	Small	Immature	None present
2	Immature	Initial enlargement	Initial rugae, reddening	Small amount near penile base
3	Initial enlargement	Continued enlargement	Increased rugae, reddening	Increased amount, distribution, coarseness, curl
4	Continued enlargement	Continued enlargement	Increased rugae, reddening	Increasing as above
5	Full adult	Full adult	Full adult	Adult amount and distribution (pubic area and medial thighs)

TABLE 2.6. Tanner Staging of Female Breasts		
Tanner Stage	**Breast**	**Areola**
1	Prepubertal	Prepubertal
2	Small breast bud	Beginning enlargement
3	Continued development	Developing, continuous with breast
4	Continued development	Projection separate from breast
5	Full adult breasts	Flattened areola and protruding nipple

Lack of a hymen does not necessarily imply sexual contact; participation in active games and sports can also rupture it.

▼ A **pelvic examination** is usually performed on sexually active teenagers or if a specific problem is suspected. In adolescent girls, the possibility of pregnancy should always be considered, even if the patient denies sexual experience.

Tanner staging of pubic hair in females is the same as in males (Table 2.5). Tanner staging of breasts is described in Table 2.6.

▼ RECTUM AND ANUS

Rule out fissures or anal prolapse. In a newborn, check for a patent anus. A digital examination is usually only performed if there are abdominal or rectal symptoms, a pelvic mass, or malformation. Check for sphincter tone, masses, and tenderness.

▼ SKIN

▼ First, assess overall **skin color.** General erythema can reflect fever, sun exposure, or atropine toxicity. Pallor may be found in children with shock, anemia, or poor local circulation. Peripheral cyanosis (evidenced by bluish discoloration of the nailbeds) can be caused by cold stress, local venous obstruction, or shock.

⚡ HINT In normal newborns, it is common for the hands and feet to be cyanotic, especially when they have been exposed to cold surroundings.

▼ Check for **skin pigmentation** (areas of generalized or localized color change). Hypopigmented lesions can be caused by tinea versicolor, vitiligo, tuberous sclerosis, or albinism. Bluish-black lesions, especially over the lower back and buttocks in infants, are often Mongolian spots.

▼ **Vascular nevi** are commonly found in infants and children. Nevus flammeus lesions occur as flat, irregular pink patches. Strawberry hemangiomas are typically soft, compressible lesions. Port wine stains are flat markings that are embedded in the skin.

▼ **Burns** are classified as first-degree (erythema only), second-degree (erythema plus blister formation), and third-degree (involving the subcutaneous tissue).

▼ **Skin puffiness** from edema (excess extracellular water and sodium) may be associated with renal, cardiac, or hepatic disease.

▼ MUSCULOSKELETAL SYSTEM
Gross Deformities and Congenital Anomalies

Deformities are most commonly caused by **fractures** but can also be **congenital** [e.g., polydactyly (extra fingers or toes), syndactyly (webbed or fused digits)].

⚕ HINT In evaluating injuries, consider child abuse if the damage is worse than accounted for by the history, if the child has multiple bruises, if there is a mixture of old and new injuries, or if there is a delay in seeking medical care.

Fingers and Toes

Observe the fingers and toes for **clubbing** (broadening and thickening of the terminal phalanges). Clubbing can be associated with many different systemic diseases, including congenital heart disease, pulmonary disease (e.g., cystic fibrosis), chronic hepatic disease, and gastrointestinal disorders (e.g., Crohn disease, ulcerative colitis).

Legs

Examine the shape of the leg bones:

▼ **Genu varum (bowleggedness)** develops routinely in infants until about 18 months of age. Severe genu varum may be an indication of rickets or a congenital abnormality.
▼ **Genu valgum (knock-knees)** is most often seen in children older than 2 years and often persists until adolescence.
▼ **Tibial torsion** is a twisting of the tibia thought to be caused by uterine pressure on the developing fetus. It often resolves spontaneously once the child begins walking.

Feet

In metatarsus adductus (inversion of the forefoot), the lateral border of the foot is "C"-shaped, instead of straight. The most serious congenital foot deformity is **clubfoot** (talipes equinovarus). This condition involves three major abnormalities: metatarsus adductus, fixed foot inversion, and equinus (or downward positioning of the foot).

⚕ HINT It is important to distinguish **rigid deformities,** which are more serious, from **flexible deformities.** With a flexible deformity, the foot can be brought to a normal position with gentle pressure.

Gait and Stance

Infants starting to walk typically have a wide-based gait that persists until approximately age 2 years.

▼ **Joints.** The joints should be examined for range of motion, warmth, redness, tenderness, and presence of effusion. In infants older than 6 months, always check for congenital hip dislocation using the Ortolani maneuver (Figure 2.4). Other useful signs of congenital hip dislocation are unequal leg length and asymmetric thigh skin folds.

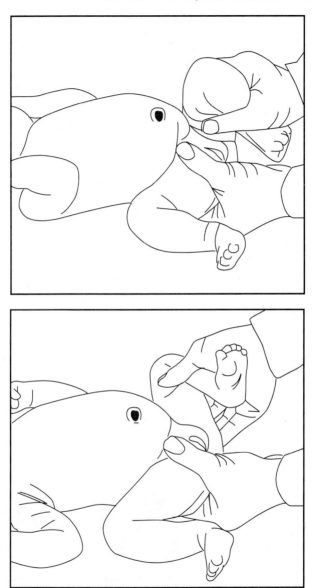

FIGURE 2.4. Ortolani maneuver to check for dislocated hip.
With your index finger over the greater trochanter and your thumb over the inner thigh, flex the hip 90° and slowly abduct it from the midline. Feel for an abnormal "clunk" as a dislocated femoral head slips into the acetabulum.

▼ **Muscles.** Examine the muscles for tone by grasping the muscle and estimating its firmness during passive range of motion. Assess muscle strength, observing for weakness or paralysis. Look for contractures (fixed deformities that often have accompanying muscle atrophy). Check muscle mass, observing for atrophy or hypertrophy.

▼ **Spine.** Inspect the spine, observing for tufts of hair, dimples, abnormal coloration, masses, or cysts. Any of these can indicate spina bifida (a limited defect in the spinal column through which spinal membranes and spinal cord tissue may protrude). A small dimple anywhere in the midline can indicate a dermoid sinus [an epidermis-lined tract leading from the skin to the spinal cord that presents a risk of central nervous system (CNS) infection]. Check for spinal masses, including meningoceles, teratomas, or lipomas.

▼ **Posture.** Observe the child's posture, checking for abnormal spinal curvatures. In lumbar lordosis, the curve is anteroposterior, with the convexity anterior. Lumbar lordosis is usually normal for children but if severe can be a sign of rickets or abdominal wall weakness. In kyphosis, the anteroposterior curve of the spine has a posterior convexity. Scoliosis refers to a lateral curvature of the spine. All school-aged children and adolescents should be examined for scoliosis. Have the child bend forward, and look for unilateral elevation of the rib cage and hip.

⚡ HINT The posture of the newborn often reflects the newborn's intrauterine position. For example, babies born breech often have very flexed hips and extended knees.

Suggested Readings

Barness LA: *Manual of Pediatric Physical Diagnosis*, 6th ed. St. Louis, Mosby, 1991.

Jones KL (ed): *Smith's Recognizable Patterns of Human Malformation*, 4th ed. Philadelphia, WB Saunders, 1997.

Pavan-Langston D (ed): *Manual of Ocular Diagnosis and Therapy*, 4th ed. Philadelphia, Lippincott-Raven, 1996.

Zitelli BJ (ed): *Atlas of Pediatric Physical Diagnosis*, 3rd ed. Philadelphia, Lippincott-Raven, 1997.

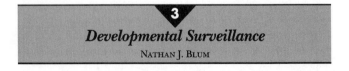

3

Developmental Surveillance

NATHAN J. BLUM

Primary care physicians play a vital role in identifying children at risk for developmental disabilities and in referring them for appropriate early intervention services. Developmental surveillance involves using information obtained from the history, physical examination, and developmental screening tests to assess development on an ongoing basis. This ongoing monitoring of development is critical for two reasons. First, **new circumstances** (e.g., medical illness, family or environmental disruption, injuries) may interfere with development. Second, as children develop, they gain **new categories of skills** that are difficult to assess at earlier points (e.g., one cannot usually detect isolated language delays in children younger than 18–24 months, the point at which children begin to develop a good repertoire of language skills).

▼ HISTORY

The following information should be elicited:

▼ **Parental concerns regarding the child's development.** In most cases, parental concerns regarding the child's language development, articulation, fine motor skills, or global development are likely to be associated with true developmental delays. Parental concerns about behavior or personal–social skills are associated with developmental delays in some cases.
▼ **Risk factors for developmental disabilities** (Table 3.1)
▼ **Attainment of developmental milestones** (Table 3.2)

▼ PHYSICAL EXAMINATION
Head Circumference

Brain growth is the principal stimulus for increasing head circumference. Therefore, a small head circumference may indicate abnormalities in brain growth that place a child at risk for developmental disabilities. A large head circumference may be a sign of hydrocephalus, a genetic syndrome, or a metabolic storage disease. However, before assuming pathology in a child, one should measure the parents' head sizes because a small or large head circumference may be a family trait.

TABLE 3.1. Risk Factors for Developmental Disabilities

Prenatal
  Maternal illness, infection, or malnutrition
  Maternal exposure to toxins, teratogens, alcohol, illicit drugs, anticonvulsants, antineoplastics, or anticoagulants
  Decreased fetal movements
  Intrauterine growth retardation
  Family history of deafness, blindness, or mental retardation
  Chromosomal abnormalities
Perinatal
  Asphyxia—Apgar scores of 0–3 at 5 minutes
  Prematurity, low birth weight
  Abnormal presentation
Postnatal
  Meningitis, encephalitis
  Seizure disorder
  Hyperbilirubinemia—bilirubin >25 mg/dl in full-term infant
  Severe chronic illness
  Central nervous system trauma
  Child abuse and neglect

TABLE 3.2. Developmental Milestones From Birth to 5 Years

Age (Months)	Adaptive/Fine Motor	Language	Gross Motor	Personal–Social
1	Grasp reflex (hands fisted)	Facial response to sounds	Lifts head in prone position	Stares at face
2	Follows object with eyes past midline	Coos (vowel sounds)	Lifts head in prone position to 45°	Smiles in response to others
4	Hands open Brings objects to mouth	Laughs and squeals Turns toward voice	Sits: head steady Rolls to supine	Smiles spontaneously
6	Palmar grasp of objects	Babbles (consonant sounds)	Sits independently Stands, hands held	Reaches for toys Recognizes strangers
9	Pincer grasp	Says "mama," "dada" nonspecifically, comprehends "no"	Pulls to stand	Feeds self Waves bye-bye
12	Helps turn pages of book	2–4 words Follows command with gesture	Stands independently Walks, one hand held	Points to indicate wants
15	Scribbles	4–6 words Follows command no gesture	Walks independently	Drinks from cup Imitates activities

Age (mo)				
18	Turns pages of book	10–20 words Points to 4 body parts	Walks up steps	Feeds self with spoon
24	Solves single-piece puzzles	Combines 2–3 words Uses "I" and "you"	Jumps Kicks ball	Removes coat Verbalizes wants
30	Imitates horizontal and vertical lines	Names all body parts	Rides tricycle using pedals	Pulls up pants Washes, dries hands
36	Copies circle Draws person with 3 parts	Gives full name, age, and sex Names 2 colors	Throws ball overhand Walks up stairs (alternating feet)	Toilet trained Puts on shirt, knows front from back
42	Copies cross	Understands "cold," "tired," "hungry"	Stands on one foot for 2–3 sec	Engages in associative play
48	Counts 4 objects Identifies some numbers and letters	Understands prepositions (under, on, behind, in front of) Asks "how" and "why"	Hops on one foot	Dresses with little assistance Shoes on correct feet
54	Copies square Draws person with 6 parts	Understands opposites	Broad-jumps 24 inches	Bosses and criticizes Shows off
60	Prints first name Counts 10 objects	Asks meaning of words	Skips (alternating feet)	Ties shoes

▼ **HINT** Microcephaly is defined as a head circumference less than the 3rd percentile; macrocephaly is defined as a head circumference greater than the 97th percentile.

Congenital Anomalies or Dysmorphic Features

Congenital anomalies or dysmorphic features are associated with many genetic syndromes that may cause mental retardation or learning disabilities. Although a karyotype is a good initial screen, syndromes associated with small deletions (e.g., Williams syndrome, Prader-Willi syndrome, velocardiofacial syndrome) will not be detected by a routine karyotype. Detecting these disorders requires the use of fluorescent in situ hybridization (FISH) technology, using a probe for the specific region of the chromosome to be investigated. Genetics consultation is indicated when considering these tests.

Dermal Lesions of Neurocutaneous Syndromes

▼ **Ash leaf spots** are hypomelanotic macules found in 90% of patients with tuberous sclerosis. Ultraviolet light may be necessary to visualize the spots. One or two hypopigmented lesions may be seen in normal individuals. Approximately 50% of patients with tuberous sclerosis have mental retardation.

▼ **Café-au-lait spots** are light brown, flat macules seen in patients with neurofibromatosis but also seen in 10% of the population. They are more common on the trunk than on the extremities. Six or more lesions, greater than 5 millimeters in diameter before puberty or 15 millimeters in diameter after puberty, should lead to investigation for other signs of neurofibromatosis. Patients with neurofibromatosis are at risk for hearing loss and learning disabilities.

▼ **Port wine nevus.** Ten percent of children with cutaneous angioma involving the upper face (forehead and eye) have an intracranial angioma (Sturge-Weber syndrome). Approximately 50% of patients with Sturge-Weber syndrome have mental retardation.

Muscle Tone

▼ **Hypertonia** (i.e., increased resistance of muscle groups to movement) may be a sign of cerebral palsy (CP), but in the first year of life children with isolated increases in muscle tone should not be diagnosed with CP because they may outgrow the problem.

▼ **Hypotonia** (i.e., decreased resistance of muscle groups to movement) occurs in infants with neuromuscular disorders or injury to the brain or spinal cord. Rarely, hypotonia is the only sign of a metabolic disorder (e.g., peroxisomal disorders, acid maltase deficiency). Hypotonia also occurs in some chromosomal disorders, such as Down syndrome. (Therefore, obtaining a karyotype should be considered if the child is dysmorphic and hypotonic.)

Primitive Reflexes

Asymmetries of primitive reflexes may help identify hemiplegias or other nerve injuries. Persistence of primitive reflexes beyond the time of usual disappearance (Table 3.3) or an obligate response may be signs of CP.

TABLE 3.3. Primitive Reflexes

Primitive Reflex	Age at Disappearance (Months)	Description
Palmar grasp	3–4	Pressing against the palmar surface of the infant's hand results in flexion of all fingers.
Rooting	3–4	Stroking the perioral skin at the corners of the mouth causes the mouth to open and turn to stimulated side.
Galant	2–3	Stroking along the paravertebral area causes lateral flexion of the trunk with the concavity toward the stimulated side.
Moro	4–6	Sudden movement of the head causes symmetric abduction and extension of the arms followed by gradual adduction and flexion of the arms over the body.
Asymmetric tonic neck	4–6	Turning the head to one side leads to extension of extremities on that side and flexion on the contralateral side, putting the infant in the "fencing" position.
Tonic labyrinthine	2–3	In the supine position, neck extension leads to shoulder retraction and trunk and lower extremity extension that is reduced by neck flexion.
Positive support	2–3	Stimulation of the ball of the foot leads to cocontraction of opposing muscle groups, allowing weight to be borne.
Placing/stepping	Variable	When the dorsal surface of one foot touches the underside of a table, the infant places the foot on the table top.

▼ HEARING ASSESSMENT
Screening

A National Institutes of Health Consensus Panel (March, 1993) and the American Academy of Pediatrics have recommended universal hearing screening during the newborn period because the risk factors for hearing loss (Table 3.4) will only identify half of infants with significant hearing impairment. Approximately half of the 50 states mandate this screening. The most cost-effective screening method is still the subject of some debate, but the currently available methods include otoacoustic emissions and auditory brainstem responses.

▼ **Otoacoustic emissions (OAE).** Otoacoustic emissions refers to sounds that are thought to originate from the hair cells of the cochlea. In individuals with an auditory threshold of 20 decibels or better, OAEs can be evoked by presenting clicking sounds to the ear. If the auditory threshold is above 30–40 decibels, the evoked OAEs are absent. The test takes 2–5 minutes to administer and is relatively inexpensive. However, fluid in the middle ear or debris in the auditory canal will interfere with the test, leading to a false-positive rate as high as 10% in the newborn period.

▼ **Auditory brainstem response (ABR).** Electroencephalogram (EEG) electrodes attached to the forehead and behind the ears detect brain activity in response to 30–40 decibel clicks presented to an ear. Absence of the expected brain activity suggests an abnormality of hearing. The test takes 5–15 minutes to perform and is significantly more expensive than OAE testing, but the false-positive rate is lower (2%–3%).

In some locations a two-step screening process is applied in which those who fail OAEs are then screened by ABRs and only those who fail both screens are referred for further evaluation. This two-step process may have the lowest false-positive rate.

⚡ HINT Expressive language milestones (e.g., laughing, cooing, babbling) can be misleading because deaf infants also exhibit these milestones in the first 4–6 months. By approximately 12 months of age, babbling decreases in deaf infants, but in hearing infants it continues to increase and sounds more like the infant is talking.

TABLE 3.4. Risk Factors For Hearing Impairment
Family history of deafness
Congenital "TORCH" infection
Congenital malformation of the head and neck
Prematurity (<1500 g at birth)
Extended stay in neonatal intensive care unit (>48 hrs)
Hyperbilirubinemia requiring exchange transfusion
Meningitis or encephalitis
Anoxia

Formal Hearing Testing

▼ **0–6 months: Auditory evoked responses (AERs).** The use of AERs as a screening test was described earlier. When the test is done by an audiologist, the intensity of the sound can be varied so that an auditory threshold can be obtained. This test is highly sensitive (false-negative results are rare), but a false-positive result is possible. Therefore, positive test results should be confirmed by audiometry when the child is old enough.

▼ **6–24 months: Visual reinforcement audiometry.** A sound is paired with a visual event (e.g., a doll's eyes light up). Once the child has learned the association, she will look toward the doll in anticipation of the visual event when a sound is heard.

▼ **2–5 years: Conditioned play audiometry.** The child is asked to engage in a play task every time a sound is heard.

▼ **Older than 6 years: Standard audiometry.**

▼ VISION ASSESSMENT

The **detection of amblyopia** is the most important reason for early vision screening—early detection of amblyopia can prevent vision loss in the "neglected" eye. The most common causes of amblyopia are **strabismus** (see Chapter 2, "The Physical Examination") and **anisometropia** (an eye with a refractive error 1.5 diopters or greater than its pair).

Visual acuity improves with age. Newborns should be able to fixate on a face; by 1–2 months of age, infants should be able to follow an object horizontally across their visual field. By 6 months of age, visual acuity is about 20/100, and at 3 years it is 20/30 to 20/40. By 5–6 years of age, children should have 20/20 vision.

Office vision screening using the Snellen chart can be performed with children who know the letters of the alphabet. Variations of this test, such as the tumbling "E" chart and the Allen chart, have been developed for younger children. When using the tumbling "E" chart, the child is asked to point in the direction of the "legs" of the letter. The Allen chart contains pictures of toys, animals, and other familiar objects.

▼ DEVELOPMENTAL SCREENING TESTS
General Development

Ages 0–6 Years: Denver II

The Denver developmental screening test (Denver II; Fig. 3.1) tests four skill areas: personal–social, fine motor–adaptive, language, and gross motor skills. 1989 norms are based on test administration to more than 2,000 children. Bars on the test sheet depict ages at which 25%, 50%, 75%, and 90% of children successfully perform each task. If a child cannot perform one task that 90% of children of the same age successfully perform (or two or more tasks that 75% of children of the same age successfully perform), further developmental evaluation is probably necessary.

Ages 0–3 Years: CAT/CLAMS

The CAT/CLAMS test assesses visual–motor and language skills and provides a developmental quotient (developmental age/chronologic age). For children older than 18 months, these scores correlate well with scores on the Bayley Mental Scales.

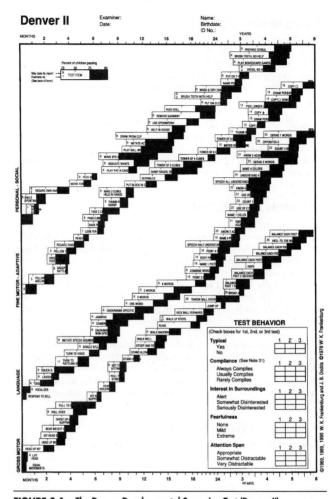

FIGURE 3.1. The Denver Developmental Screening Test (Denver II).
An explanation of how to administer the test is provided in a training manual
and videotapes available from Denver Developmental Materials Inc., P.O. Box
6919, Denver, Colorado 80206–0919; telephone (800) 419–4729. (Reprinted
with permission from Dr. Frankenburg.)

Ages 0–3 Years: Revised Gesell Developmental Schedules

The 1987 revision of the Gesell Developmental Schedules assesses five skill
areas: adaptive, fine motor, gross motor, language, and personal-social. The
Gesell Developmental Schedules contain many more items at each age level
than the CAT/CLAMS or Denver II tests. Explanations of how to administer

DIRECTIONS FOR ADMINISTRATION

1. Try to get child to smile by smiling, talking or waving. Do not touch him/her.
2. Child must stare at hand several seconds.
3. Parent may help guide toothbrush and put toothpaste on brush.
4. Child does not have to be able to tie shoes or button/zip in the back.
5. Move yarn slowly in an arc from one side to the other, about 8" above child's face.
6. Pass if child grasps rattle when it is touched to the backs or tips of fingers.
7. Pass if child tries to see where yarn went. Yarn should be dropped quickly from sight from tester's hand without arm movement.
8. Child must transfer cube from hand to hand without help of body, mouth, or table.
9. Pass if child picks up raisin with any part of thumb and finger.
10. Line can vary only 30 degrees or less from tester's line.
11. Make a fist with thumb pointing upward and wiggle only the thumb. Pass if child imitates and does not move any fingers other than the thumb.

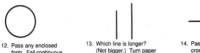

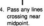

12. Pass any enclosed form. Fail continuous round motions.
13. Which line is longer? (Not bigger.) Turn paper upside down and repeat. (pass 3 of 3 or 5 of 6)
14. Pass any lines crossing near midpoint.
15. Have child copy first. If failed, demonstrate.

When giving items 12, 14, and 15, do not name the forms. Do not demonstrate 12 and 14.

16. When scoring, each pair (2 arms, 2 legs, etc.) counts as one part.
17. Place one cube in cup and shake gently near child's ear, but out of sight. Repeat for other ear.
18. Point to picture and have child name it. (No credit is given for sounds only.)
   If less than 4 pictures are named correctly, have child point to picture as each is named by tester.

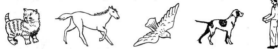

19. Using doll, tell child: Show me the nose, eyes, ears, mouth, hands, feet, tummy, hair. Pass 6 of 8.
20. Using pictures, ask child: Which one flies?... says meow?... talks?... barks?... gallops? Pass 2 of 5, 4 of 5.
21. Ask child: What do you do when you are cold?... tired?... hungry? Pass 2 of 3, 3 of 3.
22. Ask child: What do you do with a cup? What is a chair used for? What is a pencil used for?
   Action words must be included in answers.
23. Pass if child correctly places and says how many blocks are on paper. (1, 5).
24. Tell child: Put block on table; under table; in front of me, behind me. Pass 4 of 4.
   (Do not help child by pointing, moving head or eyes.)
25. Ask child: What is a ball?... lake?... desk?... house?... banana?... curtain?... fence?... ceiling? Pass if defined in terms of use, shape, what it is made of, or general category (such as banana is fruit, not just yellow). Pass 5 of 8, 7 of 8.
26. Ask child: If a horse is big, a mouse is __? If fire is hot, ice is __? If the sun shines during the day, the moon shines during the __? Pass 2 of 3.
27. Child may use wall or rail only, not person. May not crawl.
28. Child must throw ball overhand 3 feet to within arm's reach of tester.
29. Child must perform standing broad jump over width of test sheet (8 1/2 inches).
30. Tell child to walk forward, 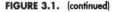 heel within 1 inch of toe. Tester may demonstrate. Child must walk 4 consecutive steps.
31. In the second year, half of normal children are non-compliant.

OBSERVATIONS:

FIGURE 3.1. (continued)

each item are provided in a manual that is available by writing to Developmental Education Materials Inc, P. O. Box 272391, Houston, Texas 77277-2391.

Language Development

Ages 0–3 Years: Early Language Milestone (ELM) Scale-2

This test assesses auditory expressive language skills, auditory receptive language skills, and visual communication skills. It can be scored using a pass-fail system or percentile scores can be obtained. Information on this test is available from Pro-ed, 8700 Shoal Creek Boulevard, Austin, Texas 78757.

Age > 2 Years: Peabody Picture Vocabulary Test-III (PPVT-III)

The PPVT-III tests receptive language skills. From a group of four pictures, the patient must select the one picture that best illustrates a specific word. A progressively more difficult sequence of words and pictures is administered until the patient is no longer identifying the correct picture at a frequency higher than chance. Scores tend to correlate well with the verbal intelligence quotient (IQ). Additional information on this test is available from the American Guidance Service, Circle Pines, Minnesota 55014.

Visual-Motor Skills

Ages 3–12 Years: Gesell Figures

Children develop the ability to draw progressively more complex figures in a predictable manner (Fig. 3.2).

Ages 3–8 Years: Draw-a-Person Test

This test assesses the child's visual–motor and conceptual skills by requiring the child to draw a picture of a person. The child receives one point for each feature of the person that he includes. The total number of points can be used to determine an age-equivalent score.

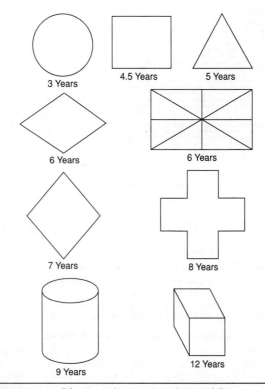

FIGURE 3.2. Gesell figures used to assess visual–motor skills.
Children are capable of drawing progressively more complex shapes.

Suggested Readings

Dworkin PH: Detection of behavioral, developmental, and psychosocial problems in pediatric primary care. *Curr Opin Pediatr* 5:531–536, 1993.

Frankenburg WK: Preventing developmental delays: is developmental screening sufficient? *Pediatrics* 93:586–593, 1994.

Frankenburg WK, Dodds J, Archer P, et al.: The Denver II: A major revision and restandardization of the Denver Developmental Screening Test. *Pediatrics* 89:91–97, 1992.

Friendly DS: Development of vision in infants and young children. *Pediatr Clin North Am* 40:693–703, 1993.

Garganta C, Seashore MR. Universal screening for congenital hearing loss. *Pediatric Annals* 29:302–308, 2000.

Gilbride KE: Developmental testing. *Pediatr Rev* 16:338–345, 1995.

Glascoe FP, Altemeier WA, Maclean WE: The importance of parents' concerns about their child's development. *Am J Dis Child* 143:955–958, 1989.

Harris DB. *Children's Drawings as Measures of Intellectual Maturity.* New York, Harcourt, Brace, & World, 1963.

Jones KL. *Smith's Recognizable Patterns of Human Malformation.* Philadelphia, WB Saunders, 1997.

Rossman MJ, Hyman SL, Rorabaugh ML, et al.: The CAT/CLAMS assessment for early intervention services. *Clin Pediatr* 33:404–409, 1994.

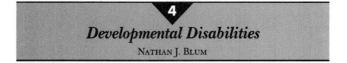

4
Developmental Disabilities
NATHAN J. BLUM

When caring for children with developmental disabilities, the physician must consider **possible causes** for the disorder, **screening** for problems associated with the disorder and **interventions** to minimize functional impairment and prevent long-term complications.

▼ CEREBRAL PALSY (CP)
Definition and Etiology

CP is a nonprogressive disorder of motion and posture that results from injury to the developing central nervous system (CNS). Epidemiologic data strongly suggest that **prenatal factors** (see Chapter 3, "Developmental Surveillance," Table 3.1) play a role in the development of CP. **Prematurity** is a significant risk factor; approximately 10%–15% of infants with a birth weight of less than 1000 grams develop CP. Although **perinatal asphyxia** was once thought to be a major cause of CP, it is now thought to cause less than 10% of cases. In fact, fewer than 20% of full-term infants with a 10-minute Apgar score of 0–3 who survive have CP (Nelson & Ellenberg, 1981). In approximately 25% of patients, **no cause** can be identified.

Classification

▼ **Spastic (pyramidal).** This form of CP is characterized by increased deep tendon reflexes and increased muscle tone with a "clasp knife" quality (i.e., initially, resistance to movement is strong but then the muscle gives way suddenly).

▼ **Choreoathetoid (extrapyramidal).** This form of CP is characterized by sudden involuntary movements of the extremities. Muscle tone is variable within the individual over time. The resistance to movement is described as "lead pipe" rigidity (i.e., persistent pressure results in slow movement of the limb).

▼ **Mixed.** Components of both spastic and choreoathetoid CP are present.

Associated Problems

▼ **Cognitive deficits**—mental retardation (50%), learning disabilities
▼ **Speech and language deficits**—communication disorders, dysarthria
▼ **Sensory deficits**—visual impairment, strabismus, hearing impairment
▼ **Gastrointestinal problems**—oral-motor dysfunction, gastroesophageal reflex disease (GRD), constipation
▼ **Urinary tract problems**—spastic bladder, recurrent urinary tract infection (UTI)
▼ **Neurologic problems**—spasticity, seizures
▼ **Musculoskeletal problems**—joint contractures, dislocated hips, scoliosis
▼ **Psychosocial and behavioral problems**

✂ HINT In most children, the diagnosis of CP will be evident in the first year of life. However, some children who have increased muscle tone in the first year of life will "grow out of it." These children, who do not have CP, may show attention deficits or learning disabilities in elementary school.

▼ MYELOMENINGOCELE

Definition and Etiology

A myelomeningocele is a sac containing meninges and a malformed spinal cord that protrudes through defective vertebrae. (In contrast, a meningocele is a sac containing only meninges; the spinal cord is normal.)

Myelomeningoceles develop approximately 28 days after conception if the neural tube fails to close. The cause of this defect is not known, but **maternal oral folic acid supplementation** prior to conception and throughout the first trimester has been shown to reduce the risk of myelomeningocele by 50%–70%. **Genetic factors** are also important; the risk of recurrence in the family of a child with a myelomeningocele is 50 times higher than in the general population.

Classification

The level of the lesion is predictive of the degree of functional impairment. Difficulties with bowel and bladder function occur with virtually all lesions.

▼ **Thoracic lesions**—flaccid paralysis of both lower extremities with weakness of the trunk musculature
▼ **L1 to L2 lesions**—flaccid paralysis of the knees, ankles, and feet with voluntary hip flexion and adduction

▼ **L3 lesions**—same as L1 to L2 lesions, but knee flexion is present as well
▼ **L4 to L5 lesions**—knee flexion and extension and ankle dorsiflexion are present, but plantar flexion and hip extension are weak or absent
▼ **Sacral lesions**—mild weakness of ankles and toes

Associated Problems

The degree and type of associated problems are also related to the level of the lesion.

▼ **Cognitive deficits**—mental retardation (33%), learning disabilities
▼ **Neurologic problems**—hydrocephalus (70%–80%), Arnold-Chiari deformity (type II)
▼ **Urinary tract problems**—incontinence, recurrent UTI, vesicoureteral reflex, kidney damage
▼ **Bowel dysfunction**—incontinence, constipation
▼ **Musculoskeletal disorders**—scoliosis, hip dislocation
▼ **Sexual dysfunction**—partial erection, retrograde ejaculation
▼ **Ophthalmologic disorders**—strabismus
▼ **Dermatologic disorders**—decubitus ulcers

HINT At a few centers fetal surgery to close the myelomeningocele is being done late in the second or earlier in the third trimester of the pregnancy. Although results are preliminary, this type of surgery seems to have the potential to greatly decrease the neurological impairment.

▼ MENTAL RETARDATION
Definition and Etiology

"Mental retardation" is a term that refers to "...substantial limitations in present functioning. It is characterized by significantly subaverage intellectual functioning, *existing concurrently with* (emphasis added) related limitations in two or more of the following applicable adaptive skill areas: communication, self-care, home living, social skills, community use, self-direction, health and safety, functional academics, leisure, and work. Mental retardation manifests before age 18 (American Association on Mental Retardation, Washington, DC, 1992).

The likelihood of identifying the cause of a patient's mental retardation depends on the severity of the retardation. A cause can be identified in approximately 50% of patients with mild mental retardation and in more than 80% of patients with severe or profound mental retardation. **Chromosomal abnormalities** (e.g., Down syndrome, fragile X syndrome) are the most commonly identified causes of mental retardation. Other causes of mental retardation include perinatal or postnatal injury, fetal alcohol syndrome, intrauterine infection, and inborn errors of metabolism.

Classification

The American Association on Mental Retardation has recommended against using intelligence quotient (IQ)–based labels (i.e., mild = an IQ of 55–69, moderate = an IQ of 40–54, severe = an IQ of 25–39, and profound = an IQ of less than 25) to classify mental retardation, but this classification scheme is still widely used. Descriptions of a child's strengths, weaknesses, and the level of support needed (intermittent, limited, extensive, pervasive) are most helpful in planning for the individual.

🎗 HINT Tests of intelligence performed during the infant and toddler years are not highly predictive of later IQ test scores. Furthermore, mental retardation cannot be diagnosed from IQ tests alone.

🎗 HINT The development quotient (DQ) equals the mental age divided by the chronologic age, multiplied by 100. A child with a DQ of less than 50 is at very high risk for mental retardation. Children with a DQ greater than 50 should not be diagnosed with mental retardation during the infant and toddler years.

Associated Problems

For children with a specific syndrome, the associated problems are related to the syndrome. In general, children with mental retardation are at increased risk for **hearing or visual deficits,** which occur in up to 25% of children with mild mental retardation and in more than 50% of children with severe mental retardation. **Seizures** and **behavior problems** ranging from hyperactivity to self-injury occur with increased frequency in this population.

🎗 HINT Physicians tend to underestimate the capabilities of children with mental retardation. Many children diagnosed with mild mental retardation function independently in the community as adults.

▼ PERVASIVE DEVELOPMENTAL DISORDER (PDD)

Definition and Etiology

PDD encompasses a variety of disorders (e.g., autistic disorder, Asperger syndrome, Rett disorder) characterized by impairments in **reciprocal social interactions, communication skills,** and **imaginative play behaviors.** Many children engage in stereotyped behaviors and have a markedly restricted range of activities and interests.

It is believed that these disorders are caused by damage to the brain or abnormal development of the brain. Genetic studies demonstrate an increased familial incidence of these disorders.

Most cases of classic Rett syndrome have recently been discovered to be caused by mutations in a gene on the X chromosome that codes for methyl-CpG-binding protein 2. Interestingly, not all females with this mutation have Rett syndrome (perhaps related to X chromosome inactivation patterns), but mutations in this gene must usually be lethal in males, as Rett syndrome is found almost exclusively in females.

Classification

▼ **Autistic disorder**—severe impairments in reciprocal social interactions, communication skills, and imaginative play behaviors

▼ **Asperger syndrome**—severe impairments in social interactions, frequent repetitive behaviors, and a restricted range of interests or activities but no significant delays in language skills or global cognitive skills

▼ **PDD–not otherwise specified (PDD–NOS)**—problems such as those described for autistic disorder and Asperger syndrome but not of sufficient severity to meet criteria for one of these diagnoses

▼ **Rett disorder**—patients have symptoms of autism but also have acquired microcephaly and the loss of purposeful hand movements

▼ **Childhood disintegrative disorder**—characterized by the loss of skills in multiple areas of functioning after at least 2 years of normal development; a diagnosis of exclusion after metabolic and neurodegenerative disorders are ruled out

---

HINT Children with autistic disorder may learn a few words and then stop using them between the ages of 12 and 24 months. However, they should not lose more complex language skills or skills in other areas.

Associated Problems

▼ **Cognitive deficits**—mental retardation (60%–70% of patients with autistic disorder), learning disabilities

▼ **Neurologic problems**—seizure disorder

▼ **Psychosocial and behavioral problems**—hyperactivity, unusual responses to sensory input, self-injurious behaviors, schizophrenia

▼ HEARING IMPAIRMENT
Definition and Etiology

Causes of hearing loss are summarized in Table 4.1.

▼ **Conductive hearing loss** is caused by damage to the external or middle ear. Hearing is decreased for sound conducted by air, but sounds conducted by bone are heard normally.

▼ **Sensorineural hearing loss** is caused by damage to the cochlea or auditory nerve. Both bone and air conduction of sound is abnormal.

▼ **Anacusis** is total hearing loss.

TABLE 4.1. Causes of Hearing Loss

Congenital
  Genetic syndromes (e.g., Waardenburg, Usher, craniofacial)
  Familial deafness (70%–80% autosomal recessive)
  Congenital "TORCH" infection
  Ototoxic drugs taken during first trimester
Acquired
  Genetic syndromes (e.g., Alport syndrome, Alström syndrome, neurofibromatosis)
  Meningitis or encephalitis
  Prematurity
  Hyperbilirubinemia requiring exchange transfusion
  Birth anoxia (Apgar score 0–3 at 5 minutes)
  Ototoxic medications
  Trauma

TABLE 4.2.   Classification of Hearing Loss

Degree of Hearing Loss	Decibel Level at Which Sounds Become Inaudible
Slight	16–25
Mild	26–40
Moderate	41–65
Severe	66–95
Profound	≥96

Classification

Degrees of hearing loss are summarized in Table 4.2. Individuals with moderate hearing loss miss most speech sounds at normal conversational levels.

Associated Problems

Associated problems largely depend on the cause of the hearing impairment and when the impairment develops. Difficulty with reading skills and behavioral disturbances are more common than in the general population.

▼ VISION IMPAIRMENT
Definition and Etiology

Most classification schemes would consider an individual visually impaired if the corrected visual acuity in the best eye was 20/60 or worse. In the United States, the legal definition of blindness is a best corrected visual acuity of 20/200 or a peripheral visual field restricted to 20° or less. Causes of vision impairment are summarized in Table 4.3.

Associated Problems

▼ **Cognitive deficits**—mental retardation (20%–25% of blind children)
▼ **Speech and language deficits**—developmental delays (imitation of mouth movements is an important component of speech development)

TABLE 4.3.   Causes of Vision Impairment

Congenital
   Congenital "TORCH" infections
   Malformations of visual system
   Cataracts
   Genetic syndromes
Acquired
   Retinopathy of prematurity
   Strabismus
   Genetic syndromes
   Macular disease
   Tumors (e.g., retinoblastoma)
   Trauma
   Infection
   Anoxia

▼ **Psychosocial and behavioral problems**—stereotypic behaviors, self-injurious behavior

---

🏅 HINT Blind children with normal intelligence have developmental delays. Gross motor skills (e.g., sitting) develop about 2 months later in blind children than in sighted children, and a blind child may begin to walk 3–7 months later than a sighted child. Signs of attachment may also occur at different times than in sighted children. Stranger anxiety occurs at approximately the same time as it does in sighted children, but separation anxiety does not develop until later.

▼ SPEECH AND LANGUAGE DISORDERS
Definition and Etiology

Speech refers to the sounds used to communicate information, and language refers to the system by which the sounds are given meaning. Language disorders are present when a child's skills at using language are significantly below her nonverbal cognitive skills.

Language disorders may be acquired through a brain injury or they may be congenital. In some cases, differences in the processing of auditory information are thought to be the cause of congenital language disorders.

🏅 HINT Always test the child's hearing.

🏅 HINT Assess verbal and nonverbal skills. For many children with mental retardation, the initial concern will be about the child's language skills.

Classification

▼ **Expressive language disorder**—the child's ability to formulate ideas into words is below her ability to understand language and perform nonverbal skills.
▼ **Mixed receptive-expressive language disorder**—the child's ability to formulate ideas into words and to understand language is below his nonverbal cognitive skills.
▼ **Phonological disorder**—the child is not able to use speech sounds that are appropriate for her age and dialect.

Associated Problems

▼ **Language-based learning disabilities**—e.g., reading, spelling, writing disorders.
▼ **Behavioral problems**

▼ LEARNING DISABILITIES
Definition and Etiology

In the Individuals with Disabilities Education Act Amendments of 1990, learning disability is defined as "a disorder in one or more of the basic psychological processes involved in understanding language, spoken or written, which may manifest itself in an imperfect ability to listen, speak, read, write, spell, or do mathematical calculations." School systems often define learning disabilities on the basis of discrepancies between expected achievement (based on IQ test results) and actual performance on achievement tests.

Learning disabilities may occur along with other conditions but are not the direct result of sensory impairments, mental retardation, social-emotional disturbance, cultural differences, or inappropriate instruction. Although the cause of learning disabilities is not known, **genetic factors** appear to play a role. Multiple members of a family often have learning disabilities, although the pattern does not follow classic Mendelian inheritance. In addition, learning disabilities occur with increased frequency in many **genetic syndromes.**

Classification

Multiple classification schemes have been suggested, but none is widely accepted. Reading learning disabilities are the most common learning disability. In the majority of cases, reading disabilities are thought to be related to deficits in phonological processing.

Associated Problems

▼ Speech and language disorders
▼ Psychosocial and behavioral problems—attention deficit hyperactivity disorder (ADHD), low self-esteem, school avoidance

---

⚡ HINT Failing a child or having him repeat a grade is not an appropriate intervention for a child with a learning disability. Physicians should insist that a psychological evaluation be performed on any child having difficulty in school. There are few situations in which repeating a grade is an appropriate intervention.

▼ ATTENTION DEFICIT HYPERACTIVITY DISORDER (ADHD)
Definition and Etiology

ADHD is characterized by developmentally inappropriate levels of **inattention, impulsivity,** and **hyperactivity.** In almost all cases, school functioning is impaired. The cause is not known. Research suggests that there may be decreased activity of frontal lobe neurons involving the dopamine and norepinephrine neurotransmitter systems. Genetic factors, prenatal exposure to environmental toxins (e.g., lead, alcohol), and postnatal brain injury (e.g., infections, inborn errors of metabolism, trauma) have been associated with some cases of ADHD, but in most patients no cause can be identified.

⚡ HINT "Developmentally inappropriate" levels of inattention or activity are difficult to define. Clinically, norm-referenced parent and teacher questionnaires are used to help make the diagnosis.

Classification

▼ Primarily inattentive type—the child is inattentive, but does not have high levels of activity or impulsivity.
▼ Primarily hyperactive—impulsive type-the child has high levels of activity and impulsivity, but not a high level of inattention.

▼ **Combined type**—the most common form of ADHD; the child has high levels of hyperactivity, impulsivity, and inattention.

Associated Problems

▼ **Cognitive–learning disabilities**
▼ **Neurologic problems**—"soft" neurologic signs
▼ **Psychosocial and behavioral problems**—oppositional defiant disorder, conduct disorder, anxiety disorder, depression, low self-esteem, poor social skills

---

✄ HINT Some children may appear to have symptoms of ADHD but really have other problems that are affecting their attention span (e.g., a chaotic or stressful home environment; unrecognized learning disabilities, sensory impairments, psychiatric disorders, or absence seizure disorder). However, children with any of these problems can have a coexisting attention deficit disorder.

Suggested Readings

Batshaw ML: *Children with Disabilities*. Baltimore, Brookes Publishing, 1997.

Curry CJ, Stevenson RE, Aughton D, et al. Evaluation of mental retardation: Recommendations of a consensus conference. *Am J Med Gen* 72:468–477, 1997.

Nelson KB, Ellenberg JH: Apgar scores as predictors of chronic neurologic disability. *Pediatrics* 68:36–44, 1981.

Percy AK. Genetics of Rett Syndrome: Properties of the newly discovered gene and pathobiology of the disorder. *Current Opin Pediatr* 12:589–595, 2000.

Shepard LA, Smith ML: Synthesis of research on grade retention. *Educational Leadership* 47(8):84–88, 1990.

5
Immunizations

▼ IMMUNIZATION SCHEDULE

The recommended childhood immunization schedule is given in Table 5.1. Important points to remember include:

▼ There are no contraindications to the simultaneous administration of multiple vaccines that are routinely recommended for infants and children. However, influenza and diphtheria-tetanus-pertussis (DTP) vaccines should be given on separate occasions because of the local and systemic reactions associated with these vaccines.

▼ A lapse in the immunization schedule does not require reinstituting the initial series. If a dose of vaccine is missed, merely give it at the next visit.

TABLE 5.1.

Recommended Childhood Immunization Schedule
United States, 2002

Vaccine ▼ / Age ▶	Birth	1 mo	2 mos	4 mos	6 mos	12 mos	15 mos	18 mos	24 mos	4-6 yrs	11-12 yrs	13-18 yrs
Hepatitis B[1]	Hep B #1	Hep B #2 (only if mother HBsAg (-))			Hep B #3						Hep B series	
Diphtheria, Tetanus, Pertussis[2]			DTaP	DTaP	DTaP		DTaP			DTaP	Td	
Haemophilus influenzae Type b[3]			Hib	Hib	Hib	Hib						
Inactivated Polio[4]			IPV	IPV		IPV				IPV		
Measles, Mumps, Rubella[5]						MMR #1				MMR #2	MMR #2	
Varicella[6]							Varicella				Varicella	
Pneumococcal[7]			PCV	PCV	PCV	PCV			PCV	PCV	PPV	
Hepatitis A[8]										Hepatitis A series		
Influenza[9]						Influenza (yearly)				Influenza (yearly)		

range of recommended ages · catch-up vaccination · preadolescent assessment

Vaccines below this line are for selected populations

TABLE 5.1. (Continued)

This schedule indicates the recommended ages for routine administration of currently licensed childhood vaccines, as of December 1, 2001, for children through age 18 years. Any dose not given at the recommended age should be given at any subsequent visit when indicated and feasible. ▨ Indicates age groups that warrant special effort to administer those vaccines not previously given. Additional vaccines may be licensed and recommended during the year. Licensed combination vaccines may be used whenever any components of the combination are indicated and the vaccine's other components are not contraindicated. Providers should consult the manufacturers' package inserts for detailed recommendations.

1. Hepatitis B vaccine (Hep B). All infants should receive the first dose of hepatitis B vaccine soon after birth and before hospital discharge; the first dose may also be given by age 2 months if the infant's mother is HBsAg-negative. Only monovalent hepatitis B vaccine can be used for the birth dose.

Monovalent or combination vaccine containing Hep B may be used to complete the series; four doses of vaccine may be administered if combination vaccine is used. The second dose of vaccine should be given at least 4 weeks after the first dose, except for Hib-containing vaccine which cannot be administered before age 6 weeks. The third dose should be given at least 16 weeks after the first dose and at least 8 weeks after the second dose. The last dose in the vaccination series (third or fourth dose) should not be administered before age 6 months.

Infants born to HBsAg-positive mothers should receive hepatitis B vaccine and 0.5 mL hepatitis B immune globulin (HBIG) within 12 hours of birth at separate sites. The second dose is recommended at age 1-2 months and the vaccination series should be completed (third or fourth dose) at age 6 months.

Infants born to mothers whose HBsAg status is unknown should receive the first dose of the hepatitis B vaccine series within 12 hours of birth. Maternal blood should be drawn at the time of delivery to determine the mother's HBsAg status; if the HBsAg test is positive, the infant should receive HBIG as soon as possible (no later than age 1 week).

2. Diphtheria and tetanus toxoids and acellular pertussis vaccine (DTaP). The fourth dose of DTaP may be administered as early as age 12 months, provided 6 months have elapsed since the third dose and the child is unlikely to return at age 15-18 months. **Tetanus and diphtheria toxoids (Td)** is recommended at age 11-12 years if at least 5 years have elapsed since the last dose of tetanus and diphtheria toxoid-containing vaccine. Subsequent routine Td boosters are recommended every 10 years.

3. Haemophilus influenzae type b (Hib) conjugate vaccine. Three Hib conjugate vaccines are licensed for infant use. If PRP-OMP (PedvaxHIB® or ComVax® [Merck]) is administered at ages 2 and 4 months, a dose at age 6 months is not required. DTaP/Hib combination products should not be used for primary immunization in infants at age 2, 4, or 6 months, but can be used as boosters following any Hib vaccine.

4. Inactivated poliovirus vaccine (IPV). An all-IPV schedule is recommended for routine childhood poliovirus vaccination in the United States. All children should receive four doses of IPV at age 2 months, 4 months, 6-18 months, and 4-6 years.

5. Measles, mumps, and rubella vaccine (MMR). The second dose of MMR is recommended routinely at age 4-6 years but may be administered during any visit, provided at least 4 weeks have elapsed since the first dose and that both doses are administered beginning at or after age 12 months. Those who have not previously received the second dose should complete the schedule by the visit at 11-12 years.

6. Varicella vaccine. Varicella vaccine is recommended at any visit at or after age 12 months for susceptible children (i.e. those who lack a reliable history of chickenpox). Susceptible persons aged ≥13 years should receive two doses, given at least 4 weeks apart.

7. Pneumococcal vaccine. The heptavalent **pneumococcal conjugate vaccine (PCV)** is recommended for all children aged 2-23 months and for certain children aged 24-59 months. **Pneumococcal polysaccharide vaccine (PPV)** is recommended in addition to PCV for certain high-risk groups. See MMWR 2000;49(RR-9):1-37.

8. Hepatitis A vaccine. Hepatitis A vaccine is recommended for use in selected states and regions, and for certain high-risk groups; consult your local public health authority. See MMWR 1999;48(RR-12):1-37.

9. Influenza vaccine. Influenza vaccine is recommended annually for children age ≥ 6 months with certain risk factors (including but not limited to asthma, cardiac disease, sickle cell disease, HIV, and diabetes; see MMWR 2001;50(RR-4):1-44), and can be administered to all others wishing to obtain immunity. Children aged ≤12 years should receive vaccine in a dosage appropriate for their age (0.25 mL if age 6-35 months or 0.5 mL if aged ≥ 3 years). Children aged ≤ 8 years who are receiving influenza vaccine for the first time should receive two doses separated by at least 4 weeks.

▼ ADMINISTRATION GUIDELINES
Sites

The preferred sites for the subcutaneous (SC) or intramuscular (IM) administration of vaccines are the anterolateral aspect of the upper thigh or the deltoid area of the upper arm. In **children younger than 1 year,** intramuscular injections should be administered in the **anterolateral aspect of the thigh.** For **children older than 1 year,** the **deltoid muscle** is the preferred site of administration. Ordinarily, the upper outer aspect of the buttocks should not be used for immunizing an infant because the gluteal region consists mainly of fat until the child has been walking for some time. Furthermore, there is a risk of damaging the sciatic nerve.

DTP Vaccine
Tetanus Toxoid, Absorbed

IM: 0.5 ml. Primary immunization consists of 3 doses; the second dose is administered 4–8 weeks after the first dose, and the third dose is given 6–12 months after the second dose. Alternatively, the Advisory Committee on Immunization Practices (ACIP) and the AAP recommends four doses for primary immunization, with the first three administered at 4- to 8-week intervals and the fourth dose 6–12 months after the third dose. A fifth dose is usually administered before school entry, at age 4–6. Subsequent boosters should be administered at 10-year intervals throughout life.

Tetanus Immune Globulin (Hyper-Tet)

IM: 250 U as a single dose for postexposure prophylaxis. For treatment of tetanus, doses of 3000–6000 U in children or adults are recommended. The immune globulin will not block the effectiveness of tetanus toxoid but should be administered at different sites.

Diphtheria Antitoxin

Intravenous by slow infusion or IM: All patients are dosed the same. Sensitivity to horse serum should be tested before administering the dose. Depending on symptoms and length of illness, 20,000–120,000 U.

Precautions

Precautions for DTP and diphtheria-tetanus-acellular pertussis (DTaP) include:

▼ Persistent, inconsolable crying or screaming for more than 3 hours after the previous dose
▼ Unusual or high-pitched crying within 48 hours of the previous dose
▼ Collapse or shock-like state within 48 hours of the previous dose
▼ Temperature higher than 40.5°C (104.9°F) unexplained by another cause within 48 hours of the previous dose
▼ Progressive neurologic disorder characterized by developmental delay or neurologic findings
▼ Personal history of convulsions

Poliovirus Vaccine [Poliovirus vaccine, live, oral, trivalent (sabin, TOPV, OPV, Orimune); Poliovirus vaccine, inactivated (Salk, IPV)]

IPV regimen (SC): Two 0.5-ml doses are administered at least 4 weeks apart, but preferably 8 weeks apart starting at 2 months of age. A third dose is administered at 12–18 months of age and a fourth dose should be given at school entry or at about 4–6 years of age.

IPV/OPV regimen (SC and orally): Two 0.5-ml doses of IPV are administered at 2 and 4 months of age with DTP or DTaP and Hib vaccines, followed by OPV doses at 12–18 months of age and again at 4–6 years of age.

Monovalent Measles and Measles-Mumps-Rubella (MMR) Vaccines [measles vaccine (Attenuvax); measles and rubella vaccine (M-R-Vax II); measles, mumps, and rubella vaccine (M-M-R II)]

SC in the outer aspect of the upper arm: 0.5 ml at age 15–18 months. A booster dose (principally for measles) is now recommended at age 4–6 years (ACIP) or 11–12 years (AAP).

Federal law requires that the date of administration, manufacturer, lot number, and expiration date of the vaccine and the name, title, and address of the person administering the dose be entered into the patient's permanent medical record. It also requires providers to distribute information on vaccines before each vaccination.

Contraindications

Contraindications to measles vaccination include pregnancy, anaphylactic reaction to neomycin, recent injection of immune globulin, and compromised immunity (except in patients with HIV).

⚔ HINT In patients who have been exposed to the measles virus, the vaccine may be given within 72 hours of exposure to provide protection. Alternatively, if given within 6 days of exposure, immune globulin (0.25 ml/kg, intramuscularly) may prevent or modify measles in a susceptible person. Children and adolescents with symptomatic HIV infections who are exposed to measles should receive immune globulin prophylaxis (0.5 ml/kg) regardless of their immunization status. The maximum dosage for all patients is 15 ml. Live measles vaccine should be given 3 months after immune globulin administration if no contraindications exist.

Varicella Virus Vaccine (Varivax)

SC (in the outer aspect of the upper arm):

Age 1–12 years: 0.5 ml single dose
Adolescents and adults: 0.5 ml/dose for two doses separated by 4–8 weeks

Pneumococcal: Pneumococcal Vaccine, Conjugate (Prevnar)

IM:

Infants: 0.5 ml/dose given at 2, 4, and 6 months of age, with a booster dose given at 12–15 months of age

Previously unvaccinated older infants and children:

7–11 months of age: A total of three doses is given with at least 2 months between doses, and the third dose is given after the first birthday

12–23 months of age: A total of two doses is given at least 2 months apart

24 months or older: A single dose is given

Pneumococcal Vaccine, Polyvalent (Pneumovax 23, Pnu-Imune 23)

SC or IM: Over age 2 years and adults: 0.5 ml. The manufacturers presently do not recommend a booster dose because of the increased incidence and severity of adverse effects. The AAP and ACIP presently recommend revaccination in those patients at greatest risk (asplenia, sickle cell, and organ transplant).

Revaccination should be considered in children after age 3–5 if they will be older than age 10 at the time of revaccination, and in adults after 6 or more years since the last vaccination.

Hib

Haemophilus b Conjugate Vaccine (ActHIB, HibTITER, OmniHIB, PedvaxHIB, ProHIBIT)

Depends on the product used. If possible, the patient's immunization should be completed with the same vaccine because information on the interchangeability of the vaccines is lacking. In situations in which the brand of vaccine used previously is not known, the primary objective in infants age 2–6 months should be to assure that three doses of conjugate vaccine have been administered. Administer 0.5 ml of the vaccine IM in the outer aspect of the vastus lateralis or deltoid. The following doses are listed by age at first vaccination and by product.

ActHIB, HibTITER, OmniHIB

Age 2–6 months: Three injections given at about 2-month intervals and a booster dose after age 15 months

Age 7–11 months: Two injections given at about 2-month intervals and a booster dose after age 15 months, but not less than 2 months after the second injection

Age 12–14 months: One injection and a booster dose after age 15 months, but not less than 2 months after the first injection

Age 15 months and older: A single injection

PedvaxHIB

Age 2–6 months: Two injections given at about 2-month intervals and a booster at age 12 months

Age 7–11 months: Two injections given at about 2-month intervals and a booster dose after age 15 months, but not less than 2 months after the second injection

Age 12–14 months: One injection and a booster dose after age 15 months, but not less than 2 months after the first injection

Age 15 months and older: A single injection

ProHIBiT

Age 15 months and older: A single injection

Haemophilus b Conjugate Vaccine with Hepatitis B Vaccine (Comvax)

IM: Previously unvaccinated infants: 0.5 ml at 2, 4, and 12–15 months of age. Infants vaccinated with a single dose of hepatitis B vaccine shortly after birth may be vaccinated using Comvax on the schedule listed above. Patients who have received more than one dose of hepatitis B vaccine may receive Comvax at any time they are scheduled to receive doses of the two vaccines.

Hep A Vaccine (Havrix, VAQTA)

Havrix (IM)

Children and adolescents: 360 ELISA U/0.5 ml dose with two doses given about 1 month apart
Age 18-adults: 1440 ELISA U/1 ml dose as a single dose

A booster dose is recommended to be given 6–12 months later to ensure adequate titers.

VAQTA (IM)

Children and adolescents: 25 U/0.5 ml dose as a single dose
Adults: 50 U/1 ml dose as a single dose

A booster dose given 6–12 months after the initial dose ensures adequate titers.

Hep B Vaccine

Hep B Immune Globulin (H-BIG, Hep-B-Gammagee, HyperHep)

IM (anterolateral thigh in children, deltoid in adults): Two different products are available. Interchangeability of the vaccines has not been documented, but Engerix-B may be used to complete a series that was initiated with Recombivax-HB.

Engerix B

Infants born to HBsAg-positive mothers: 10 μg (0.5 ml) on the first day of life, at age 1 month, and at age 6 months
Infants born to HBsAg-negative mothers: 10 μg (0.5 ml) on the first or second day of life, at age 1 month, and at age 6 months or at age 1–2 months, at age 4 months, and at age 6–18 months
Under age 11 years: 10 μg (0.5 ml) for a three-dose series at 0, 1, and 6 months or a four-dose series at 0, 1, 2, and 12 months
Over age 11 years–adults: 20 μg (1 ml) for a three-dose series at 0, 1, and 6 months or a four-dose series at 0, 1, 2, and 12 months
Dialysis or immunocompromised patients: 40 μg (2 ml) administered as two 1-ml doses at separate sites for a four-dose series at 0, 1, 2, and 6 months
IM (anterolateral thigh in children, deltoid in adults): If H-BIG and hepatitis B vaccine are administered at the same time, use different sites for each injection.

Neonates born to Hep B surface antigen (HBsAg)–positive mothers: 0.5 ml within 12 hours of birth

Postexposure prophylaxis: 0.06 ml/kg to a maximum of 5 ml as soon as possible, but within 7 days of exposure. A second dose should be administered 28–30 days after exposure.

Recombivax-HB

Infants born to HbsAg-positive mothers: 5 μg (0.5 ml) on the first day of life, age 1 month, and age 6 months

Infants born to HBsAg-negative mothers and children under age 11: 2.5 μg (0.25 ml or 0.5 ml) at 0, 1, and 6 months. In infants, the series may be started at birth or at age 1–2 months.

Age 11–19: 5 μg (0.5 ml) for a three-dose series at 0, 1, and 6 months

Adults: 10 μg (1 ml) for a three-dose series at 0, 1, and 6 months

Dialysis and immunocompromised patients: 40 μg (1 ml) of the special dialysis formula at 0, 1, and 6 months

Revaccination (booster) doses are not generally recommended except in dialysis patients whose antibody levels have fallen to < 10 mIU/ml. Levels should be tested in vaccinated individuals who are exposed to HBsAb-positive blood. If levels are inadequate, a dose of H-BIG and a booster dose of vaccine should be administered at the same time in separate sites.

▼ SPECIAL CIRCUMSTANCES

Premature Infants and Infants with Medical Problems

Premature infants should be immunized **at the usual age** with the usual dose. Reducing or dividing doses of vaccines is not recommended.

Infants who have had an **intraventricular hemorrhage** or other neurologic event soon after birth but are **stable at age 2 months** should also be **immunized.** Infants who are still in the hospital at age 2 months can also receive immunizations. The administration of **OPV to hospitalized infants should be avoided** (to avoid transmitting the virus in the nursery), but it is acceptable to administer IPV to these patients. If the infant has a history of **chronic respiratory disease,** the **split virus influenza vaccine** should be administered at 6 months of age; family members and caretakers should also be vaccinated.

Immunodeficient and Immunosuppressed Children

Patients being **treated with corticosteroids** may need to be considered immunocompromised. Live-virus vaccines or **live-bacteria vaccines should not be given** to patients with congenital disorders of immune function. IPV should be used for the patient and the family. Table 5.2 summarizes recommendations for HIV-infected children.

Asplenic Children

Children who have undergone splenectomy, children with functional asplenia (sickle cell disease), and children with congenital asplenia have an increased risk of fulminant bacteremia, which is associated with a high mortality rate. Important pathogens in asplenic children include *Streptococcus pneumoniae, Neisseria meningitidis, Haemophilus influenzae* type B, and *Escherichia coli.*

TABLE 5.2. Recommendations for Routine Immunization of HIV-Infected Children in the United States

Vaccine	Known Asymptomatic HIV Infection	Symptomatic HIV Infection
Hepatitis B	Yes	Yes
DTaP (or DTP)	Yes	Yes
IPV*	Yes	Yes
MMR	Yes	Yes†
Hib	Yes	Yes
Pneumococcal‡	Yes	Yes
Influenza§	Yes	Yes
Varicella‖	No	No

DTP = diphtheria and tetanus toxoids and pertussis vaccine; DTaP = diphtheria and tetanus toxoids acellular pertussis vaccine; IPV = inactivated poliovirus vaccine; MMR = live-virus measles, mumps, and rubella; Hib = *Haemophilus influenzae* type b conjugate. (Adapted from the American Academy of Pediatrics. In Peter G, ed. *1997 Red Book: Report of the Committee on Infectious Diseases.* 24th ed. Elk Grove Village, IL: American Academy of Pediatrics, 1997.)

* Only inactivated polio vaccine (IPV) should be used for HIV-infected children, HIV-exposed infants whose status is indeterminate, and household contacts of HIV-infected patients.

† Severely immunocompromised HIV-infected children should not receive MMR vaccine.

‡ Pneumococcal vaccine should be administered at 2 years of age to all HIV-infected children. Children who are older than 2 years of age should receive pneumococcal vaccine at the time of diagnosis. Revaccination after 3 to 5 years is recommended in either circumstance.

§ Influenza vaccine should be provided each fall and repeated annually for HIV-exposed infants 6 months of age and older, HIV-infected children and adolescents, and for household contacts of HIV-infected patients.

‖ Varicella vaccine is not currently indicated for HIV-exposed or HIV-infected patients, but studies are in progress to determine safety and possible indication.

Polyvalent pneumococcal vaccine and quadrivalent meningococcal polysaccharide vaccine should be given to all asplenic children older than 2 years. *H. influenzae* type B vaccine should be **initiated in infancy** as for otherwise healthy children. **Daily antimicrobial prophylaxis** is also recommended for asplenic children regardless of their vaccination status.

Children with Personal or Family History of Seizures

A family history of convulsive disorders is neither a contraindication to immunization with DTP or measles vaccine nor a reason to postpone immunization. **Pertussis immunization** in infants with **recent seizures** should be **postponed** until a progressive neurologic disorder is excluded or the cause of the seizure is determined.

Children with Chronic Disease

In general, children with chronic disease should receive the **same immunizations recommended for healthy children.**

TABLE 5.3. Guide to Tetanus Prophylaxis in Routine Wound Management

History of Absorbed Tetanus Toxoid (Doses)	Clean, Minor Wounds		All Other Wounds*	
	Td†	TIG‡	Td†	TIG‡
Unknown or < 3	Yes	No	Yes	Yes
≥ 3§	No‖	No	No#	No

Adapted from the American Academy of Pediatrics. In Peter G, ed. *1997 Red Book: Report of the Committee on Infectious Diseases.* 24th ed. Elk Grove Village, IL: American Academy of Pediatrics, 1997.

Td = adult-use tetanus and diphtheria toxoids; TIG = tetanus immune globulin (human).

* Such as, but not limited to, wounds contaminated with dirt, feces, soil, or saliva; puncture wounds; avulsions; and wounds resulting from missiles, crushing, burns, or frostbite.

† For children < 7 years, diphtheria and tetanus toxoids and acellular pertussis (DTaP) or diphtheria-tetanus-pertussis (DTP) is recommended; if pertussis vaccine is contraindicated, diphtheria-tetanus toxoid (DT) is given. For persons ≥ 7 years of age, Td is recommended.

‡ Equine tetanus antitoxin should be used when TIG is not available.

§ If only 3 doses of fluid toxoid have been received, a fourth dose of toxoid, preferably an adsorbed toxoid, should be given.

‖ Yes, if more than 10 years since the last dose.

Yes, if more than 5 years since the last dose. (More frequent boosters are not needed and can accentuate side effects.)

Children with immunologic disorders should not receive live vaccines. However, patients who are **HIV-positive** should receive the measles vaccine.

Children with certain chronic diseases (e.g., cardiac, pulmonary, hematologic, metabolic, or adrenal disorders; cystic fibrosis) are more **prone to the complications of influenza and pneumococcal infections** and should receive the **appropriate vaccines.**

Children with Wounds

The treatment of a wound depends on the nature of the wound and on the patient's immunization history. Guidelines for tetanus prophylaxis are given in Table 5.3.

▼ COMMON MISCONCEPTIONS REGARDING CONTRAINDICATIONS TO IMMUNIZATION

Many misconceptions exist regarding contraindications to immunization (Cody et al, 1981). **The following are not appropriate contraindications to immunization:**

▼ A mild acute illness characterized by a low-grade fever or mild diarrhea in an otherwise well child

▼ Antimicrobial therapy or being in the convalescent phase of an illness

▼ A reaction to a previous DTP dose that involved only soreness, redness, or swelling in the immediate vicinity of the vaccination site or a temperature of less than 105°F (40.5°C)
▼ A household contact who is pregnant
▼ Recent exposure to an infectious disease
▼ Breast-feeding (does not interfere with immunization with OPV)
▼ A history of nonspecific allergies or relatives with allergies
▼ Allergies to penicillin (none of the vaccines licensed in the United States contains penicillin)
▼ Allergies to duck meat or duck feathers (no vaccine available in the United States is produced in substrates containing duck antigens)
▼ Family history of convulsions (it is permissible to administer pertussis and measles vaccinations to patients with a family history of convulsions)
▼ Family history of sudden infant death syndrome (DTP vaccination is permissible in these patients)
▼ Family history of an adverse event, unrelated to immunosuppression, following a vaccination
▼ Malnutrition

▼ OTHER SOURCES OF INFORMATION

The **schedule** for the immunization of children is **constantly changing.** The following publications are excellent sources of up-to-date information:

▼ *2000 Red Book: Report of the Committee on Infectious Diseases,* 25th ed. This reference is published at 2- to 3- year intervals by the Committee on Infectious Diseases of the AAP.
▼ *Pediatrics.* Statements of the Committee on Infectious Diseases of the American Academy of Pediatrics (AAP) are published in this monthly journal.
▼ *Morbidity and Mortality Weekly Report* (**MMWR**). Http://www.mmr.org. This report is published weekly by the Centers for Disease Control and Prevention (CDC) and contains current vaccine recommendations.
▼ *Health Information for International Travel.* This monograph is published annually by the CDC and contains guidelines for specific immunizations required for international travel. It can be purchased from the Superintendent of Documents, United States Government Printing Office, Washington, DC, 20402.
▼ **http://www.aap.org.** This is the web site for the American Academy of Pediatrics.

Suggested Readings

Cody DL, Baraff LJ, Cherry JD, et al.: Nature and rates of adverse reactions associated with DTP and DT immunizations in infants and children. *Pediatrics* 68:650–660, 1981.

2000 Red Book: Report of the Committee on Infectious Diseases, 25th ed. Elk Grove Village, IL, American Academy of Pediatrics, 2000.

http://www.cdc.gov/nip/links.htm. CDC National Immunization Program.

http://www.cdc.gov/od/nvpo/. National Vaccine Program Office.

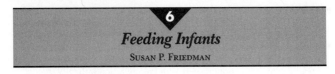

Feeding Infants

SUSAN P. FRIEDMAN

▼ NUTRITIONAL NEEDS OF HEALTHY, FULL-TERM INFANTS

The nutritional needs of a healthy, full-term infant are summarized in Table 6.1.

⚡ HINT   Contraindications to both breast- and bottle-feeding:
▼ Respiratory rate > 80 breaths/min
▼ An infant with poor suck/swallow
▼ An absent gag reflex
▼ Symptoms of sepsis or asphyxia
▼ Poorly tolerated feeding with sterile water

▼ BREAST-FEEDING

Breast-feeding is the optimal choice for feeding normal infants, and breast milk is the gold standard on which many infant formulas are based.

Contraindications to Breast-Feeding

The following are contraindications to breast-feeding:

▼ Inborn error of metabolism (e.g., galactosemia)
▼ Poor suck/swallow
▼ Maternal AIDS
▼ Active (untreated) tuberculosis
▼ Maternal drug or alcohol abuse or cigarette smoking
▼ Breast cancer (currently under treatment)
▼ Maternal prolactinoma
▼ Maternal psychosis
▼ History of breast reduction surgery involving ligation of the milk ducts (may breast-feed if supplements are provided as needed)

TABLE 6.1. Nutritional Needs of Healthy, Full-Term Infants	
Nutritional Element	**Daily Requirement**
Calories	Approximately 100 kcal/kg/day
Fluids	Approximately 150 ml/kg/day*
Carbohydrates	37%–44% of calories
Protein	10%–12% of calories
Fat	40%–50% of calories; 3% from linoleic acid

* Of formula or breast milk, to provide adequate calories.

▨ **HINT**   Maternal hepatitis B is not a contraindication to breast-feeding, provided the infant receives hepatitis vaccination and hepatitis immunoglobulin shortly after birth.

▼ Maternal use of medications that are contraindicated with breast-feeding, as per the findings of the American Academy of Pediatrics Committee on Drugs

Patient Counseling

Drug Use During Lactation

The nursing mother should be counseled to **avoid all drugs,** including over-the-counter and herbal medications, **until she has consulted her physician.** Cigarettes and significant alcohol intake should be avoided. An occasional glass of beer or wine may aid in milk let-down if the mother is tense. Cigarette smoking is no longer considered an absolute contraindication to breast-feeding, but the mother should be counseled regarding the dangers of nicotine to the infant.

Nutrition and Rest

Nursing mothers need an **extra 500–600 calories per day** of nutritious foods and **enough fluids** to satisfy thirst, usually several extra glasses per day. **Supplemental calcium** should be obtained by continuing to take prenatal vitamins. **Adequate rest** is also important (it is ideal if the mother can nap when the infant naps).

Breast-Feeding Technique

It is neither necessary nor desirable to wash the nipples, but **clean hands are important.** The mother should be comfortable—it may be helpful to place extra pillows under her elbows and on her lap. The baby should be positioned on his side in the mother's arms, facing the mother.

The mother should support the breast, taking care to keep her fingers away from the areola. Tickling the baby's lower lip with the nipple will induce him to open his mouth wide, at which point he should be drawn close to the mother's body. The mother should ensure that the baby takes the breast at least 1 inch beyond the protruding part of the nipple.

Both breasts should be offered at each feeding, for a minimum of 10 minutes on each breast. The starting breast should be alternated. **Nipples should be allowed to air dry** or patted down before covering them at the end of the feeding.

Feeding Frequency and Intake

Feedings for the first few weeks should take place **at least every 2–3 hours. No supplemental water or formula** should be given **during the first 2 weeks,** unless medically indicated. (Table 6.2 summarizes nutrition supplementation for full-term, breast-fed infants.)

Management of Problems

Engorgement

Engorgement may occur on the third or fourth postpartum day and can cause significant discomfort for the mother. It is important to reassure the

TABLE 6.2. **Nutrition Supplementation for Full-Term, Breast-Fed Infants**	
Formula or water	Not recommended during the first 2 weeks unless medically indicated
Fluoride	0.25 mg/day, starting at 6 months (if tap water is not fluoridated)
Vitamin D	400 IU/day
Iron	Vitamins with iron or iron-fortified cereal, starting at 4–6 months

mother that a high level of engorgement typically lasts only 24–48 hours. Management strategies include:

▼ Continuing to nurse frequently
▼ Application of hot compresses or taking a hot shower before nursing to alleviate discomfort
▼ Application of ice packs to the breasts after nursing
▼ Administration of acetaminophen (possibly with a small dose of codeine)
▼ Pumping only a small amount of milk to avoid increased milk production (if a breast pump is being used)

Sore, Cracked, or Hemorrhagic Nipples

▼ The infant's position on the nipple should be reevaluated; an infant that latches on to an inadequate amount of the nipple is the most common cause of sore nipples. The mother should be sure that the infant's lower lip is furled outward.
▼ Exposure of the nipples to air is important. In addition, applying expressed breast milk to cracked nipples and allowing it to air dry has resulted in dramatic healing in some patients.
▼ Mothers should be advised to nurse the baby on the least affected side first. Prefeeding with milk that has been manually expressed may appease the overly vigorous nurser. In severe cases, breast-feeding on the affected side should be temporarily terminated, and a breast pump should be used.
▼ Administration of acetaminophen 20 minutes before nursing (but only every 4 hours) may alleviate discomfort.

Galactocele

A galactocele (**plugged milk duct**) presents as a persistent, hard, round or linear lump, usually in the lateral and inferior quadrants of the breast. **Warm, moist heat** should be applied to the breast for 20 minutes before each nursing, and the **breast should be massaged** from the body toward the nipple, concentrating on the involved area. Mothers should be advised to **nurse the baby frequently** (i.e., every 1.5–2 hours) for at least 10 minutes on each side. The **affected side should be offered first,** and the infant should be positioned with his chin toward the affected area, which will facilitate emptying of the affected quadrant. It may take several nursing sessions to empty the plugged duct.

Mastitis

Lactating mothers with mastitis present with **fever, shaking chills, and malaise,** followed by **localized breast erythema and pain.** Mothers should be advised to continue to nurse frequently. Treatment is with oral ampicillin, the application of warm compresses, rest, and pain medication (if necessary).

Poor Early Weight Gain

Breast-fed, full-term infants may **lose as much as 10% of their birth weight** during the first several days of life, but they should regain it by 2 weeks of age. A phone call or visit within 48 hours after discharge is important to catch any problems early. The mother should be questioned regarding:

▼ The frequency and duration of nursing sessions
▼ Signs of established lactation (i.e., diminished breast fullness after nursing, leaking, cessation of nipple discomfort after latching on, uterine cramps during nursing)
▼ Normal infant voiding (minimum of 6–8 times per day, pale urine). Note: The baby may void twice between diaper changes so the number of voidings may vary.
▼ Normal infant defecation (3–4 loose stools per day on days 3–4, 4–6 loose stools per day on days 4–6, 8–10 loose stools per day on weeks 2–4)
▼ Infant response to feeding (e.g., sleepy, satisfied)

An abnormal response to any of these questions should prompt an immediate office visit. If the infant is discharged within 48 hours of birth, an office visit within 2–3 days is important.

According to Lawrence (1984), the most common factors associated with poor early weight gain are:

▼ Ineffective breast-feeding technique
▼ Infrequent or inappropriately short feedings (e.g., excessive nighttime intervals)
▼ Water supplementation
▼ Maternal problems that inhibit milk letdown

▼ BOTTLE-FEEDING
Patient Counseling

Bottle-Feeding Technique

Sterile water is offered first to check for adequate suck/swallow, regurgitation, and a patent upper gastrointestinal tract. Glucose water is as irritating as formula if aspirated and therefore should not be used for this purpose.

If the initial feeding is tolerated, the infant can be offered full-strength formula. The bottle should be held so that no air enters the nipple, and the bottle should never be "propped."

Feeding Frequency and Intake

Formula can be given **every 3–4 hours.** A small-for-gestational-age infant may require small, frequent feedings until his gastric capacity increases, whereas a large-for-gestational-age infant of a diabetic mother should be given early and frequent feedings, and his blood sugar should be monitored carefully.

The typical full-term neonate will drink only 15–30 ml (0.5–1 oz) per feeding during the first few days of life. The mother should be assured that this is sufficient because of in utero–acquired stores. She should be told to expect an **intake of 3–4 oz per feeding** (approximately every 3–4 hours) **by the end of the first week.**

Formula Types

The specific compositions of many commonly available infant formulas are listed in Table 6.3. Whole cow's milk should not be introduced until 1 year of age.

Cow's Milk–based [Full-term (Standard)] Formulas

Full-term (standard) formulas, which provide 20 kcal/oz, are generally suitable for infants with **birth weights higher than 2000 g**, most **full-term small-for-gestational-age** infants, and some **preterm infants once they reach term** (usually close to the time of hospital discharge).

Soy-based (Lactose-free) Formulas

Soy-based formulas are indicated for infants with **temporary or chronic lactose intolerance** and for infants with **galactosemia.** They are also often used when intolerance to cow's milk protein is suspected. However, the use of soy-based formula in this situation is not generally recommended because of a significant antigenic crossover between cow's milk protein and soy protein. Soy-based formulas are **not recommended for prolonged use in preterm infants** because the phytase content may lead to hypophosphatemia and rickets.

Preterm Formulas

These formulas, which provide 24 or 27 kcal/oz, are specially designed to meet the needs of **preterm infants.** They should be used until the infant reaches 40 weeks gestation (or longer, if the infant's birth weight is less than 1000 g).

Dietary Supplementation

Calories

Caloric supplements are often required for infants with higher-than-usual caloric needs, decreased oral intake, decreased fluid tolerance, or a combination of these factors (e.g., preterm infants, infants with bronchopulmonary dysplasia, infants with congestive heart failure). Care should be taken to maintain the **correct balance of nutrients.**

Carbohydrate

Carbohydrate supplements (e.g., Polycose, Karo syrup, rice cereal, infant oatmeal) are **well-tolerated** and **inexpensive** but **low in caloric density.** Polycose and Karo syrup may cause diarrhea if more than 2 ml/oz of formula are given. Rice cereal can cause constipation, especially if more than 1–2 tsp/4 oz of formula are added (it may be advisable to substitute infant oatmeal for the rice cereal).

Fat

Fat supplements are **high in caloric density.** The **best-tolerated forms** [microlipids or medium-chain triglyceride (MCT) oil, 1 ml/oz of formula] are **more expensive** and **lower in caloric density** than inexpensive, less well-tolerated vegetable oil, which may cause diarrhea. Vegetable oil is also harder to keep mixed with the formula. Microlipids supply 4.5 kcal/ml, MCT oil supplies 7.6 kcal/ml, and vegetable oil supplies 9 kcal/ml.

Protein

Protein supplements are generally **well tolerated** but of relatively **low caloric density.**

Fluoride

Fluoride supplementation (0.25 mg/day) is indicated **after 6 months** of age for **all breast-fed infants** who live in an area with **nonfluoridated water,** as well as for **formula-fed infants** who are given formula that is reconstituted using nonfluoridated water or who are fed ready-to-feed formula.

Vitamins

Vitamin supplementation is **not required** for healthy, full-term infants with normal formula volume intake. Infants with specific medical problems, such as malabsorption, may require vitamin supplementation.

▼ SOLID FOODS

Solid foods are typically introduced to the infant's diet at **4–6 months of age.** Foods can be introduced earlier if the infant seems to require more than 32 oz/day of formula.

Initially, small volumes of solid foods are provided once daily. The volume is gradually increased, and the frequency is increased to three times daily with some snacks. **Formula or breast milk** remains an important part of the infant's diet **throughout the first year** of life and should be maintained at 24–32 oz/day.

The order in which foods are introduced varies widely across cultural groups and is based more on tradition than on science. Table 6.4 offers a suggested schedule for introducing solid foods.

▓ HINT   Certain foods (e.g., raisins, nuts, popcorn, hard candy, hot dogs, and grapes) should be avoided because of the risk of choking.

▼ SPECIAL CONSIDERATIONS FOR PRETERM INFANTS
Calorie Requirements

Healthy preterm infants usually grow well with a diet that provides **110–130 kcal/kg/day.** Infants with **complications** (e.g., pulmonary bronchodysplasia, congestive heart failure) frequently require **130–200 kcal/kg/day** to achieve adequate growth.

To increase caloric intake, it is necessary to increase the feeding volume (if fluid restriction is not a concern), the caloric density of the feedings, or both. If it is necessary to increase the feeding volume but the infant is unable to consume the increased volume, supplemental feedings can be provided through a nasogastric or orogastric tube.

Most preterm infants initially require a caloric density of at least 24 kcal/oz (the density of most preterm formulas). Caloric density can be increased by concentrating the formula until it provides 24–27 kcal/oz; additional increases in caloric density can be achieved by adding caloric supplements (e.g., microlipids, MCT oil, Polycose).

TABLE 6.3. Composition of Infant Formulas (per 100 kcal)

Name (Manufacturer)	Kcal/oz	CHO (% of cal/type)	Fat (% of cal/type)	PRO (% of cal/type)	FE (mg)	Vit D (IU)	mg Ca/mg PO
Cow's milk–based standard formulas							
Enfamil (Mead Johnson); with/without iron	20*	44% Lactose	43% Palm olein, coconut oil, soy oil, sunflower oil	8% Cow's milk	1.8/0.7	60	78/53
Similac (Ross); with/without iron	20*	43% Lactose	49% Soy oil, coconut oil	8% Cow's milk	1.8/0.22	60	78/42
Good Start (Carnation)†	20‡	44% Lactose, corn malto-dextrin	46% Palm oil, safflower oil, coconut oil	10% Whey and whey protein	1.5	60	64/36
Soy-based standard formulas							
Isomil (Ross)	20	41% Corn syrup, sucrose	49% Coconut oil, soy oil, high-oleic safflower oil	10% Soy protein isolate, L-methionine	1.8	60	105/75
Prosobee (Mead Johnson)	20	42% Corn syrup solids	48% Coconut oil, soy oil, palm oil, sunflower oil	10% Soy protein isolate, L-methionine	1.8	60	105/83

Preterm formulas

Formula		Carbohydrate	Fat	Protein			
Similac Special Care (Ross)	24§	42% Lactose (50%), corn syrup solids (50%)	49% MCT oil (50%), soy oil (30%), coconut oil (20%)	11% Nonfat milk whey (60%), casein (40%)	1.8/0.37	150	180/100
Enfamil Premature (Mead Johnson); with/without iron	24§	44% Lactose (50%), corn syrup solids (50%)	46% MCT oil (40%), soy oil (40%), coconut oil (20%)	12% Nonfat milk whey (60%), casein (40%)	1.8/0.25	270	165/83
Similac Neosure (Ross)‖	22	41% Lactose (50%), glucose polymers (50%)	49% MCT oil (25%), LCT oil (75%)	10% Whey (50%), casein (50%)	1.8	70	105/62
EnfaCare (Mead Johnson)	22	43% Lactose (40%), glucose polymers (60%)		High oleic sunflower oil (35%), soy oil(30%), MCT oil (20%), coconut oil (15%)	47		

Special formulas#

Formula		Carbohydrate	Fat	Protein			
Nutramigen (Mead Johnson)	20	44% Modified corn starch, corn syrup solids	45% Palm olein, soy oil, coconut oil, sunflower oil	11% Casein hydrolysate and amino acids	1.8	60	94/63

Continued

TABLE 6.3.   Composition of Infant Formulas (per 100 kcal) (continued)

Name (Manufacturer)	Kcal/oz	CHO (% of cal/type)	Fat (% of cal/type)	PRO (% of cal/type)	FE (mg)	Vit D (IU)	mg Ca/mg PO
Pregestimil (Mead Johnson)	20	41% Corn syrup solids, modified cornstarch, dextrose	48% MCT oil (55%), corn oil (10%), soy oil (25%), safflower oil (10%)	11% Casein hydrolysate, amino acids	1.8	50	115/75
Portagen (Mead Johnson)	20	46% Corn syrup solids, sucrose, citrates	40% MCT oil (85%), corn oil, lecithin	14% Sodium caseinate	1.7	53	64/47
Alimentum (Ross)‖	20	41% Sucrose, modified tapioca starch	48% MCT oil (50%), safflower oil (40%), soy oil (10%)	11% Casein hydrolysate, amino acids	1.8	45	105/75
Lactofree (Mead Johnson)	20	43% Corn syrup solids	48% Palm olein, soy oil, coconut oil, sunflower oil	9% Cow's milk protein isolate	1.8	60	82/55

| Neocate (Scientific Hospital Supplies, Inc.) | 20 | 47% Corn syrup solids, dextrose, maltose, maltotriose, oligosaccharides | 41% Hybrid safflower oil, coconut oil, soy oil | 12% Synthetic free amino acids | 1.85 | 87 | 124/93 |

CHO = carbohydrate; CF = cystic fibrosis; FE = iron; LCT = long-chain triglyceride; MCT = medium-chain triglyceride; PRO = protein.

* Also available as 24 kcal/oz and 27 kcal/oz.
† Formula with a low renal solute load.
‡ Also available as 24 kcal/oz.
§ Also available as 20 kcal/oz.
‖ Available only as ready-to-feed.

Indications for Special Formulas

Name	Indications
Nutramigen	Cow's milk allergy, severe or multiple food allergies, severe or persistent diarrhea, galactosemia
Pregestimil	Malabsorption, intestinal resection, severe or persistent diarrhea, food allergies
Portagen	Steatorrhea secondary to CF, intestinal resections, pancreatic insufficiency, biliary atresia, lymphatic anomalies, celiac disease
Alimentum	Problems with digestion or absorption, severe or prolonged diarrhea, CF, steatorrhea, food allergies, intestinal resection
Lactofree	Lactose intolerance *without* cow's milk protein intolerance
Neocate	Cow's milk allergy, soy and protein hydrolysate intolerance, multiple food protein intolerance

TABLE 6.4.	Suggested Schedule for Introducing Solid Foods
Baby's Age	Appropriate Solid Foods
4–5 months	Iron-fortified infant cereal mixed with breast milk, water, or juice to a mustard-like consistency and offered on a small spoon (not in a bottle); rice, oatmeal, and barley varieties should be introduced before the mixed type Strained fruits and vegetables*
6 months	Plain yogurt mixed with strained fruit
7–9 months	Pureed meats†
8–10 months	Soft "finger foods" (e.g., banana chunks, cooked carrots), Cheerios
> 12 months	Foods with higher allergenic potential (e.g., egg whites, citrus fruits, chocolate, berries)

* The order is not important, as long as there is a 2- to 3-day interval between new foods to identify any food intolerances.

† Most infants dislike pureed meats (a good source of iron, protein, and calories) and will accept them only if mixed with other foods.

Breast Milk

Breast milk provides a low renal solute load and excellent digestibility and absorption. **In preterm infants, supplementation of breast milk is necessary.** Breast-milk fortifiers developed for supplementation include Enfamil Human Milk fortifier (Mead Johnson) and Similac Natural Care (Ross). Both increase the calories, protein, minerals (particularly calcium and phosphorus), and vitamins of human milk to the levels required for preterm infants. These fortifiers are expensive and difficult to obtain outside of the hospital.

HINT An inexpensive alternative for the infant who still requires a caloric density of 24 kcal/oz after hospital discharge is to supplement breast milk with powdered full-term formula [1 tsp formula powder to 3 oz of breast milk or EnfaCare (Mead Johnson)], preterm formula powder (1 tsp powder to 3 oz breast milk), or Neosure (Ross). Breast-milk feedings can also be alternated with 24 or 27 kcal/oz formula feedings.

Formula

Preterm infant formulas (see Table 6.3) should be used for **all preterm infants with a birth weight of less than 2000 g who are not breast-fed** until the infant reaches the 40 weeks' postconception mark. EnfaCare (Mead Johnson) or Neosure, special formulas designed to be consumed by the preterm infant from the time of hospital discharge until the postconceptional (adjusted) age of 9 months to 1 year, provides the extra calories and minerals these infants need.

Solid Foods

Assuming the baby's oral motor skills are normal, solid foods can be introduced to the preterm infant following the **same recommendations as those for full-term infants,** using the postconceptional (adjusted) age. Abnormal oral motor skills and other feeding disorders are relatively common in the preterm population; therefore, the baby's **feeding skills should be assessed** carefully for both liquid and solid feedings.

References for Breast-Feeding Mothers

Dana N, Price A: *The Working Woman's Guide to Breast Feeding.* Deep Haven, MN, Meadowbrook, 1987.

Eiger MS, Olds SW: *The Complete Book of Breast-Feeding.* New York, Workman Publishing, 1972.

Suggested Readings

American Academy of Pediatrics, Committee for Quality Improvement and Subcommittee on Hyperbilirubinemia: Practice parameters: management of hyperbilirubinemia in the healthy term newborn. *Pediatrics* 94(4): 558–565, 1994.

American Academy of Pediatrics, Committee on Drugs: The transfer of drugs and other chemicals into human breast milk. *Pediatrics* 108(3):776–789, 2001.

American Academy of Pediatrics, Committee on Nutrition. *Pediatric Nutrition Handbook,* 3rd ed. Elk Grove Village, IL, American Academy of Pediatrics, 1998.

American Academy of Pediatrics, Committee on Nutrition: Nutrition and lactation. *Pediatrics* 68(3):435–443; 1981.

American Academy of Pediatrics, Committee on Nutrition: Soy protein based formulas: recommendations for use in infant feeding. *Pediatrics* 101(1):148–153, 1998.

American Academy of Pediatrics, Work Group on Breastfeeding: Breastfeeding and the use of human milk. *Pediatrics* 100(6): 1035–1039, 1997.

Bernbaum JC, Hoffman-Williamson M: *Primary Care of the Preterm Infant.* St. Louis, Mosby, 1991.

Gartner LM (ed): Breast-feeding in the hospital. *Semin Perinatol* 18:475, 1994.

Gartner LM: Neonatal jaundice. *Pediatr Rev* 15(11):422–431, 1994.

Laurence RA: *Breastfeeding: A Guide for the Medical Profession,* 4th ed. St. Louis, Mosby, 1994.

Lemons P, Stuart M, Lemons JA: Breast-feeding the premature infant. *Clin Perinatol* 13:111–122, 1994.

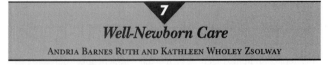

7
Well-Newborn Care
ANDRIA BARNES RUTH AND KATHLEEN WHOLEY ZSOLWAY

▼ INTRODUCTION

The birth of a new baby is a marvelous time for each family, full of excitement as well as some uncertainty as the amazing journey of child rearing begins. The well-newborn visits are an opportunity for parents to ask questions regarding the health and development of their baby. These visits enable the physician to **assess the baby's health, growth, and development** and offer guidance to parents throughout their baby's early years. Parents are often given **reassurance** about many aspects of normal newborn physical findings and development. This chapter describes the concerns most frequently encountered during the well-newborn visits.

▼ NEWBORN SCREENING TESTS

Blood is drawn from the infant's heel prior to discharge from the hospital. This blood is sent for newborn screening tests, which look for a variety of **metabolic and genetic disorders.** The specific tests vary by state and may include biotinidase deficiency, branched-chain ketoaciduria (maple syrup urine disease), congenital adrenal hyperplasia (CAH), congenital hypothyroidism, cystic fibrosis (CF), galactosemia, homocystinuria, PKU, sickle cell disease, toxoplasmosis, and tyrosinemia. The results of these tests should be discussed at one of the early visits.

▼ SKIN
Generalized Rashes

Neonatal rashes are a common cause of concern for parents. A full discussion of rashes occurring in infancy is provided in Chapter 67, "Rashes."

Diaper Dermatitis (Diaper Rash)

Diaper dermatitis is a common problem presenting in infancy. Multiple conditions can predispose an infant to diaper rash, including sensitive skin, moisture trapped by a diaper, and the acid-base balance of stool and urine. Parents should be advised that **prevention is the best cure.** The diaper area should be kept as dry as possible; frequent diaper changes have been shown to decrease the occurrence of diaper dermatitis. Leaving the perineal area open to air as much as possible and applying a barrier cream to protect against local irritation have also proved beneficial.

Physical examination allows for the diagnosis of some of the more common skin irritations in the diaper area.

▼ **Irritant contact dermatitis** appears as erythema with shallow ulcerations predominantly located on the buttocks, thighs, abdomen, and perianal area, sparing the creases. The diagnosis is made clinically and treatment involves elimination of the irritant, use of a barrier cream, and exposure of the area to air as much as possible.

▼ **Candidal diaper dermatitis** can appear at any age and is characterized by beefy red, scaly plaques with satellite lesions, papules, and pustules. Diagnosis is most often made clinically on the basis of the characteristic appearance of the skin; however, a potassium hydroxide (KOH) preparation would demonstrate the presence of yeast. Treatment involves application of a topical antifungal agent (e.g., nystatin ointment or clotrimazole 1%) and exposure of the perineal area to air.

Mongolian Spots (Congenital Dermal Melanocytosis)

Mongolian spots are **blue-gray macules** that are most commonly seen in Asian, Hispanic, and African-American infants. They are typically a few centimeters in diameter and are located on the buttocks and lumbosacral area; less commonly, they may be much larger or located on the face or extremities.

They typically disappear by the age of 7–13 years, but some lesions (particularly the larger ones) persist into adulthood.

Salmon Patch (Nevus Simplex, Telangiectatic Nevus)

A salmon patch is a congenital vascular abnormality that involves the eyelids, glabella, forehead, or occiput. It consists of **smooth pink or red macular lesions,** often accompanied by telangiectasia. Salmon patches on the glabellar region or upper eyelids (angel kisses) usually disappear by age 1. The "stork bite" on the nape of the neck occurs in 22% of all infants and persists in 50% of these infants.

Café-au-Lait Macules

Café-au-lait macules are **pale brown macules with irregular margins** that range in size from 2 ml to 2 cm. They may appear at birth or in early childhood. Isolated café-au-lait macules occur in 10%–20% of the normal population. The presence of six or more café-au-lait macules may be a sign of neurofibromatosis.

▼ CRANIUM
Fontanelles

There are commonly two palpable fontanelles, the **anterior fontanelle** and the **posterior fontanelle.** The anterior fontanelle may minimally increase in size immediately after birth but then gradually decreases in size and is generally closed by 6–18 months of age. The posterior fontanelle is generally smaller than the anterior fontanelle and is usually closed to palpation by 4 months but may be closed at birth.

Caput Succedaneum

A caput succedaneum is a **diffuse swelling of the soft tissue of the scalp,** usually involving the presenting portion of the head during a vertex delivery. The edema, which is evident during the first few hours of life, crosses suture lines and may cross the midline. In uncomplicated cases of caput succedaneum, no specific treatment is needed; the swelling resolves during the first few days of life. Molding of the head and overriding of the parietal bones is often associated with a caput succedaneum; however, these conditions resolve during the first few weeks of life.

In rare instances, a hemorrhagic caput may occur and cause shock secondary to loss of circulating blood volume. In this instance, blood transfusion and circulatory support are needed. Extensive ecchymoses may result in hyperbilirubinemia, necessitating phototherapy.

Cephalohematoma

A cephalohematoma is a **subperiosteal hemorrhage** that results in swelling that is limited in distribution to one cranial bone (i.e., the swelling does not cross suture lines). Subperiosteal bleeding is a slow process; therefore, the cephalohematoma may not be evident until several hours after birth. A skull fracture, usually linear, may be an associated finding. Most cephalohematomas are resorbed between the ages of 2 weeks and 3 months of age. In some cases, a bony protuberance remains for years. Despite this residual calcification, no specific treatment is recommended.

✂ HINT The presence of pulsations, evidence of increased pressure with crying, and a bony defect on skull films can differentiate cranial meningocele from
cephalohematoma.

Molding

Asymmetry in the appearance of the cranium (molding) results from the
gentle application of asymmetric pressure on the cranial bones, which
occurs when an infant spends a significant portion of time in the same
position. Molding can be managed by repositioning the infant to eliminate
asymmetric pressure. In severe cases, a special helmet may be prescribed to
diminish the asymmetry.

Molding needs to be differentiated from **craniosynostosis (premature closure of a suture),** which may cause progressive asymmetry of the head. When
the diagnosis is not apparent clinically, radiographs are indicated to differentiate molding from craniosynostosis. In some instances, a three-dimensional
computed tomography (CT) scan may be needed to demonstrate the distinction. In the event of craniosynostosis, neurosurgical intervention is indicated
because of the possibility of asymmetric brain growth and compression of intracranial structures.

▼ EYES
Eye Color

Eye color is a frequent question posed by parents. Eye color is usually established by 3–6 months of age; however, additional iris pigmentation continues
throughout the first year of life. Depth of eye color may not be evident until
the first birthday.

Strabismus

During the newborn period, the eyes frequently wander. However, the **wan-
dering should diminish** (until it eventually disappears) within the first 2
months. If the eyes remain fixed in a certain position (e.g., one eye turning
inward), referral to an ophthalmologist is warranted. Even transient crossing
of the eyes beyond the age of 3 months is considered pathologic and warrants
an evaluation by an ophthalmologist.

Blocked Lacrimal Duct

The lacrimal system develops fully over the first 3–4 years of life. The lacrimal
glands begin to produce tears by the third or fourth week of life. In approximately 1% of newborns, one or both of the lacrimal ducts is blocked,
preventing drainage of tears.

Affected children appear to have **excessive tearing.** Therapy entails gentle
massage of the lacrimal duct and the use of a warm, wet washcloth to wipe
the collection of tears and mucus from the eye. Most blocked lacrimal ducts
open spontaneously by the first birthday. Children with persistent lacrimal
duct obstruction beyond 12 months should be evaluated by an ophthalmologist. Parents should be cautioned to call the pediatrician if the conjunctiva
becomes red, if the eye discharge becomes purulent, or if the area surrounding the eye or the medial aspect of the nose becomes swollen. These physical
findings may indicate conjunctivitis, ophthalmia neonatorum, or dacryocystitis (see Chapter 68, "Red Eye").

▼ EARS
Hearing

Significant bilateral hearing loss (> 35 db) is present in 1 to 3 per 1000 well newborns and in 2 to 4 per 1000 infants in the intensive care unit. If undetected, significant hearing loss will impede speech, language, and cognitive development. The American Academy of Pediatrics recommends that **universal hearing screening** occur in the newborn period, with appropriate follow-up so that all infants with significant hearing loss can be identified by 3 months of age and have necessary interventions implemented by 6 months of age.

▼ ORAL CAVITY
Teeth

Primary teeth eruption typically occurs at the age of 6 months (range 3–16 months). Natal teeth are teeth present at or shortly after birth. These teeth are generally poorly formed with thin enamel and poor attachments and are often located at the end of a stalk of uncalcified tissue. The **natal teeth often are primary teeth that have erupted early.** If removed, spacing of the secondary teeth may be affected; therefore, removal of the natal teeth is recommended only if they are a significant irritant to the tongue or if they present a danger of aspiration secondary to their poor attachment.

Dental Lumina Cysts, Bohn Nodules, and Epstein Pearls

Dental lumina cysts are clear or bluish fluid-filled sacs located bilaterally or quadrilaterally on the gum surfaces. These cysts are generally not painful, do not interfere with feeding, and are not associated with surrounding erythema. They disappear within a few weeks and do not require any intervention.

Yellowish-white cysts composed of islands of epithelial cells are termed **Bohn nodules** when they are located on the alveolar ridge and **Epstein pearls** when they are located near the midpalatal raphe at the junction of the hard and soft palate. These cysts require no treatment and commonly disappear within a few weeks.

Thrush

White patches in the mouth of an infant may indicate the presence of thrush, a fairly common infection caused by *Candida albicans*. Unlike residual breast milk or formula, these white patches cannot be easily wiped from the oral mucosa or tongue surface. When thrush is removed from the oral mucosa, the exposed mucosa is typically red and raw and may bleed. Treatment consists of the use of a topical antifungal agent (e.g., nystatin oral suspension). Care should be taken to avoid reinfection from contaminated nipples and pacifiers.

▼ CHEST
Breast Hypertrophy and Galactorrhea

Breast buds are present in most term infants (both male and female) and in preterm infants beyond 36 weeks gestational age.

▼ **Hypertrophy** results from the passage of maternal hormones across the placenta during gestation.

▼ **Galactorrhea** occurs in up to 6% of normal-term infants and typically occurs in infants with larger breast nodules. The thin, milky discharge ("witch's milk") may be caused by maternal estrogen or neonatal prolactin.

Generally, both breast hypertrophy and galactorrhea resolve within several weeks, but occasionally galactorrhea can persist for several months and breast hypertrophy can persist into early childhood.

Mastitis

Primary infection of the breast may occur in newborns when bacteria invade the already hypertrophied breast tissue, resulting in cellulitis and abscess. *Staphylococcus aureus* is most frequently the involved organism, but 5%–10% of infections are caused by gram-negative enteric bacteria.

Typically, the breast bud is erythematous, enlarged, warm, and tender; purulent drainage from the nipple may be present. Infants are usually well-appearing, with only 25% presenting with fever or ill appearance. Treatment consists of the intravenous administration of oxacillin and gentamicin after obtaining appropriate cultures (including culture of the purulent nipple drainage). Occasionally, a fluctuant abscess forms, requiring surgical drainage.

▼ UMBILICUS
Normal Umbilicus

The umbilical cord is composed of two umbilical arteries and one umbilical vein. After birth, the cord is clamped, cut, and treated topically (e.g., with triple dye, alcohol, bacitracin, silver sulfadiazine, or povidone-iodine) to decrease bacterial colonization. The remnant of the cord is then left exposed to dry.

The cord generally falls off on its own in 7–28 days, but it may take longer. Parents should be reassured that the presence of **oozing, a few drops of blood, or a mild odor are normal.** Indications for concern are significant redness of the skin (especially circumferential), significant malodorous discharge, or bleeding that is not stopped by gentle pressure.

Umbilical Hernia

Umbilical hernia, which is caused by failure of a central fascial defect below the umbilicus to close, presents as a **bulge at the umbilicus** that is more prominent with crying or straining. Umbilical hernia is more common in African-American infants, premature infants, and infants with congenital hypothyroidism.

Most defects close spontaneously by the age of 4 or 5 years and incarceration or strangulation rarely occurs, so reassurance is most appropriate. Generally, the **likelihood of closure is inversely related to the size of the hernia,** with most small- to moderate-sized hernias closing spontaneously. Hernias with a diameter greater than 2 cm are less likely to close spontaneously. Repair is usually indicated if the hernia persists beyond 5 years. Traditional remedies (e.g., umbilical bands, taping coins over the umbilicus) do not hasten closure of the hernia and may irritate the surrounding skin.

Omphalitis

Infection of the umbilical cord and surrounding tissues results when bacteria colonize and invade the umbilical cord stump. Once a major cause of neonatal mortality, omphalitis is now **rare in developed countries.** Complications include sepsis, hepatic abscess, peritonitis, and portal vein thrombosis.

The condition typically presents with purulent, foul-smelling drainage from the umbilical cord and erythema (frequently circumferential) that progresses to induration and erythema of the abdominal wall. Symptoms include lethargy, irritability, poor feeding, and fever.

Treatment consists of the intravenous administration of oxacillin and gentamicin to treat *S. aureus,* group A streptococci, group B streptococci, and enteric gram-negative rods.

Umbilical Granuloma

Umbilical granuloma results when an **excessive amount of granulation tissue,** which is not covered by epithelium, accumulates after the separation of the umbilical cord. A small, pink mass with persistent weeping and crusting is found at the base of the umbilicus. It is important to differentiate this relatively common and benign condition from patent omphalomesenteric duct and urachal remnant (see next section).

Treatment consists of the application of silver nitrate to the granulation tissue. Care should be taken to avoid the normal, surrounding skin, which can be burned by the silver nitrate. Serial applications frequently are required.

Patent Omphalomesenteric Duct and Patent Urachus

The **omphalomesenteric duct** is a connection between the intestinal tract and the placenta that forms during fetal development. It normally involutes, but if it remains patent, a tubular attachment persists between the ileum and the umbilicus through which intestinal contents can drain. A patent omphalomesenteric duct may be demonstrated by inspection and probing of the tract that is visible at the surface of the umbilicus.

If the **urachus** persists after birth, there is a free connection between the urinary bladder and the abdominal wall through which urine may pass. Signs may include a constantly wet umbilicus or the patient may develop a urinary tract infection (UTI).

For both conditions, the treatment is prompt surgical repair.

▼ GENITALIA

Boys

Normal Care of the Penis

In **uncircumcised** boys, the foreskin is generally not retractable at birth. Parents should attempt to keep the foreskin clean, avoiding attempts at forcible retraction of the prepuce, which may result in scarring. The foreskin gradually becomes retractable over time with growth and with the gentle stretching that is involved with washing. In **circumcised** boys, the exposed glans should be coated with petroleum jelly with each diaper change until it is epithelialized.

Hypospadias and Epispadias

In **hypospadias,** the urethral meatus is abnormally located ventral to the tip of the glans. Classification of the type of hypospadias is based on the anatomic location of the urethral meatus (i.e., glanular, coronal, midshaft, distal shaft, penoscrotal, or perineal). There is usually an associated abnormality of the foreskin as well as associated chordee (ventral curvature of the penis). The abnormality of the foreskin is usually a clue that hypospadias may be present. In patients with suspected hypospadias, circumcision should be deferred because the presence of the foreskin facilitates the subsequent repair of hypospadias.

Epispadias, in which the urethra opens on the dorsum of the penis, is a more severe lesion that is usually associated with exstrophy of the bladder. Incontinence is a commonly associated finding.

Cryptorchidism (Undescended Testicle)

Cryptorchidism is found in 3.4%–5.8% of full-term boys and may be unilateral or bilateral. Most testes that are not descended at birth spontaneously descend during the first 3 to 6 months; few testes descend after this time. The incidence of cryptorchidism at the age of 1 year is approximately 0.8%.

The treatment for cryptorchidism is **orchiopexy,** which is optimally performed by 1 year of age to decrease the risk of infertility, malignancy, and testicular torsion. Because timing is critical, all infants with unilateral or bilateral undescended testes at the 4- or 6-month visit should be referred to a urologist for evaluation.

Inguinal Hernia and Hydrocele

Both hernias and hydroceles result from failure of the processus vaginalis to undergo fusion and obliteration during fetal life.

▼ **Inguinal hernia** occurs in 1%–5% of children, is ten times more common in boys than in girls, and may occur in up to 30% of premature infants born before 36 weeks gestation.

▼ **Indirect inguinal hernia** presents as a bulge in the inguinal canal that may be present at rest or may only be appreciated during straining or crying, as a loop of intestine descends into the hernia sac. Appropriate therapy consists of referral for surgical repair within a short time of diagnosis to minimize the risk of incarceration or strangulation.

▼ A **hydrocele** represents persistence of the processus vaginalis with partial closure proximally, which allows fluid to pass into the scrotal sac. The condition is evidenced by the presence of scrotal swelling, which transilluminates in the absence of a hernia. Hydroceles in infants may communicate with the peritoneal cavity, or they may be noncommunicating. Hydroceles are often associated with inguinal hernias or they may be an isolated finding. Most infants with isolated hydrocele undergo spontaneous closure of the processus vaginalis with resolution of the hydrocele, so reassurance is most appropriate. Referral to a surgeon is indicated for patients with hydroceles that persist beyond the age of 6 months to 1 year (surgeons have different preferences for timing of surgery) or that wax and wane in size, indicating communication with the peritoneal cavity and the associated risk of hernia.

Girls

Vaginal Discharge and Bleeding

Normal newborn girls have well-estrogenized vaginal mucosa because of the transplacental passage of maternal hormones; therefore, a thick, white vaginal discharge is a normal finding in a newborn girl. Many newborns also have a scant amount of vaginal bleeding in the first week of life due to withdrawal of maternal estrogen. Parents should be reassured that both findings are normal.

▼ URINATION AND DEFECATION

Urate Crystals ("Pink Diaper Syndrome")

Parents may notice a **pink crystalline substance** in the diaper or a **salmon-pink residue** on the surface of the diaper, resulting from the deposition of urate crystals. Urate crystals are usually easily distinguished from blood on the basis of appearance, but occult blood testing can also be performed. Urate crystals are typically found in the setting of concentrated urine and **may indicate dehydration,** so a careful assessment for hydration status is warranted (including frequency of wet diapers, vital signs, and presence of a sunken fontanelle or dry mucous membranes). Parents should be counseled to increase the frequency and amount of feedings if there are concerns about an infant's hydration.

Meconium, Transitional Stool, and Typical Stool

Passage of some amount of **meconium** usually occurs within the first 12 hours of life, with 99% of all term infants and 95% of preterm infants passing meconium within the first 48 hours of life. **Transitional stools** follow the passage of meconium until the passage of the typical stool of the newborn is established. Typically, the stool is described as yellow and seedy in breast-fed infants and yellow or brown in formula-fed infants.

Failure to pass meconium can occur as a result of imperforate anus, functional intestinal obstruction (i.e., Hirschsprung disease), illness, or hypotonia. Failure to pass transitional stools following the passage of meconium may be indicative of a volvulus or malrotation. Any newborn who fails to pass meconium or fails to progress to passing **typical stools** should be evaluated in a timely fashion to rule out the presence of intestinal obstruction.

Establishment of a Bowel Pattern and Constipation

In each newborn, the establishment of a **normal bowel pattern** occurs over time and varies as the newborn grows. The typical breast-fed baby will pass a bowel movement after each feeding initially, but by the age of 1 month, normal patterns vary from a bowel movement after each feeding to one every 1–7 days. The typical formula-fed baby has a bowel movement every 1–3 days.

Constipation (difficulty in passing stool) can occur at any age. It is important to discuss with the parents of a newborn the fact that the consistency and regularity of the passing of stool varies over time. Parents should be advised to contact the physician if the infant develops abdominal distention, vomiting, refusal to eat, bloody stools, or extremely hard stools. These clinical signs and symptoms may indicate pathology, including many of the entities discussed in Chapter 22, "Constipation."

▼ COMMON CONCERNS

Recommended Sleeping Position

The American Academy of Pediatrics (AAP) recommends placing healthy, term infants to sleep in a nonprone position. **Sleeping supine confers the lowest risk of sudden infant death syndrome (SIDS)** and is preferred. This recommendation is based on analysis of a number of studies from around the world that demonstrate an association between the prone sleeping position and an increased risk of SIDS. In the United States, there has been a reduction in prone sleeping from 70% to 20% of infants since 1992, with a concomitant 40% reduction in the rate of SIDS.

In addition, parents should be instructed not to put infants to sleep on waterbeds, sofas, or soft mattresses. They should not place any soft objects (such as pillows, quilts, sheepskins, or stuffed toys) in an infant's sleeping environment, and they should recognize that loose bedding may also present a hazard to a small infant. Overheating and overbundling should be avoided.

Hiccups

Many babies hiccup. The precise cause is unknown, although many feel it is a reflection of an immature nervous system. If hiccups persist for 5–10 minutes and are distressing to those caring for the baby, nursing or a few sucks on a bottle of sugar water may relieve the hiccups.

Sneezing and Coughing

In babies, sneezing and coughing can be a protective mechanism to clear material from the respiratory passages. Therefore, intermittent sneezing or coughing should not be of concern. Persistent coughing or sneezing may be a sign of a problem and requires evaluation by a physician.

Chin Quivering

A baby's chin may intermittently quiver. This motion is a reflection of an immature nervous system and the quivering stops as the nervous system matures.

Suggested Readings

American Academy of Pediatrics, Task Force on Infant Sleep Position and Sudden Infant Death Syndrome. Changing Concepts of Sudden Infant Death Syndrome: Implications on Infant Sleep Environment and Sleep Position. *Pediatrics* 105(3):650–655, 2000.

American Academy of Pediatrics, Task Force on Newborn and Infant Hearing. Newborn and Infant Hearing Loss: Detection and Intervention. *Pediatrics* 103(2):527–530, 1999.

Avery GB, Fletcher MA, MacDonald MG: *Neonatology: Pathophysiology and Management of the Newborn.* Philadelphia, Lippincott Williams and Wilkins, 1999.

Gill B, Kogan S: Cryptorchidism. Current Concepts. *Pediatr Clin North Am* 44(5):1211–1227, 1997.

Hurwitz S: *Clinical Pediatric Dermatology: A Textbook of Skin Disorders of Childhood and Adolescence.* Philadelphia, WB Saunders, 1993.

Kendig JW. Care of the Normal Newborn. *Pediatr Rev* 13:262–268, 1992.

Scheree LR, Grosfels JL: Inguinal hernia and umbilical anomalies. *Pediatr Clin North Am* 40(6):1121–1131, 1993.

Shusterman S: Pediatric dental update. *Pediatr Rev* 15:311–319, 1994.

Singalavanija S, Frieden IJ: Diaper dermatitis. *Pediatr Rev* 16:142–154, 1995.

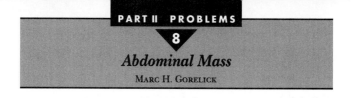

Abdominal Mass

MARC H. GORELICK

▼ INTRODUCTION

In children, abdominal masses present in variable ways. **Some produce symptoms or signs,** while **others remain silent** even when large. An abdominal mass may be discovered by a parent or caregiver, or it may be an incidental finding during physical examination. The **age of the child is an important factor** in the differential diagnosis—most masses discovered in neonates are benign, whereas up to 50% of masses in older children are malignant (Table 8.1). The most common sites of origin of abdominal masses according to the age of the patient are given in Table 8.2.

⚴ HINT In newborns, the bladder is an abdominal organ.

⚴ HINT An abdominal mass in a neonate is usually renal in origin—ureteral pelvic obstruction and multicystic kidney are the most common causes of abdominal mass in neonates.

▼ DIFFERENTIAL DIAGNOSIS LIST

Infectious Causes

Appendiceal abscess
Tubo-ovarian abscess
Hepatic abscess
Perinephric abscess

Neoplastic Causes

Malignant

Wilms tumor (nephroblastoma)
Neuroblastoma
Lymphoma
Rhabdomyosarcoma
Ovarian tumor

Benign

Ovarian teratoma
Sacrococcygeal teratoma
Mesonephric blastoma

Traumatic Causes

Perinephric hematoma
Pancreatic pseudocyst
Adrenal hematoma

TABLE 8.1. Common Abdominal Masses

Neonates	Infants	Older Children
Hydronephrosis	Hydronephrosis	Constipation
Ureteropelvic obstruction	Wilms tumor	Wilms tumor
Multicystic kidney	Neuroblastoma	Neuroblastoma
Distended bladder	Distended bladder	Hydronephrosis
Ectopic kidney	Multicystic kidney	Appendiceal abscess
Hydrometrocolpos	Pyloric stenosis	Ovarian cyst
Gastrointestinal duplication	Intussusception	
	Hydrometrocolpos	

Congenital or Vascular Causes

Cysts—ovarian, choledochal, hepatic, mesenteric, urachal
Hydronephrosis
Polycystic or multicystic kidney
Ectopic or horseshoe kidney
Posterior urethral valves
Gastrointestinal (bowel) duplication
Pyloric stenosis
Hydrometrocolpos or hematocolpos
Anterior myelomeningocele
Renal vein thrombosis

Miscellaneous Causes

Constipation
Distended bladder
Intestinal distention—intussusception, imperforate anus, Hirschsprung disease, volvulus, meconium ileus
Gallbladder hydrops
Pregnancy (intrauterine or ectopic)

▾ DIFFERENTIAL DIAGNOSIS DISCUSSION

Constipation

Constipation is discussed in Chapter 22, "Constipation."

Intussusception

Intussusception is discussed in Chapter 9, "Abdominal Pain, Acute."

TABLE 8.2. Sites of Origin of Abdominal Masses

	Renal	Other Retroperitoneal	Gastrointestinal	Genital
Neonates	20%	15%	55%	10%
Infants and older children	55%	23%	18%	4%

Appendiceal Abscess

Etiology

Untreated acute appendicitis leads to perforation with abscess formation.

Clinical Features

A child with an appendiceal abscess appears generally ill. **Fever and abdominal pain** are common symptoms. Although many children have a history highly suggestive of appendicitis (see Chapter 9, "Abdominal Pain, Acute"), others have an atypical history characterized by a subacute course, with symptoms present for days to weeks.

⚕ HINT Patients (especially young children) with appendiceal abscess may not show typical abnormalities associated with appendicitis, such as anorexia and peritoneal signs.

Evaluation

A **tender mass** is located in the **right lower quadrant,** and signs of peritoneal irritation are often, but not invariably, present. The mass may be palpable on rectal examination. In **postpubertal females, a pelvic examination** is important to exclude pelvic inflammatory disease.

Leukocytosis with a left shift is a helpful supportive finding. If the diagnosis of appendicitis is clear, additional studies are unnecessary. In difficult cases, an abdominal radiograph may provide confirmatory evidence [e.g., a fecalith (present in less than 10% of cases), free intraperitoneal air, or a right lower quadrant mass effect with ileus]; however, **ultrasound** is the diagnostic study of choice.

Treatment

Urgent surgical consultation is necessary. Preoperatively, patients should receive broad-spectrum parenteral **antibiotics** to cover gram-negative and anaerobic organisms.

Distended Bladder

Etiology

A palpably distended bladder results from **obstruction** (e.g., posterior urethral valves in boys, extrinsic mass, stricture), **neurologic dysfunction** (e.g., spinal cord injury, myelomeningocele, anticholinergic medication), or **voluntary retention** (as a result of dysuria).

Evaluation

The history should include questions about urinary frequency, dysuria, and the quality of the stream as well as bowel function, which may also be affected in cases of neurogenic bladder.

Palpation of the abdomen reveals a **smooth suprapubic mass,** which may be somewhat tender if the abdomen is grossly distended. The mass is cystic to percussion. Look for evidence of urethral or vaginal irritation and evaluate **neurologic function.** The innervation of the bladder is S2–S4, the same area as the sacrum, so **testing the anal wink** identifies those patients with disruption of bladder innervation.

An **ultrasound** confirms that the mass is the bladder, and a **voiding cystourethrogram** may help identify the cause of the distention. **Urinalysis** should be performed if dysuria suggests cystitis.

Treatment

Urethral catheterization relieves the distention. Definitive treatment depends on the underlying cause of the obstruction, but usually referral to a urologist is required.

Hydronephrosis

Etiology

Hydronephrosis **(dilatation of the renal collecting system)** results from **partial or complete obstruction of urine flow.** Causes include ureteropelvic junction obstruction, posterior urethral valves, vesicoureteral reflux, ureterocele, and duplication of the collecting system.

Clinical Features

Many children with hydronephrosis are **asymptomatic;** others present with **abdominal pain** (often chronic or recurrent) or, in rare cases, evidence of **renal failure.**

Evaluation

Abdominal examination reveals a **palpable unilateral or bilateral smooth flank mass,** especially in infants. **Any palpable kidney in a child older than 3 years** of age is suspicious, as is **asymmetry in younger children.**

Ultrasound is diagnostic.

Treatment

Most causes of hydronephrosis are treated with **surgical repair.**

Wilms Tumor (Nephroblastoma)

Etiology

Wilms tumor, the **most common intra-abdominal malignancy in children,** accounts for virtually all pediatric renal neoplasms. Wilms tumor is associated with certain **congenital anomalies:** genitourinary malformations, hemihypertrophy, and sporadic aniridia. There is also a **familial form** of Wilms tumor.

Clinical Features

Peak incidence is at **3 years** of age. Most patients present with an **asymptomatic abdominal mass** or **abdominal distention.** This diagnosis should be considered in any young child with a large abdomen. Occasional symptoms include abdominal pain, vomiting, hematuria, and hypertension.

Evaluation

The mass is **smooth and firm,** rarely crossing the midline; in 5%–10% of patients, masses are **bilateral.** In some cases, the mass is so large (mean diameter of 11 cm at the time of diagnosis in one study) that **diffuse distention,** rather than a discrete mass, is felt.

Although it may show microscopic hematuria, urinalysis is too nonspecific to be helpful. An **abdominal sonogram** or **computed tomography (CT) scan** shows a solid, intrarenal mass.

Treatment

Wilms tumor is treated with a combination of **surgical resection (nephrectomy)** and **chemotherapy.** Success rates depend on the extent of disease and the clinical stage at the time of diagnosis.

Neuroblastoma

Etiology

A malignancy arising from neural crest cells, neuroblastoma is the **second most common solid tumor of childhood.** In approximately two-thirds of patients, the primary site is in the **abdomen** (usually adrenal); the **thoracic region** is the next most common site.

Clinical Features

Like Wilms tumor, neuroblastoma may present as an **asymptomatic mass.** However, patients tend to be somewhat **younger** (median age, 2 years) and they appear **more ill**—an indication of the high incidence of metastatic disease at diagnosis (approximately 60%).

Associated symptoms may include **abdominal pain, urinary obstruction, diarrhea** (caused by tumor secretion of vasoactive intestinal peptide), **anorexia, malaise,** and **site-specific symptoms** from metastases to the bone, skin, liver, or central nervous system. Although most tumors produce catecholamines, rapid metabolism makes symptoms of hypertension and irritability rare.

⚡ HINT Opsomyoclonus, consisting of myoclonic jerks, ataxia, and jerky eye movements ("dancing eyes, dancing feet") is a unique paraneoplastic syndrome associated with neuroblastoma. Findings suggestive of opsomyoclonus should prompt a search for an occult neuroblastoma, even in the absence of an abdominal mass.

Evaluation

A **firm, irregular, nontender mass** is palpable in the **abdominal region.** Other physical examination findings include **pallor, subcutaneous nodules,** and **hepatomegaly.**

⚡ HINT Neuroblastoma is one of the few causes of massive hepatomegaly.

Urinary levels of catecholamine metabolites (i.e., vanillylmandelic acid, homovanillic acid, and metanephrine) were used for screening in the past, but abdominal ultrasound or CT is the current diagnostic procedure of choice. Identification of a solid adrenal or paraspinal mass, which is calcified in 80% of patients, strongly suggests neuroblastoma. Findings usually produce biliary tract obstruction with jaundice and acholic stools.

Treatment

Treatment may include **bone marrow transplantation, chemotherapy, radiation therapy,** and **surgical debulking or resection.** The prognosis depends on the stage of the disease, the age of the patient, the site of the primary tumor, and the findings on histologic evaluation. Patients with stage IV-S disease, which often presents in the first few months of life, may experience spontaneous regression of the primary tumor.

Cysts

Etiology

Cysts may arise as **developmental variants** from any number of structures.

Clinical Features

Symptoms are **variable** and depend on the site of the cyst; **nonspecific abdominal pain** is most common. An ovarian cyst may cause cyclic pain in menarchal girls, while a choledochal cyst usually produces biliary tract obstruction with jaundice and acholic stools.

Evaluation

Many cysts are palpable on abdominal or pelvic examination as a **smooth, soft or firm mass** at the site of the organ of origin.

A **sonogram** is the optimal diagnostic tool.

Treatment

Ovarian or mesenteric cysts discovered as an incidental finding may be followed; cysts causing **significant symptoms** require **excision.**

Renal Cystic Disease

Types of Renal Cystic Disease

▼ **Multicystic dysplastic renal disease** is one of the most common causes of abdominal masses in neonates. The affected kidney consists of a mass of cysts with little or no identifiable renal tissue; bilateral cases are associated with renal failure.

▼ **Polycystic renal disease.** In polycystic renal disease, one or both kidneys contain multiple cortical and medullary cysts consisting of dilated tubules. The more common autosomal dominant form usually presents in adulthood but is sometimes diagnosed in children. The autosomal recessive form, which is more severe, usually manifests itself in infancy. Both forms are uncommon in children.

⚡ HINT The majority of infants with autosomal recessive polycystic kidney disease also have hepatic cysts, sometimes leading to severe liver disease.

Clinical Features

Except for those with bilateral involvement, infants with multicystic dysplastic kidney present with an **asymptomatic flank mass** that is irregular and nontender. Infants with bilateral cystic kidneys may have a history of **oligohydramnios** and, in severe cases, findings of **Potter syndrome.** Children with multicystic dysplastic kidney have a high incidence of **associated urinary tract anomalies** and require **complete urologic evaluation.**

Patients with polycystic kidney disease often have concomitant **hematuria** (gross or microscopic) or **hypertension,** but renal failure is rare. Again, a **unilateral or bilateral flank mass** is palpated.

Evaluation

In all cases, **ultrasound** confirms the diagnosis.

Treatment

Patients with renal cystic disease require close follow-up to monitor for signs of **renal insufficiency** or **hypertension.**

Gastrointestinal (Bowel) Duplication

Etiology

Occurring in any part of the gastrointestinal tract, but most commonly in the **region of the ileocecal valve,** duplication cysts result from a **morphogenetic defect.** The cyst usually does not communicate with the true intestinal lumen, producing a closed cystic mass. Gastrointestinal (bowel) duplication is the **most common cause of neonatal gastrointestinal masses.**

Evaluation

Bowel duplications may be **asymptomatic** or they may cause **intestinal obstruction.** They are typically compressible and mobile and are either round or tubular. The diagnosis is made by **ultrasound** or a **gastrointestinal contrast study.**

🎗 HINT The mucosa of the cyst may arise from any part of the gastrointestinal tract, regardless of location; when gastric mucosa is included, ulceration or perforation may result.

Treatment

Surgical resection is generally curative.

Hydrometrocolpos and Hematocolpos

Etiology

Imperforate hymen leads to accumulation of secretions in the vagina; if undetected until puberty, accumulated menstrual blood causes hematocolpos.

Clinical Features

The distended vagina may **interfere with voiding or defecation,** but infants are otherwise **asymptomatic.**

Evaluation

The **mass is smooth, suprapubic,** and **frequently palpable** on rectal examination. The imperforate hymen may also be seen bulging externally.
   An **ultrasound** shows the dilated, fluid-filled vagina.

Treatment

Resection of the imperforate hymen is required.

▼ EVALUATION OF ABDOMINAL MASS
Patient History

The following items should be noted:

▼ Symptoms (e.g., fever, abdominal pain, vomiting, jaundice)
▼ Stooling pattern (frequency, consistency)
▼ Voiding pattern
▼ History of trauma

▼ Menstrual history
▼ History of abdominal surgery or umbilical catheterization

Physical Examination

The following should be noted or sought on physical examination:

▼ Size and location of mass
▼ Presence of tenderness
▼ Findings on percussion
▼ Blood pressure
▼ Presence of scleral icterus
▼ Evidence of dehydration

Laboratory Studies

The choice of laboratory studies is guided by the type of symptoms and signs that are involved. Studies to be considered include:

▼ Urinalysis
▼ Complete blood cell count
▼ Blood urea nitrogen and creatinine
▼ Electrolytes
▼ Hepatic transaminases and bilirubin

Diagnostic Modalities

▼ **Ultrasound.** The diagnostic study of choice in most cases of abdominal mass is ultrasound. Exceptions include clinically diagnosed constipation, intrauterine pregnancy, and appendicitis, where further studies are generally unnecessary, or intussusception, where a contrast enema is both diagnostic and therapeutic. Ultrasound examination provides information regarding the location and character (cystic versus solid, homogeneous versus heterogeneous, calcified) of the abdominal mass and should be the initial study in most cases.

▼ **Abdominal radiographs,** while frequently obtained, provide little information in a relatively asymptomatic child. An exception is the use of radiographs to detect calcifications in a mass, which may help narrow the differential diagnosis (Table 8.3).

▼ **Abdominal CT,** which provides more detailed anatomic information than ultrasound, should be reserved for further delineation of certain masses but may be a substitute when ultrasound is unavailable.

TABLE 8.3. Abdominal Masses Commonly Associated with Calcification

Neuroblastoma
Teratoma
   Ovarian
   Sacrococcygeal
Adrenal hematoma
Hepatic hemangioma
Meconium peritonitis

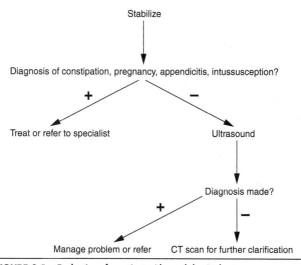

FIGURE 8.1. Evaluation of a patient with an abdominal mass.
CT = computed tomography.

▼ **Intravenous urography,** once the initial study of choice, has now been supplanted by the preceding methods.

▼ APPROACH TO THE PATIENT (FIGURE 8.1)

The work-up of an abdominal mass should be accompanied by **supportive care** and **resuscitation** in an ill-appearing child, including **fluid therapy** in the presence of dehydration, **supplemental oxygen** and **assisted respiration** in patients with respiratory compromise, and **control of blood pressure** in patients with symptomatic hypertension. The initial study in these patients is an **abdominal series** (flat and upright) to evaluate for obstruction or perforation. Once the child is stabilized, additional studies may be undertaken.

Suggested Readings

Cass DL, Hawkins E, Brandt ML, et al.: Surgery for ovarian masses in infants, children, and adolescents: 102 consecutive patients treated in a 15-year period. *J Pediatr Surg* 36(5):693–699, 2001.

Caty MG, Shamberger RC: Abdominal tumors in infancy and childhood. *Pediatr Clin North Am* 40:1253–1271, 1993.

Kuppermann N, O'Dea T, Pinckney L, et al.: Predictors of intussusception in young children. *Arch Pediatr Adolesc Med* 154(3):250–255, 2000.

Merten DF, Kirks DR: Diagnostic imaging of pediatric abdominal masses. *Pediatr Clin North Am* 32:1397–1425, 1985.

Morrison SC: Controversies in abdominal imaging. *Pediatr Clin North Am* 44(3):555–574, 1997.

Neville HL, Ritchey ML: Wilms' tumor. Overview of National Wilms' Tumor Study Group results. *Urol Clin North Am* 27(3):435–442, 2000.

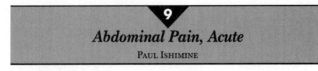

9
Abdominal Pain, Acute
PAUL ISHIMINE

▼ INTRODUCTION

The evaluation of acute abdominal pain in a child can challenge the diagnostic capabilities of any clinician. A **common chief complaint,** the spectrum
of etiologies ranges from benign to life-threatening. An ordered approach to
evaluation is required, guided by the history and physical examination with
selected laboratory and imaging studies. In many cases, a definitive diagnosis
may not be made on a single patient encounter, and **repeated evaluation** is
required.

▼ DIFFERENTIAL DIAGNOSIS LIST
Gastrointestinal

Appendicitis/appendiceal abscess
Peptic ulcer disease/gastritis
Esophagitis/gastroesophageal reflux
Cholecystitis
Pancreatitis/pancreatic pseudocyst
Hepatitis
Gastroenteritis
Constipation
Bowel obstruction/volvulus
Incarcerated hernia
Intussusception
Hirschsprung disease
Inflammatory bowel disease
Primary peritonitis
Necrotizing enterocolitis
Mesenteric adenitis
Abdominal trauma: duodenal hematoma, splenic/liver contusion
Foreign body ingestion

Genitourinary

Urinary tract infection
Renal calculus
Nephrotic syndrome
Pregnancy: intrauterine, ectopic
Pelvic inflammatory disease
Ovarian cyst/ovarian torsion
Mittelschmerz
Dysmenorrhea
Endometriosis
Hematocolpos/hydrometrocolpos
Testicular torsion/torsion of the appendix testis
Orchitis
Epididymitis

Respiratory

Pneumonia
Streptococcal pharyngitis
Asthma

Oncologic

Wilms tumor
Neuroblastoma
Leukemia
Lymphoma
Hepatoblastoma
Ovarian tumor
Teratoma
Typhlitis
Rhabdomyosarcoma

Systemic Disorders

Diabetic ketoacidosis
Vasculitis/Henoch-Schönlein purpura
Collagen vascular disease: lupus, polyarteritis nodosa
Kawasaki disease
Hemolytic uremic syndrome
Infectious mononucleosis
Sickle cell disease
Cystic fibrosis
Porphyria

Miscellaneous

Functional
Colic
Toxins: caustic ingestion, black widow spider bite
Inborn errors of metabolism
Orthopedic: septic arthritis/osteomyelitis/discitis
Abdominal migraine
Aortic aneurysm
Herpes zoster
Heat cramps

Any of the causes of chronic abdominal pain can present with an acute exacerbation.

▼ DIFFERENTIAL DIAGNOSIS DISCUSSION

Acute Gastroenteritis

Acute gastroenteritis is discussed in Chapter 27, "Diarrhea, Acute."

Constipation

Constipation is discussed in Chapter 22, "Constipation."

Colic, Peptic Disease, and Functional Abdominal Pain

Colic, peptic disease, and functional abdominal pain are discussed in Chapter 10, "Abdominal Pain, Chronic."

Appendicitis

Etiology

Appendicitis is a common cause of abdominal pain, occurring in children of all ages. Appendicitis is typically caused by obstruction of the appendiceal lumen, resulting in appendiceal distention, inhibition of lymphatic and vascular drainage, edema, and perforation.

Clinical Features

The **classic symptoms** of appendicitis are periumbilical abdominal pain, followed by fever, anorexia, and vomiting. As the disease progresses, pain localizes to the right lower quadrant (McBurney point). However, patients with appendicitis often present atypically and with **nonspecific symptoms.** An appendix situated in the lateral colonic gutter may cause flank pain, while an appendix positioned more medially may irritate the bladder and cause dysuria and suprapubic pain. Alternatively, an appendix positioned in the pelvis may cause diarrhea if the inflamed appendix irritates the sigmoid colon. Patients may prefer to lie still because of the peritoneal irritation caused by an inflamed appendix.

⚠ HINT Diarrhea (9%–46%), constipation (5%–28%), and dysuria (4%–20%) are frequently found in patients with appendicitis. The diagnosis of appendicitis must be considered before attributing a child's abdominal pain solely to these conditions.

Unfortunately, making the diagnosis of appendicitis can be challenging, especially in preverbal children in the early stages of the disease process. As a result, patients frequently present after the appendix has **perforated.** These patients may report transient improvement of their pain immediately after perforation but soon complain of diffuse abdominal pain from peritonitis.

Evaluation

The physical examination will frequently reveal a slight fever and tenderness in the right lower quadrant, although tenderness may be found in the flank or elsewhere in the abdomen, depending on the location of the appendix. The following three signs may be seen with appendicitis:

▼ **Rovsing sign**—pain in the right lower quadrant with palpation of the left lower quadrant
▼ **Iliopsoas sign**—pain in the right lower quadrant with flexion of the thigh against resistance
▼ **Obturator sign**—pain in the right lower quadrant when the flexed thigh and knee are held and the hip is rotated internally

A rectal examination may reveal irritation of the rectal wall by an inflamed appendix. If the appendix has perforated and the child has developed **peritonitis,** he or she may have diffuse abdominal tenderness, rebound tenderness, and abdominal wall rigidity. These children will also have signs of systemic toxicity, such as a higher fever, tachycardia, and tachypnea.

Laboratory studies can be helpful in cases where the history and physical examination are equivocal. A **complete blood cell (CBC) count** often reveals a mild leukocytosis with an increasing left shift as the appendix becomes more gangrenous or ruptures; however, a normal white blood cell count does not rule out appendicitis. **Electrolytes** are usually not helpful unless significant dehydration exists. A few white blood cells in the urine may be found if the appendix lies near the bladder or the ureter. **Radiographs** of the abdomen may occasionally reveal an appendicolith (13%–22%). More commonly, however, the x-ray findings are non-specific. Diagnostic accuracy is enhanced in equivocal patients by the use of either **abdominal ultrasound and/or abdominal computed tomography scan.**

✄ HINT Appendicitis is primarily a clinical diagnosis, and normal laboratory values and imaging studies do not exclude the diagnosis. If a child has normal studies but a worrisome history or examination, he or she should undergo a period of close observation with serial abdominal examinations.

Treatment

The treatment for appendicitis is **appendectomy,** and therefore surgical consultation should be requested promptly once the diagnosis of appendicitis is suspected. Pain management and supportive care should be provided while awaiting operative intervention. Antibiotic therapy should be initiated prior to surgery in patients with suspected perforation.

Intussusception

Etiology

Intussusception occurs when a **proximal segment of bowel telescopes into a distal portion of intestine,** causing edema, lymphatic obstruction, and vascular compromise. Intussusception is typically ileocolic, but may also be ileoileal or colocolic. If a diagnosis is not made in a timely fashion, this ischemic portion of bowel becomes gangrenous and eventually perforates, leading to peritonitis. Most cases are idiopathic; however, intussusception may arise from an **intestinal lead point.** In infants, hypertrophied lymph nodes may create a lead point, while in older children tumors, polyps, Meckel diverticula, duplications, or intestinal lesions associated with Henoch-Schönlein purpura are most often identified as lead points.

Intussusception is the most common cause of **intestinal obstruction** in young children and occurs most commonly in patients 4 to 12 months of age. The classic symptoms of intussusception are episodic abdominal pain, vomiting, and "currant jelly" stools. Periods of severe pain, often causing the child to pull up his legs, are followed by periods of no obvious discomfort or lethargy. Eventually, the child begins to vomit and develops more consistent pain as the intestine becomes more edematous and ischemic. This circulatory compromise causes sloughing of the intestinal mucosa, which results in passage of "currant jelly" stools.

Evaluation

Patients with intussusception may look **generally well** or may be quite ill-appearing with **unstable vital signs.** Abdominal examination may reveal distention because of either partial or complete obstruction. Occasionally, a sausage-like mass can be palpated, most often in the right upper quadrant. Rectal examination may reveal heme-positive stool. Laboratory studies should include a CBC, electrolytes, blood urea nitrogen, creatinine, and crossmatch. Abdominal radiographs may show varying degrees of small bowel obstruction. A soft tissue mass (the lead point of the intussusception) may be visible. Rarely, free air may be noted because of intestinal perforation. These radiographic findings are helpful if present, but frequently the plain film shows a **non-specific gas pattern.**

Treatment

Intravenous fluids should be provided for presumed dehydration and a nasogastric tube should be placed to decompress the stomach and intestines. The administration of **broad-spectrum antibiotics** is recommended prior to attempted reduction. An **air or barium contrast enema** can be both a diagnostic and a therapeutic maneuver in suspected intussusception. If barium enema or air insufflation is unsuccessful, or if the child appears systemically toxic prior to the enema, **operative reduction** is necessary. Because of the potential need for emergent surgery, surgical consultation is mandatory when intussusception is suspected. The recurrence rate after successful nonoperative reduction is reported to be 5%–10%; recurrence is more common in an older child with a lead point.

Testicular Torsion

Etiology (See Chapter 78, "Thermal Injury")

Testicular torsion is an important cause of acute scrotal pain and frequently results in referred abdominal pain. Torsion occurs in a testicle that is inadequately fixed to the scrotal wall. The pain from testicular torsion is caused by twisting of the spermatic cord, resulting in testicular ischemia.

Clinical Features

Boys report **sudden onset of scrotal pain** that often radiates to the abdomen. Often there is a misleading history of minimal trauma. The boy typically looks very uncomfortable, and physical examination reveals a swollen, tender, elevated testicle.

Evaluation

Testicular torsion is a **urologic emergency,** and the rate of testicular salvage is inversely related to the time to detorsion. Thus, if the clinical suspicion for torsion is high, these children are often taken directly to the operating room without confirmatory testing. In less obvious cases, the diagnosis can be confirmed with testicular ultrasound or a testicular nuclear perfusion scan to differentiate testicular torsion from torsion of the appendix testis and epididymitis.

Treatment

In equivocal cases, once the diagnosis is confirmed, these patients are taken to the **operating room for detorsion.** Attempts can be made at manual detorsion; however, even if non-surgical detorsion is successful, these boys must be taken to the operating room for exploration and orchiopexy, albeit less emergently.

Respiratory Tract Infections

Group A Streptococcal Pharyngitis (See Chapter 75, "Sore Throat")

Patients with group A streptococcal pharyngitis sometimes present with abdominal pain with or without throat pain, fever, and cervical adenopathy. A rapid streptococcal antigen detection test or throat culture can be helpful in making the diagnosis, although a positive result may also indicate a carrier state.

Lower Lobe Pneumonia

Children with lower lobe pneumonia may present with respiratory symptoms and abdominal pain. Evidence for a pneumonia may be as subtle as an increased respiratory rate or unexplained high fevers. Lower lobe pneumonias are sometimes discovered incidentally on abdominal x-rays taken for evaluation of abdominal pain. Treatment is with analgesics and appropriate antibiotics for pneumonia.

Henoch-Schönlein Purpura

Henoch-Schönlein purpura is discussed in Chapter 18, "Bleeding and Purpura."

Toxin Exposures and Foreign Body Ingestions

Although many substances can cause nausea and vomiting when ingested, some **toxins** are more commonly associated with abdominal pain. Examples include iron, aspirin, caustic ingestions, strychnine, lead, and other heavy metals. Specific antidotes (e.g., deferoxamine for iron toxicity) can be given in addition to activated charcoal and other gastrointestinal decontamination measures as indicated. Treatment of the patient who has a toxic ingestion should be coordinated with a **poison control center. Swallowed foreign bodies** such as needles or disc batteries can also cause abdominal pain by irritating or perforating the gastrointestinal mucosa. Although most swallowed foreign bodies travel through the gastrointestinal tract without difficulty, foreign bodies that cause symptoms should be removed by a gastroenterologist, otolaryngologist, or surgeon, depending on the location of the foreign body. A unique toxic exposure causing abdominal pain is a **black widow spider bite.** Venom from the black widow spider (*Latrodectus mactans*) can cause severe abdominal cramping and can cause cardiovascular collapse in young children. Black widow spider antivenin may be indicated in the presence of systemic symptoms.

Trauma

Etiology

The history is an important consideration in evaluating a child with abdominal trauma. Abdominal trauma is categorized as either **blunt** or **penetrating,** and most children with abdominal trauma have blunt trauma. Common mechanisms of injury include falls, motor vehicle-related injuries, and child abuse. While the history is crucial in evaluating children with abdominal trauma, children injured because of child abuse may have inaccurate or deceptive histories.

> 🏛 **HINT**   Consider child abuse in patients whose caretakers seek evaluation late after the onset of symptoms.

Clinical Features

Abdominal symptoms may be subtle immediately after an injury and may be further limited by distracting injuries and alterations in mental status. A high index of suspicion for abdominal injury is appropriate in the evaluation of the patient with trauma.

Evaluation

Patients with abdominal trauma must be thoroughly examined.

▼ Tachycardia—initial symptom with blood loss
▼ Hypotension—a late sign, developing only after significant bleeding
▼ Tachypnea and shallow respirations—an attempt to minimize abdominal pain associated with breathing
▼ Pain and tenderness—focal due to a solid organ injury, or diffuse because of peritoneal irritation from a perforated viscus or intraperitoneal blood
▼ Gross blood on rectal examination—a hollow viscus injury

Further evaluation of the patient's abdominal pain depends on the results of the history and physical examination. In a child in whom the suspicion of injury is low, **observation** and a **repeat physical examination** are appropriate. However, in patients with worrisome findings, **immediate evaluation** is warranted. Laboratory abnormalities may be found on complete blood cell count, liver function tests, pancreatic function tests, or urinalysis; however, normal values do not rule out intra-abdominal injury. With the exception of a pelvis x-ray to look for fracture, x-rays are of limited value in the evaluation of abdominal trauma. The imaging study of choice is an **abdominal computed tomography (CT) scan** with oral and intravenous contrast. The sensitivity for detecting solid organ injury is excellent. The CT scan is less sensitive in detecting hollow viscus and pancreatic injury. **Diagnostic peritoneal lavage (DPL)** is performed in select circumstances (e.g., when a patient is too unstable to go to the CT scanner). While DPL is even more sensitive than CT scan, the DPL is less specific in determining the need for surgical repair because many solid injuries that cause a positive DPL are managed non-operatively. Although abdominal ultrasound is being used more extensively in adult trauma patients, its role in the evaluation of the pediatric trauma patient is less clear. **Immediate surgical consultation** is indicated for patients with significant abdominal trauma.

Treatment

Patients with abdominal trauma should have their **life-threatening conditions** addressed first. After the patient's airway, breathing, circulation and cervical spine have been stabilized, the patient's abdominal injuries can then be addressed. Penetrating trauma of the abdomen represents a **surgical emergency,** and wounds that violate the peritoneal cavity are generally explored in the operating room. Patients with solid organ injury are frequently **managed non-operatively,** but these management decisions should be directed by a surgeon. For those patients who do not have any obvious injuries after initial evaluation with persistent post-traumatic abdominal pain, **close observation** is indicated.

▼ EVALUATION OF ACUTE ABDOMINAL PAIN

The differential diagnosis of acute abdominal pain in a child is extensive, and determining the etiology of a patient's abdominal pain challenges a physician's diagnostic abilities.

History

Type and Location of Pain

▼ **Visceral pain** is caused by stretching of the nerve fibers surrounding an abdominal organ and is a poorly localized, aching pain.
  ▼ **Epigastric pain** originates from structures derived from the foregut (e.g., the stomach, duodenum, pancreas, liver, and biliary tree).
  ▼ **Periumbilical pain** arises from involvement of the midgut structures (e.g., the jejunum, ileum, and large intestine up to the splenic flexure).
  ▼ **Suprapubic pain** is produced by hindgut structures (e.g., the distal colon and rectum) and bladder.
▼ **Somatic pain** occurs when pain fibers in the parietal peritoneum are irritated either by inflammation of the peritoneum itself or by an adjacent, inflamed organ. Somatic pain is better localized than visceral pain and is typically worsened by movement.
▼ **Referred pain** to the lower neck and shoulders is associated with phrenic nerve irritation from pancreatitis, splenic pathology, or hepatobiliary disease.

Characteristics of Pain

▼ **Sudden onset** suggests perforation of a visceral organ or ischemia.
▼ **Gradual onset** suggests inflammation, such as pain associated with appendicitis.
▼ **Colicky spasms** of pain suggest pain from a hollow viscus, such as kidney stones or gallstones.

Associated Symptoms

Ask about the following:

▼ **Fever or chills**
▼ **Nausea or vomiting** (specifically if there is bile or blood in the emesis)
▼ **Abdominal distention**
▼ **Stool irregularities** (e.g., constipation, diarrhea, hematochezia, melena, or mucus in the stools)
▼ **Other complaints,** such as sore throat, dyspnea, cough, dysuria or urinary frequency, and extra-abdominal pain
▼ **Sexual history**—for adolescent boys and girls
▼ **Menstrual history, vaginal bleeding, or discharge**—for adolescent girls
▼ **Past medical history and medications**

Physical Examination

A complete physical examination should be performed on patients with abdominal pain prior to examining the abdomen itself, with emphasis on:

▼ **Vital signs and general appearance**
▼ **HEENT**—eyes and mucus membranes should be checked for icterus, and the pharynx should be inspected.
▼ **Lungs and heart**

The abdomen should be examined in the following order:

▼ **Inspection**—look for scars, masses, distention, and peristalsis.
▼ **Auscultation**—may reveal high-pitched bowel sounds typical of bowel obstruction or the absence of bowel sounds as seen in a patient with an ileus.

TABLE 9.1.   Differential Diagnosis of Acute Abdominal Pain by Age and Location

	< 2 years	2–5 years	5–12 years	Adolescence
Localized pain	Appendicitis (late) Incarcerated hernia Urinary tract infection	Appendicitis (late) Urinary tract infection Sickle cell disease	Appendicitis (late) Urinary tract infection Infectious mononucleosis Peptic ulcer disease	Appendicitis (late) Urinary tract infection Infectious mononucleosis Peptic ulcer disease Cholecystitis Pelvic inflammatory disease Ovarian cyst / torsion Pregnancy / ectopic
Diffuse pain	Appendicitis (early or perforated) Intussusception Volvulus / malrotation Colic Food allergy Constipation Hemolytic-uremic syndrome Necrotizing enterocolitis Gastroenteritis Henoch-Schönlein purpura Hirschsprung disease	Appendicitis (early or perforated) Constipation Gastroenteritis Ingestion Pharyngitis Pneumonia Henoch-Schönlein purpura Diabetic ketoacidosis Asthma Sickle cell disease Inflammatory bowel disease	Appendicitis (early or perforated) Diabetic ketoacidosis Pharyngitis Pneumonia Gastroenteritis Constipation Functional Inflammatory bowel disease Testicular torsion Asthma Sickle cell disease	Appendicitis (early or perforated) Dysmenorrhea Mittelschmerz Functional Inflammatory bowel disease Diabetic ketoacidosis Testicular torsion Gastroenteritis

▼ **Palpation**—In a verbal child, ask the patient which part of his or her abdomen hurts the most; this should be the last area palpated. Palpation may reveal masses or guarding.

▼ A **rectal examination** and **genital examination** are important for both males and females. A pelvic examination should be considered in all post-pubertal females.

Laboratory Studies

The following laboratory tests may be helpful:

▼ Complete blood cell count and erythrocyte sedimentation rate may be abnormal in the setting of infection.

▼ Electrolytes, blood urea nitrogen, and creatinine are of limited diagnostic utility but may help in the management of fluid repletion.

▼ A glucose level is helpful in patients suspected of having diabetic ketoacidosis.

▼ Liver function tests and amylase and lipase levels should be sent when hepatic or pancreatic disease is suspected.

▼ Blood type and crossmatch should be sent if transfusion is a possibility.

▼ Urinalysis may reveal infection or hematuria.

▼ A urine pregnancy test should be done in all pubertal females with abdominal pain.

▼ Throat, stool, cervix, and urine cultures should be done if infection is suspected.

Imaging Modalities

Various imaging studies can be used in evaluation of the patient:

▼ **Plain abdominal radiographs**—an abdominal obstruction series is more helpful than a single film of the abdomen and may reveal a bowel obstruction, ileus, fecalith, renal or biliary calculi, free air, or a mass. A chest x-ray may reveal thoracic pathology causing abdominal pain.

▼ **Fluoroscopy with contrast** is used when looking for malrotation or intussusception.

▼ **Ultrasound** can help evaluate right upper quadrant pain, the kidneys, gynecologic causes of abdominal pain, and suspected appendicitis.

▼ **Abdominal CT** is helpful in the evaluation of abdominal masses and solid organ injury. CT is also being used more frequently in the evaluation of appendicitis.

▼ APPROACH TO THE PATIENT (TABLE 9.1)

See Table 9.1

Suggested Readings

Garcia-Peña SM, Mandl KD, Kraus SJ, et al.: Ultrasonography and limited computed tomography in the diagnosis and management of appendicitis in children. *JAMA* 282(11): 1041–1046, 1999.

Irish MS, Pearl RH, Caty MG, Glick PL: The approach to common abdominal diagnoses in infants and children. *Pediatr Clin North Am* 45(4): 729–772, 1998.

Mason JD: The evaluation of acute abdominal pain in children. *Emerg Med Clin North Am* 14(3): 629–643, 1996.

Pearl RH, Irish MS, Caty MG, Glick PL: The approach to common abdominal diagnoses in infants and children, part II. *Pediatr Clin North Am* 45(6): 1287–1326, 1998.

Rothrock SG, Pagane J: Acute appendicitis in children: emergency department diagnosis and management. *Ann Emerg Med* 36: 39–51, 2000.

Ruddy RM: Pain-abdomen. In *Textbook of Pediatric Emergency Medicine*, 4th ed. Edited by Fleisher GR, Ludwig S. Philadelphia, Lippincott Williams and Wilkins, 2000, 421–428.

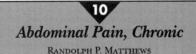

10

Abdominal Pain, Chronic

RANDOLPH P. MATTHEWS

▼ DIFFERENTIAL DIAGNOSIS LIST

Infectious Causes

Abscess, appendiceal or other abdominal
Giardia lamblia enteritis and other parasitic infections
Helicobacter pylori-mediated esophagitis, gastritis, and peptic ulcer disease
Hepatitis
Lower lobe pneumonia
Mesenteric adenitis
Pelvic inflammatory disease, tubo-ovarian abscess, and/or Fitz-Hugh-Curtis syndrome
Urinary tract infection
Vertebral infection—discitis, osteomyelitis

Inflammatory Causes

Celiac disease
Cholecystitis
Collagen vascular disease
Henoch-Schönlein purpura
Inflammatory bowel disease
Milk-protein allergy and/or eosinophilic gastroenteritis
Non-*H. pylori*-mediated esophagitis, gastritis, and peptic ulcer disease (reflux, nonsteroidal anti-inflammatory drugs, corticosteroids, etc.)
Pancreatitis, with or without pseudocyst

Metabolic Causes

Acute intermittent porphyria
Carbohydrate intolerance/malabsorption
Cystic fibrosis
Diabetes mellitus

Anatomic/Mechanical Causes

Appendiceal colic
Bezoar

Choledochal cyst
Cholelithiasis
Constipation
Foreign body
Hernia
Intermittent intussusception
Intestinal duplication
Intestinal pseudo-obstruction
Malrotation with intermittent volvulus (from a Meckel diverticulum, Ladd band, etc.)
Nephrolithiasis
Ureteropelvic junction obstruction

Hematologic/Oncological Causes

Abdominal tumor—Wilms, neuroblastoma
Hereditary angioedema
Leukemia
Lymphoma, including gastrointestinal (GI) tract lymphomas
Sickle cell disease
Spinal column tumor—e.g., leukemia, osteosarcoma

Gynecologic Causes

Dysmenorrhea
Endometriosis
Hematometrocolpos
Mittelschmerz
Ovarian cyst/teratoma

Neurologic/Psychiatric Causes

Abdominal epilepsy
Abdominal migraine
Conversion reaction
Depression
School phobia

Toxic Causes

Aspirin
Chronic corticosteroid use
Lead poisoning

Traumatic Causes

Abdominal muscle strain
Intra-abdominal hematoma

Causes of Unclear Etiology

Functional abdominal pain
Nonulcer dyspepsia
Irritable bowel syndrome
Colic

▼ DIFFERENTIAL DIAGNOSIS DISCUSSION

Chronic abdominal pain is one of the **most common and difficult diagnoses** in pediatrics. Prevalence studies indicate that as many as 20% of middle and high school students experience frequent abdominal pain. Approximately 90% of these children have **functional or nonorganic abdominal pain,** pain that cannot be explained by any infectious, inflammatory, anatomic, or biochemical mechanism. The remainder of the patients have **organic abdominal pain,** the most common causes of which are described in detail as follows.

Organic Causes of Abdominal Pain

Chronic Constipation

Constipation is discussed in Chapter 22, "Constipation."

Peptic Disease

Etiology

Peptic disease is a term that encompasses **esophagitis, gastritis, duodenitis,** and **ulcer disease** in these locations. The most typical **causes vary with age,** with infants most likely having esophagitis resulting from gastroesophageal reflux. In children, reflux remains a cause of esophagitis, although gastritis from other causes, such as nonsteroidal anti-inflammatory drug or corticosteroid exposure, extensive burns, or head trauma, may occur. In older children and adolescents, *Helicobacter pylori* infection becomes relatively more common and duodenitis becomes more prevalent, although the other conditions persist at a much lower incidence. Often this group will have a positive family history of ulcer disease.

Evaluation

The **symptoms** of peptic disease also **vary with age. Infants,** in whom reflux is the typical cause, **may have regurgitation or failure to thrive** associated with the disease. Often the parents describe the pain as crying or arching of the back after feeds. In **younger children** with peptic disease, **pain** is generally present **in the mid to upper abdomen** and has no temporal relation to eating. In contrast, peptic disease in the **older child** is characterized by **epigastric pain,** occasionally associated with vomiting, occurring after meals and in the early morning. Relief of pain during eating is not a characteristic sign of peptic disease in children. In any age child, **occult blood loss** from inflammation may lead to melena or occult blood in the stool. Diagnosis is established by **endoscopy,** although milder cases may be inferred as positive by successful therapeutic trial of medication. A **pH probe** may be helpful to document reflux-associated pain. **Breath tests for *H. pylori*** may be helpful to establish the diagnosis, but are not widely available.

Treatment

Peptic disease is treated with **acid blockade,** either an **H2 receptor antagonist or a proton pump inhibitor.** If reflux is a concern, a prokinetic agent such as **metoclopramide** may be tried after an upper GI series has been obtained to rule out an anatomic cause of reflux such as malrotation. Treatment for *H. pylori* **infection** involves **acid blockade** using a proton pump inhibitor as well as **double antibiotic therapy** with amoxicillin, clarithromycin, or metronidazole.

Carbohydrate Intolerance

Etiology

Malabsorption of lactose is by far the **most common type of carbohydrate intolerance** that produces abdominal pain. **Sorbitol** is also a frequent offender, while malabsorption of other sugars may occur in rare disease states. Intolerance of lactose is caused by deficiency of the enzyme lactase, an inhabitant of the small intestinal brush border. Congenital deficiency of lactase is extraordinarily rare, and the **most common causes of true lactase deficiency** are a **genetic late-onset lactase deficiency or mucosal injury.** The genetic form of late-onset lactase deficiency is least common in those of Scandinavian and Northwest European descent and most common in those of Native American, Southeast Asian, Turkish, Italian, and African descent. Mucosal injury occurs after gastroenteritis, particularly that caused by rotavirus, parasitic infections such as *Giardia*, celiac disease, Crohn disease, and radiation or drug exposure. **Sorbitol** is found in **many sugar-free items,** and has been shown to cause abdominal pain in some children.

Evaluation

The typical course following ingestion of lactose-containing food involves nausea and fullness progressing to **periumbilical abdominal pain, cramps, increased flatulence,** and finally **watery diarrhea.** Occasionally in adolescents there may be vomiting. Diagnosis may be made by history alone, although a **lactose breath test** is the gold standard of diagnosis. In this test, patients are fed lactose and breath is collected for hydrogen gas produced by fermentation of undigested lactose by colonic bacteria.

Treatment

Treatment involves **avoidance** of the offending sugar. There are multiple dairy products, including formula, that do not contain lactose. In addition, **dietary supplements of lactase** can predigest the lactose before consumption. Avoidance of other carbohydrates is more difficult, although there are special formulas and nutritional supplements for many types of carbohydrate intolerance.

Inflammatory Bowel Disease

Inflammatory bowel disease is discussed in Chapter 34, "Gastrointestinal Bleeding, Lower."

Chronic Pancreatitis

Etiology

Chronic pancreatitis, more correctly termed **recurrent acute pancreatitis, is typified by recurrent bouts of abdominal pain with periods of intervening wellness** that **may progress to pancreatic insufficiency.** The etiology of chronic pancreatitis in children is often unclear. Hereditary pancreatitis accounts for its presence in some of these children, while other causes include congenital or acquired pancreatic duct anomalies, cystic fibrosis, hypocalcemia, organic acidemias, and various hyperlipidemia syndromes. Occasionally, chronic pancreatitis is associated with pseudocyst formation.

Evaluation

Symptoms of chronic pancreatitis include **midepigastric pain** that may be **associated with stress or a large fatty meal.** Pain may radiate to the back, and **nausea and vomiting** are frequently associated. The episode usually **resolves within 1 week.** Occasionally, symptoms are associated with pancreatic insufficiency or diabetes mellitus. Diagnosis is based on history and laboratory findings of **elevated amylase and lipase.** Amylase typically peaks 3 days after the onset of pancreatitis; the timing of the elevation of lipase is variable. **Abdominal ultrasound or computerized tomography (CT) scan** may show enlargement or inflammation of the pancreas. Endoscopic retrograde cholangiopancreatography is useful in patients in whom gallstones are suspected (unusual in children) or in whom there is a concern for anatomic abnormalities.

Treatment

Treatment of pancreatitis involves **bowel rest and pain control.** Occasionally, the problem persists long enough for patients to require **parenteral nutrition.** For those children in whom pancreatic insufficiency is suspected, **pancreatic enzyme supplementation** may be helpful. **Drainage or removal of a pseudocyst** is indicated if present to prevent possible infection or rupture.

Ureteropelvic Junction Obstruction and Other Genitourinary Disorders

Ureteropelvic junction obstruction refers to a **kink in the ureter at the outlet from the renal pelvis.** Ureteral obstruction leads to abdominal pain and occasional renal damage in children. The condition is **more common in males** and tends to be **left-sided.** Symptoms vary with age. **Infants** often present with an **abdominal mass or pyelonephritis,** while in **children** the presentation is more frequently **abdominal pain.** The pain is crampy and intermittent, occasionally as infrequent as twice per week, and may radiate to the groin or flank. **Older children** may have a **palpable abdominal mass or abnormalities on urinalysis** such as hematuria, but the absence of these findings does not rule out an obstruction. Diagnosis is made by **renal ultrasound or CT scan** of the abdomen. Treatment involves **surgical relief** of the obstruction.

Other genitourinary disorders may cause abdominal pain as well. **Nephrolithiasis** may present as recurrent bouts of abdominal and/or groin pain, occasionally associated with hematuria. **Cystic teratoma of the ovary** may lead to chronic or recurrent abdominal pain, generally in the lower quadrants or pelvic region. As with ureteropelvic junction obstruction, **ultrasound** is the diagnostic method of choice for both of these entities. Treatment of nephrolithiasis in children is **supportive** although further diagnostic evaluation for a cause may be indicated, especially in young children.

Appendiceal Abscess

Appendiceal abscess is discussed in Chapter 8, "Abdominal Mass."

Parasitic Infections

Etiology

The most common parasitic infection associated with chronic abdominal pain is **giardiasis,** caused by the protozoan *Giardia lamblia.* This infection is most frequently associated with **drinking contaminated fresh water,** although in children, **day care** may be a source.

Evaluation and Treatment

Symptoms usually **resolve over weeks,** but **occasionally children develop chronic symptoms** of diffuse, crampy abdominal pain, nausea, abdominal distention and increased flatulence, watery diarrhea, and weight loss from malabsorption. Diagnosis may be made by collecting the stool specifically to **look for the cysts or trophozoites,** or if these are negative and the suspicion is high, examination of **duodenal aspirates or biopsy specimens** may be revealing. Treatment is with **metronidazole.**

Infection with other parasites such as *Ascaris lumbricoides* or *Trichuris trichiura* may lead to abdominal pain if the parasite load is very high. Associated symptoms include anorexia, diarrhea, rectal prolapse, and occasionally small bowel obstruction. Diagnosis is made by screening the stool for ova and parasites. Treatment of these helminths is **pyrantel pamoate and mebendazole for ascariasis** and **mebendazole alone for trichuriasis.** Improvement of sanitation is necessary for population-wide eradication.

Chronic Intestinal Pseudo-Obstruction

Etiology

Chronic intestinal pseudo-obstruction refers to a **heterogeneous set of disorders** that results in **symptoms consistent with obstruction** but **without an actual mechanical blockage.** These diseases appear to **result from decreased contractility of the intestinal smooth muscle** and are generally caused by a multitude of conditions that result in **myopathy or neuropathy,** either localized to the viscera or systemic diseases such as muscular dystrophy.

Evaluation and Treatment

Symptoms include pain similar to the pain of true obstruction: **vomiting, abdominal distention, constipation,** and **early satiety.** Diagnosis is difficult and requires exclusion of the causes of obstruction but may be suggested by **scintigraphic studies of motility. Intestinal manometry** may be helpful as well, although these tests are not done frequently in children. Treatment is often **supportive** and may include **enteral feeding** into the jejunum if more proximal feeds are not tolerated. Pharmacological treatment has not been shown to be helpful.

Nonorganic Causes of Abdominal Pain

Functional Abdominal Pain

Functional abdominal pain is defined as pain that occurs **at least once per month for at least three consecutive months without a clear organic etiology.** Between 10% and 20% of school-aged children are believed to have some variety of functional abdominal pain. The mean age of onset is **between 5 and 8 years,** with males and females affected equally until the age of 9 years, at which point more females are affected. Onset **after the age of 14 years** is usually associated with symptoms more consistent with **irritable bowel syndrome,** while onset **before the age of 5 years** suggests an **organic etiology.** Although psychological factors are important, there is no correlation of functional abdominal pain with personality traits such as perfectionism or chronic worrying; these children are of average intelligence and are not superintellects or overachievers.

Etiology

The factors that produce functional abdominal pain are not entirely clear, although correlation with various psychosocial factors has been described. **Family stress** appears to be important. Often there is a family history of alcoholism, behavioral problems, abdominal pain, or migraine headaches. The **family dynamic in response to the pain** is important as well, as often there is positive reinforcement for having abdominal pain, ranging from emotional support to excusing from school or household chores. Pathophysiologic studies have focused on the autonomic nervous system and gastrointestinal motility, suggesting a possible role for altered gastric motility and heightened sensitivity to intestinal contractions in individuals with functional abdominal pain.

Evaluation

Functional abdominal pain is categorized on the basis of the location of pain using the Rome criteria shown in Table 10.1.

▼ **Periumbilical pain** is by far the most common and is classified as true functional abdominal pain.
▼ **Chronic epigastric pain** is defined as nonulcer dyspepsia.
▼ **Pain in the infraumbilical region** is thought to represent a childhood presentation of irritable bowel syndrome.

These latter two conditions are believed to be caused by altered gastrointestinal motility of the stomach and large bowel, respectively. The pain of functional abdominal pain is **recurrent and paroxysmal** in nature, varying in

TABLE 10.1. Rome Criteria for the Diagnosis of Functional Abdominal Pain in Children with Pain of at Least 12 Weeks Duration over the Past 12 Months

Functional Abdominal Pain	Nonulcer Dyspepsia	Irritable Bowel Syndrome
Continuous abdominal pain in child age 5–15 years AND	Persistent or recurrent pain or discomfort in the epigastric area AND	Abdominal pain or discomfort with at least two of the following: relief with defecation, onset associated with a change in frequency or appearance of stool AND
Minimal or no relationship of pain with eating, defecation, or menses AND	No evidence (including gross visualization or biopsy) that organic disease explains the symptoms AND	No structural or biochemical abnormalities to explain the symptoms AND
The pain is not factitious AND	No evidence that dyspepsia is relieved by defecation or a change in stool pattern.	Associated with abnormal stool frequency (<3/week or >3/day), alternating stool character, straining, urgency, passing mucus, bloating, and distention.
The child does not satisfy criteria for another type of functional abdominal pain.		

TABLE 10.2. Clinical Features of Abdominal Pain of Organic Etiology

Age less than 5 years
Family history of inflammatory bowel disease or peptic ulcer disease
Pain not in the midline
Pain awakening the child from sleep
Pain that is referred to the back, chest, shoulder, or extremities
Associated joint pain or swelling
Dysuria, flank pain, hematuria, or dark-colored urine
Dyspareunia or vaginal discharge
Constitutional symptoms such as fever, weight loss, growth deceleration, rash, or
   night sweats
Emesis, especially if grossly bloody or bilious
Diarrhea, constipation, or fecal incontinence
Gross or occult blood in the stool
Perianal disease (tags, fissures, fistulae)
Decreased energy or sleepiness after pain attacks

severity but not waking the child up at night. There is typically **a clustering of the pain episodes** within days or weeks that waxes and wanes over the course of months. The pain is often difficult for the child to describe and is often not associated with eating or other activities but frequently occurs at the **same time of day.** The presence of symptoms such as weight loss, melena, and other red flags listed in Table 10.2 suggests the presence of an **organic etiology** to the pain.

As with all diagnoses in medicine, a **thorough and careful history** is the most helpful tool in the diagnosis of functional abdominal pain. In addition to screening for organic causes, the clinician should work with the family to track the course of the pain and to attempt to gain a psychosocial understanding of the child and the family. A **pain diary** kept by the family is often a useful diagnostic and even occasionally therapeutic tool. Despite the clear influence of stress and other psychosocial factors in this disease, it is important that this diagnosis not be arrived at as a last resort, after "more serious" causes of abdominal pain have been "ruled out." It may be helpful to have a **psychologist or psychiatrist** as part of the diagnostic team, even if the cause is organic, because abdominal pain of any nature causes stress on the child and the family. Early involvement of such professionals also avoids the problem of addressing these issues late in the work-up, which can give the impression to the family that "it's all in his/her head" and therefore not a "real" disease. Clearly, the clinician should use the tools available to identify the cause of abdominal pain, while attempting to avoid overreliance on elaborate tests and unnecessary referrals to specialists.

The physical examination of the child with functional abdominal pain should be normal. Although indiscriminate testing of these children is unwarranted, **normal screening laboratory tests** will reassure the clinician and family that there is no organic cause of the abdominal pain. **Laboratory testing** should include complete blood cell count, erythrocyte sedimentation rate, liver function tests including aminotransferases and albumin, urinalysis, and examination of the feces for ova and parasites. **Upper endoscopy** is indicated in patients with **dyspepsia pain. Lactose breath test** is helpful if lactose intolerance is a concern, and **abdominal ultrasound** may be helpful if the child is difficult to examine or if there is concern for an anatomic problem.

Treatment

▼ **Functional abdominal pain.** Treatment begins with making the diagnosis and letting the family understand that this is a real entity and not a wastebasket term. The goal of therapy is to allow the child to function with pain or to eliminate the pain if possible. Generally this involves **addressing the stressors** that seem to be contributing to the pain and **reversing the positive reinforcement** the child may be receiving. **School attendance is critical** to breaking the cycle, and school health officials must be instructed of the need for negative reinforcement. Involvement of **mental health professionals,** as stated earlier, may be helpful for many families in particularly stressful situations. Drug therapy for functional abdominal pain is generally not indicated, and hospitalization should be avoided.

▼ **Irritable bowel syndrome.** The mainstay of treatment for adults is a high-fiber diet; results in children, however, are less convincing. Antispasmodics such as hyoscyamine, which act through anticholinergic mechanisms to cause smooth muscle relaxation, may be helpful. However, these drugs have significant side effects and are only rarely used in children. Much of the therapy for irritable bowel syndrome in children relies on **reassurance and education,** with psychological or behavioral support added if necessary.

Colic

Although not technically a form of functional abdominal pain, colic may be thought of as **functional abdominal pain of infancy.** As with the conditions described earlier, this disease has no clear organic basis and is affected by psychosocial issues in the family. Furthermore, there is no clear evidence that colic pain is gastrointestinal pain; however, because the two are linked in many family's and physician's minds, we will discuss colic at this point.

Etiology

Colic, when referring to the prolonged crying seen in infancy, is technically defined as colic syndrome. Although features of this syndrome vary depending on who is defining it, Wessel has established a "rule of threes"—that is, crying for **more than 3 hours per day for more than 3 days per week for more than 3 weeks.** The **etiology of colic is not well understood,** and the mechanisms proposed to cause it are at best vague. The **immaturity of the infant nervous system** may play a role, particularly the transitioning to a more awake state. The gradual decrease in colic symptoms does coincide with the acquisition of skills such as the social smile and hand coordination sufficient for thumb sucking—skills that enable the infant to more adequately maintain a calm awake state. Other proposed etiologies include **intolerance to cow's milk,** although there is little evidence that children with colic have true milk protein intolerance and the symptoms of that disorder do not include colic-like symptoms.

Evaluation

The **crying** noted in colic typically **peaks in the evening** and peaks at the **age of 2 months,** generally tapering off by 3–4 months of age. Other features include movements and facial features interpreted as being consistent with pain, as well as **gastrointestinal symptoms** such as gas and abdominal distention. Clearly, these criteria are loose and may fall within the realm of normal infant behavior, albeit at one end of the curve. Physical and laboratory examinations of children with colic are uniformly normal.

Treatment

Treatment of colic is designed to **relieve the parents' stress.** Infants in this age range are targets of abuse, and preventing overstressed parents from harming these children is an important goal. Advice to parents of an infant with colic should always include suggestions on how to manage the stress, such as relief to take a brief break from caregiving. **Reassurance** that the crying will stop eventually is helpful. **Changes in caregiving and in the environment** that facilitate the awake state and reduce crying may be helpful, such as increasing carrying and rocking, using a pacifier, increasing background white noise with a vacuum cleaner or washing machine, or taking a ride in the car or stroller. Dicyclomine is not indicated for use in infants because it is associated with respiratory distress and apnea. Changing from breast- to formula-feeding is not indicated, and switching formulas should only be done if there is a suggestion of a true milk protein intolerance.

▼ APPROACH TO THE PATIENT

The diagnosis of chronic abdominal pain does not easily lend itself to a simple flow chart because many of the conditions have overlapping symptoms.

History: Important Questions

- ▼ How long has the pain lasted?
- ▼ Where exactly is the pain and does it radiate?
- ▼ Is the pain made worse or better by eating or stooling?
- ▼ Is there any association of the pain with menses?
- ▼ Does the pain wake you up at night?
- ▼ Is there any fever, weight loss, joint pain, or rash?
- ▼ Has there been any vomiting? If so, is it bilious?
- ▼ Has there been any diarrhea? Any bloody or melenotic stool?
- ▼ Any ingestion of toxins such as aspirin or lead?
- ▼ Any exposure to untreated fresh water? Attending day care?
- ▼ Any family history of inflammatory bowel disease, peptic ulcer disease, functional abdominal pain, migraines?

Physical Examination: Important Clues

- ▼ Vital signs, general appearance
- ▼ Weight and height percentile
- ▼ Mouth: Well-hydrated? Ulcers?
- ▼ Abdominal exam: Distended? Tender? If so, location? Rebound? Mass or stool palpable?
- ▼ Rectal exam: Perianal disease? Hard stool? Grossly bloody or occult blood?
- ▼ Skin: Jaundice? Rash?
- ▼ Musculoskeletal: Joint swelling, redness, or tenderness?

TABLE 10.3. Distinguishing Characteristics of Various Causes of Chronic Abdominal Pain

Diagnosis	Historical Clues	Physical Exam Clues	Lab/Diagnostic Study Clues
Functional abdominal pain	▶ Periumbilical pain ▶ Duration >3 months ▶ Pain not associated with eating or stooling ▶ Pain does not awaken child	Normal exam	Normal lab findings
Nonulcer dyspepsia	▶ Epigastric pain ▶ Duration >3 months ▶ Pain not associated with stooling ▶ Pain does not awaken child	Normal exam	Normal labs and studies, including endoscopy
Irritable bowel syndrome	▶ Infraumbilical pain ▶ Duration >3 months ▶ Pain relieved by defecation or associated with a change in bowel pattern ▶ Pain does not awaken child	Normal exam	Normal labs
Chronic constipation	▶ Diffuse, vague pain ▶ Decreased stool frequency, hard or voluminous stool common ▶ May have withholding or encopresis	Often hard stool on rectal exam	▶ Normal labs ▶ Abdominal radiograph may show abundant stool
Peptic disease	▶ Epigastric pain ▶ Reflux and poor weight gain possible, especially in infants ▶ Often but not always after meals ▶ Family history of ulcers possible	▶ May have epigastric tenderness ▶ Hemepositive stools may be present	▶ Anemia possible ▶ pH probe may be helpful ▶ Endoscopy shows esophagitis, gastritis, duodenitis, or ulcers ▶ *Helicobacter pylori* studies may be positive

Carbohydrate intolerance	▶ Diffuse, crampy pain after meals ▶ Watery diarrhea typical ▶ May have poor weight gain ▶ May be postinfectious ▶ More common in certain ethnic groups	Usually normal	Breath tests for the offending sugar are the tests of choice
Inflammatory bowel disease	▶ Pain is diffuse or localized ▶ Constitutional symptoms such as fever, weight loss, rash, joint pain common ▶ Diarrhea or bloody stool may be present ▶ Vomiting possible ▶ Mouth ulcers or perianal disease may be present	▶ Fever, tachycardia ▶ Abdominal tenderness ▶ Hemepositive stools frequent ▶ Rash or joint findings possible	▶ Elevated erythrocyte sedimentation rate, anemia, hypoalbuminemia are common ▶ Upper GI/small bowel series may show strictures in Crohn disease ▶ Endoscopy and biopsy needed for diagnosis
Chronic pancreatitis	▶ Midepigastric pain ▶ May radiate to back ▶ May have vomiting or loss of appetite ▶ May have malabsorptive symptoms	▶ May be ill-appearing or cachectic ▶ Midepigastric tenderness common	▶ Elevated amylase and lipase ▶ May have enlargement of pancreas by ultrasound or CT
Ureteropelvic junction obstruction	▶ Diffuse pain that may radiate to groin or flank ▶ May have hematuria ▶ May have vomiting ▶ May be intermittent	▶ May have palpable abdominal mass ▶ May have costovertebral angle tenderness	Ultrasound or CT scan shows anomaly
Nephrolithiasis	▶ Severe intermittent crampy pain in abdomen and/or flank, occasionally radiating to groin ▶ May have hematuria ▶ Vomiting possible	May have abdominal or costovertebral angle tenderness	Ultrasound or CT scan may show presence of stone

Continued

TABLE 10.3. Distinguishing Characteristics of Various Causes of Chronic Abdominal Pain (continued)

Diagnosis	Historical Clues	Physical Exam Clues	Lab/Diagnostic Study Clues
Ovarian teratoma	▸ Intermittent lower quadrant pain, often one sided ▸ Vomiting possible	Lower-quadrant fullness, tenderness	▸ Ultrasound or CT scan will show anomaly ▸ Ultrasound can also determine blood flow
Giardiasis	▸ Diffuse, crampy pain ▸ Weight loss or poor weight gain possible ▸ Nausea, watery diarrhea, bloating, increased flatulence common ▸ Exposure through day care or contaminated fresh water	Abdominal distention common	▸ Stool examination may show cysts ▸ May need to perform duodenal aspirates or endoscopy
Biliary colic	▸ RUQ or midepigastric crampy pain after meals, especially fatty foods ▸ May have vomiting ▸ May be obese or have concurrent illness	RUQ or midepigastric tenderness possible	▸ May have elevated bilirubin or transaminases ▸ Ultrasound shows gallstones or thickened gallbladder wall
Partial small bowel obstruction	▸ Intermittent crampy pain, vomiting, and decreased flatus ▸ Vomiting may be bilious ▸ May have history of previous abdominal surgery	▸ Abdominal distention and tenderness ▸ May have scars from previous surgery on abdomen	Abdominal radiograph frequently shows fixed air-fluid levels with decreased air distally
Dysmenorrhea	▸ Crampy lower abdominal pain, occurring during menses ▸ Often a family history of dysmenorrhea	Normal exam	Normal studies, although some may have endometriosis

Condition	History/Symptoms	Physical Examination	Laboratory/Diagnostic
Pelvic inflammatory disease	▶ Suprapubic or generalized abdominal pain ▶ History of sexual activity ▶ May have vaginal discharge	▶ Fever ▶ Usually have lower abdominal tenderness ▶ Cervical discharge ▶ Positive cervical motion or adnexal tenderness	▶ Positive cervical cultures or ligase chain reactions ▶ Often have elevated erythrocyte sedimentation rate and WBC count ▶ Ultrasound may show tuboovarian abscess
Lead poisoning	▶ Diffuse pain ▶ Often a history of pica ▶ In high-risk exposure area	Usually normal	▶ Elevated serum lead level ▶ Microcytic anemia ▶ May see basophilic stippling
Sickle cell disease	▶ Diffuse or localized pain, often periumbilical ▶ May be typical for child's vasoocclusive crisis pain	▶ May have fever ▶ May have tenderness, splenomegaly	▶ Sickled red cells ▶ Anemia
Abdominal epilepsy	▶ Intermittent severe pain ▶ May be associated with seizures	Normal exam	▶ EEG is abnormal ▶ May respond to antiepileptic drugs
Abdominal migraine	▶ Intermittent severe pain ▶ May be associated with headache, vomiting ▶ Family history of migraine	Normal exam	May respond to antimigraine medications

CT = computed tomography; EEG = electroencephalogram; GI = gastrointestinal; RUQ = right upper quadrant; WBC = white blood cell.

Laboratory Studies

▼ Complete blood cell count
▼ Erythrocyte sedimentation rate
▼ Liver function tests: aminotransferases, albumin, bilirubin
▼ Amylase and lipase
▼ Urinalysis
▼ Electrolytes, blood urea nitrogen, creatinine

Diagnostic Tests: Based on Clinical Suspicion

▼ Abdominal two-view radiograph
▼ Abdominal ultrasound
▼ Lactose or other breath tests
▼ Endoscopy

Table 10.3 displays distinguishing characteristics of the different causes of chronic abdominal pain. The determination of the exact cause of a child's abdominal pain may require some time, and parents may need to bring the child back to the physician for multiple visits. Occasionally, referral to a specialist is indicated. It is critical that all involved work as a team and address all of the factors that have produced chronic abdominal pain in the child.

Suggested Readings

Barr RG: Colic and gas. In *Pediatric Gastrointestinal Disease: Pathophysiology, Diagnosis, Management,* 3rd ed. Edited by Walker WA, Durie PR, Hamilton JR, et al. Hamilton, On, BC Decker, 2000.

Boyle JT: Abdominal pain. In *Pediatric Gastrointestinal Disease: Pathophysiology, Diagnosis, Management,* 3rd ed. Edited by Walker WA, Durie PR, Hamilton JR, et al. Hamilton, On, BC Decker, 2000.

Boyle JT: Recurrent abdominal pain. *Pediatr Rev* 18:310–320, 1997.

Broussard DL: Pseudo-obstruction. In *Clinical Pediatric Gastroenterology.* Edited by Altschuler SM, Liacouras CA. Philadelphia, Churchill Livingstone, 1998.

Hyams JS: Crohn disease. In *Pediatric Gastrointestinal Disease,* 2nd ed. Edited by Wyllie R, Hyams JS. Philadelphia, WB Saunders, 1999.

Kirschner BS (ed): Management of abdominal pain. *Pediatr Ann* 30:12–47, 2001.

Liquornik K, Liacouras CA: *Helicobacter pylori* in pediatrics. In *Clinical Pediatric Gastroenterology.* Edited by Altschuler SM, Liacouras CA. Philadelphia, Churchill Livingstone, 1998.

Markowitz, JF: Ulcerative colitis. In *Pediatric Gastrointestinal Disease,* 2nd ed. Edited by Wyllie R, Hyams JS. Philadelphia, WB Saunders, 1999.

Semeao E, Altschuler SM: Irritable bowel syndrome. In *Clinical Pediatric Gastroenterology.* Edited by Altschuler SM, Liacouras CA. Philadelphia, Churchill Livingstone, 1998.

Wenner WJ: Constipation and encopresis. In *Clinical Pediatric Gastroenterology.* Edited by Altschuler SM, Liacouras CA. Philadelphia, Churchill Livingstone, 1998.

Wyllie R, Mahajan LA: Chronic abdominal pain of childhood and adolescence. In *Pediatric Gastrointestinal Disease,* 2nd ed. Edited by Wyllie R, Hyams JS. Philadelphia, WB Saunders, 1999.

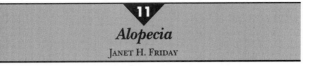

11
Alopecia
JANET H. FRIDAY

▼ INTRODUCTION

Tinea capitis, trichotillomania, alopecia areata, and **telogen effluvium** account for more than 95% of cases of alopecia in children. The growth cycle of hair consists of an **active growth phase (anagen),** a **transition phase (catagen),** and a **resting phase (telogen).** After the telogen phase, the hair is shed and replaced by a new anagen bulb. On a normal scalp, approximately 85%–90% of the hair is in the anagen phase. There are 100,000 hairs on the normal scalp. Hair loss is only clinically apparent when a person has lost 25%–50% of his hair.

▼ DIFFERENTIAL DIAGNOSIS LIST
Infectious Causes

Tinea capitis
Secondary syphilis

Toxic Causes

Cytotoxic agents
Anticonvulsants
Radiation
Hypervitaminosis A
Anticoagulants

Neoplastic Causes

Histiocytosis

Traumatic Causes

Trichotillomania
Traction alopecia
Friction alopecia

Congenital Causes

Aplasia cutis congenita
Nevus sebaceous
Epidermal nevus
Hemangioma
Loose anagen syndrome
Ectodermal dysplasia
Hair shaft defects

Metabolic or Genetic Causes

Androgenic alopecia
Acrodermatitis enteropathica

Anorexia nervosa
Malnutrition
Hypo- or hyperthyroidism
Hypopituitarism
Diabetes mellitus

Inflammatory Causes

Alopecia areata
Systemic lupus erythematosus
Scleroderma

Miscellaneous Causes

Atopic dermatitis
Seborrheic dermatitis
Psoriasis
Telogen effluvium
Anagen effluvium

▼ DIFFERENTIAL DIAGNOSIS DISCUSSION
Tinea Capitis
Etiology

Caused by dermatophyte infection of the scalp hairs, tinea capitis is respon-sible for **more than 50% of cases of hair loss** in children. Currently, the most prevalent fungus causing tinea capitis is *Trichophyton tonsurans*.

Clinical Features

Tinea capitis is seen most commonly in school-age children. The infection causes **patchy hair loss** that may or may not be accompanied by **scale.** Some areas may seem completely bald and indistinguishable from alopecia areata, but on closer examination the scalp contains **very short hairs,** called "**black-dot**" **tinea capitis.**

Evaluation

Unlike *Microsporum canis*, which caused epidemic outbreaks of tinea capitis during the 1940s, *T. tonsurans* does not show immunofluorescence under Wood lamp examination. Diagnosis can be confirmed using a **potassium hydroxide (KOH) preparation** and by **fungal culture** of the hair and scale. A KOH preparation reveals organisms inside the hair shaft.

Treatment

Oral griseofulvin dosed at 15 mg/kg once daily for 6–8 weeks is the standard therapy for tinea capitis in children. It is best absorbed when taken with **fatty foods.** The medication is **safe in children;** it is not necessary for the patient to undergo laboratory testing before initiating drug therapy. Newer antifungal medications such as **fluconazole, itraconazole,** and **terbinafine** may also be effective and require a shorter course of therapy. A **2.5% selenium shampoo** may hasten resolution in combination with systemic antifungal medication. An effort should be made to identify and treat infected household contacts to avoid reinfection.

✍ HINT The infection may be accompanied by a hypersensitivity reaction called a kerion, which is a boggy, inflammatory mass. The surface may contain pustules, and cervical lymphadenopathy is usually present. Although it may appear to be superinfected, the lesion can usually be successfully treated with griseofulvin and oral prednisone.

✍ HINT Tinea capitis mimics many other conditions and should be considered to be the diagnosis of exclusion in all cases of acquired localized alopecia.

Alopecia Areata

Etiology

Alopecia areata is the **second most common cause** of alopecia in children and may appear insidiously in an otherwise healthy school-age patient. Multiple factors are implicated in the pathophysiology, including genetic, organ-specific autoimmune, and nonspecific immune components.

Clinical Features

The hair loss occurs in **variably sized patches** completely **devoid of hair.** Hairs surrounding the area of alopecia may demonstrate a narrow waist on microscopic examination ("exclamation point" hairs). The **entire scalp is involved in alopecia totalis,** and the **entire body** is **involved in alopecia universalis.** Accompanying features may include **pitting** or a **scotch-plaid pattern** on the **nails.** Other autoimmune disorders may occur in these patients, such as Hashimoto thyroiditis, diabetes mellitus, vitiligo, Addison disease, and inflammatory bowel disease.

Evaluation

Hair pluck with microscopy should be performed to look for classic **"exclamation point" hairs,** which confirm the diagnosis of alopecia areata.

Treatment

Treatment for this disorder is less than straightforward. Modalities such as topical and systemic steroids, minoxidil, and anthralin have been used; unfortunately, none have proved effective in reversing the course of disease. In **one-third of patients,** the **condition regresses spontaneously** within 6 months. More extensive cases are less likely to resolve. A frank discussion with the patient and family and **close follow-up** are mandatory. A **wig or hairpiece** may be necessary to counteract the psychological trauma of this disease. **Referral to a pediatric dermatologist** should be considered in all cases in which aggressive therapy seems warranted.

Trichotillomania

Etiology

Seen more commonly in children than in adults, trichotillomania is an **uncontrollable urge to pull out one's own hair.** Adolescent girls are most commonly afflicted; however, in children younger than 6 years, it is more common in boys.

Clinical Features

The hair-pulling results in **ill-defined areas of baldness** in **unusual distributions.** The diagnosis is usually made clear by the presence of **many broken hairs of various lengths.** The sites involved are varied, although a predilection

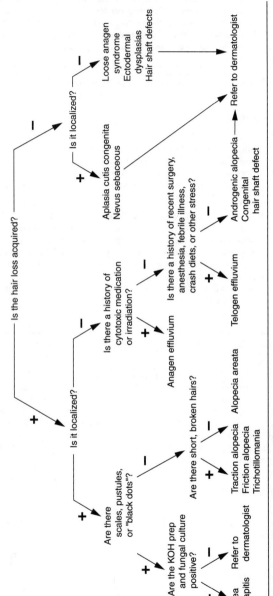

FIGURE 11.1. Evaluation of a patient with alopecia.
KOH prep = potassium hydroxide preparation.

for the side of handedness may be seen. The periphery of the scalp is usually spared. Other body hair may also be involved in severe cases. Often, nail biting, thumb sucking, and **other compulsive behaviors** are also present.

Evaluation

Hair pluck should be performed to rule out alopecia areata. A **scalp biopsy** may be necessary to confirm the diagnosis.

Treatment

The largest obstacle to treatment of the disorder is often **acceptance of the diagnosis by the family.** Treatment consists largely of **behavior modification** and in severe cases may be augmented by **clomipramine. Referral to a psychiatrist** may be warranted.

Telogen Effluvium

Telogen effluvium occurs when a **large percentage of scalp hairs enter the resting phase** after a **stressful event** and are shed 2–4 months later. The precipitant may be childbirth, major surgery, anesthesia, febrile illness, crash dieting, or psychological trauma. The hallmark of telogen effluvium is **diffuse acute hair loss** that **spontaneously resolves** over several months. Hair pluck reveals a disproportionate number of hair follicles in the telogen phase. Eventually, **full recovery** of hair growth ensues and no treatment is necessary.

Traction Alopecia and Friction Alopecia

Tension on the hair shaft can cause hair loss in areas most affected (traction alopecia). Tight braiding of the hair, ponytails, cornrows, and hot combs are the worst culprits. In a similar fashion, hair in **areas of pressure,** such as the occiput in a supine infant, may exhibit hair loss, although the scalp is functionally normal (friction alopecia). Hair loss occurs in a **classic distribution.** Diagnosis is made on a clinical basis. If the alopecia fails to respond to conservative management, the diagnosis should be re-evaluated. The hairstyle or positioning should be altered. Normal hair growth should follow.

Anagen Effluvium

Like telogen effluvium, anagen effluvium is characterized by **diffuse acute hair loss.** In anagen effluvium, hair loss results from **disruption of the normal hair growth cycle** following a toxic insult to the hair follicle. The causes are usually cytotoxic agents such as vincristine and cyclophosphamide. Heavy metal toxicity, hypothyroidism, and severe malnutrition have also been implicated. If the cause is not apparent, hair pluck will differentiate anagen effluvium from telogen effluvium. The **hair will regrow following removal of the offending agent,** although the color and texture of the new hair may be different.

▼ EVALUATION OF ALOPECIA

Patient History

The elements of the history most crucial to the diagnosis of alopecia disorders are as follows:

▼ **Time of onset**—congenital versus acquired
▼ **Associated stressors**—childbirth, recent surgery, toxic exposures, seizures, and febrile illnesses
▼ **Any abnormal behaviors**—e.g., thumb sucking, nail biting

Physical Examination

Physical examination should focus on **distribution of hair loss, presence of scale, presence of broken hairs,** and **nail findings.** A magnifying glass and good lighting aid in detection of subtle scalp findings.

Laboratory Studies

A **KOH preparation** is important when the diagnosis of tinea capitis is suspected, and **fungal culture** should be obtained. A **hair pluck** is used to diagnose telogen effluvium or alopecia areata. **Morphological examination of the hair shaft** allows detection of structural defects.

⚡ HINT If a diagnosis is still unclear after an initial evaluation, referral to a dermatologist may be warranted.

▼ APPROACH TO THE PATIENT (FIGURE 11.1)

Suggested Readings

Atton AV, Tunnessen WW: Alopecia in children: the most common causes. *Pediatr Rev* 12(25):25–30, 1990.

Friedlander SF, Suarez S: Pediatric anti-fungal therapy. *Dermatol Clin* 16(3):527–537, 1998.

Levy ML: Disorders of the hair and scalp in children. *Pediatr Clin North Am* 38(4):905–919, 1991.

Madani S, Shapiro J: Alopecia areata update. *J Am Acad Dermatol* 42(4):549–566, 2000.

Raimer SS: New and emerging therapies in pediatric dermatology. *Dermatol Clin* 18:1, 2000.

Verbov J: Hair loss in children. *Arch Dis Child* 68:702–706, 1993.

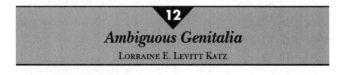

12
Ambiguous Genitalia

LORRAINE E. LEVITT KATZ

▼ INTRODUCTION

Genitalia are defined as ambiguous when it is not possible to categorize the gender of the child based on outward appearances. Ambiguous genitalia may be associated with genotypic **females who are virilized,** genotypic **males who are undermasculinized,** and problems of **gonadal differentiation.**

Sexual Differentiation

Management of patients with sexual ambiguity requires an understanding of normal sexual differentiation. The primitive gonad is bipotential, containing both ovarian (cortical) and testicular (medullary) components. Sexual differentiation is determined by the genetic information contained in the sex chromosomes, as well as by hormonal factors.

Male Sexual Differentiation

The SRY gene (i.e., the sex-determining region) on the short arm of the Y chromosome is the **primary testis-determining factor (TDF).** Additional genetic factors that are important to sexual differentiation include DAX-1, SOX-9, and WT1. The TDF induces the bipotential gonads to develop as testes by 6–7 weeks' gestation. At 7–8 weeks' gestation, Sertoli cells in the testes secrete müllerian-inhibiting substance (MIS), which causes regression of the müllerian ducts in the male fetus.

Human chorionic gonadotropin (HCG) and fetal pituitary gonadotropin stimulate the Leydig cells in the fetal testes to secrete **testosterone,** which causes the wolffian structures to develop into the vas deferens, epididymis, and seminal vesicles. Testosterone is converted locally to dihydrotestosterone (DHT) by 5α-reductase. DHT is necessary for the development of the scrotum and phallus from the labial scrotal folds and the genital tubercle.

Although the formation of the male genitals is complete by 12 weeks' gestation, MIS stimulates abdominal descent of the testes in the second trimester. During the second and third trimesters, further testicular descent and penile growth are stimulated by testosterone.

Female Sexual Differentiation

The differentiation of the bipotential gonad into an ovary by 10 weeks' gestation requires that two X chromosomes be present and that the Y chromosome (i.e., the SRY gene) be absent. Because MIS is not produced, the müllerian ducts develop into the uterus, the fallopian tubes, and the upper two thirds of the vagina. In the **absence of androgens,** the wolffian ducts degenerate, the external genitalia differentiates as the clitoris and labia, and the urogenital sinus becomes the lower third of the vagina and urethra.

▼ DIFFERENTIAL DIAGNOSIS LIST

Virilized Female

Pseudohermaphroditism

Congenital adrenal hyperplasia (CAH)—21-hydroxylase deficiency, 3β-hydroxysteroid dehydrogenase deficiency, 11-hydroxylase deficiency
Maternal androgen exposure—exogenous, excess androgen production
Associated anatomic anomalies

Chromosomal Aberrations

XO/XY
XX/XY

True Hermaphroditism

Idiopathic

Undervirilized Male

Pseudohermaphroditism

CAH—17,20-desmolase deficiency, 3β-hydroxysteroid dehydrogenase deficiency, 17α-hydroxylase deficiency
Other androgen synthesis defects—17-lyase deficiency, 17-ketosteroid reductase deficiency, 5α-reductase deficiency

Partial androgen receptor defects
Associated anatomic abnormalities

Gonadal (Testicular) Dysgenesis

Leydig Cell Hypoplasia

True Hermaphroditism

Idiopathic

▼ DIFFERENTIAL DIAGNOSIS DISCUSSION
Gonadal (Testicular) Dysgenesis

Etiology

▼ In **pure gonadal dysgenesis,** dysgenesis of the genital ridges results in gonads that are hypoplastic. The condition may be inherited or caused by teratogenic agents.

▼ In **partial gonadal dysgenesis,** teratogenic factors or vascular accidents may damage the gonads following differentiation into testes (in genetic males).

▼ In **mixed gonadal dysgenesis,** individuals with the mosaic genotypes XO/XY and XX/XY have gonads that contain both medullary and cortical elements.

Clinical Features

▼ In **pure gonadal dysgenesis,** the phenotype is that of a normal female.

▼ In **partial gonadal dysgenesis,** MIS has been secreted and the müllerian structures have degenerated, but the development of male external genitalia (which depends on the conversion of testosterone to DHT) does not occur. External genitalia are phenotypically female or ambiguous, but there are no gonads or müllerian structures. Testicular damage that occurs during the second and third trimesters may be less severe and may result in micropenis (i.e., a normally formed, appropriately positioned phallus with a length less than 2.5 standard deviations below the appropriate mean for the patient's age) or cryptorchidism.

▼ In **mixed gonadal dysgenesis,** external genitalia may be normal female, intersex, or normal male. Patients with XO/XY mosaicism often have many of the classic features of Turner syndrome. The presence of testicular tissue in patients with mixed gonadal dysgenesis increases the likelihood of androgenic hormonal function and the presence of wolffian duct structures.

Evaluation

The diagnosis is made by chromosomal analysis. In some cases, gonadal biopsy is indicated.

Treatment

Individuals with mixed gonadal dysgenesis have an increased risk of malignant degeneration of gonadal tissues, and gonadectomy is recommended.

True Hermaphroditism

True hermaphrodites possess both ovarian and testicular elements. They may have a separate ovary and a testis on the contralateral side or a combination of the two gonads ("ovotestes").

Etiology

True hermaphrodites include patients with mixed gonadal dysgenesis as well as those with the karyotype 46,XX and (less commonly) 46,XY. The differentiation of the internal duct structures corresponds to the amount of testicular tissue present in the gonad on the same side. Müllerian duct structures may develop on the side of an ovary with contralateral wolffian duct structures, thus indicating that MIS acts locally.

Clinical Features

The degree of functioning testicular tissue determines the appearance of the external structures.

Evaluation

After ruling out hormonal causes of ambiguous genitalia, the definitive diagnosis can be made by gonadal biopsy demonstrating both ovarian and testicular tissue.

Treatment

Ovotestes and dysgenetic testes should be removed because of the risk for malignant degeneration.

Female Pseudohermaphroditism

Pseudohermaphroditism occurs when the external genitalia do not correspond to the chromosomal or gonadal sex (i.e., an XX female who is masculinized, or an XY male who is inadequately masculinized). The internal genitalia develop normally.

Etiology

Virilization of the genotypic female fetus is usually caused by **androgens** produced by the fetus or transferred across the placenta. Androgen exposure before 12 weeks' gestation results in interference of septation of the urogenital sinus and some degree of labial scrotal fusion. After 12 weeks' gestation, androgen exposure can cause clitoral enlargement but not labial scrotal fusion. The following are sources of androgen exposure:

▼ **CAH.** 21-Hydroxylase, 11-hydroxylase, and 3β-hydroxysteroid dehydrogenase deficiencies are associated with the production of excessive amounts of adrenal androgens and are the most common causes of virilization in newborn females. 21-Hydroxylase deficiency represents 90% of cases of CAH.
▼ **Exogenous androgens.** The use of progestational agents in the first trimester of pregnancy for prevention of spontaneous abortion has been associated with female virilization; as a result, the use of these agents has been decreased.
▼ **Exposure to maternal androgens.** The production of androgens by the mother, either as a result of poorly controlled CAH or as a result of an ovarian or adrenal tumor, may also cause masculinization of the female fetus.
▼ **Idiopathic.** Anomalies of the gastrointestinal and urinary tract may be associated with virilization of the female external genitalia without exposure to androgens. Rarely, female pseudohermaphroditism may occur independently of anatomic abnormalities or androgen exposure.

Clinical Features

The external genitalia are virilized. Patients with 21-hydroxylase or 3-hydroxylase deficiencies may present with salt-losing crises within a few weeks of birth.

Evaluation

In patients with pseudohermaphroditism caused by CAH (i.e., 21-hydroxylase deficiency, 3β-hydroxysteroid dehydrogenase deficiency, or 11-hydroxylase deficiency), the diagnosis can be made by obtaining baseline steroid measurements and steroid measurements following adrenocorticotropic hormone (ACTH) administration (Tables 12.1 through 12.3). Baseline and stimulated steroid levels will be elevated.

In patients with other causes of pseudohermaphroditism, the androgen levels are not elevated and the diagnosis can usually be made on the basis of the patient's history and physical examination.

Treatment

Patients with pseudohermaphroditism caused by CAH should receive cortisol and mineralocorticoid replacement as needed. Cosmetic surgical repair may be appropriate for all patients.

Male Pseudohermaphroditism

Etiology

Inadequate masculinization of the genotypic male fetus can be caused by enzyme disorders of testosterone synthesis or a lack of responsiveness to testosterone action (androgen resistance syndromes).

▼ **CAH** can result in undervirilization of the male fetus when the adrenal enzymes necessary for testosterone synthesis (i.e., 3 β-hydroxysteroid, 17α-hydroxylase, cholesterol desmolase) are also deficient in the testes. 3β-Hydroxysteroid dehydrogenase plays an important role in the early biosynthetic pathway of glucocorticoids, mineralocorticoids, and sex steroids. 17α-Hydroxylase deficiency is a rare disorder that results in the inability to produce sex steroids. Cholesterol desmolase deficiency results in insufficient mineralocorticoid, glucocorticoid, and androgen synthesis.

TABLE 12.1. Clinical and Biochemical Features of Congenital Adrenal Hyperplasia (CAH)

Enzyme Defect	Sexual Ambiguity Female	Sexual Ambiguity Male	Additional Clinical Manifestations	Predominant Steroids
Desmolase	−	+	Salt wasting	. . .
3β-Hydroxysteroid dehydrogenase	+	+	Salt wasting	17-OH-Pregnenolone, DHEA
21-Hydroxylase	+	−	Salt wasting	17-OH-Progestone, androstenedione
11-Hydroxylase	+	−	Hypertension	11-Deoxycortisol
17-Hydroxylase	−	+	Hypertension	DOC, corticosterone

DHEA = dehydroepiandrosterone; DOC = deoxycorticosterone.

TABLE 12.2. Normal Serum Adrenal Steroid Levels in Newborn Infants

Steroid	Preterm Sick 24–28 weeks	Preterm Sick 31–35 weeks	Preterm Well 31–35 weeks	Full Term
Cortisol (μg/dl)	7.5 ± 4	6 ± 2.7	6.9 ± 3.8	6.2 ± 3.9
17-OH-Preg (ng/dl)	1794 ± 1818	1395 ± 694	942 ± 739	245 ± 291
17-OH-Pro (ng/dl)	651 ± 661	373 ± 317	169 ± 95	36 ± 13*
11-deoxycortisol (ng/dl)	662 ± 548	294 ± 239	111 ± 62	87 ± 42
DHEA (ng/dl)	1872 ± 4038	675 ± 502	920 ± 1227	286 ± 238
DHEAS (μg/dl)	467 ± 312	459 ± 209	341 ± 93	162 ± 88
Androstenedione (ng/dl)	479 ± 1032	206 ± 86	215 ± 134	149 ± 67

Data based on information in Lee MM, Rajabapalan L, Berg G, et al: Serum adrenal steroid concentrations in premature infants. *J Clin Endocrinol Metab* 69:1133–1136, 1989, and in Wiener D, Smith J, Dahlem S, et al: Serum adrenal steroid levels in healthy term 3-day-old infants. *J Pediatr* 110(1):122–124, 1987.

17-OH-Preg = 17-OH-pregnenolone; 17-OH-Pro = 17-OH-progesterone; DHEA = dehydroepiandrosterone; DHEAS = dehydroepiandrosterone sulfate.

*17-OH-Pro values in full-term sick newborns may be double or triple the baseline values. No data are available for other steroid hormones in sick full-term infants.

TABLE 12.3. Serum Adrenal Steroid Levels in Infants 1-Hour Post-ACTH Administration

Steroid	Preterm Sick (24–28 weeks)	Well Infants (2–12 months)* Female	Well Infants (2–12 months)* Male
Cortisol (μg/dl)	18.3 ± 6.8	40 ± 8.1	38.2 ± 4.4
17-OH-Preg (ng/dl)	5730 ± 4461	1610 ± 800	1242 ± 753
17-OH-Pro (ng/dl)	968 ± 876	142 ± 50	196 ± 85

Data based on information in Hingre RV, Gross SJ, Hingre KS, et al: Adrenal steroidogenesis in very low birth weight preterm infants. *J Clin Endocrinol Metab* 78(2): 266–270, 1994, and in Lashansky G, Saenger P, Fishman K, et al: Normative data for adrenal steroidogenesis in a healthy pediatric population: age- and sex-related changes after adrenocorticotropin stimulation. *J Clin Endocrinol Metab* 73:674–686, 1991.

ACTH = adrenocorticotropic hormone; 17-OH-Preg = 17-OH-pregnenolone; 17-OH-Pro = 17-OH-progesterone.

* No post-ACTH steroid data are available for full-term newborns.

▼ **Other androgen synthesis defects.** 17-Ketosteroid reductase deficiency in the testes prevents the conversion of androstenedione to testosterone. 17-Lyase is necessary for the conversion of C21 steroids to C19 androgenic steroids in the testes. 5α-Reductase deficiency prevents conversion of testosterone to DHT, which is necessary for the development of the male external genitalia.

▼ **Syndromes of androgen resistance** result from abnormalities in the androgen receptors or post-receptor defects. Testicular feminization is the classic

X-linked androgen resistance syndrome. Affected patients have normal female external genitalia with absent wolffian and müllerian structures.

Clinical Features

Patients with male pseudohermaphroditism may show micropenis, hypospadias, a poorly developed scrotum, or undescended testes. Alternatively, a normal female phenotype may be present.

▼ **CAH.** Patients with 3β-hydroxysteroid dehydrogenase deficiency or cholesterol desmolase deficiency exhibit severe salt wasting in addition to ambiguity of the external genitalia. 17α-Hydroxylase–deficient individuals may be hypertensive because this disorder also results in increased mineralocorticoid production.

▼ **Other androgen synthesis defects.** Individuals with 17-ketosteroid reductase deficiency and 17-lyase deficiency have variable degrees of undervirilization. Patients with 5α-reductase deficiency have a blind vaginal pouch, small phallic structure, and severe hypospadias; some infants are assigned a female sex at birth. Because the testis produces both MIS and testosterone, regression of the müllerian ducts and normal development of wolffian structures occur. With increasing testosterone concentrations at puberty, individuals develop penile enlargement, testicular descent of inguinal testes into the labial scrotal folds, and secondary sexual characteristics (e.g., pubic hair, increased muscle mass).

▼ **Syndromes of androgen resistance.** Patients with incomplete forms of androgen resistance often present with sexual ambiguity, whereas individuals with complete androgen resistance appear phenotypically female. A blind vaginal pouch (caused by MIS secretion by the testes) is present. Testes may be located in the abdomen, inguinal canal, or in an inguinal hernia. There is no virilization at puberty, and breasts develop as the result of peripheral conversion of high levels of testosterone to estradiol. Most affected patients develop little or no pubic hair.

Evaluation

▼ **CAH.** The diagnosis can be made by measuring elevated steroids in the serum at baseline and after ACTH stimulation (see Tables 12.1 through 12.3).

▼ **17-Ketosteroid reductase deficiency** can be diagnosed by an abnormal ratio of androstenedione to testosterone, either at baseline or after stimulation with HCG.

▼ **17-Lyase deficiency** is suggested by low androgen levels and increased gonadotropin levels.

▼ **5α-Reductase deficiency.** The testosterone:DHT ratio is normally less than 16 basally and following HCG stimulation; a ratio greater than 30 suggests the diagnosis of 5α-reductase deficiency. The diagnosis is confirmed by finding reduced 5α-reductase activity in fibroblasts in genital skin samples.

▼ **Syndromes of androgen resistance.** Patients have an XY karyotype, no müllerian structures, and elevated testosterone and LH levels in the newborn period.

Treatment

Patients with CAH should receive cortisol and mineralocorticoid replacement as needed. Cosmetic surgical repair may be necessary.

Other Defects in Male External Genital Development

Hypospadias may be a finding in various intersex disorders. Although isolated first-degree hypospadias is usually not associated with endocrine abnormalities, the incidence of associated intersex disorders increases as the severity of the hypospadias increases, and with the presence of bilateral undescended testes. **Micropenis** may occur with congenital hypopituitarism, isolated gonadotropin deficiency (Kallman syndrome), testicular dysfunction, or partial androgen resistance.

▼ EVALUATION OF AMBIGUOUS GENITALIA

Patient History

The following information should be sought:

▼ A careful maternal obstetric history that focuses on drug ingestion and exposure to teratogens or infections during the pregnancy, particularly during the first trimester
▼ A careful family history, focusing on any androgenic changes in the mother or anything suggestive of CAH in other family members (e.g., neonatal death, virilization, or precocious adrenarche)

Physical Examination

The following information needs to be noted:

▼ Palpable gonads, which imply the presence of Y chromosome material
▼ The length and diameter of the penis (Table 12.4) and the position of the urethra
▼ The existence of a vagina, the degree of fusion of the labia, and the length of the clitoris (Table 12.4)
▼ Other dysmorphic features, especially those involving the urinary tract and anus

TABLE 12.4. Penile and Clitoral Length in the Newborn Infant

	Gestational Age	Length
Males*		
	30 weeks	2.5 ± 0.4 centimeters
	34 weeks	3.0 ± 0.4 centimeters
	Term	3.5 ± 0.4 centimeters
Females†		
	Term‡	4.0 ± 1.24 millimeters

Data based on information in Feldman KW, Smith DW: Fetal phallic growth and penile standards for newborn male infants. *J Pediatr* 86:395, 1975, and in Oberfield S, Mondok A, Shanrivar F, et al: Clitoral size in full-term infants. *Am J Perinatol* 6(4):453, 1989.

* Measure from the pubic ramus to the tip of the glans with gentle pressure applied.

† Measure with the labia majora separated and the prepuce skin retracted.

‡ The clitoris achieves full size by 27 weeks' gestation and may appear more prominent in premature infants relative to the labia.

TABLE 12.5. Normal Laboratory Values for Serum Testosterone and Dihydrotestosterone (DHT)

	Testosterone (ng/dl)		DHT (ng/dl)	
	Male	Female	Male	Female
Cord blood	13–55	5–45	< 2–8	< 2–8
26–28 weeks' gestation	59–125	5–16	. . .	. . .
31–35 weeks' gestation	37–198	5–22	10–53	2–13
Full term	75–400*	20–64†	5–60‡	< 2–15§

Data provided by the Esoterix Endocrinology Laboratory, Los Calabasas Hills, California.

* Levels decrease to 20–50 ng/dl during week 1, and then increase to 60–400 ng/dl at 20–60 days. Levels decrease to prepubertal values by 7 months.

† Levels decrease to < 10 ng/dl during the first month and remain at that level until puberty.

‡ Levels decrease during week 1, and then increase to 12–85 ng/dl by 30–60 days. Levels decrease to prepubertal values by 7 months.

§ Levels decrease to < 3 ng/dl during the first month and remain at that level until puberty.

Laboratory Studies

▼ **Karyotyping.** Blood and bone marrow samples should be submitted for karyotyping. Some laboratories can have a karyotype result from a bone marrow specimen available within 6 hours. A standard chromosome analysis should be performed as well because bone marrow karyotyping can miss mosaicism.

▼ **Serum levels** of **17-hydroxyprogesterone, 17-hydroxypregnenolone, dehydroepiandrosterone, testosterone, DHT, 11-deoxycortisol,** and **androstenedione** should be obtained. Normal values for serum testosterone and DHT are given in Table 12.5. Recall that adrenal steroid levels are elevated in premature infants, particularly when the child is ill and under stress (see Tables 12.2 and 12.3).

▼ **Serum levels** of **luteinizing hormone (LH)** and **maternal androgens** may be appropriate to obtain.

▼ **Biopsy samples.** A gonadal biopsy or skin biopsy to evaluate testosterone metabolism may be indicated.

Diagnostic Imaging Studies

▼ **Pelvic ultrasound** can demonstrate a uterus and gonads.

▼ **Vaginogram.** The injection of contrast dye into urethral or vaginal openings will demonstrate müllerian ducts (if any are present). The absence of a müllerian system implies functioning testicular tissue early in gestation and the secretion of MIS.

▼ **Radiologic studies,** such as intravenous pyelography (IVP), bone age, or a barium enema, may be indicated.

▼ APPROACH TO THE PATIENT (FIGURE 12.1)

Ambiguous genitalia in the neonate should be treated as a **medical emergency** and the diagnostic evaluation undertaken as soon as possible. A team

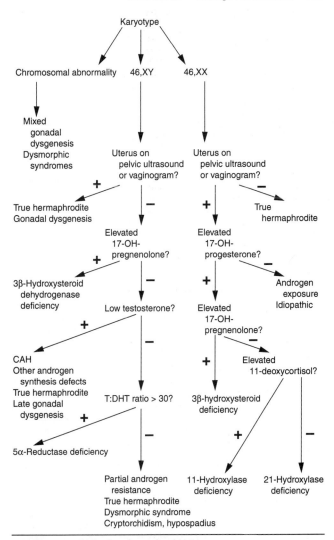

FIGURE 12.1. Evaluation of sexual ambiguity.
T:DHT ratio = testosterone:dihydrotestosterone ratio.

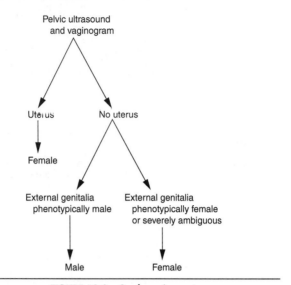

FIGURE 12.2. Gender assignment.

approach with consultations from endocrinology, urology, and psychiatry is useful.

Often, it is advisable for parents to delay naming or announcing the birth of their child until the definitive gender is assigned. The parents should be informed that the definitive gender will be determined within 48–72 hours. **Gender assignment** usually can be made on the basis of the physical examination, karyotype, and internal pelvic structures while awaiting the results of serum studies; however, karyotype should not be the major factor in gender determination because gonadal function and future sexual function are more important. In addition, the size of the phallus and the degree of hypospadias need to be considered (Figure 12.2). For families known to carry CAH mutations, prenatal diagnosis and treatment may help to reduce virilization of the female fetus.

☝ HINT Females with CAH, even when severely virilized, should be raised as females because cosmetic repair can be managed surgically, and patients have good future potential for sexual function and reproduction.

Suggested Readings

Carlson AD, Obeid JS, Kanellopoulou N, Wilson RC, New MI: Congenital adrenal hyperplasia: update on prenatal diagnosis and treatment. *J Steroid Biochem Mol Bio* 69(1-16):19–29, 1999.

Coran AG, Polley TZ: Surgical management of ambiguous genitalia in the infant and child. *J Pediatr Surg* 26:812–820, 1991.

White PC, Speiser PW: Congenital Adrenal Hyperplasia due to 21-Hydroxylase Deficiency. *Endocrine Reviews* 21(3):245–291, 2000.

Vaiman D, Pailhoux E: Mammalian sex reversal and intersexuality: deciphering the sex-determination cascade. *Trends in Genetics* 16 (11):488–94, 2000.

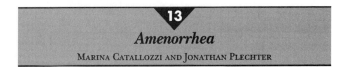

13
Amenorrhea
MARINA CATALLOZZI AND JONATHAN PLECHTER

▼ INTRODUCTION

Amenorrhea is defined as the **absence of menses** and is common during adolescence. Determining the underlying cause of amenorrhea necessitates an understanding of the normal menstrual cycle. Although the broad differential diagnosis includes genetic, endocrine, structural, environmental, and psychological disorders, **pregnancy should always be considered.** Evaluation should begin soon after amenorrhea is noted because underlying pathological conditions can cause tremendous physical and emotional sequelae.

Menarche, a pivotal event of puberty, requires intact and functioning interactions between the hypothalamus, pituitary, ovaries, and uterine endometrial lining. Successful menstrual cycles also require the presence of an unobstructed uterus, cervix, and vagina. The body must have an adequate amount of fat and not be under any extremes of stress (e.g., extreme exercise, emotional stress). Normal cycles indicate the presence of ovulation. **Menarche is one of the latest signs of puberty in females,** occurring at Tanner stage (or sexual maturity rating) IV in the majority of adolescents. Menarche generally occurs 2–2.5 years after thelarche and 1 year after the growth spurt. In the United States, 12.8 years is the average age of menarche for white females (the range is 9–16 years, and the average age is slightly lower for black females). Race, nutritional status, body fat, and maternal age at menarche all influence an individual's age of menarche. Ovulation can be delayed for as long as 2 years after menarche. Normal menstrual cycles have 21- to 45-day cycles (depending on the individual), have flow lasting 2–7 days, and have an average blood loss of between 30 and 40 ml.

⚕ HINT Although the arbitrary age of primary amenorrhea is 16.5 years, if a girl 14 years or older presents with absence of breast budding, diagnostic evaluation should be performed immediately, because it is unlikely that she will menstruate within the next 2 years.

The menstrual cycle begins with pulsatile release of gonadotropin-releasing hormone from the hypothalamus, causing secretion of follicle-stimulating hormone (FSH) and luteinizing hormone (LH) from the pituitary. Ovarian follicles grow and develop under the influence of FSH. Theca cells produce androgens that are converted to estrogen by granulosa cells. This increased estrogen not only inhibits the pituitary release of FSH, causing follicles to involute, but it also stimulates breast budding, uterine development, and endometrial growth. In the first part of the cycle, increased estrogen leads to decreased FSH release. Midcycle, FSH results in LH surge and ovulation. In **early adolescence,** although estrogen levels are high, the feedback patterns are not mature, and **menses are anovulatory,** representing sloughing of a proliferative endometrium rather than shedding secondary to the luteal phase of an ovulatory cycle.

Primary amenorrhea is the **absence of menarche (with normal pubertal development) by 16 years of age, 14 years** of age **(without normal pubertal development),** or **2 years after completion** of **sexual maturation. Secondary amenorrhea** is the **absence of menstruation for three cycle lengths** (usually between 6 and 12 months, depending on whether the patient was oligomenorrheic). Although primary and secondary amenorrhea are helpful in describing menstrual cycle interruption in terms of timing, the terms do not indicate an underlying cause or offer information about treatment or prognosis. Although the differential diagnosis of amenorrhea can be presented on the basis of timing, since several of the processes that cause amenorrhea can present as primary or secondary, the evaluation and diagnostic strategy is based on pubertal physiology and sexual development.

▼ DIFFERENTIAL DIAGNOSIS LIST

Amenorrhea with Delayed Puberty

Constitutional delay

Hypergonadotropic hypogonadism—Turner syndrome (45XO), pure gonadal dysgenesis, autoimmune oophoritis, Addison disease, medications, tuberculosis

Hypogonadotropic hypogonadism—Kallmann syndrome, chronic illness, weight loss, exercise, stress, marijuana use

Endocrine—thyroid disease, diabetes, hyperprolactinemia

Anorexia nervosa

Hypothalamic or pituitary disorders—pituitary adenoma, head trauma

Genital tract anomalies—androgen insensitivity or testicular feminization, congenital absence of the uterus, obstruction of the outflow tract

Amenorrhea with Normal Puberty

Pregnancy

Lactation

Menopause

Hyperandrogenism—polycystic ovarian syndrome, late-onset congenital adrenal hyperplasia, Cushing disease, ovarian or adrenal tumors, hyperthecosis (hypertrophy of ovarian stroma)

Immaturity of the hypothalamic–pituitary–ovarian axis (anovulatory cycles)

Hyperprolactinemia—lactation, pituitary tumor, renal failure, psychoactive drugs (e.g., Haldol–renal failure)

Thyroid disease

Anorexia nervosa

▼ DIFFERENTIAL DIAGNOSIS DISCUSSION

🏋 HINT Pregnancy is the most common cause of secondary amenorrhea in women of reproductive age, and this possibility should always be ruled out first.

Hypergonadotrophic Hypogonadism

Etiology

Gonadal failure (i.e., **lack of ovarian estrogen production**) is the **most common cause of primary amenorrhea,** accounting for almost 50% of cases. It is usually caused by a **chromosomal disorder or deletion of all or part** of an **X chromosome.** The chromosomal disorders that cause gonadal failure are usually the result of a **random** meiotic or mitotic **abnormality** (i.e., they are not inherited). If the chromosomes are normal [46,XX or 46,XY (pure gonadal dysgenesis)], a gene disorder may be the cause of the primary amenorrhea. Because two X chromosomes are necessary for normal ovarian development, patients with **Turner syndrome** (45,X), **mosaicism** involving an X chromosome, **or an abnormal X chromosome** may develop **streak ovaries,** which are masses of fibrous tissue located in the normal anatomic position of the ovary. These streak ovaries **do not produce estrogen;** therefore, estrogen-induced negative feedback inhibition of the hypothalamic–pituitary axis fails to occur.

Evaluation

An **FSH level greater than 40 mIU/ml** suggests a lack of functioning ovarian follicles, confirming the diagnosis of gonadal failure.

Hypothalamus:Pituitary Disorders

Etiology

Patients with **normal female internal genitalia** but **absent secondary sex characteristics** as a result of a central nervous system (CNS)–hypothalamus–pituitary disorder have **low levels of estrogen** and **gonadotropin.** Any **anatomic lesion** of the hypothalamus or pituitary gland can cause low gonadotropin production. These lesions can be **congenital** (e.g., aqueductal stenosis or absence of the sellar floor) or **acquired** (e.g., tumors). The most common tumors are **pituitary adenomas,** which result in **elevated levels of prolactin.** (Most, but not all, pituitary tumors secrete prolactin; chromophobe adenomas are the most common non–prolactin-secreting pituitary tumors.)

Evaluation

Patients with suspected CNS–hypothalamic–pituitary disorders should undergo **computed tomography** or **magnetic resonance imaging** of the hypothalamic–pituitary region to rule out the presence of a lesion. Pituitary adenoma can be detected by finding an elevated **serum prolactin level.**

Congenital Absence of the Uterus

Etiology

Congenital absence of the uterus (uterine agenesis, uterovaginal agenesis, Rokitansky-Kuster-Hauser syndrome) is the **second most common cause of**

primary amenorrhea, after gonadal failure. **Congenital** absence of the uterus accounts for approximately 15% of cases of primary amenorrhea, and occurs in 1 of every 4000–5000 female births. Congenital absence of the uterus is an accident of development and is only rarely genetically inherited. Patients have no underlying endocrine abnormality, but are amenorrheic because of absence of the end organ.

Clinical Features

Patients have normal breasts and pubic and axillary hair, but the **vagina is shortened or absent** and the **uterus is absent.** The ovaries are present and function normally, with ovulation occurring cyclically. Approximately 33% of patients with congenital absence of the uterus have **congenital renal abnormalities,** and 12% have **skeletal abnormalities. Cardiac and other congenital abnormalities** occur with increased frequency.

Androgen Insensitivity (Testicular Feminization)

Etiology

Androgen insensitivity is a syndrome caused by the **absence of a gene on the X chromosome** for the testosterone receptor. It is inherited in an **X-linked recessive** or sex-limited autosomal dominant fashion with transmission **through the mother.** Patients are **genetically normal males** with a 46,XY karyotype and normally functioning testes that produce normal male levels of testosterone and dihydrotestosterone. Because there are no testosterone receptors, there is **no development of external or internal male genitalia.** In the absence of sex steroids, **female development** occurs. The fetal testes produce müllerian-inhibiting substance, which causes müllerian-duct regression (explaining the absence of the uterus).

Clinical Features

Patients have **normal female external genitalia** and a **short or absent vagina. Pubic and axillary hair is absent or scanty** because of the lack of androgen receptors, but **breast development is normal or excessive** because there is no androgenic opposition to the small amounts of estrogen produced by the testes and adrenals. The **gonads** in these patients are **abnormal,** and 20% develop a **malignancy** (gonadoblastoma or dysgerminoma).

✄ HINT Patients with testicular feminization can be differentiated from patients with uterine agenesis by the absence of normal pubic hair.

Treatment

Patients with testicular feminization are **phenotypically female** and have been raised as such. They should be told that they are **sterile** because of a missing piece of the X chromosome, and that the **gonads must be removed** because they are at risk of developing a malignancy. These malignancies rarely occur before age 20 years; therefore, it is recommended that the gonads be left in place until after puberty to allow normal sexual maturity.

▼ EVALUATION OF AMENORRHEA
Patient History

Delayed or absent menstruation can be very anxiety provoking. Be sensitive to the parent and adolescent's level of concern during the history. Review of growth and development, detailed menstrual history (e.g., menarche, dysmenorrhea, duration, and flow), history of illnesses, and medications can all be discussed with the patient and parent. To obtain accurate information, the **sexual history, psychosocial assessment,** and **substance use** history should be **obtained privately with the patient.** Questions regarding diet, physical activity (duration and intensity), weight change and body image can give an indication if there is an eating disorder. Review of symptoms should focus on:

▼ New-onset virilizing symptoms
▼ Vasomotor symptoms (associated with low circulating estrogens)
▼ Galactorrhea (hyperprolactinemia)
▼ Cyclic pain, bloating or breast changes (vaginal outlet obstruction)
▼ Palpitations, fatigue, or nervousness (hyperthyroidism)

Physical Examination

Height, weight, body habitus, and vital signs (**hypertension** may indicate some of the causes of hyperandrogenicity such as Cushing disease) should be measured. Signs of **anorexia nervosa** include bradycardia, hypotension, and hypothermia. Thorough funduscopic and neurologic exam can help to rule out **pituitary or other CNS lesions.** Other areas of focus should include the **thyroid,** the **breasts** (for Tanner staging and galactorrhea), and the **genital area** (Tanner stage and hyperandrogenism, virilization, consider pelvic exam to rule out ovarian mass). **Pelvic exam** is not necessary if the patient has never

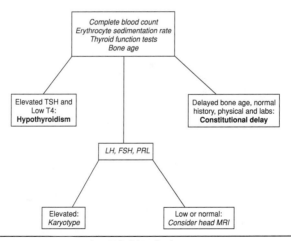

FIGURE 13.1. Amenorrhea with delayed puberty.
(Modified from Pletcher JB, Slap GB: Menstrual disorders. Amenorrhea. *Pediatr Clin North Am* June;46(3):505–518, 1999.)

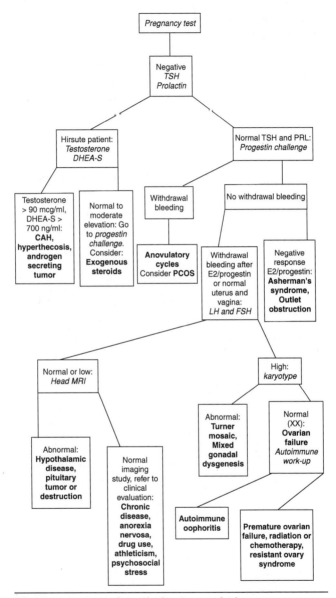

FIGURE 13.2. Amenorrhea with otherwise normal puberty.
(Modified from Pletcher JB, Slap GB: Menstrual disorders. Amenorrhea. *Pediatr Clin North Am* June;46(3):505–518, 1999.)

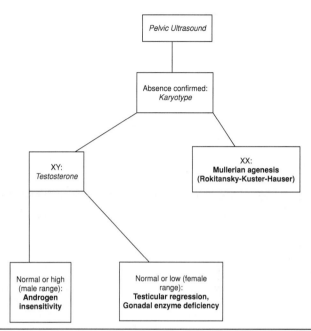

FIGURE 13.3. Genital tract anomalies.
(Modified from Pletcher JB, Slap GB: Menstrual disorders. Amenorrhea. *Pediatr Clin North Am* June;46(3):505–518, 1999.)

been sexually active and genital anomalies are not suspected. Otherwise, pelvic exam can help to evaluate for imperforate hymen and the presence of uterus and ovaries. Laboratory work-up is dependent on the pubertal development. See Figures 13.1 through 13.3 for step-wise work-up.

▼ TREATMENT OF AMENORRHEA

Apart from specific therapies with regard to the diagnoses listed in the differential diagnosis list, the principles behind management of amenorrhea are the same regardless of the etiology:

1. Restore ovulatory cycles to ensure good long-term prognosis.
2. If ovulatory cycles do not occur spontaneously, estrogen–progestin therapy is indicated.
3. Reassure the patient and parent.
4. Re-evaluate frequently.

Suggested Readings

Folch M, Pigem I, Konje JC: Mullerian agenesis: etiology, diagnosis, and management. *Obstet Gynecol Surv* 55(10):644–649, 2000.

Golden NH, Jacobson MS, Schebendach J et al: Resumption of menses in anorexia nervosa. *Arch Pediatr Adolesc Med* 151(1):16–21, 1997.

McIver B, Romanski SA, Nipploldt TB: Evaluation and management of amenorrhea. *Mayo Clin Proc* 72(12):1161–1169, 1997.

Mishell DR: Primary and secondary amenorrhea: etiology, diagnostic evaluation and management. In *Comprehensive Gynecology*, 3rd ed. Edited by Mishell DR, Stenchever MA, Droegemueller W, et al. St. Louis, Mosby-Year Book, 1997.

Pletcher JR, Slap GB: Menstrual disorders. Amenorrhea. *Pediatr Clin North Am* 46(3):505–518, 1999.

Speroff L, Glass RH, Kase NG: Amenorrhea. In *Clinical Gynecologic Endocrinology and Infertility*, 5th ed. Edited by Speroff L, Glass RH, Kase NG. Baltimore, Williams & Wilkins, 1994.

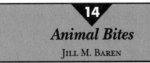

14
Animal Bites
JILL M. BAREN

▼ INTRODUCTION

Humans have contact with animals in a variety of occupational and recreational settings, and over half of households in the United States have at least one pet. **Animal and human bite wounds are frequent** in the pediatric population and are seen in primary care offices and emergency departments. As a result, all pediatric practitioners should become familiar with evaluation and management of the most common animal bite wounds. The complex microbiology of animal bite wounds makes management a challenging clinical problem, and therapy is often empiric.

▼ DIFFERENTIAL DIAGNOSIS LIST

Local bacterial wound infection—mouth flora vary by species (Table 14.1)
Rabies—many animals, especially dogs, cats, bats, foxes, raccoons, skunks
Tularemia—many animals, especially rabbits, cats, squirrels, pigs, sheep, coyotes, ticks
Rat-bite fever
Cat-scratch disease (CSD)
Herpes B virus—monkeys
Leptospirosis—rodents, dogs, livestock

▼ DIFFERENTIAL DIAGNOSIS DISCUSSION
Dog and Cat Bites

Dog and cat bites make up the **majority of bite wounds.** Because of their inquisitive nature, children are bitten by dogs and cats more frequently than adults, with most bites occurring in the 5–9-year-old age group. Their size relative to an animal causes children to sustain **more facial bites,** resulting in greater severity of **laceration, infection, disability,** and **death,** especially when large dogs are involved. **Cat bite wounds** are typically **puncture wounds** that involve the hand or extremity. Because of the sharp and slender nature of cat teeth, they are able to **penetrate bones,** which may lead to greater morbidity from complicated wounds.

TABLE 14.1. Organisms Commonly Associated with Bite Wounds

Animal	Organism	Special Considerations
Dog and cat	*Pasteurella multocida* *Streptococcus* species *Staphylococcus aureus* *Neisseria* species *Eikenella* *Capnocytophage canimorsus* (dogs) Anaerobes: *Bacteroides, Fusobacterium*	Rabies prophylaxis based on immunization status, ability to observe animal, local epidemiology
Horse	Similar to dog and cat	Crush injury, osteomyelitis
Pig and sheep	Dog and cat flora + *Francisella tularensis* and others	
Rat	Dog and cat flora + *Streptobacillus moniliformis, Leptospira*	Rabies prophylaxis generally not needed
Ferret and gerbil	Rat flora + *Acinetobacter anitratus*	Antipseudomonal penicillin
Raccoon, bat, fox	High risk for rabies	RIG, HDCV
Squirrel	*Francisella tularensis*	Gentamicin
Aquatic	*Aeromonas hydrophila, Vibrio, Enterobacter, Pseudomonas*	
Avian	*Staphylococcus, Clostridium, Aspergillus, Bacteroides, Pseudomonas*	
Human	Many aerobic and anaerobic bacteria, especially *Streptomyces, Staphylococcus, Eikenella corrodens, Corynebacterium, Bacteroides, Clostridium*	Hand injuries high risk
Monkey	Human flora + *Herpes B*	Antiviral therapy

This table is not an exhaustive list of organisms.
HDCV = human diploid cell vaccine; RIG = rabies immune globulin.

Dog bites have an infection rate of approximately 5%–15%, the lowest of all mammalian bites. **Cat bites become infected more frequently** (20%–50%). Wound characteristics often determine the risk of infection. Puncture wounds, wounds on the hands or feet, those involving joints, tendons, or other deep structures and those in hosts with comorbid illness or immunosuppression are at higher risk for infection. The microbiology of infected dog and cat bite wounds has been well studied (see Table 14.1). Most bite wound infections are **polymicrobial** with an average of three to five isolates per bite wound.

Humans Bites

Following dog and cat bites, **human bites** are the **next most common** types of mammalian bite injuries. Human bites are most commonly seen in **teenage or young adult males** and are often related to **aggressive behavior, sports,** and **sexual activity. Wound infections** occur in about 10% of human bites although up to 50% of bites to the hand may become infected. **Delays in care,** which are common as a result of the circumstances of injury, **have a direct effect on infection rates and prognosis. Simple bites** that occur from occlusion of the teeth on skin, such as bites occurring in daycare, **rarely become infected.** Human bite infections are **polymicrobial** with a mixture of anaerobes and aerobes (see Table 14.1). *Eikenella corrodens* deserves special mention, as it is present in 25% of isolates from clenched fist injuries. It has also exhibited synergistic growth with other aerobic organisms.

⚡ HINT When a bite occurs as the result of a direct blow of the victim's hand into the biter's mouth, there is typically a puncture wound overlying one of the metacarpal–phalangeal joints on the dorsum of the hand (clenched-fist syndrome). Penetration of the joint capsule may occur with tendon, nerve, or bone damage. These wounds may appear mild at first, but are deceiving and can result in extensive infection that requires surgical exploration, debridement, and intravenous antibiotics.

Other significant infectious diseases like *Herpes* virus, syphilis, tuberculosis, actinomycosis, tetanus, and hepatitis B and C have also been documented as occurring through human bites. Although there have been no definitive cases of HIV transmission from this route, detection of HIV in saliva makes this an unlikely but possible way to acquire HIV infection.

Complications

Local Wound Infection

Characteristics of infected bite wounds include **erythema, warmth, fluctuance, purulent drainage,** and **tenderness** at the site, with **surrounding edema** and **regional adenitis.** Local wound infections can also be accompanied by **mild systemic symptoms** such as **fever, chills,** and **malaise,** and may be associated with **serum leukocytosis.**

Various clinical syndromes may help to differentiate the type of organism that predominates in a bite-wound infection. Infection caused by *Pasteurella* species may evolve rapidly with intense cellulitis and lymphangitis within 24 hours. Cellulitis due to *Staphylococcus* or *Streptomyces* species usually evolves more slowly. *Pasteurella* may also cause more **serious infections** such as **osteomyelitis** or **septic arthritis** after direct inoculation into deeper tissues or by localized extension of cellulitis. **Immunocompromised hosts** can present with local or systemic infections and are at **higher risk for invasive disease** with *Pasteurella.*

Rabies

Individuals often seek medical care after an animal bite wound because of the concern for rabies. In the United States there are only about one to three documented cases per year, and **rabies prophylaxis recommendations vary by the geographic area and the type of animal** involved. Large metropolitan areas have had long periods without report of rabies from a domesticated animal. In other parts of the United States, bats, skunks, and foxes serve as the primary reservoirs of rabies, and bats are responsible for the majority of cases. When traveling outside the US in areas like Mexico, dog rabies is much more common. There are approximately 35,000 cases worldwide annually. Rabies is caused by a *Lyssavirus* and is **transmitted via the saliva of an infected animal through a bite or scratch.**

⚴ HINT   Many rabies cases do not have a definitive history of contact with any animal, and not all rabid animals will foam at the mouth or behave aggressively. Therefore, rabies infection should be considered in any individual who presents with signs and symptoms of rapidly progressive encephalitis.

The clinical syndrome of rabies is characterized by **fever, malaise, headache,** and **anxiety** in the early stages. This is followed by **progressive neurologic symptoms** including muscle spasm, autonomic instability, altered mental status with hallucinations, respiratory muscle paralysis, lacrimation, salivation, perspiration, and coma. Infection can be confirmed with **specific serologic testing.** Despite supportive care, rabies is **usually fatal** as there is no known effective treatment.

Tularemia

Tularemia, caused by infection with *Francisella tularensis*, is primarily a **tick-borne disease** but may be transmitted by **bites from animals** such as rabbits, cats, squirrels, pigs, sheep, and coyotes. The clinical syndrome is characterized by an **abrupt onset of fever, chills, headache, anorexia, malaise,** and **fatigue. Cough** and **gastrointestinal symptoms** may also occur. At the site of the bite there may be a **tender ulcer** associated with **tender local adenopathy.** The diagnosis can be confirmed with **serologic testing,** and treatment is usually with **streptomycin or gentamicin.**

Rat-Bite Fever

Rat-bite fever is caused by *Streptobacillus moniliformis*. The organism is found in the oral flora of **wild, pet, and laboratory rats** and is transmitted by **bites, scratches, and handling dead rats.** There is a 3–10-day incubation period after exposure, followed by **acute onset of fever, chills, headache, myalgias,** and **maculopapular rash,** which often involves the **palms** and **soles.** The rash may take on other forms such as petechiae, purpura, vesicles, or desquamation. There also may be associated **septic polyarthritis,** and more rarely endocarditis, pericarditis, and brain abscess.

The organism can be **cultured from blood, synovial fluid,** and **vesicle fluid,** and the receiving laboratory should be informed that *Streptobacillus moniliformis* is the organism of interest. *Streptobacillus* is **sensitive to penicillin,** and therapy should be initiated with this drug. Alternative drugs are ampicillin, cefuroxime, cefotaxime, and doxycycline. **Recovery is excellent.**

Cat-Scratch Disease

Cat-scratch disease (CSD) is caused by *Bartonella henselae,* a rickettsia-like organism. It is transmitted primarily to individuals who have close contact with a cat via **bites, scratches, ticks,** and **cat flea bites.**

Patients with uncomplicated CSD will develop a **nontender papule** at the site of inoculation followed by **regional lymphadenopathy** that **persists for weeks to months.** The most common involved nodes are axillary, cervical, submandibular, and inguinal. Nodes may suppurate and be accompanied by symptoms such as **fever, malaise, anorexia,** and **headache.** Complicated CSD is more common in **immunosuppressed patients** and may cause **neurologic symptoms** such as encephalopathy, peripheral neuropathy, or vision loss, as well as **pneumonia, endocarditis,** and **osteomyelitis.**

Many cases of CSD **resolve spontaneously** without specific therapy, but all of the following **antimicrobials** have been noted to produce a clinical response: rifampin, ciprofloxacin, gentamicin, and trimethoprim/sulfamethoxazole. **Macrolides** have also recently been used with success in **AIDS patients with CSD. Routine antimicrobial treatment is not recommended** for otherwise healthy individuals with regional lymphadenitis. When nodes become painful and fluctuant, aspiration may provide symptomatic relief.

▼ EVALUATION OF ANIMAL BITES

Patient History

Unstable patients should be **evaluated immediately for massive blood loss and wounds that interfere with a patent airway** (tracheal or laryngeal location) **or breathing** (pneumothorax). Important facts to elicit when taking a history from a bitten individual include **type of animal, provoking factors** for the bite, **allergies, medications,** and **comorbid conditions,** especially those associated with immune suppression. Obtain a history of **tetanus immunization** as well as any previous bites or rabies immunizations.

Physical Examination

The following items should be noted during examination of a bite wound:

▼ Body location,
▼ Depth of the wound,
▼ Range of motion of the affected part
▼ Type of wound—puncture, crush, laceration, abrasion
▼ Involvement of deeper structures—tendon, nerve, vessel, bone
▼ Function of tendons and nerves
▼ Signs of inflammation or infection—edema, erythema, odor, exudates, foreign debris

The **physical examination** may need to take place **after local anesthesia** to maximize the ability to explore the wound. **Photographs or diagrammatic drawings** of wounds are helpful.

Imaging

When **fractures** or **foreign bodies** such as tooth fragments are suspected, a radiograph should be obtained.

Laboratory Evaluation

Routine wound cultures are not needed for animal or human bites that do not have any signs of infection. As a general rule, most bite wounds at this point will be more likely to reflect the indigenous flora of the animal's mouth and are not predictive of future infection. **Older wounds** or those with **evidence of infection** should be cultured for both **aerobic and anaerobic organisms** after superficial crusts are removed. It is imperative to **notify the laboratory of the source of a bite wound culture** and of any suspected organisms.

▼ TREATMENT OF ANIMAL BITES

Wound Management

Experts advocate **copious irrigation** of bite wounds as well as **surface cleaning.** The fluid of choice is **normal saline** (1% povidone–iodine may be added) using a volume of at least 250 ml. Irrigation should be performed **under pressure** with an 18- or 19-gauge catheter attached to a syringe, and **devitalized tissue should be débrided. Puncture and other small wounds should never be injected** as this may inoculate bacteria into deeper structures, increasing tissue trauma and the risk of infection.

The decision to primarily suture a bite wound is made on a case-by-case basis and depends on many factors including the length of time between the bite and presentation, the location of the wound, the appearance of the wound and comorbidities of the patient. Studies have suggested that carefully selected bite wounds are safe for primary closure. **Wounds that are candidates for primary closure** are those to the **head and face** and wounds in other **low-risk areas** such as the proximal extremities and the trunk.

It is generally agreed that all **bites older than 24 hours, bites to the hand, and bites with evidence of infection should not be sutured.** Wounds that are **high risk** should have **delayed primary closure** 72 hours after antimicrobial prophylaxis has begun. Aftercare should consist of explicit **instructions for wound cleansing, dressing changes, and antibiotic use** (topical or oral as indicated), as well as **signs and symptoms of possible infection. Large wounds or those over joint surfaces** should be **splinted and elevated.** Appropriate **analgesics** should be prescribed for several days. **Close follow-up** should be arranged for all bite wounds.

Anti-microbial Prophylaxis

Prophylactic antimicrobial therapy is generally recommended for the following:

▼ All human bites
▼ Most cat bites
▼ Bites presenting 8 hours or more after injury
▼ All bites to the hand
▼ Deep puncture wounds
▼ Wounds with moderate-to-severe tissue destruction (crush)
▼ Facial wounds
▼ Wounds to patients with comorbid conditions or immunosuppression.

Duration of therapy should be 3–5 days. **Amoxicillin–clavulanate** is the drug of choice for prophylaxis of an animal bite wound, with an appropriate spectrum of activity against common flora in the mouths of dogs, cats, and humans. Alternatives for penicillin-allergic patients are few. Erythromycin is inadequate empiric therapy, because it has poor activity against both *Pasteurella* and *Eikenella* species. The newer macrolides have only slightly better activity against *Pasteurella* and moderately increased activity against *Eikenella*. Postpubertal, nonpregnant patients may receive **doxycycline** or **tetracycline; clindamycin plus trimethoprim/sulfa** is the most reasonable choice in penicillin-allergic patients who are too young for these agents.

Antimicrobial Treatment for Infected Wounds

Infected wounds that have **failed outpatient therapy** require **hospitalization.** *Pasteurella multocida* should be considered in any patient with a wound infection **following a dog or cat bite.** Ampicillin/sulbactam is appropriate empiric intravenous therapy. If *Pasteurella* has been definitively isolated, **penicillin** is the drug of choice. Alternatives for penicillin-allergic patients are **ciprofloxacin** or **tetracycline** if appropriate for age, and **selected cephalosporins** (cefpodoxime, cefuroxime).

Tetanus Prophylaxis

Tetanus immunization should be given according to standard Centers for Disease Control and Prevention (CDC) recommendations when patients are **deficient in immunization status** or in cases of **high-risk wounds.**

Rabies Prophylaxis

Prompt and thorough wound irrigation with soap or iodine solution is an important first step in preventing rabies. Immediate active and passive prophylaxis is indicated for wild animals known to carry rabies and domestic animals with symptoms of rabies; these **animals should be euthanized and the brain examined** in a qualified laboratory. Passive immunization with **rabies immune globulin (RIG)** in a dose of 20 IU/kg should be given as follows: **half of the dose at the site of the bite wound and the other half at a separate intramuscular location.** In **children** the recommended site is the **anterolateral thigh.** Active immunization with the **human diploid cell vaccine (HDCV)** must be initiated and **repeated on days 3,7,14, and 28** after the injury. The dose of the vaccine is 1.0 cc intramuscularly given at a site distant from the immune globulin. **Local inflammatory reactions** may occur and should respond to ice packs and analgesics. Occasionally **mild systemic responses** may also occur (myalgias, nausea) and are usually self-limited.

Domestic animals with an unknown rabies immune status may be **observed for 10 days.** RIG and HDCV should be initiated at the first sign of rabies symptoms in the animal. Cases in which the animal is unavailable should be treated as recommended by local health officials.

▼ **HINT** Animal bites should be reported to the local health department for surveillance as indicated by local jurisdiction. The risk of rabies differs geographically and appropriate treatment may vary. Reports to law enforcement agencies may also be necessary to facilitate observation of animals for rabies.

HIV Prophylaxis for Human Bites

The risk of HIV transmission from a human bite is controversial but **thought to be rare.** Bites from a **person known to be infected with HIV** or bites from a person in which there was **visibly blood-tainted saliva** should be **treated prophylactically** with **oral antiviral agents** according to standard CDC recommendations. In all other instances, postexposure prophylaxis should be determined on a case-by-case basis, but **baseline and 6-month HIV testing** of the victim is prudent. All human bite wounds should be **thoroughly cleansed with a virucidal agent** as soon as possible to lessen any risk of HIV transmission.

▼ PREVENTION OF ANIMAL BITES

Since bites frequently lead to infection, efforts to reduce the risk of infection should be aimed primarily at prevention. Adults, especially pet owners, should become familiar with the psychology of cats and dogs and teach children to avoid provoking behaviors. When handling other animals, appropriate precautions should be taken, such as **wearing gloves** and other **protective garments.**

Suggested Readings

Bunzli WF, Wright DH, Hoang AD, et al.: Current management of human bites. *Pharmacotherapy* 18(2):227–234, 1998.

Chen E, Hornig S, Shepherd SM, et al.: Primary closure of mammalian bites. *Acad Emerg Med* 7:157–161, 2000.

Glaser C, Lewis P, Wong S: Pet- animal-, and vector-borne infections. *Pediatr Rev* 21(7):219–232, 2000.

Goldstein EJ: Current concepts on animal bites: bacteriology and therapy. *Curr Clin Top Infect Dis* 19:99–111, 1999.

Griego RD, Rosen T, Orengo IF, et al.: Dog, cat, and human bites: a review. *J Am Acad Dermatol* 33:1019–1029, 1995.

Moore DA, Sischo WM, Hunter A, et al.: Animal bite epidemiology and surveillance for rabies postexposure prophylaxis. *J Am Vet Med Assoc* 217:190–194, 2000.

Weber DJ, Rutala WA: Zoonotic infections. *Occup Med* 14(2):247–284, 1999.

Wiley JF: Mammalian bites: review of evaluation and management. *Clin Pediatr* 29(5):283–287, 1990.

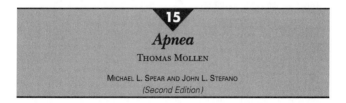

15

Apnea

Thomas Mollen

Michael L. Spear and John L. Stefano
(Second Edition)

▼ INTRODUCTION

The National Institute of Health's (NIH) *1986 Consensus Statement on Infantile Apnea and Home Monitoring* describes an apparent life-threatening event (ALTE) as "an episode that is frightening to the observer and is characterized by some combination of apnea (central or occasionally obstructive), color change (usually cyanotic or pallid but occasionally erythematous or plethoric), marked change in muscle tone (usually marked limpness), choking, or gagging...in some cases, the observer fears that the infant has died...previously used terminology such as 'aborted crib death' or 'near-miss SIDS' should be abandoned because it implies a possibly misleading close association between this type of spell and SIDS."

▼ DIFFERENTIAL DIAGNOSIS LIST

Infectious Causes

Sepsis
Pneumonia
Respiratory syncytial virus (RSV) infection
Meningitis

Toxic Causes

Drug-induced apnea
Postanesthesia ALTE

Neoplastic Causes

Central nervous system (CNS) tumor

Traumatic Causes

Intracranial hemorrhage (subdural, subarachnoid)
Munchausen by proxy syndrome
Child abuse

Congenital or Vascular Causes

CNS arteriovenous malformation (AVM)
Congenital heart disease

Metabolic or Genetic Causes

Inborn errors of metabolism
Hypoglycemia
Hyponatremia

Anatomic Causes

Arnold-Chiari deformity
Vascular ring
Structural lung malformation
Diaphragmatic hernia
Cystic adenomatoid malformation

Miscellaneous Causes

Apnea of prematurity
Mild periodic breathing during sleep
Central hypoventilation syndromes (Ondine curse)
Anemia

Seizures
Arrhythmia (prolonged QT interval)
Vocal cord paralysis
Tracheoesophageal fistula
Occasional choking during feeding
Upper airway obstruction
Gastroesophageal reflux disease (GRD)

▼ DIFFERENTIAL DIAGNOSIS DISCUSSION
Infection

Clinical Features

Although apnea can be the only initial symptom of infection, untreated sepsis progresses rapidly, and the infant will develop other signs and symptoms that suggest this diagnosis. **Pneumonia** caused by RSV can be **associated with life-threatening apnea** and is a **primary cause of infant mortality** among **premature infants** after hospital discharge, especially during the **winter months.**

Evaluation

In an infant who presents with acute apnea, a **careful history** and **physical examination** should be performed in an attempt to elucidate the presence of an acute infection. Depending on the history and physical examination findings, appropriate **laboratory tests** can be ordered.

Treatment

Treatment depends on the underlying infection. Effective **antibacterial therapies,** and some **antiviral therapies,** are available. **Prompt diagnosis and treatment are essential.**

Apnea of Prematurity

Premature infants have a much **higher risk for ALTE** and **sudden infant death syndrome (SIDS)** than do infants who were born at or near term gestation (37 weeks or longer).

Clinical Features

Apnea of prematurity is characterized by **pauses in respiration** that last **longer than 20 seconds.** Accompanying **bradycardia** (defined by age) may also be present.

Only some of these episodes are detected by hospital personnel or parents. In a study involving tracings of asymptomatic premature infants' respiratory patterns, heart rates, nasal air flow, and oxyhemoglobin saturations, almost 50% of the infants had prolonged apnea and other findings defined as abnormal.

Treatment

Several strategies have been proposed to address **home monitoring** of premature infants. The NIH consensus report to the American Academy of Pediatrics recommends against the routine evaluation of premature infants before discharge with a standard two-channel pneumogram (thoracic impedance and heart rate monitoring) because this test has a high rate of false-positive and false-negative results and is not a reliable predictor of infants who will suffer an ALTE or succumb to SIDS.

One accepted approach is to monitor **all premature infants up to and beyond the postnatal age associated with the highest rate of SIDS** (i.e., 2–4 months). If the infant is stressed (e.g., by an upper respiratory tract illness), it is speculated that the "normal" pauses in respiration can become pathological and present as an ALTE.

⚡ HINT Periodic breathing (i.e., short intervals of apnea interspersed between short intervals of respirations) can appear pathological to the parent. However, **isolated periodic breathing** in a premature infant is **not predictive** of ALTE or SIDS.

⚡ HINT Many premature infants have mild GRD and a history of choking during feeding. It can be extremely difficult to determine when these episodes are truly ALTEs and when they are merely normal variations. If the episode is associated with the factors listed in the NIH's definition of ALTE (i.e., apnea, color change, marked change in muscle tone), then the infant should be admitted for a more complete evaluation.

Obstructive Apnea

Etiology

Obstructive apnea is the **inability to effectively oxygenate, ventilate, or both,** despite adequate central respiratory drive. Causes include:

▼ **GRD.** The most common cause of obstructive apnea is GRD; as many as 20% of premature infants with apnea have an obstructive component.
▼ **Prematurity.** The incomplete development of cartilaginous structures in a premature infant's airway can lead to kinking of the airway and obstructive apnea.
▼ **Laryngeal webs** or **laryngomalacia** can also present as obstructive apnea.

Clinical Features

The parents describe the baby as **regurgitating formula or milk,** either during feeding or afterward. Infants may have **"awake apnea,"** which is most commonly caused by GRD. Alternatively, infants may **struggle during feeding,** with **exaggerated respiratory effort.**

Evaluation

If GRD is suspected, a **barium swallow with video** capabilities allows the radiologist and the speech therapist to assess both reflux and swallowing function to determine appropriate therapy. Other causes of obstructive apnea require evaluation by an **otolaryngologist.**

Treatment

Thickened formula, and **metoclopramide** have been used to treat GRD. **Prone positioning** after feeds, with the infant's head elevated to a 45° angle, has also been effective. Patients with obstructive apnea caused by a condition other than GRD may require **tracheostomy.**

Trauma

Etiology

Birth trauma (e.g., intracranial or subgaleal hemorrhage, rather than a caput or cephalohematoma) and **child abuse** (including physical abuse and Munchausen by proxy syndrome) can be associated with apnea.

⚔ HINT Munchausen by proxy syndrome is among the differential diagnoses for recurrent apnea; parents with this psychological disorder can interfere with the proper functioning of home monitoring. In addition, parentally induced suffocation can lead to true apnea; the associated hypoxia can be detected with a monitor capable of storing and downloading the data for physician interpretation.

Evaluation

A **careful history** and **imaging studies** help in confirming the diagnosis of child abuse or birth trauma. Often the information stored in the **home apnea monitor** can help in determining if events at home are real, and when they occurred.

Neurologic Disorders

Seizures, CNS structural abnormalities (e.g., AVM, Arnold-Chiari deformity), CNS tumors, and **intracranial hemorrhage** can be associated with an ALTE initially. **Persistent idiopathic apnea** is the **hallmark of central hypoventilation disorders,** the most well known of which is Ondine curse.

Clinical Features

The apnea may be associated with **seizures** or symptoms of **increased intracranial pressure.** If a neurologic diagnosis is suspected, then appropriate **CNS imaging studies,** an **electroencephalogram (EEG),** and **laboratory blood tests** are indicated.

Treatment

Treatment depends on the underlying cause. Either **anticonvulsant therapy** or **surgical intervention** may be necessary. Patients with central hypoventilation syndromes may require **nighttime mechanical ventilation.**

Cardiac Disease

⚔ HINT An infant with an ALTE rarely has cardiac disease.

The most common life-threatening cardiac abnormality is **cardiac arrhythmia.** A prolonged QT interval has been noted in infants who have died of SIDS. On rare occasions, **congenital heart disease** presents as an ALTE.

Clinical Features

In addition to apnea, infants with heart disease usually have more obvious signs of heart failure, such as **failure to thrive** or **cyanosis.** A **vascular ring** can be associated with **inspiratory stridor.**

Evaluation

When congenital heart disease is suspected, the initial evaluation usually includes an **electrocardiogram (ECG), chest radiograph,** and an **echocardiogram.**

Treatment

Treatment depends on the underlying pathological condition; **medical therapy** is useful for some arrhythmias, and **surgical therapy** may be required by patients with structural heart disease.

Respiratory Abnormalities

Clinical Features

Often, an infant with apnea caused by a structural lung abnormality is **tachypneic** and **cyanotic,** and he uses the **accessory respiratory muscles.** An **abnormal cry** or **inspiratory stridor** is present in patients with vocal cord paralysis. **Choking during feeding** is seen with tracheoesophageal fistula.

Evaluation

A **chest radiograph** is helpful initially. Often, **flexible laryngoscopy or bronchoscopy** will be needed.

Treatment

Some structural lung abnormalities (e.g., cystic adenomatoid malformation, diaphragmatic hernia) are **surgically correctable.** Vocal cord paralysis may improve **spontaneously.**

▼ EVALUATION OF APNEA

There are several approaches to evaluating an infant who has experienced an ALTE.

Some regional health care centers perform a **routine battery of tests** on every patient with an admitting diagnosis of ALTE. These tests include:

- ▼ EEG
- ▼ ECG
- ▼ Chest radiograph
- ▼ Complete blood cell count
- ▼ Serum electrolyte panel
- ▼ Serum calcium level
- ▼ Serum glucose level
- ▼ Blood urea nitrogen and creatinine level
- ▼ Multichannel recordings of the heart rate
- ▼ Thermistor nasal air flow
- ▼ Respiratory rate
- ▼ Pulse oximetry
- ▼ Esophageal pH

Other institutions rely on a **carefully obtained history** and **physical examination** to guide the evaluation more cost effectively. Because the physical examination at the time of admission is often normal, the history is of paramount importance.

▼ TREATMENT OF APNEA

As many as 50% of infants admitted with the diagnosis of ALTE are discharged without determining the cause. Regardless of whether a diagnosis is determined, **home monitoring** and **cardiopulmonary resuscitation training** are indicated.

Evaluation of home-monitoring records or diaries or use of the newer documented home-monitoring technologies allows the physician to determine whether the episodes are recurrent. The newer devices provide a more precise description of the ALTE, allowing the clinician to embark on a more focused evaluation of the problem. Some investigators rely on **analysis of pneumograms** created by the home monitor; others **download the record of alarms** stored in the monitor's memory (a "memory monitor"). The **"memory monitor"** allows physicians to examine **longitudinal data** to aid in the process of home monitoring. However, much of these data are **false-positive alarms** caused by movements or a shallow amplitude signal and must be interpreted with caution.

The criteria for discontinuation of home monitoring vary. The most common approach is to **stop monitoring after 1–2 months of no alarms or after the child has undergone some stress** (e.g., an upper respiratory tract infection or diphtheria–tetanus–pertussis immunization) without an incident of apnea. **Discontinuation** of home monitoring is, understandably, often **difficult for the parents** of an infant who has experienced an ALTE. A common approach is to **eliminate monitoring during naps,** and then to **eliminate it during overnight sleep.**

Suggested Readings

Finer NN, Barrington KJ, Hayes B: Prolonged periodic breathing: significance in sleep studies. *Pediatrics* 89:450–453, 1992.

National Institutes of Health: *Infantile Apnea and Home Monitoring.* Washington, DC, National Institutes of Health, 1986.

United States Department of Health and Human Services publication NIH 87-2905.

Ramanathan R, Corwin MJ, Hunt CE, et al. The Collaborative Home Infant Monitoring Evaluation (CHIME) Study Group: Cardiorespiratory events recorded on home monitors: comparison of healthy infants with those at increased risk for SIDS. *JAMA* 285(17):2199–2207, 2001.

Southall DP, Richards JM, deSwiet M, et al.: Identification of infants destined to die unexpectedly during infancy: evaluation of predictive importance of prolonged apnea and disorders of cardiac rhythm or conduction. *Br Med Bull* 286:1092, 1983.

Marcus CL: Advances in management of sleep apnea syndromes in infants and children. *Pediatr Pulmonol* 18(Suppl):188–189, 1999.

Wenzl TG, Schenke S, Peschgens T, et al.: Association of apnea and nonacid gastroesophageal reflux in infants: Investigations with the intraluminal impedance technique. *Pediatr Pulmonol* 31(2):144–149, 2001.

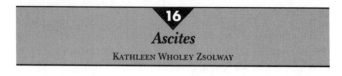

16
Ascites
Kathleen Wholey Zsolway

▼ INTRODUCTION

Ascites is the **pathological accumulation of fluid** in the **peritoneal cavity.** It can be caused by **decreased plasma oncotic pressure, obstructed lymphatic or venous drainage,** or **irritation of the peritoneum** (e.g., as a result of infection, trauma, or neoplasia).

▼ DIFFERENTIAL DIAGNOSIS LIST

Infectious Causes

Bacterial peritonitis
Chronic tuberculous peritonitis
Congenital toxoplasmosis, other, rubella, cytomegalovirus, and herpes simplex virus (TORCH) infection

Neoplastic Causes

Hodgkin disease
Intraperitoneal tumor

Congenital or Vascular Causes

Hepatic vein occlusion (Budd-Chiari syndrome)
Portal vein obstruction
Renal vein thrombosis
Congestive heart failure
Thoracic duct obstruction (chylous ascites)

Metabolic or Congenital Causes

Lysosomal storage disease

Inflammatory Causes

Chronic adhesive pericarditis
Peritonitis—rheumatic, meconium, bile

Miscellaneous Causes

Cirrhosis
Nephrotic syndrome
Perforation of the urinary tract
Obstructive uropathy
Acute glomerulonephritis
Chronic renal failure
Protein-losing enteropathy (PLE)
Pancreatitis
Systemic lupus erythematosus
Familial Mediterranean fever
Maternal diabetes

Enlarged lymph node
Pulmonary lymphangiectasia
Malnutrition

▼ DIFFERENTIAL DIAGNOSIS DISCUSSION
Cirrhosis

In children other than neonates, cirrhosis is the **most common cause** of ascites.

Etiology

Cirrhosis is a process characterized by **increased fibrous tissue** and **nodule formation following necrosis of the hepatocyte** within the liver. It represents **irreversible distortion** of the intrahepatic vascular and biliary structures. Cirrhosis may develop in association with chronic active hepatitis, galactosemia, cystic fibrosis, Wilson disease, and structural abnormalities of the biliary system.

The ascites of hepatic cirrhosis is a consequence of **hypoalbuminemia** (secondary to failure of protein synthesis) and **excess salt and water retention.** Cirrhosis commonly causes **peripheral edema** after the presence of ascites has become evident.

Clinical Features

The physical examination may demonstrate a **firm liver with irregular margins (hepatomegaly)** or a **small liver, spider angiomata, palmar erythema, and splenomegaly,** depending on the degree of cirrhosis.

The two major sequelae of cirrhosis are **portal venous hypertension** and **hepatocellular failure.** The main signs of portal hypertension are **splenomegaly, hematemesis** (as a result of bleeding from esophageal varices), and **bloody stools** as a result of bleeding from hemorrhoids. **Hepatic coma** may also occur.

Evaluation

Liver function tests, serum albumin levels, prothrombin time, and **blood ammonia levels** are often ordered to assess liver function. A **complete blood cell (CBC) count** may reveal anemia, thrombocytopenia, and leukopenia as a result of hypersplenism. Various imaging options are available: **ultrasound** may reveal increased echogenicity; **radioisotope scanning** may reveal decreased uptake, increased flow to the spleen, and irregular hepatic texture; a **computed tomography** scan is sensitive for detection of abnormal liver texture, size, and vascular appearance. A **liver biopsy** is often needed to identify the cause of the cirrhosis.

Treatment

Management entails the **prevention and treatment** of **life-threatening complications. Liver transplantation** is considered standard therapy for patients with advanced cirrhosis.

Dietary and drug regimens should be initiated in a controlled hospital environment. The diet should provide adequate calories for growth. **Fat intake** should be **reduced** and the diet supplemented with **calcium** and **vitamins A, D, E, and K. Diuretics** and **decreased sodium** content in the diet may improve the ascites and edema.

Portal hypertension may require management with a shunt to divert portal blood flow to the systemic circulation; however, shunt procedures are associated with increased morbidity and mortality.

Infectious Peritonitis

Etiology

▼ **Primary peritonitis** is an infection in the peritoneal cavity secondary to microorganism invasion via the blood or lymphatics. Causative organisms include pneumococci, group A streptococci, and less commonly, gram-negative bacilli and viruses.

▼ **Secondary peritonitis** is an infection in the peritoneal cavity that occurs through rupture of an intra-abdominal viscus or extension of an abscess. In children, the most common cause of secondary peritonitis is appendicitis. Other causes include gangrenous bowel, necrotizing enterocolitis, and idiopathic gastric or bowel perforation. The causative organisms are the normal flora of the gastrointestinal tract. Secondary peritonitis may also occur as a complication of a ventriculoperitoneal shunt and in patients receiving peritoneal dialysis. *Staphylococcus epidermidis* can be the causative agent in these patients.

Evaluation

Typically, the history includes the **rapid onset of abdominal pain, fever,** and **vomiting** (e.g., over the course of **48 hours**). Physical examination reveals either diffuse or lower quadrant **severe abdominal tenderness. Bowel sounds** are **hypoactive or absent,** and **abdominal rigidity** may be present. The **patient prefers** to lie in a **supine position** and feels severe discomfort with motion or palpation.

Abdominal radiographs of patients with peritonitis often reveal intestinal dilatation, edema of the small intestine, peritoneal fluid, and absence of the psoas shadow. Patients with intestinal perforation have radiographic evidence of free air in the peritoneal cavity.

Needle aspiration of the peritoneal fluid should be performed if peritonitis is suspected or if the patient has an unexplained fever and fluid in the abdomen. Analysis of the peritoneal fluid from a patient with infectious peritonitis typically reveals an **elevated protein level** and an **elevated white blood cell count** (i.e., greater than 300 cells/mm^3), of which more than 25% are polymorphonuclear leukocytes. A **Gram stain** and **culture** of the fluid should be performed to help guide antimicrobial therapy.

Treatment

In patients with peritonitis, careful attention must be paid to **fluid and electrolyte status.** In addition, parenteral **antimicrobial therapy** should be initiated. Combination therapy with ampicillin, gentamicin, and clindamycin provides appropriate initial coverage. Antimicrobial therapy should be modified based on culture and Gram stain results. **Surgical evaluation** should occur early because surgical exploration may be necessary to evaluate for a perforated viscus.

Protein-Losing Enteropathy (PLE)

Etiology

PLE, the **loss of proteins across the gastrointestinal mucosa,** occurs in a variety of disease states (Table 16.1).

Evaluation

The patient's **history** reflects the underlying disease state. **Edema** may be the presenting physical examination finding, although symptoms of a disturbance in bowel function may be elicited in a careful history.

The primary method of diagnosing enteric protein loss is the **detection of elevated α_1-antitrypsin (α_1-AT) in the stool.** α_1-AT is a protein that is not actively secreted, absorbed, or digested by the gastrointestinal tract. Quantification can be performed on a spot stool sample or on stool samples that have been collected over several days. Spot sample results appear to correlate well with those obtained from samples collected over a period of time.

TABLE 16.1. Diseases Associated with Enteric Protein Loss

Loss from intestinal lymphatics
  Intestinal lymphangiectasia
    Primary
    Secondary (i.e., resulting from cardiac disease)
      Constrictive pericarditis
      Congestive heart failure
      Cardiomyopathy
  Obstructive lymphatic disorders
    Malrotation
    Lymphoma
    Tuberculosis
    Sarcoidosis
    Radiation therapy and chemotherapy
    Retroperitoneal fibrosis or tumor
    Arsenic poisoning
Loss from an abnormal or inflamed mucosal surface
  Ménétrier disease
  Eosinophilic gastroenteritis
  Milk- and soy-induced enterocolitis
  Celiac disease
  Tropical sprue
  Ulcerative jejunitis or colitis
  Radiation enteritis
  Graft-versus-host disease
  Necrotizing enterocolitis
  Crohn disease
  Hirschsprung disease
  Systemic lupus erythematosus
  Bacterial overgrowth
  Giardiasis
  Bacterial and parasitic infections
  Common variable immunodeficiency

Modified from Proujansky R: Protein-losing enteropathy. In *Pediatric Gastrointestinal Disease*, 2nd ed. Edited by Walker WA, Durie PR, Hamilton JR, et al. Philadelphia, BC Decker, 1996.

Treatment

Treatment addresses the **underlying cause** of PLE. **Reduction in dietary fat** intake can aid in decreasing the enteric protein loss.

▼ APPROACH TO THE PATIENT (FIGURE 16.1)

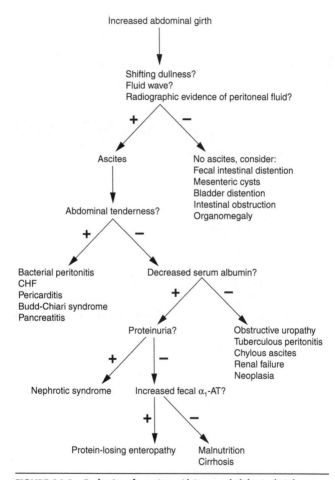

FIGURE 16.1. Evaluation of a patient with increased abdominal girth. α_1-AT = α_1-antitrypsin; CHF = congestive heart failure. (Modified with permission from Simon JE: Abdominal distension. In *Textbook of Pediatric Emergency Medicine*, 3rd ed. Edited by Fleisher GR, Ludwig S. Baltimore, Williams & Wilkins, 1993, p 102.)

Suggested Readings

Cronan KM, Norman ME: Renal and electrolyte emergencies. In *Textbook of Pediatric Emergency Medicine*, 4th ed. Edited by Fleisher GR, Ludwig S. Baltimore, Williams & Wilkins, 2000, pp 811–858.

Kelsch RC, Sedman AB: Nephrotic syndrome. *Pediatr Rev* 14:30–38, 1993.

Proujansky R: Protein-losing enteropathy. In *Pediatric Gastrointestinal Disease*, 2nd ed. Edited by Walker WA, Durie PR, Hamilton JR, et al. Philadelphia, BC Decker, 1996, pp 812–817.

Reynolds TB: Ascites. *Clin Liv Dis* 4(1):151–168, vii, 2000.

Runyon BA: Care of patients with ascites. *N Engl J Med* 330:337–342, 1994.

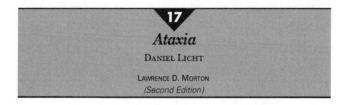

17

Ataxia

DANIEL LICHT

LAWRENCE D. MORTON
(Second Edition)

▼ INTRODUCTION

Ataxia is a **disturbance of muscle coordination** that is **not accompanied by a disturbance of muscle strength.** Ataxia is characterized by **errors of motor activity** with regard to rate, range, direction, timing, duration, and force.

▼ DIFFERENTIAL DIAGNOSIS LIST

The major causes of acute ataxia differ significantly from those of chronic ataxia (Table 17.1).

Acute Ataxia

Infectious Causes

Encephalitis

Postinfectious immune disorder—acute cerebellar ataxia, Miller Fisher syndrome, multiple sclerosis, myoclonic encephalopathy, Kawasaki disease

TABLE 17.1. Causes of Ataxia

Form of Ataxia	Major Causes	Other Causes
Acute ataxia	Ingestion	Migraine
	Postinfectious cerebellitis	Neuroblastoma
Acute recurrent ataxia	Migraine	. . .
	Metabolic disease	
Chronic ataxia	Congenital disorders with mental deficiency	. . .
Chronic progressive ataxia	Brain tumors	Ataxia–telangiectasia
	Neuroectodermal tumors	Friedreich ataxia

Toxic Causes

Ethanol
Anticonvulsants
Antihistamines

Neoplastic Causes

Brain-stem tumor
Cerebellar tumor

Paraneoplastic Causes

Opsoclonus–myoclonus syndrome (the syndrome of dancing eyes and dancing feet)

Metabolic or Genetic Causes

Dominant recurrent ataxia
Carnitine acetyltransferase deficiency
Hartnup disease
Maple syrup urine disease
Episodic ataxia type 1 (paroxysmal ataxia and myokymia)
Episodic ataxia type 2 (SCA 6, familial hemiplegic migraine)
Pyruvate decarboxylase deficiency

Psychosocial Causes

Conversion disorder

Miscellaneous Causes

Migraine headache (benign paroxysmal vertigo)
Trauma

Chronic or Progressive Ataxia

Neoplastic Causes

Neuroectodermal tumor
Posterior fossa tumor
Glioma
Astrocytoma
Ependymoma
Medulloblastoma

Metabolic or Genetic Causes

Ataxia—telangiectasia
Ataxia—oculomotor apraxia
Friedreich ataxia
Refsum disease
Progressive myoclonic epilepsy (formerly known as Ramsay Hunt syndrome)

Miscellaneous Causes

Fixed-deficit ataxia—ataxic cerebral palsy, congenital malformations
Acquired diseases—e.g., systemic lupus erythematosus, hypothyroidism

▼ DIFFERENTIAL DIAGNOSIS DISCUSSION
Acute Ataxia

Brain Tumor

Brain-stem or cerebellar tumors that **grow rapidly, acutely hemorrhage,** or **shift** can cause **hydrocephalus,** which causes acute decompensation of the brain stem, leading to acute ataxia.

⚡ HINT   Cerebellar hemispheric dysfunction leads to limb ataxia on the same side of the lesion.

Conversion Disorder

Conversion disorder is characterized by **involuntary alteration or limitation of physical function** as a result of a **psychological conflict.** The disorder is most common in older children and adolescents, and the findings typically do not match the expected physiology. For example, some patients are able to sit down without difficulty, but will lurch or stagger when they attempt to stand up. This is incongruent because sitting requires better balance and would therefore be difficult for someone with a true coordination or balance disturbance. When this gait is extreme, it is termed astasia–abasia.

Encephalitis

Some agents commonly implicated in brain-stem encephalitis include:

▼ Epstein-Barr virus
▼ poliomyelitis
▼ ECHO virus
▼ coxsackievirus
▼ varicella-zoster virus
▼ *Mycoplasma*
▼ *Borrelia burgdorferi* (the agent responsible for Lyme disease)

Ataxia occurs, often in association with other types of cranial nerve dysfunction, in patients who have **diffuse encephalitis with altered awareness and seizures.** Most children completely recover, although some are left with significant neurologic impairment.

Genetic Disorders

▼ **Dominant recurrent ataxia** is characterized by recurrent bouts of ataxia without an identifiable metabolic cause. Ataxic symptoms, some of which are associated with cerebellar hypoplasia, become apparent in patients before the age of 3 years.
▼ **Hartnup disease** is a rare disorder in which defective amino acid transport in the cells of the proximal renal tubules and the small intestine leads to massive aminoaciduria. Patients are developmentally delayed and have a borderline intelligence quotient (IQ). They are photosensitive and develop pellagra-like rashes when exposed to sunlight. Episodic ataxia is frequently reported, sometimes with delirium and emotional lability. The ataxia is triggered by intercurrent infections.
▼ **Maple syrup urine disease (intermittent form),** an amino acidemia caused by deficiency of a branched-chain decarboxylase, leads to bouts of ataxia

and encephalopathy. Between attacks of ataxia, the patient's physical examination and IQ are typically normal. During attacks, the blood and urine exhibit elevated levels of branched-chain amino acids.

▼ **Episodic ataxia type 1 (paroxysmal ataxia and myokymia) and episodic ataxia type 2,** an autosomal dominant disorder, is characterized by attacks of ataxia that last from minutes to hours. The average age of onset is 5–7 years. Patients with this disorder usually respond to acetazolamide therapy.

▼ **Pyruvate decarboxylase deficiency.** Most patients with this deficiency have episodic ataxia, dysarthria, and mild developmental delays (although some develop normally). Triggers for attacks of ataxia include infection and a high carbohydrate load. The disorder becomes apparent once the child reaches preschool age. Patients have elevated lactate and pyruvate levels during attacks and occasionally following an oral glucose load. Treatment includes a ketogenic diet and the administration of acetazolamide. The prognosis varies and is related to the percentage of preserved enzyme activity.

Postinfectious Immune Disorders

▼ **Acute cerebellar ataxia** is characterized by the sudden onset of ataxia 2–3 weeks after an upper respiratory tract infection. Children between the ages of 1 and 5 years appear most sensitive. Generally, there is a good outcome within several days to weeks; however, when the ataxia is associated with opsoclonus or myoclonus, persistent neurologic sequelae can occur. Corticosteroids are of unproven benefit in the treatment of acute cerebellar ataxia.

▼ **Miller Fisher syndrome** is a rare syndrome characterized by the acute onset of ataxia, ophthalmoparesis, and hyporeflexia after an upper respiratory tract infection. Complete recovery within several weeks is the rule.

▼ **Multiple sclerosis** (rare in children) is a demyelinating disease characterized by recurrent bouts of neurologic symptoms involving different parts of the central nervous system. Magnetic resonance imaging shows numerous white matter "plaques." Currently, acute flairs are treated with high-dose corticosteroids.

▼ **Myoclonic encephalopathy with neuroblastoma (opsoclonus myoclonus syndrome)** is generally characterized by the triad of myoclonus, opsoclonus, and ataxia in patients with a neuroblastoma. The outcome varies widely.

Trauma

Cerebellar hematoma is a postconcussion syndrome, and **ataxia can persist for weeks.** Trauma can also produce basilar or vertebral artery occlusion accompanied by occipital headache and other cranial nerve dysfunction.

Chronic or Progressive Ataxia

Congenital Disorders (Fixed-Deficit Ataxia)

Several congenital disorders produce **chronic ataxia,** and most are associated with some degree of **mental deficiency.** Onset usually occurs in infancy or childhood but can be delayed until the patient reaches adulthood. In one recognized variant of cerebral palsy, ataxia is the prominent feature and patients may be hypotonic and hyporeflexic.

Neoplasia

In a child with progressive ataxia, brain tumors are an important consideration:

▼ **Neuroectodermal tumors** are the second most common childhood malignancy.

▼ **Posterior fossa tumors** are most common in children younger than 8 years.

▼ **Gliomas** generally present with cranial nerve findings and ataxia as a later symptom.

▼ **Astrocytomas, ependymomas,** and **medulloblastomas** frequently present with symptoms of increased intracranial tumors. Medulloblastomas generally grow rapidly.

Hereditary Disorders

▼ **Ataxia–telangiectasia** is a multisystemic disease that most prominently affects the nervous and immune systems. Truncal ataxia usually develops before the first birthday. Drooling and dysarthria are common. Telangiectatic lesions, most commonly affecting the conjunctivae and ears, develop after the age of 2 years. Complications include frequent sinopulmonary infections (as a result of deficient immunoglobulin E and immunoglobulin A) and an increased incidence of neoplasia, especially Hodgkin disease, leukemia, and lymphomas. α-Fetoprotein and carcinoembryonic antigen levels are elevated, while immunoglobulin levels are decreased. Treatment usually entails vigorous antibiotic support for infections. There is currently no effective therapy for the neurologic symptoms.

▼ **Ataxia–oculomotor apraxia** is clinically related to ataxia–telangiectasia. It is autosomal recessive and has the neurologic features of ataxia–telangiectasia, but symptoms start after the age of 1 year, and patients have a normal immunologic status.

▼ **Friedreich ataxia** is a multisystemic disorder affecting the peripheral nerves, spinal cord, heart, and carbohydrate metabolism. The ataxia usually begins in childhood. Limb ataxia is worse than truncal ataxia. Kyphoscoliosis is common, and there is early loss of position, light touch sensation, and deep tendon reflexes. Diabetes mellitus occurs in 10%–40% of patients. Cardiomyopathy occurs in all patients, and most die from its complications.

▼ **Refsum disease** is an inborn error of phytanic acid metabolism characterized by retinitis pigmentosa, recurrent polyneuropathy, and ataxia. Elevated serum levels of phytanic acid are found. Treatment is usually dietary, but acute cases with significant cardiac involvement can be treated with plasmapheresis.

▼ **Progressive myoclonic epilepsy (Ramsay Hunt disease)** [progressive degeneration of the dentate nucleus and superior cerebellar peduncle] is characterized by ataxia, myoclonus, and seizures. Although this disease is usually autosomal recessive, autosomal dominant and mitochondrial cases have also been described. Seizures and myoclonus may resolve with valproate therapy.

▼ **Other hereditary disorders** that may present with ataxia include Wilson disease, biotinidase deficiency, adrenoleukodystrophy (X-linked), hypobetalipoproteinemia, juvenile sulfatide lipidosis, sea-blue histiocytosis, Leigh disease, Leber optic neuropathy, and multiple sclerosis.

▼ APPROACH TO THE PATIENT

There are two major **pitfalls** involved with diagnosing ataxia:

The first is **confusing ataxia with other gait disturbances,** such as dizziness, vertigo, and conversion disorders. Misdiagnosis can be avoided by obtaining a careful history of symptoms, noting evidence of cerebellar dysfunction on neurologic examination, and observing other findings related to ataxia (e.g., dysmetria, an intention tremor, dysdiadochokinesia).

The second is **misidentifying chronic progressive ataxia as acute ataxia.** Usually, the causes of and possible treatments for acute and chronic ataxia are very different; therefore, so distinguishing between the two is important.

The approach to a patient with acute ataxia is illustrated in Figure 17.1.

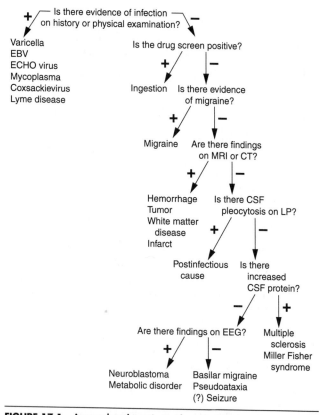

FIGURE 17.1. Approach to the patient with acute ataxia.
CSF = cerebrospinal fluid; *CT* = computed tomography; *EBV* = Epstein-Barr virus; *EEG* = electroencephalogram; *LP* = lumbar puncture; *MRI* = magnetic resonance imaging.

⚠ HINT Mild chronic ataxia may be improperly dismissed as clumsiness.

Suggested Readings

Fenichel GM: *Clinical Pediatric Neurology: A Signs and Symptoms Approach*, 4th ed. Philadelphia, WB Saunders, 2001, pp 223–242.

Menkes JH: *Textbook of Child Neurology*, 5th ed. Baltimore, Williams & Wilkins, 1995.

Swainman KF, Ashwal S: *Pediatric Neurology: Principles and Practice.* St Louis, Mosby, 1999, pp 787–800.

Tunnessen WW: *Signs and Symptoms in Pediatrics*, 3rd ed. Philadelphia, Lippincott-Raven, 1999, pp 747–758.

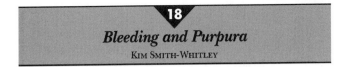

18

Bleeding and Purpura
KIM SMITH-WHITLEY

▼ INTRODUCTION

Purpura [i.e., **petechiae and ecchymoses (bruises)**] and excessive bleeding are caused by disruptions in one or more of the three stages of normal hemostasis:

▼ **Vascular phase**—vasoconstriction
▼ **Platelet phase (primary hemostasis)**—platelet plug formation
▼ **Plasma phase (secondary hemostasis)**—fibrin thrombus formation

Vascular abnormalities are characterized by **purpuric lesions;** laboratory tests demonstrate **normal platelet number and function** as well as **normal coagulation.** Disorders of primary hemostasis **(platelet disorders)** are also characterized by **purpuric lesions,** but **laboratory test results are not normal.** Disorders of secondary hemostasis **(coagulation disorders)** are characterized by **hemarthroses** and **deep bleeding.**

▼ DIFFERENTIAL DIAGNOSIS LIST
Disorders of Increased Platelet Destruction

Immune-Mediated Thrombocytopenia

Idiopathic thrombocytopenic purpura (ITP)
Evans syndrome
Neonatal, isoimmune, and autoimmune
Posttransfusion purpura
Drug related
HIV infection
Systemic lupus erythematosus (SLE)

Microangiopathic Hemolytic Anemia

Hemolytic-uremic syndrome

Miscellaneous Causes of Platelet Destruction

Central venous catheter thromboses
Type 2B and platelet-type von Willebrand disease (vWD)
Asphyxia
Persistent pulmonary hypertension
Postexchange transfusion
Drug therapy—e.g., heparin

Disorders of Decreased Platelet Production

Congenital amegakaryocytic thrombocytopenia
Thrombocytopenia with absent radii (TAR)

Generalized Bone Marrow Depression

Fanconi anemia
Aplastic anemia
Vitamin B_{12} or folate deficiency
Viral infection—varicella-zoster virus, measles virus, rubella, cytomegalo-
virus, Epstein-Barr virus
Drugs—e.g., chemotherapeutic agents

Bone Marrow Infiltration

Leukemia
Malignancy metastatic to bone marrow
Myelofibrosis
Osteopetrosis
Histiocytosis
Infection—e.g., tuberculosis

Disorders of Platelet Sequestration

Splenomegaly
Large hemangiomas (Kasabach-Merritt syndrome)

Disorders of Platelet Function

Bernard-Soulier disease
Glanzmann thrombasthenia
Wiskott-Aldrich syndrome
Platelet granule defects
Drug-induced abnormalities—e.g., aspirin, ibuprofen
Systemic disease—e.g., uremia

Vascular Abnormalities

Autoimmune Vascular Purpuras

Henoch-Schönlein purpura and other allergic purpuras
Purpura fulminans

Infection

Bacterial—e.g., *Neisseria meningitidis,* streptococcal toxins
Viral—e.g., measles, influenza

Rickettsial—Rocky Mountain spotted fever
Parasitic—malaria

Structural Malformations

Telangiectasia syndromes—ataxia-telangiectasia, hereditary hemorrhagic telangiectasia (Rendu-Osler-Weber syndrome)
Connective tissue disorders—Ehlers-Danlos syndrome, osteogenesis imperfecta, vitamin C deficiency
Trauma—accidents, child abuse, factitious purpura
Miscellaneous—Kaposi sarcoma, toxins (e.g., snake venom), emboli (e.g., septic, tumor), thrombocytosis

Coagulation Disorders

vWD

Factor Deficiencies

Intrinsic factor deficiencies—factors VIII (hemophilia A), IX (hemophilia B), XI
Extrinsic factor deficiencies—factor VII
Common pathway factor deficiencies—factors I (fibrinogen), II (prothrombin), V, X
Multiple factor deficiencies—disseminated intravascular coagulation (DIC), liver disease, vitamin K deficiency
Factor XIII deficiency

Drug- or Toxin-Induced Coagulation Disorders

Heparin or warfarin therapy
Toxicity—e.g., ingestion of warfarin-containing rat poisons

▼ DIFFERENTIAL DIAGNOSIS DISCUSSION I: BLEEDING AND PURPURA IN CHILDREN

Idiopathic Thrombocytopenic Purpura (ITP)

ITP, the **most common cause of low platelet counts** in childhood, can be categorized as **acute** (thrombocytopenia resolves within 6 months of diagnosis) or **chronic.** Although ITP can occur at any age, the **peak incidence** in children is **between** the ages of **2 and 6 years.**

Etiology

The exact cause of ITP is unknown, but the disorder is thought to be **immune-mediated.** A **viral illness** may precede ITP.

Clinical Features

The child with ITP appears otherwise well but has a **rapid onset of purpuric lesions.** ITP is rarely associated with significant bleeding episodes, but **epistaxis** occurs in about one-third of patients. Clinical findings of lymphadenopathy and hepatosplenomegaly should alert the physician to a diagnosis other than ITP (e.g., malignancy, metabolic disorder).

Evaluation

Laboratory evaluation should include a **reticulocyte count,** a **direct antibody test (DAT),** and an **antinuclear antibody screen** when appropriate, in addition to a **complete blood cell (CBC) count. Other causes** of thrombocytopenia (e.g., SLE) **should be considered,** particularly in **older girls.**

✂ HINT Evans syndrome—autoimmune hemolytic anemia with thrombocytopenia—is evidenced by a positive DAT and an elevated reticulocyte count and usually requires more intensive intervention than does acute ITP.

Routine **bone marrow aspiration** to evaluate acute ITP is controversial; however, the procedure should be considered **before initiating steroid therapy** to avoid partially treating an unusual presentation of acute leukemia. **Increased platelet precursors** (megakaryocytes) are seen on **histologic examination** of bone marrow aspirate in patients with ITP.

Treatment

Many believe that treating patients with acute ITP is often **unnecessary.** If a child experiences **significant blood loss, treatment is warranted.** Treatment options include **intravenous immunoglobulin** (800 mg/kg), steroids (2 mg/kg/day for 1–4 weeks), and, in Rh-positive children, **anti-D immune globulin** (50–75 μg/kg). Intravenous immunoglobulin administration is associated with a more rapid increase in platelet count than steroid therapy. If a patient with known ITP requires therapy, then it is best to use whatever therapy has been beneficial for that patient in the past.

Intracranial hemorrhage and **life-threatening hemorrhage,** although rare in patients with ITP, may be fatal. Therefore, **treatment is mandatory** if the ITP patient has **head trauma,** an **abnormal neurologic examination,** or **copious blood loss. High-dose steroid therapy** with intravenous immunoglobulin administration should be initiated rapidly before more detailed evaluations. In patients with ongoing life-threatening bleeding, **continuous platelet transfusions, emergent splenectomy, or both** may be necessary.

Disseminated Intravascular Coagulation (DIC)

Etiology

DIC is a **consumptive coagulopathy** that is characterized by **uncontrolled activation of coagulation** and **fibrinolysis** associated with an underlying disease (Table 18.1).

✂ HINT The acute critically ill child should be considered septic until proven otherwise.

TABLE 18.1. Causes of Disseminated Intravascular Coagulation (DIC)

Infection—bacterial, viral, fungal, rickettsial
Cardiovascular disorder—shock
Toxins—snake bites
Tumors—myeloid leukemia
Trauma—massive generalized or head trauma
Hematologic disorder—hemolytic transfusion reactions
Miscellaneous causes—burns, purpura fulminans, severe asphyxia

Clinical Features

Children with DIC usually **appear ill** and **bleed from multiple sites.** In neonates, DIC usually manifests as **gastrointestinal bleeding** or **oozing from skin puncture sites.**

Evaluation

In patients with DIC, laboratory values show a **normal or decreased platelet count, increased prothrombin time (PT) and partial thromboplastin time (PTT), decreased fibrinogen,** and **increased fibrin split products.** A peripheral blood smear is significant for **schistocytes, fragmented red blood cells (RBCs),** and **normal or decreased platelets.**

Treatment

Treatment is directed toward managing the underlying disorder and **replacing coagulation factors and platelets.**

Hemolytic-Uremic Syndrome

Hemolytic-uremic syndrome is discussed in Chapter 79, "Urine Output, Decreased."

Kasabach-Merritt Syndrome

Clinical Features and Evaluation

Kasabach-Merritt syndrome is characterized by **hemangiomas** and a **consumptive thrombocytopenia.** The hemangiomas are generally large with a cavernous component and are found on the **neck, trunk, or extremities;** however, the **lesions can be small** and located on visceral organs, making the diagnosis difficult.

Laboratory findings include **thrombocytopenia** and, at times, **schistocytes** on the peripheral blood smear. The **PT and PTT may be prolonged,** suggesting a consumptive coagulopathy.

Treatment

Treatment entails management of the hemangioma. If **surgery** is planned, the physician should be aware that manipulating these lesions **can exacerbate the thrombocytopenia,** the **consumptive coagulopathy, or both.**

Wiskott-Aldrich Syndrome

Etiology

Wiskott-Aldrich syndrome is an **X-linked recessive disorder** characterized by **severe eczema, immunodeficiency,** and **thrombocytopenia** with small platelets. The thrombocytopenia is caused by poor marrow production and immune destruction.

Evaluation

Diagnosis is confirmed by **immunologic** as well as **hematologic testing.**

Treatment

Splenectomy improves the thrombocytopenia but **increases the patient's risk of sepsis.**

Henoch-Schönlein Purpura

Etiology and Incidence

Henoch-Schönlein purpura is an **acquired inflammatory vascular disorder.** The exact **cause is unknown;** however, Henoch-Schönlein purpura is thought to be an **immune process** and the disease is often referred to as **allergic or anaphylactoid purpura.** The age range is 6 months to 16 years, but Henoch-Schönlein purpura is **most common in early childhood,** with most patients presenting in the first decade of life.

Clinical Features

Diffuse inflammation of the small vessels causes **abdominal pain, arthritis,** and **palpable purpura.** Renal involvement occurs in 50% of patients. Most patients have a **prodromal upper respiratory infection** 1–3 weeks before the onset of illness. The **hallmark** of this disorder on physical examination is a **symmetric pattern of purpura,** primarily involving the **buttocks and lower extremities.** In some patients, purpura are also found on the extensor surfaces of the arms. The palms, soles, and genitalia are spared.

Evaluation

Hematuria, proteinuria, and **cellular casts on urinalysis** confirm nephritis in patients with Henoch-Schönlein purpura. The CBC, PT, and PTT are normal unless major gastrointestinal blood loss has occurred, in which case the **hemoglobin may be low.**

Treatment

Henoch-Schönlein purpura, a **self-limited disorder,** usually resolves in 1–6 weeks. Treatment primarily involves supportive therapy. **Corticosteroids** are used to alleviate gastrointestinal and, less often, musculoskeletal symptoms.

von Willebrand Disease (vWD)

Etiology

vWD, the **most common inherited bleeding disorder,** is characterized by an **abnormal von Willebrand factor (vWF)–factor VIII complex.** The complex is either quantitatively or qualitatively abnormal. Patients with vWD can be classified as having **type 1, type 2, type 3, or platelet-type** vWD, according to the clinical history and laboratory test results. Approximately 65%–80% of vWD patients have type 1 vWD. The mild form of this inherited disease is primarily autosomal dominant, although the severe variant is autosomal recessive.

Clinical Features

Children with vWD present with **mucocutaneous bleeding. Epistaxis, gum oozing, menorrhagia,** and **easy bruising** are common complaints. Patients with type 3 (severe) vWD may develop **joint and intramuscular bleeding.**

Evaluation

Laboratory findings are significant for a **prolonged PTT,** a **prolonged bleeding time, or both,** although these screening tests may be normal at times in some patients with vWD. **Additional laboratory evaluation,** including ristocetin cofactor, factor VIII–related antigen (vWF), and factor VIII:coagulant (factor VIII:C) evaluation, should be done by a **hematologist.** Patients with vWD may have decreased factor VIII:C activity, decreased vWF, decreased ristocetin cofactor, or a combination of the three findings.

Treatment

Multiple treatment options are available for patients with vWD, depending on the type of vWD, as well as the safety and cost effectiveness of particular therapies. **Desmopressin acetate,** an analog of vasopressin, is often used to treat or prevent bleeding episodes in patients with **type 1** vWD, although its use is controversial in patients with type 2B and platelet-type vWD. **Type 2B and type 3 patients** can receive **factor VIII concentrate** with retained vWF activity and those with **platelet-type vWD** may need **platelet transfusions,** depending on their past experience with blood products.

Hemophilia A and B (Factor VIII and Factor IX Deficiencies)

Etiology and Incidence

Factor VIII deficiency (hemophilia A) occurs in 1 of every 10,000 live male births, and factor IX deficiency (hemophilia B) occurs in 1 of every 40,000 live male births. Most patients have a **family history of bleeding disorders,** but spontaneous mutations are responsible for about 30% of cases of hemophilia.

Clinical Features

Children with factor VIII and factor IX deficiencies develop similar clinical features depending on the severity of the factor deficiency. In **infancy,** there can be **excessive bleeding after circumcision or bruising at injection sites.** Later in **childhood** patients develop **easy bruisability, large hematomas,** and **hemarthroses or intramuscular hemorrhages** (the hallmarks of hemophilia). Patients with severe factor deficiencies can experience **bleeding episodes spontaneously** or **following trauma.** Patients with moderate or **mild factor deficiencies** rarely have spontaneous hemorrhages, but are at risk for **posttraumatic bleeding** and bleeding after **surgical procedures.** The **most common cause of morbidity is recurrent hemarthroses.**

Evaluation

Laboratory evaluation should include a **platelet count,** a **PT,** a **PTT,** and a **bleeding time.** In patients with factor VIII or IX deficiency, the PTT is prolonged, but the PT is normal. Therefore, in patients with an isolated prolonged PTT, levels of factors VIII and IX should be measured. Severe factor VIII or IX deficiency is classified by factor activity levels of less than 1%. Patients with moderate disease have levels of 1%–5%, and those with mild disease have levels of 5%–20%.

Treatment

The most **serious hemorrhages** in patients with hemophilia are **intracranial, retropharyngeal, retroperitoneal,** and those involving the **airway.** The goal of treatment in these circumstances is to achieve a factor activity level of 100% and to offer appropriate supportive therapy.

▼ **Intracranial hemorrhage.** In patients with severe factor deficiency, intracranial hemorrhage may be spontaneous; therefore, any patient with severe factor deficiency who has a change in mental status or other neurologic findings should be treated for an intracranial hemorrhage until radiologic studies prove negative. Intravenous access and factor replacement should occur before obtaining a head computed tomography (CT) scan. Factor VIII and IX deficiencies cause poor secondary clot formation, so that bleeding usually occurs hours after the initial trauma. Therefore, a negative head CT scan does not exclude a slowly developing intracranial hemorrhage. Many clinicians admit children following head trauma, particularly those who have severe factor deficiency, to inpatient wards for observation, with frequent neurologic examinations.

▼ **Intramuscular bleeding** can be massive, leading to shock. The muscles of the thigh and the iliopsoas muscle in particular can accommodate large volumes of blood. Patients with hemophilia should be admitted to the hospital for close monitoring and bed rest if bleeding occurs in these areas. Extensive intramuscular bleeding can compromise vascular blood flow and cause compartment syndromes. Tingling, numbness, or loss of pulses in an extremity requires immediate factor replacement to 100% and an orthopedic evaluation.

▼ **Joint bleeds (hemarthroses)** require treatment with factor products and immobilization to avoid chronic complications (e.g., decreased mobility, contractures). The goal of factor replacement for hemarthroses depends on the child's individual bleeding history, but in general, factor replacement should be aimed at obtaining an activity level of 30%–50% for 1–2 days. If recurrent hemarthroses have developed in the affected joint (the so-called 'target' joint), then higher factor activity levels should be obtained. Today, many patients receive factor on a regular or "prophylactic" schedule to prevent recurrent joint bleeds. This approach to hemophilia treatment requires the guidance of a hematologist or a hemophilia specialist.

▼ **Moderate hemorrhages** involving muscles, hematomas, or lacerations usually require treatment to reach a peak factor activity level of 30%. Oral mucosa bleeding may require factor correction and α-aminocaproic acid therapy. α-Aminocaproic acid therapy decreases mouth bleeding by inhibiting clot breakdown and is contraindicated in patients with hematuria or DIC.

▼ **Hematuria** can occur spontaneously in patients with severe hemophilia, or after trauma in patients with moderate-to-mild disease. Treatment is directed toward cessation of bleeding while avoiding obstruction, which could lead to an obstructive uropathy. Factor replacement, hydration, and bed rest are recommended.

▼ **Replacement therapy for dental or surgical procedures.** Patients with factors VIII and IX deficiencies must receive replacement therapy before dental, surgical, or other general procedures, including laceration repair, suture removal, or spinal tap. The patient's hematologist should be consulted before initiating any procedures.

▼ **Factor inhibitors.** Of patients with factor VIII deficiency, about 10%–25% develop factor inhibitors (i.e., antibodies to factor VIII). Patients who do not improve clinically after receiving the appropriate dosage of factor and who have complied with supportive care measures (e.g., splinting, avoidance of weight bearing with hemarthroses) should be evaluated for the presence of a factor inhibitor. Patients with factor inhibitors require alternative treatment options.

Factor XI Deficiency

Factor XI deficiency is an autosomal disorder primarily affecting persons of **Ashkenazi descent.** This bleeding disorder is **mild,** including **epistaxis, menorrhagia,** and **postoperative bleeding.** The **PTT is prolonged** in these patients and the diagnosis is confirmed by a factor-specific assay.

Factor XII Deficiency

This deficiency is characterized by a **prolonged PTT** with a **normal PT and bleeding time.** Factor XII-deficient patients are **not at risk for increased bleeding.**

Infection-Related Purpura

An **acute febrile illness** associated with a **petechial rash** may indicate a **benign, self-limited viral process** or a **severe, life-threatening bacterial illness** (e.g., meningococcal infection). Therefore, ill-appearing **children with fever and petechiae should be considered septic until proven otherwise.**

Infections can cause purpura by a wide variety of mechanisms. Severe bacterial infections are often associated with DIC. Viral illness can be associated with thrombocytopenia from increased platelet destruction (e.g., ITP) or from decreased production. In addition to causing thrombocytopenia, bacterial, fungal, and viral illnesses can cause **platelet dysfunction** and **vascular abnormalities.**

Drug-Related Purpura

Drug-induced thrombocytopenia in the hospital setting is most often caused by **chemotherapeutic agents** that suppress bone marrow activity. **Heparin, quinidine, digoxin, penicillin,** and **seizure medications** (e.g., valproic acid) can cause immune-mediated thrombocytopenia, which generally **reverses when the drug is discontinued.** Some drugs, such as H_2 **blockers,** are associated with **idiopathic thrombocytopenia.**

Drug-induced platelet dysfunction as a result of cyclooxygenase enzyme inhibition is seen with **aspirin-containing compounds** and to a lesser degree with **nonsteroidal anti-inflammatory drugs** such as ibuprofen. **Penicillins** and **cephalosporins** can also cause platelet dysfunction, particularly in children with systemic disease. Platelet function should **return to normal 7–10 days** after the offending drug is discontinued.

▼ DIFFERENTIAL DIAGNOSIS DISCUSSION II: BLEEDING AND PURPURA IN NEONATES

Bleeding and purpura in the neonate presents a slightly different differential diagnosis than bleeding in the child.

⚡ HINT Patients whose mothers took aspirin, phenytoin, warfarin, or thiazide diuretics are at increased bleeding risk during the neonatal period.

Vitamin K Deficiency (Hemorrhagic Disease of the Newborn)

Etiology

In the past, vitamin K deficiency was **primarily a disease of breast-fed infants** because cow's milk contains four to ten times the amount of vitamin K found in human breast milk. As a result, vitamin K prophylaxis is recommended for all newborns at birth to prevent hemorrhagic disease in the high-risk breast-fed group.

Clinical Features and Evaluation

Presently, vitamin K deficiency is most common in breast-fed infants who have missed their vitamin K prophylaxis. Affected infants may present with **excessive bleeding at 2–5 days of age.** The infant will have **PT and PTT elevations above the normal range** for gestational age.

---

𝟐 HINT Ill neonates who are transferred from other institutions may not have received vitamin K before transport. Infants of mothers taking phenobarbital are at increased risk for hemorrhagic disease of the newborn.

Treatment

Treatment is the administration of **1 mg vitamin K_1 parenterally.**

Neonatal Alloimmune (Isoimmune) Thrombocytopenia

Etiology

Neonatal alloimmune (isoimmune) thrombocytopenia is characterized by **moderate-to-severe isolated thrombocytopenia.** This **antibody-mediated destruction of platelets** is analogous to hemolytic disease of the newborn and occurs when **maternal antibodies** that are directed against paternal antigens found on the patient's platelets cross the placenta, entering the patient's circulation. These antibodies cause increased platelet destruction in the neonate. The most common offending antigen is PLA-1. Thrombocytopenia will persist as long as the maternal antibodies are found in the patient's circulation, usually **21 days or less.**

Clinical Features

The infant with neonatal alloimmune (isoimmune) thrombocytopenia is generally well appearing, but may have **petechiae, ecchymoses,** and **mucosal membrane bleeding** within the **first 48 hours of life,** depending on the platelet count. Petechiae and ecchymoses can be found at **injection sites** as well as at pressure points, such as the **extensor surfaces of the knees** and on the **abdomen** where diapering causes pressure. **Intracranial hemorrhage** has been reported in 10%–15% of patients.

Evaluation

Thrombocytopenia **can be severe,** with a platelet count of less than $20,000/mm^3$. The mother's platelet count is normal. **Finding maternal antibodies to paternal platelets** strongly suggests this diagnosis. The diagnosis is confirmed by isolating alloantibodies in the mother's serum, but the results are often negative.

Treatment

In the absence of bleeding, many recommend keeping the platelet count greater than $30,000/mm^3$ for the first few weeks of life. **If bleeding is severe or signs of intracranial hemorrhage are present, treatment is critical. Transfusing the infant with the mother's washed, irradiated platelets** increases the platelet count because the mother's platelets are missing the antigen against which the antibody is aimed. **Intravenous immune globulin** (IVIg) and corticosteroids can increase the infant's counts and some clinicians prefer the pharmacological approach to therapy. In **emergent situations, PLA-(–) platelets or single-donor platelets** can be used if maternal platelets are not available.

Neonatal Autoimmune Thrombocytopenia

Etiology

This type of thrombocytopenia is **secondary to an autoimmune disorder in the mother** (e.g., ITP, SLE, lymphoproliferative disorder, hyperthyroidism). Antibodies are found to maternal and patient platelets in patients with this condition.

Clinical Features and Evaluation

Infants are well-appearing and may develop **petechiae within the first 2 days of life.** The diagnosis is made by the clinical presentation of the mother and infant. The infant should have a **low platelet count with a normal PT and PTT.**

Treatment

IVIg should be administered to **patients showing signs of bleeding.** Steroid therapy should be considered in **patients who do not respond to immunoglobulin.** Life-threatening hemorrhage should be treated with **high-dose steroids** and **continuous platelet transfusion.**

Nonimmune Causes of Thrombocytopenia

Consumptive coagulopathies (e.g., DIC) and coagulopathies associated with **sepsis, asphyxia, respiratory distress, or necrotizing enterocolitis** are the most common nonimmune causes of thrombocytopenia in ill neonates. Thrombocytopenia **secondary to thrombus formation from renal vein thrombosis or catheter-related thrombi** is also a frequent occurrence. Thrombocytopenia after exchange transfusion or extracorporeal membrane oxygenation is a normal finding. Nonimmune causes of thrombocytopenia in the sick neonate also include **congenital viral infections** and **hyperbilirubinemia treated with phototherapy. Kasabach-Merritt syndrome** should be considered in neonates with thrombocytopenia and hemangioma.

✄ HINT Patients of diabetic mothers are at increased risk of polycythemia and renal vein thromboses.

✄ HINT If congenital anomalies are present on physical examination of a neonate with purpura or abnormal bleeding, TAR, Wiskott-Aldrich syndrome, Fanconi anemia, Chédiak-Higashi syndrome, and trisomy 21 should be considered.

Treatment is directed toward treating the underlying problem, factor replacement with fresh frozen plasma and cryoprecipitate, and platelet transfusions (if needed).

▼ EVALUATION OF BLEEDING AND PURPURA

Patient History

When evaluating a child with abnormal bleeding, a careful history and physical examination can direct the approach to patient management (Table 10.2). Important questions to ask pertain to the following:

▼ **Time frame.** The time frame over which the petechiae or bruises developed is important. Prior intermittent episodes of bruising or bleeding in an ill-appearing child may indicate a chronic process associated with systemic illness or malignancy. However, the well-appearing patient who experiences a rapid onset of bruising and petechiae most likely has an acquired condition, such as ITP.

▼ **Prior bleeding or bruising episodes.** The physician should ask questions about bleeding or bruising episodes since birth, such as epistaxis, menses, or excessive bleeding after surgical procedures (e.g., circumcision, tonsillectomy, dental extractions). These questions should be made in reference to family members as well as the patient. A child who presents with repeated hemarthroses and a history of requiring a blood transfusion after an uncomplicated surgical procedure most likely has a congenital bleeding disorder, whereas normal hemostasis after major surgical procedures (e.g., a tonsillectomy) makes the diagnosis of an inherited disorder of hemostasis unlikely. An exception is patients with severe hemophilia—50% who are circumcised in the newborn period without factor replacement do not have excessive hemorrhage.

⚡ HINT Remember that children may not have been exposed to situations such as surgery that would reveal a disorder of hemostasis.

▼ **Location.** The location of the bleeding is important. Unilateral epistaxis in a child who frequently traumatizes his nasal mucosa is usually normal. However, prolonged bilateral epistaxis in a child covered with bruises and petechiae is abnormal.

▼ **Medication history.** Certain drugs, especially aspirin and ibuprofen, are associated with platelet dysfunction. Some drugs can exacerbate bleeding in a patient with an underlying bleeding disorder. Children with vWD may bruise more easily after taking cough preparations or antihistamines.

Physical Examination

The physical examination should include the **skin, mucous membranes,** and **fundi.** The type of lesions, pattern of lesions, and the location, size, and stage of resolution of the lesions should be documented.

Types of Lesions

▼ **Petechiae** are small (less than 3 mm in diameter), macular, nonblanching erythematous lesions. They are most common on the face and chest, but may involve any skin area.

TABLE 18.2.   Clinical Evaluation of Pediatric Patients with Suspected Bleeding Disorders

Question	If the Answer is "Yes," Consider …
History	
When the child bleeds from an injury, does the bleeding stop and then resume?	Coagulation disorder
When the child bleeds from a superficial cut, is the bleeding profuse?	Platelet disorder
Does the patient have a history of fever?	Infection
Does the patient have a history of fever and neurologic manifestations?	Meningococcemia, TTP
Is there a history of a viral prodrome?	Hemolytic-uremic syndrome, ITP
Has the patient had repeated episodes of bleeding gums, prolonged bleeding from cuts, or massive bleeding from surgical procedures? Has the patient developed large hematomas at vaccination sites? Did the patient experience prolonged bleeding as a result of circumcision?	Congenital disorder
Do other family members have problems with easy bruising or abnormal bleeding?	Congenital disorder
Does the patient have a known chronic illness?	Coagulation or platelet disorder associated with systemic illness
Is the patient currently taking aspirin, ibuprofen, antibiotics, antihistamines, steroids, or oral contraceptives?	Drug-related purpura
Has the patient received multiple blood or platelet transfusions in the past as well as recently?	Posttransfusion purpura and alloimmunization
Could the child have ingested rat poison?	Warfarin toxicity
Does the patient have a history of delayed wound healing, rebleeding episodes, or umbilical stump bleeding?	Factor XIII deficiency
If the patient is a neonate, have there been multiple catheter placements or catheter complications?	Consumptive coagulopathy, thrombocytopenia, or both
If the patient is a neonate, is there a history of a difficult or traumatic delivery? Did the infant have a low APGAR score?	DIC or other consumptive coagulopathy
If the patient is a neonate, did the mother take phenytoin?	Vitamin K deficiency
Physical examination	
Are predominant findings on examination large ecchymoses or hemarthroses?	Coagulation disorder
Are predominant findings on examination petechiae or ecchymoses?	Platelet disorder
Are purpura symmetric and predominantly located on the legs and buttocks?	Henoch-Schönlein purpura
Are ecchymotic lesions extensive and in various stages of resolution?	Physical abuse
Is there lymphadenopathy with hepatosplenomegaly?	Leukemia, lymphoma, infection
Are there palpable purpura with a history of minimal trauma?	Platelet disorder, coagulation disorder
Is there umbilical stump bleeding?	Factor XIII deficiency
Is there jaundice and bruising?	Hepatic disease (factor deficiency)
Laboratory studies: Does the patient have a:	
Low platelet count with a normal PT and PTT?	Thrombocytopenia
Normal platelet count, PT, and PTT, but an abnormal bleeding time?	Platelet function abnormality
Normal platelet count, PT, PTT, and bleeding time?	Vascular disorder, vWD, factor XIII deficiency

Continued

TABLE 18.2. Clinical Evaluation of Pediatric Patients with Suspected Bleeding Disorders (continued)

Question	If the Answer is "Yes," Consider ...
Normal platelet count, PTT, and bleeding time, but a prolonged PT?	Factor VII deficiency
Normal platelet count, PT, and bleeding time, but a prolonged PTT?	Factor VIII, IX, or XI deficiency, vWD, or heparin effect
Normal platelet count but a prolonged PT and PTT?	DIC, vitamin K deficiency, hepatic disease, quantitative or qualitative fibrinogen disorder, warfarin or heparin effect, lupus anticoagulant
Normal PT and PTT, but a low platelet count and prolonged bleeding time?	vWD (type 2B, platelet-type), Bernard-Soulier disease, Chédiak-Higashi syndrome, platelet granule defects
Markedly low platelet count and small platelets?	Wiskott-Aldrich syndrome
Markedly low platelet count and large platelets?	ITP, Bernard-Soulier disease
Low platelet count, prolonged PT and PTT, and schistocytes?	DIC, microangiopathic process

DIC = disseminated intravascular coagulation; ITP = idiopathic (immune) thrombocytopenic purpura; PT = prothrombin time; PTT = partial thromboplastin time; TTP = thrombotic thrombocytopenic purpura; vWD = von Willebrand disease.

▼ **Ecchymotic lesions** are large and can be macular, tender, or raised. Recent injuries are usually purple, fading over time to yellowish-brown. Palpable ecchymotic lesions (raised lesions with a central nodule) are rarely a normal finding in children but are found often in boys with hemophilia.

▼ **Purpura fulminans** (purplish-black, well-demarcated, stellate lesions with central necrosis) are usually associated with DIC. They can be extensive and painful.

Findings Suggestive of a Bleeding Disorder

A child who meets any of the following criteria should be screened for a bleeding disorder:

▼ Excessive purpura involving many sites, particularly areas not normally traumatized (e.g., flexor surfaces of the arms or the axillary and inguinal regions)
▼ Many purpuric lesions of the same stage
▼ Palpable ecchymotic lesions
▼ Observed purpura or bleeding that exceeds what is expected for the child's activity level
▼ Purpura, excessive bleeding, or both in an ill-appearing child

Laboratory Evaluation

The diagnosis of a bleeding disorder in a child may not be straightforward. Children with abnormal laboratory values may not be at risk for excessive bleeding, whereas those with normal laboratory values may be. Children with **factor XII deficiency or lupus anticoagulants** are **not at risk for increased**

bleeding although their PTT values are prolonged. Conversely, children with **factor XIII deficiency or vasculitic disorders** have normal laboratory values but are at **increased risk for bleeding.**

A laboratory screening evaluation includes the following:

▼ **CBC with a platelet count.** Thrombocytopenia is a platelet count less than 150,000/mm³. Thrombocytopenia determined by automated systems should be confirmed by peripheral blood smear examination.

▼ **PT and PTT.** Normal values for PT and PTT vary according to the patient's age and the testing system used in the coagulation laboratory. PT measures the activity of factors II, V, VII, and X. PTT measures factors V, VIII, IX, X, XI, and XII. The PT reflects the extrinsic and common pathways of coagulation, whereas the PTT evaluates the intrinsic and common pathways.

⚡ **HINT** Blood for PT and PTT analysis must be obtained from a blood vessel large enough to provide free-flowing blood. Blood obtained for PT and PTT via "difficult sticks" may falsely decrease the laboratory values.

▼ **Peripheral blood smear.** Platelet, RBC, and white blood cell morphology can be helpful in narrowing the differential diagnosis. Large platelets are seen in ITP, Bernard-Soulier syndrome, and May-Hegglin anomaly. Small platelets are seen in Wiskott-Aldrich syndrome. Schistocytes accompanying a decreased platelet count suggest a microangiopathic process. WBC blasts on the peripheral blood smear suggest leukemia.

▼ **Bone marrow aspirate and biopsy.** A bone marrow aspirate and biopsy are often obtained to clarify the cause of the thrombocytopenia (i.e., increased platelet destruction or decreased platelet production). Increased megakaryocytes on a bone marrow aspirate and biopsy suggest increased peripheral destruction of platelets, whereas decreased megakaryocytes suggest decreased production.

▼ **Bleeding time.** If the initial laboratory evaluation of a patient with significant purpura, bleeding, or both is negative, then a bleeding time should be performed. Bleeding times reflect platelet quantity and the quality of platelet function. Results vary according to the experience of the laboratory technician, particularly with children. If the CBC, PT, PTT, and bleeding time are normal, a vascular abnormality or normal posttraumatic purpura is the most probable diagnosis. However, the diagnosis of vWD cannot be eliminated unless repeated evaluations are negative.

▼ TREATMENT OF BLEEDING AND PURPURA

For patients without a known diagnosis who are experiencing **life-threatening bleeding, treatment** must be initiated before a specific diagnosis can be established. **Blood products** should be used to stabilize the patient, particularly if active bleeding cannot be controlled by pressure or other mechanical means. At least 5 ml of blood should be placed in a sodium citrate tube before blood-product transfusion for coagulation studies, a CBC, a PT, and a PTT.

TABLE 18.3. Treatment of Common Childhood Bleeding Disorders

Bleeding Disorder	Treatment	Potential Complications of Therapy
Idiopathic (immune) thrombocytopenic purpura (ITP)*	Intravenous immunoglobulin	Headaches, neutropenia, volume overload, aseptic meningitis, allergic reactions, virus transmission
	Steroids	Partial treatment of leukemia, psychosis, fluid imbalance, hypertension
	Anti-D immune globulin	Hemolysis, virus transmission, allergic reactions
	Continuous platelet transfusion (for life-threatening hemorrhage)	Virus transmission, transfusion reactions
Disseminated intravascular coagulation (DIC)	Fresh frozen plasma	Virus transmission, allergic reactions
	Platelet and packed red blood cell (RBC) transfusion	Virus transmission, transfusion reactions
	Cryoprecipitate	Virus transmission
Henoch-Schönlein purpura	Steroids†	Fluid imbalance, psychosis, hypertension
Neonatal isoimmune thrombocytopenia	Transfusion of mother's washed, irradiated or PLA-1 negative platelets, IVIg, or steroids	...
Platelet function abnormalities	Platelet transfusion (for life-threatening hemorrhage)	Virus transmission, transfusion reactions
von Willebrand disease (vWD)	Desmopressin acetate (DDAVP)	Thrombocytopenia in patients with type 2B or platelet-type vWD
Type 2B and platelet-type vWD	Platelet transfusion or cryoprecipitate administration	...

* The necessity of treating acute ITP is controversial.

† Considered for patients with gastrointestinal or joint symptoms.

If the **bleeding is not life threatening,** a **diagnosis should be established before treatment.** Once a diagnosis is made, treatment (using the most specific, safest, and cost-effective product) should be initiated in conjunction with a **hematologist** (Table 18.3).

▼ APPROACH TO THE PATIENT (FIGURE 18.1)

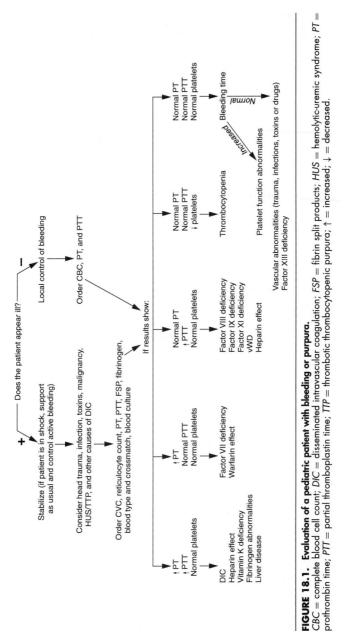

FIGURE 18.1. Evaluation of a pediatric patient with bleeding or purpura.
CBC = complete blood cell count; *DIC* = disseminated intravascular coagulation; *FSP* = fibrin split products; *HUS* = hemolytic-uremic syndrome; *PT* = prothrombin time; *PTT* = partial thromboplastin time; *TTP* = thrombotic thrombocytopenic purpura; ↑ = increased; ↓ = decreased.

Suggested Readings

Bell WR Jr: Long-term outcome of splenectomy for idiopathic thrombocytopenic purpura. *Semin Hematol* 37(1 suppl 1):22–25, 2000.

Bolton-Maggs PH: Idiopathic thrombocytopenic purpura. *Arch Dis Child* 83(3):220–222, 2000.

Katsanis E, Luike KJ, Hsu Li M, et al.: Prevalence and significance of mild bleeding disorders in children with recurrent epistaxis. *J Pediatr* 113:73–76, 1988.

Manno CS: Difficult pediatric diagnoses: bruising and bleeding. *Pediatr Clin North Am* 38:637, 1991.

Medeiros D. Buchanan GR: Idiopathic thrombocytopenic purpura: beyond consensus. *Curr Opin Pediatr* 12(1):4–9, 2000.

Ochs HD: The Wiskott-Aldrich syndrome. *Clin Rev Allergy Immunol* 20(1):61–86, 2001.

Pramanik AK: Bleeding disorders in neonates. *Pediatr Rev* 13:163, 1992.

Saulsbury FT: Henoch-Schonlein purpura. *Curr Opin Rheumatol* 13(1):35–40, 2001.

Saulsbury FT: Henoch-Schonlein purpura in children. Report of 100 patients and review of the literature. *Medicine* 78(6):395–409, 1999.

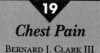

19

Chest Pain

BERNARD J. CLARK III

▼ INTRODUCTION

Chest pain in children is **common** and produces a **high level of anxiety** in parents because of its perceived association with heart disease. However, with the exception of a few uncommon, serious conditions, **chest pain in children is not related to cardiac disease.** Nearly 0.5% of all pediatric patient visits to the emergency room involve chest pain as a primary or secondary complaint. Patients seen in the office with this complaint tend to have subacute or chronic chest pain of a sporadic or episodic nature. In long-term studies, idiopathic chest pain is by far the most common diagnosis. For these reasons, the work-up of chest pain is directed toward **ruling out serious causes** and then instituting a period of **close observation.** Like chest pain, **syncope** in children is **common** and is usually benign and self-limited. There are, however, **uncommon cardiac causes** that should be considered, especially in the child who presents with **recurrent syncope** or syncope and a **family history of syncope or sudden cardiac arrest.**

▼ DIFFERENTIAL DIAGNOSIS LIST

Cardiac Causes

Myocarditis

Pericarditis

Aortic stenosis
Subaortic stenosis
Hypertrophic cardiomyopathy
Coronary artery anomalies
Arrhythmia
Mitral valve prolapse

Noncardiac Causes

Idiopathic
Musculoskeletal problems
Costochondritis
Pneumonia or Pleurisy
Asthma
Cough or upper respiratory infection
Gastrointestinal reflux

▼ DIFFERENTIAL DIAGNOSIS DISCUSSION

The differential for cardiac chest pain in children includes **inflammation** of the myocardium or pericardium, **arrhythmias,** and **structural abnormalities** such as aortic stenosis, subaortic stenosis, coronary artery anomalies, or coronary arteritis and mitral valve prolapse. A normal **electrocardiogram (ECG)** and **chest radiograph (CXR)** can rule out many of these possibilities.

Myocarditis and Pericarditis

In patients referred to a pediatric cardiologist for evaluation of chest pain, the most common serious causes of cardiac chest pain are myocarditis and pericarditis.

▼ **Myocarditis usually follows a viral illness.** Patients typically present with symptoms of **shortness of breath, nonspecific chest pain, anorexia,** or **malaise.** A physical examination may reveal the presence of an **S3 or gallop rhythm.** The CXR typically reveals **cardiomegaly,** although early in the illness it may reveal normal heart size. The **ECG reveals** changes, most typically **ST segment depression** and **T-wave abnormalities,** especially in the inferior leads (II, III, AVF, V6, V7). In these patients, the myocardium is directly affected. Therefore, they should be referred to a pediatric cardiologist for echocardiographic assessment of ventricular function. The inflammation that causes myocarditis can also directly affect the conduction system. Therefore, patients with myocarditis may present with **arrhythmias.** These arrhythmias tend to improve when inflammation resolves. In patients who develop persistent cardiomyopathy, arrhythmias may persist.

▼ **Pericarditis** more frequently presents with an **acute onset of sharp chest pain,** which is **lessened by leaning forward.** Pericarditis can result from **infectious** or **autoimmune disorders.** A physical examination reveals **neck vein distention, pulsus paradoxus,** and the presence of a **friction rub,** occasionally with both a systolic and diastolic component. These findings are caused by pericardial fluid collection, resulting from inflammation of the pericardium. In the presence of a large pericardial effusion, an ECG often reveals **low-voltage QRS complexes.** The ECG can also reveal **ST-T wave changes,** as in myocarditis. When a patient presents with these symptoms, a CXR demonstrating cardiomegaly, or an ECG showing the abnormalities mentioned, referral to a **cardiologist** is warranted.

Myocarditis and pericarditis occur after an inflammatory process that is usually an **ECHO virus** and is **most often coxsackie B.** Viral titers can help to determine the specific cause. Since Lyme disease may cause myocarditis, for a patient who presents with chest pain and a history of tick bite in an endemic area, **Lyme titers** should be obtained. Other inflammatory causes include **autoimmune disorders,** such as lupus erythematosus.

Aortic and Subaortic Stenosis

A history of chest pain in a child who also has a significant murmur may suggest **left ventricular outflow tract obstruction** caused by **aortic valve stenosis** or stenosis below the aortic valve, as in idiopathic hypertrophic subaortic stenosis (IHSS). In these patients, chest pain is equivalent to ischemic pain. **Pain occurs during exercise** because the ability to increase cardiac output is limited by the left ventricular outflow obstruction. The limited cardiac output, coupled with a fall in systemic vascular resistance during exercise, results in **coronary underperfusion** and subsequent **myocardial ischemia.**

Physical findings in patients with aortic stenosis can include a **systolic ejection click,** a **harsh systolic ejection murmur** over the base of the heart that radiates to the carotid arteries, and, frequently, a **palpable thrill in the suprasternal notch.** These patients can have normal ECGs or ECGs that suggest left ventricular hypertrophy. A patient with a significant murmur and chest pain should be referred for an **echocardiogram.**

Hypertrophic Cardiomyopathy

Another variation of **left ventricular outflow tract obstruction** is **hypertrophic cardiomyopathy.** Because IHSS can be an autosomal dominant disorder, a **thorough family history** is helpful. These patients have a **systolic murmur** that is **enhanced on standing or subjection to the Valsalva maneuver.** These maneuvers decrease left ventricular volume and thus increase the degree of outflow obstruction. Patients with a history of chest pain and a systolic murmur should be referred to a **cardiologist.**

Coronary Artery Anomalies

Anomalies of the coronary arteries, such as anomalous left coronary artery or coronary arteritis, are **uncommon.** When they present, however, the **ECG** is almost invariably **abnormal** with evidence of **left ventricular hypertrophy** and **abnormal ST segments or inverted T waves** in the left precordial leads. Most patients with anomalous left coronary artery present as **infants in a shock-like state.** This anomaly is unusual in childhood. When a young child presents with chest pain, it is important to inquire about **previous Kawasaki disease.** Of all patients with this diagnosis, 15% develop **coronary artery aneurysms** in the subacute phase of the illness about 3 to 6 weeks after diagnosis. Half of all aneurysms resolve spontaneously.

Arrhythmia

Patients who present with symptoms of **chest pain** or chest pain and **dizziness** with or without syncope may experience arrhythmias. Younger children may perceive palpitations as chest pain, and the additional symptoms of dizziness or syncope suggest an arrhythmia and require evaluation. All patients suspected of having arrhythmias should have an **ECG** during initial evaluation. In addition to obtaining a rhythm strip to assess for rhythm disturbances, all baseline intervals should be **assessed for heart block** and for **prolonged QTc syndrome.** This interval can be prolonged secondary to electrolyte imbalance (hypocalcemia), medications (class I antiarrhythmics, such as quinidine and procainamide, antidepressants, antipsychotics), or because of the long QTc syndrome. Patients with prolonged QTc syndrome are **prone to ventricular arrhythmias** and should be referred to a **cardiologist** for further evaluation and therapy.

Sinus Arrhythmia

Arrhythmias can also present as **isolated chest pain.** In sinus arrhythmia, **normal in children,** the **heart rate slows during inspiration** because of increased venous filling of the heart and thus larger volume for cardiac output. Then the **heart rate increases during expiration** because of the reduced venous return. School-age children, who have increased body awareness, may perceive this arrhythmia as abnormal.

Supraventricular Arrhythmia

The **most frequent pathological arrhythmia** in infancy and childhood has a supraventricular origin. This includes **premature atrial contractions** and **supraventricular tachycardia (SVT).** Patients who present to the emergency room with tachycardia should first have a **12-lead ECG.** Supraventricular and ventricular arrhythmia can generally be distinguished on the basis of the QRS and P-wave morphology and the rate of tachycardia. SVT is usually a **narrow complex tachycardia** with rates of approximately **200 beats per minute,** depending on the age of the patient. Patients who present with SVT can return to sinus rhythm with **vagal maneuvers,** which include Valsalva, ice to the face, inducing the diving reflex, and standing on one's head.

Intermittent Tachycardia

Frequently, patients present with intermittent tachycardia not present at the time of evaluation in the office or emergency room. If the 12-lead ECG is normal but the symptomatology suggests intermittent tachycardia, a **transtelephonic monitor** can be used. The goal of using this device is to correlate symptoms with heart rate. Transtelephonic monitoring allows the user to capture a **digital tracing of a single-lead ECG when the patient has symptoms.** This digital recording can then be transferred to the referral center for the cardiologist to interpret. If tachycardia is frequent, a **24-hour Holter monitor** may be sufficient to document the type of arrhythmia. Compared with a transtelephonic monitor, which is an event recorder, Holter monitoring is a continuous 24-hour recording of the ECG.

Ventricular Tachycardia

Patients with ventricular tachycardia (VT) can also present with **chest pain.** VT generally is noted as a side QRS tachycardia with a rate of **120 to 240 beats per minute,** generally not as rapid as SVT for the same age range. When present, VT is a **medical emergency** because this rhythm can rapidly **deteriorate into ventricular fibrillation.** For patients who appear **hemodynamically stable,** an attempt at **intravenous access** and medical conversion to sinus rhythm with **lidocaine** should be attempted. For patients who are **not hemodynamically stable** or who present with mental status changes, **cardioversion** is the treatment of choice. The cause of VT is often difficult to delineate. A new onset of VT is occasionally associated with **myocarditis** and, thus, a recent viral illness. Other causes of VT include **long QTc, exercise-induced VT,** and **benign ventricular tachycardia** of the newborn.

Patients with VT require evaluation by a pediatric **cardiologist. Exercise testing** has been extremely helpful in defining the therapeutic limit in patients with exercise-induced VT. These patients are often treated with **beta-blockers** and then undergo exercise testing again to determine if VT recurs during maximal exercise.

Mitral Valve Prolapse

Mitral valve prolapse (MVP) and associated chest pain is a common finding in adults. In some studies, up to 15% of a normal population have mitral valve prolapse on echocardiography. However, in the pediatric population, chest pain occurs equally in the normal population and those with MVP. In children, the incidence of MVP is approximately 6%.

The diagnosis of MVP is best made on **physical examination** and confirmed by **echocardiography.** Physical findings include a **mid-to-late systolic click** and possibly a **short systolic murmur** resulting from mild mitral regurgitation. The **click is accentuated** by **standing** or with the **Valsalva maneuver,** which both decrease ventricular filling and move the click from late to midsystole.

Patients suspected of MVP should be referred to a pediatric **cardiologist** for an **echocardiogram** to confirm the diagnosis. In patients without mitral regurgitation, subacute bacterial endocarditis prophylaxis is not required.

Because patients with MVP have a small but finite incidence of arrhythmias, patients with chest pain who are found to have MVP should be considered for **work-up for arrhythmia.**

▼ EVALUATION OF CHEST PAIN
Patient History

In all patients with a chief complaint of chest pain, it is important to elicit a **thorough history** of events surrounding the onset of chest pain as well as any **aggravating and relieving factors.** Important **general questions** will define the type, location, duration, and sequence of onset of the pain. Does the pain awaken the child from sleep? Further questions should be directed to separating out the **specific organ system** most responsible for the symptoms. Pain that **worsens with respiration** or deep breathing may suggest bronchospastic, or pleuritic pain. Patients with an associated **history of cough and fever** are most likely to have pneumonic or bronchospastic chest pain. A **pleural catch** is a sharp sudden pain that limits respiration and can be relieved with a deep breath. **Musculoskeletal chest pain** can be produced with movement, should be well localized, and is reproducible by specific movement or palpation. **Costochondritis** produces pain on palpation of the costochondral joints. **Gastrointestinal pain** can be diffuse, is often pre- or postprandial, and may present as a deep or burning pain.

Physical Examination Findings

The physical exam in the child with chest pain should include complete **cardiac, respiratory,** and **upper body musculoskeletal examination. Vital signs** should include blood pressure recordings from the **right arm** and **at least one lower extremity.** The **heart rate and rhythm** should be assessed. Is it regular or irregular? Is the respiratory effort normal? In reference to the cardiac exam, findings of an **organic murmur,** an **irregular heart rate,** or **additional heart sounds** other than S1 and a split S2 would warrant **further investigation** and may prompt referral to a pediatric **cardiologist.** Respiratory examination should be directed toward the **symmetry of respiratory effort** and the presence of **abnormal sounds.** The musculoskeletal system should be assessed for **palpable abnormalities** or **pain on motion** or palpation.

Laboratory Studies

If one is evaluating a child with a chief complaint of **chest pain** and a specific diagnosis is not strongly suspected or confirmed by history and physical examination, then a **PA, lateral CXR,** and a **12-lead ECG** should be done. If the history suggests an **arrhythmia,** then, in addition, a **Holter monitor** should be used.

▼ APPROACH TO THE PATIENT

Chest pain is a common complaint in the pediatric group, but the incidence of heart disease in this group is low. The diagnostic approach is to pursue associated signs or symptoms suggestive of cardiac disease (Figure 19.1). These include:

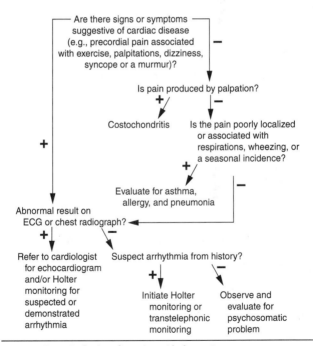

FIGURE 19.1. Evaluation of a patient with chest pain.
ECG = electrocardiogram.

▼ A history suggestive of myocarditis, such as a recent viral illness, fever, and malaise
▼ Suspicion of arrhythmia
▼ Syncope with chest pain
▼ ECG abnormalities
▼ Cardiomegaly on CXR
▼ A significant cardiac murmur.

If any of these findings is present with chest pain, further investigation and referral to a pediatric cardiologist are warranted. In patients with respiratory-type chest pain, especially pain brought on by exercise or that limits exercise, referral to a pediatric **pulmonologist** may be useful to establish a diagnosis of **exercise-induced asthma.** In the asymptomatic child with a **normal ECG and CXR, close observation** without referral is prudent.

Suggested Readings

Bachman DT, Srivastava G: Emergency department presentations of Lyme disease in children. *Pediatr Emerg Care* 14(5):356–361, 1998.
Bink-Boelkens MT: Pharmacologic management of arrhythmias. *Pediatr Cardiol* 21(6):508–515, 2000.
Jacobs W, Chamoun A, Stouffer GA: Mitral valve prolapse: a review of the literature. *Am J Med Sci* 321(6):401–410, 2001.
Kocis KC: Chest pain in pediatrics. *Pediatr Clin North Am* 46(2):189–203, 1999.

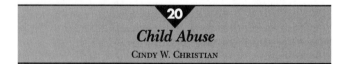

20
Child Abuse
CINDY W. CHRISTIAN

▼ INTRODUCTION

Physicians are responsible for **identifying cases of suspected abuse and reporting them** to the proper authorities for investigation. Diagnosing physical abuse can be challenging. The history provided is often misleading, and the injuries may not be pathognomonic. The presentation varies according to the injury sustained. Possible presentations include single or multiple injuries, unusual or unexplained bruising, a change in mental status, an acute life-threatening event (ALTE), respiratory distress, an inability to use an extremity, nonspecific complaints of gastrointestinal disease, and unexpected cardiorespiratory arrest.

▼ DIFFERENTIAL DIAGNOSIS LIST

Child abuse injuries can result in various physical findings that are also observed in children with physical diseases.

Infectious Diseases

Meningitis
Sepsis

Osteomyelitis
Congenital syphilis
Dermatitis herpetiformis
Impetigo
Staphylococcal scalded skin syndrome
Erysipelas
Purpura fulminans
Disseminated intravascular coagulation (DIC)

Metabolic or Genetic Diseases

Osteogenesis imperfecta
Ehlers-Danlos syndrome
Scurvy
Rickets
Glutaric aciduria type I
Copper deficiency

Congenital or Vascular Diseases

Congenital indifference to pain
Unusual skeletal variants
Arteriovenous malformation (AVM)
Aneurysm
Vasculitis—e.g., Henoch-Schönlein purpura

Hematologic Diseases

Idiopathic thrombocytopenic purpura (ITP)
Leukemia
Vitamin K deficiency
Coagulopathies

Dermatologic Disorders

Mongolian spots
Epidermolysis bullosa
Erythema multiforme
Contact dermatitis, including phytophotodermatitis
Cultural practices—cao gio (coining), cupping, moxibustion

Neoplastic Disorders

Brain tumor

Miscellaneous Disorders

External hydrocephalus

▼ COMMON PRESENTATIONS

Bruises

Differential Diagnosis

Abuse should be **suspected in a child** with a given **history of minor trauma** who has **extensive bruises or bruises on multiple body planes.** Bruises that are in **different stages of resolution, centrally located,** or **patterned** (e.g., loop marks, finger marks, belt marks) also suggest abuse. Bruises in **young infants** who are not yet cruising are also suspicious.

Many conditions can mimic inflicted bruises:

▼ **Accidental bruises** are usually found over bony prominences and are distally located. They are few to moderate in number.

▼ **Mongolian spots,** most commonly found in infants with dark complexions, are often located over the buttocks and lower back (but may be found in other locations).

▼ **Hematologic disorders** (e.g., ITP, leukemia, vitamin K deficiency, coagulopathies, DIC). Children with coagulopathies can have bruising that varies from mild to severe. The distribution of bruises in children with a bleeding diathesis should not be isolated to unusual locations.

▼ **Dermatologic disorders** [e.g., erythema multiforme, contact dermatitis (including phytophotodermatitis from lime or lemon juice)] can be associated with or resemble bruises.

▼ **Cultural practices** can also be associated with patterned bruises. It is useful to be familiar with the cultural practices of subpopulations in the community.

▼ **Genetic diseases** (e.g., Ehlers-Danlos syndrome, osteogenesis imperfecta) are usually associated with other physical stigmata.

▼ **Henoch-Schönlein purpura** is associated with lesions that are typically located on the buttocks and legs; in addition, joint, abdominal, renal, or central nervous system (CNS) manifestations are usually present.

Evaluation

If child abuse is suspected, the **size, location, shape, and color of the bruises** should be **carefully documented.**

When a **bleeding diathesis** is suspected, a **complete blood cell (CBC) count with platelet count,** a **prothrombin time (PT),** a partial thromboplastin time (PTT), and a **von Willebrand panel** serve as thorough screens.

Treatment

Most bruises require **no specific treatment** and resolve over days to weeks, depending on their size. Severe beatings, especially over the buttocks or thighs, can result in **myoglobinuria and acute renal failure.** Myoglobinuria is treated with **hydration.**

Burns

Differential Diagnosis

Abusive burns are **most common in infants and toddlers.** Some burn patterns (e.g., immersion burns) are highly specific for inflicted injury. **Immersion burns** are associated with toilet accidents or other behaviors (e.g., vomiting) that require "cleaning" the child. The pattern of burn distribution often identifies the cause—the feet, lower legs, buttocks, and genitals are burned with clear lines of demarcation, but the knees, upper legs, and other parts of the body that were not submerged are spared.

Many conditions can mimic abusive burns:

▼ **Accidental burns** include burns from hot liquid spills, burns resulting from contact with a clothes iron or curling iron, car-seat buckle burns, chemical burns, and sunburns. Accidental burns are common pediatric injuries, and most pediatric burns are accidental. The history should be compatible with the distribution and severity of the burn.

▼ **Infection** (e.g., staphylococcal scalded skin syndrome, impetigo, erysipelas) may be associated with fever and an ill appearance. Impetigo can be misidentified as cigarette burns.

▼ **Cultural rituals** may be associated with burn-like lesions.

Evaluation

Record areas of **partial and full-thickness burns** on an **anatomic chart** and **calculate the percentage of body area burned** using age-appropriate estimates (see Chapter 79, "Thermal Injury"). Additional injuries should be sought. Children **younger than 2 years** with suspicious burns should have a **skeletal survey** to assess for occult skeletal trauma.

Treatment

Detailed treatment recommendations are provided in Chapter 78, "Thermal Injury."

Fractures

Differential Diagnosis

Although most pediatric fractures are accidental, abuse should be suspected when **unexplained fractures** are identified. Virtually any bone can be injured in cases of child abuse, and no single type of fracture is diagnostic of abuse.

The following are the most commonly seen skeletal injuries:

▼ **Diaphyseal fractures** are the most common type of fracture in both abusive and accidental trauma cases. This type of fracture should cause more concern for abuse in nonambulatory infants.

▼ **Spiral fractures** are associated with twisting of the limb. These fractures can be accidental in ambulatory toddlers and children. They should cause more concern for abuse in young infants, especially if the humerus or femur is involved.

▼ **Metaphyseal fractures** are subtle injuries, most commonly identified by a skeletal survey. These fractures are associated with abusive head trauma. Although metaphyseal fractures are highly suspicious for abuse, the possibility of healing rickets or congenital syphilis should be considered. These fractures are difficult to date radiographically and usually heal without casting.

▼ **Rib fractures** are common with abusive head trauma and are seen in infants and young children in association with abuse. Only rarely do they result from direct blows to the chest, minor accidental trauma, cardiopulmonary resuscitation, and metabolic bone diseases. Multiple, bilateral, posterior fractures are very specific for child abuse. Rib fractures are difficult to identify acutely.

▼ **Skull fractures** may be accidental. In cases of severe abuse, they may be associated with severe CNS injury. Complex, multiple, bilateral fractures are more common in abused children. Most skull fractures are best identified using plain skull radiographs.

▼ **Other fracture areas** include the clavicle, vertebrae, pelvis, and face (i.e., the mandible, maxilla, or zygoma).

In addition to accidental and inflicted trauma, other causes of fractures must be considered:

▼ **Birth trauma.** Fractures of the clavicle, humerus, or femur are occasionally seen with difficult or emergency deliveries, large infants, or breech presentations. By 2 weeks of age, birth fractures should show radiographic signs of healing.

▼ **Physiologic periosteal changes.** Periosteal new bone formation of the long bones (which is seen with healing fractures) may also represent a physiologic process. Physiologic periosteal changes involve multiple bones, are symmetric, and are typically seen in the first 2–3 months of life. They should not be associated with fracture lines.

▼ **Osteogenesis imperfecta.** Most forms of osteogenesis imperfecta are identifiable on the basis of the patient history, the family history, and the physical examination. Type IV osteogenesis imperfecta is most apt to be confused with abuse. Blue sclerae, hearing impairment, dentinogenesis imperfecta, wormian bones, osteopenia, hypermobility of joints, easy bruising, short stature, a tendency toward bowing and angulation of healed fractures, and progressive scoliosis suggest osteogenesis imperfecta. Definitive diagnosis is made by biochemical analysis of cultured skin fibroblasts.

▼ **Congenital syphilis.** The osteochondritis, epiphysitis, and periostitis of congenital syphilis can mimic the metaphyseal fractures and periosteal new bone formation associated with child abuse. Pseudoparalysis of affected limbs and swelling and tenderness of the ends of involved bones suggest the diagnosis of syphilis. In addition, other manifestations are often present. Syphilis can be diagnosed by serologic testing.

▼ **Rickets.** Vitamin D deficiency, renal and hepatic disease, certain medications (e.g., antacids, anticonvulsants, furosemide), and some rare diseases cause rickets, which predisposes bones to fractures. The diagnosis of rickets depends on clinical suspicion, laboratory data (i.e., calcium, phosphorus, and alkaline phosphatase levels) and radiographic evaluation.

▼ **Osteomyelitis** is usually diagnosed on the basis of the patient's history, physical examination, erythrocyte sedimentation rate, and results of blood or bone aspirate cultures.

Evaluation

The evaluation for suspected fractures usually involves obtaining **skeletal radiographs**. A **skeletal survey** is used to **detect occult or healing fractures** and is recommended for **all children 2 years or younger** who have injuries suspicious for abuse. The skeletal survey is a less sensitive test in children 2–5 years of age, and is not generally a useful study in children older than 5 years.

Treatment

Most fractures require **casting**. Some (e.g., **rib fractures, metaphyseal fractures**) usually **do not require specific treatment**.

Abdominal Trauma

Abusive abdominal injuries are **underrecognized and underreported.** Severe abdominal trauma is the **second leading cause of death as a result of abuse.** Injuries are usually caused by **blunt trauma** and most often affect the liver and small intestine.

Differential Diagnosis

The **history** is almost always **misleading.** Children who have suffered abdominal trauma as a result of abuse may present with **nonspecific complaints** related to the **gastrointestinal tract** (e.g., bilious vomiting, abdominal pain, anorexia), complaints associated with **peritonitis** (e.g., fever, abdominal pain, lethargy), or **unexplained cardiorespiratory arrest** (as a result of blood loss or sepsis). Approximately 50% of victims have no **external soft tissue evidence** of abdominal injury. Children with minor injuries can be **asymptomatic** yet have laboratory evidence of trauma. The following conditions must be ruled out:

▼ **Accidental trauma.** Victims of severe accidental abdominal trauma tend to be older with injuries to a single, solid organ. These accidental injuries occur more often outside the home.

▼ **Infection.** Gastroenteritis, peritonitis from a perforated viscus, hepatitis, pancreatitis, and appendicitis must be ruled out.

Evaluation

A simple **hematologic work-up** can be used to screen physically abused children for associated abdominal trauma, and may reveal abdominal trauma in asymptomatic children. A CBC, liver function tests, amylase and lipase levels, and urinalysis are recommended. **Abdominal imaging** is recommended for children with significantly abnormal laboratory results.

Treatment

Solid organ injuries, unless severe, are **managed conservatively,** and usually do not require surgery. **Hollow viscus tears and severe solid organ injuries** require **surgery.** The outcome is generally favorable if the child survives the acute injury.

Head Trauma and Shaking-Impact Syndrome

Head injury, either as a result of blunt trauma, shaking with sudden deceleration forces, or both, is the **leading cause of mortality and morbidity from child abuse.** Victims of inflicted head injury are most **often infants and toddlers.** Older children who die of CNS injury more often have signs of blunt impact to the head.

Differential Diagnosis

Children with head trauma as a result of abuse often present with a **change in mental status, respiratory distress, irritability, lethargy, seizures, ALTE,** or an **increasing head circumference.** Variable degrees of **cerebral edema** may be present initially. The following disorders could also account for these findings and need to be ruled out:

▼ **Accidental trauma** (e.g., motor vehicle accidents, falls out of windows). Common childhood falls (e.g., falls down the stairs or from the couch or changing table) rarely result in life-threatening head injury.

▼ **Infection.** Sepsis and meningitis can be differentiated on the basis of the history, physical examination findings, and culture results. Bloody cerebrospinal fluid may be caused by lumbar puncture technique or a subarachnoid hemorrhage. In the latter case, the amount of blood in the fluid will not change significantly from the beginning to the end of the procedure.

▼ **Gastroesophageal reflux disease (GRD)**, central or obstructive apnea, and **inborn errors of metabolism** can be associated with ALTE, but are usually distinguished from abuse by a lack of associated traumatic findings. Some physicians advocate a retinal examination as a screen for head trauma in infants who present with ALTEs.

▼ **Intracranial vascular anomalies** (e.g., AVM, ruptured aneurysm) are usually identified by magnetic resonance imaging scan, but may not be evident immediately after they hemorrhage.

▼ **Glutaric aciduria type I**, a rare inborn error of amino acid metabolism, can present with acute encephalopathy and chronic subdural hematomas in infancy. Skeletal or other injuries should not be found. Diagnosis is made by finding increased urinary excretion of glutaric acid.

Evaluation

External physical injuries are **usually absent** and do not rule out the diagnosis of abusive head trauma. **Subtle bruises** may be of significance and should be documented. A **computed tomography (CT) scan** of the brain shows **subdural hemorrhage,** often in the posterior interhemispheric fissure. For infants with suspected abusive head trauma, a **complete ophthalmologic examination** and **skeletal survey** are essential.

Treatment

Treatment is aimed at **maintaining cerebral perfusion** and **limiting cerebral edema.** For severely injured children, intubation, hyperventilation, osmotic diuresis, and intracranial-pressure monitoring may be indicated. Despite aggressive therapy, children with severe injuries often have **poor outcomes.**

Munchausen by Proxy Syndrome

In Munchausen by proxy syndrome, the **parent fabricates or causes a child's illness.** The child is repeatedly presented for medical care, and the parent denies knowing the cause of the "disease." Acute symptoms abate when the parent is separated from the child. Common complaints include apnea, ALTE, gastrointestinal bleeding, hematuria, seizures, recurrent fevers, or recurrent infections.

Diagnosing Munchausen by proxy syndrome requires **eliminating** with reasonable accuracy any **diseases** that may account for the reported symptoms. **Delays are almost universal** because the **perpetrator** (usually the mother) commonly **appears devoted and capable.** The perpetrator is usually alone with the child at the onset of symptoms. The **history** of the acute illness is **often much more severe than the findings** on physical examination.

▼ EVALUATION OF CHILD ABUSE
Patient History

Although many victims of child physical abuse are preverbal, older abused children can often provide a history of abuse, and efforts should be made to **interview an older child alone.** Certain factors in the history given by the caregiver raise the suspicion of abuse:

▼ A history of trauma that does not correlate with the injuries sustained
▼ A history that specifically denies trauma to a child with obvious injuries

▼ A history of injury that does not correlate with the child's development (i.e., the child is developmentally incapable of injuring himself in the manner described)

▼ A history that changes as more injuries are discovered

▼ An unexpected or unexplained delay in seeking treatment

Physical Examination

Emphasis should be placed on **detecting subtle signs of injury, neglect, or alternative diagnoses.** Some injuries are pathognomonic of abuse. In these cases, the diagnosis can be made even in the absence of a history. The following areas should be covered in the physical examination:

▼ **Growth.** Plot all growth parameters, and compare with previous points if possible.

▼ **Skin.** Describe any bruises, burns, scars, or rashes in detail (i.e., size, location, pattern, color). The precise location of burns should be noted, including small splash marks, lines of demarcation, and identifiable patterns. Photographs are often used to document injuries but should not replace careful documentation, because they may not reflect accurately the characteristics of the injuries.

▼ **Head.** Palpate for areas of swelling or bogginess, for step-offs or depressions overlying fractures, and for cephalohematomas. Inspect the scalp for avulsed hair and bruises. Scalp bruising is often difficult to see because of the overlying hair.

▼ **Ears.** Look for bruises on the pinna. Battle sign (caused by a basilar skull fracture) may be noted. Examine the middle ear for blood behind the tympanic membrane.

▼ **Eyes.** Note edema, scleral hemorrhage, hyphema, and bruises. A funduscopic examination is essential for infants or young toddlers with suspected CNS injury.

▼ **Mouth and oropharynx.** Examine for evidence of trauma. Frenulum lacerations are pathognomonic of child abuse in young infants and are often associated with forced feeding. Examine the teeth for trauma and caries.

▼ **Chest.** Feel for evidence of healing rib fractures.

▼ **Heart and lungs.** Assess for tachycardia, which may be a sign of acute blood loss.

▼ **Abdomen.** Assess for signs of trauma, including bruising, abdominal tenderness, guarding, and rebound tenderness.

▼ **Back.** Look for bruises and unusual midline masses, which can represent vertebral injuries.

▼ **Genitalia, anus,** and **rectum.** Assess for signs of trauma (see Chapter 72, "Sexual Abuse").

▼ **Extremities.** Assess for soft tissue swelling, point tenderness, and function.

▼ **Neurologic examination,** including rating of the patient according to the Glasgow coma scale, is especially indicated for children with suspected head trauma.

Laboratory Studies

The following laboratory studies may be appropriate:

▼ **Hematologic evaluation.** A CBC with platelet count, PT, and PTT are indicated for children who present with bleeding or bruising. A von Willebrand panel is sometimes included in the screening process.

▼ **Toxicology screens** are indicated for infants or children with unexplained neurologic symptoms (e.g., seizures, lethargy, altered mental status, coma). Standard toxicologic screens vary.

▼ **AST, ALT, amylase, and/or lipase levels** may be elevated with acute liver or pancreatic injury and are recommended for acutely injured young children in whom the abdominal examination may not be a sensitive indicator of injury.

▼ **Urinalysis** is used as a screen for renal or bladder trauma, and it can also detect myoglobinuria and hemoglobinuria. Abused children occasionally develop myoglobinuria as a result of severe muscle injury. Urinalysis shows blood by dipstick but no red blood cells microscopically. An elevated creatine phosphokinase level supports the diagnosis of myoglobinuria and muscle injury in these patients.

Diagnostic Imaging Studies

The following studies are commonly ordered for children with suspected abuse-related injuries:

▼ A **roentgenographic skeletal survey** is indicated for all infants and children younger than 2 years who are suspected of being physically abused.

▼ A **radionuclide bone scan** is sensitive for detecting rib fractures that are less than 7–10 days old, subtle diaphyseal fractures, and early periosteal elevation. This test is most often used when the skeletal survey is negative but the physician still suspects abuse.

▼ A **CT scan** is the method of choice for diagnosing acute intracranial, pulmonary, and solid abdominal organ injuries in a seriously injured child. Significant elevations of AST and ALT should be evaluated with an abdominal CT scan.

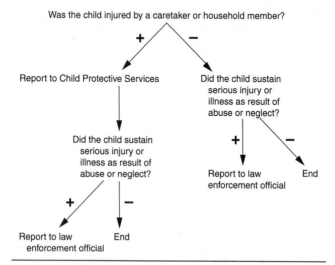

FIGURE 20.1. Reporting child abuse to officials.

▼ TREATMENT OF CHILD ABUSE

Medical treatment is guided by the diagnosed injuries. Hospitalization is required for patients with serious injuries or illnesses from abuse. Occasionally, patients require **hospitalization if a safe environment cannot be guaranteed** at the time of initial diagnosis.

▼ APPROACH TO THE PATIENT

All cases of *suspected* (not proven) **physical abuse** must be **reported to Child Protective Services** (if abuse is committed by a household member or caretaker), **law enforcement officials** (when the injuries are serious or involve a person outside the home), **or both** (Figure 20.1).

The criteria for reporting suspected child physical abuse depends on the history, examination, and laboratory findings. In some cases, the **injuries alone** are so suggestive of abuse that historical and laboratory data are not needed to reach the threshold for reporting. In other cases, the decision to report is reached only after **considering all factors.** Each state has laws that

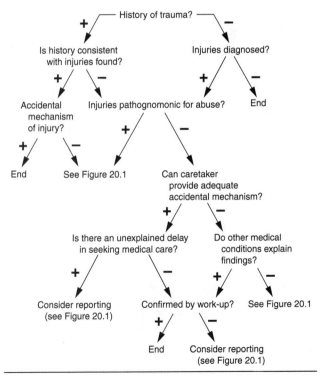

FIGURE 20.2. Approach to initiating the civil and criminal investigation of suspected abuse.

define child physical abuse, and physicians should be **aware of the laws that apply** in their state of practice.

Figure 20.2 provides a basic approach to initiating the civil and criminal investigation of suspected abuse. Individual state and institutional policies vary and may differ from this general approach. Each case must be weighed individually, with the **safety and well-being of the child** always central to the decision to report.

Suggested Readings

American Academy of Pediatrics Committee on Child Abuse and Neglect: Addendum: distinguishing sudden infant death syndrome from child abuse fatalities. *Pediatrics* 108(3):812, 2001.

American Academy of Pediatrics Committee on Child Abuse and Neglect: Shaken baby syndrome: inflicted cerebral trauma. *Pediatrics* 92:872–875, 1993.

American Academy of Pediatrics Committee on Child Abuse and Neglect: Shaken baby syndrome: rotational cranial injuries—technical report. *Pediatrics* 108(1):206–210, 2001.

American Academy of Pediatrics Section on Radiology: Diagnostic imaging of child abuse. *Pediatrics* 87:262–264,1991.

Block RW: Child abuse—controversies and imposters. Curr Probl Pediatr 29:249–272, 1999.

Cooper A, Floyd TF, Barlow B, et al.: Major blunt abdominal trauma due to child abuse. *J Trauma* 28:1483–1486, 1988.

Duhaime AC, Christian CW, Rorke LB, et al.: Nonaccidental head injury in infants: the "shaken baby syndrome." *New Engl J Med* 338:1822–1829, 1998.

Jenny C, Hymel K, Ritzen A, et al.: Analysis of missed cases of abusive head trauma. *JAMA* 281:621–626, 1999.

Johnson CF: Inflicted injury versus accidental injury. *Pediatr Clin North Am* 37:791–814, 1990.

Kleinman PK: *Diagnostic Imaging of Child Abuse.* St. Louis, Mosby Yearbook, 1998.

Nimkin K, Kleinman PK: Imaging of child abuse. *Radiol Clin North Am* 39(4):843–864, 2001.

Purdue GF, Hunt JL, Prescott PR: Child abuse by burning—an index of suspicion. *J Trauma* 28:221–224, 1988.

Reece R, Ludwig S (eds): *Child Abuse Medical Diagnosis and Management.* Philadelphia, Lippincott, Williams and Wilkins, 2001.

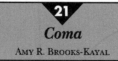

21

Coma

Amy R. Brooks-Kayal

▼ INTRODUCTION

Coma is a state of **unresponsiveness** in which the patient cannot purposefully respond to even vigorous stimuli. Less severe alterations in consciousness include **confusion** (reduced awareness manifested by slow, impaired cognition), **delirium** (increasing unawareness of environment, often associated with delusions and agitation), and **stupor** (a state of unawareness from which the patient can only be aroused by vigorous stimuli). The Glasgow Coma Scale (GCS; Table 21.1), a more precise and objective scale of consciousness, is useful for predicting neurologic outcome as well as for detecting signs of neurologic deterioration. In young infants (< 2 years old), a pediatric coma scale such as the "Infant Face Scale" can also be used.

Consciousness, or the awareness of one's self and environment, depends on the integrity of the cerebral hemispheres and the **reticular activating system (RAS)** in the brain stem. Central nervous system (CNS) lesions that alter consciousness, therefore, must produce damage or dysfunction in both the cerebral hemispheres, the subcortical white matter, or the upper thalamus, or more localized damage or dysfunction in the RAS in the brain stem. Selective destruction of the RAS may result from displacement or compression of the brain stem by a focal mass lesion in one of the cerebral hemispheres.

▼ DIFFERENTIAL DIAGNOSIS LIST
Infectious Causes

Meningitis
Encephalitis—viral encephalitis, cat-scratch disease
Toxic shock syndrome
Rocky Mountain spotted fever
Hemorrhagic shock and encephalopathy syndrome
Subdural empyema

TABLE 21.1. Glasgow Coma Scale (GCS) for Adults and Children and Modified Score for Infants

	Glasgow Coma Score (Adults/Older Children)		Modified Glasgow Coma Score (Infants)
Eye opening	Spontaneous	4	Spontaneous
	To verbal stimuli	3	To speech
	To pain	2	To pain
	None	1	None
Best verbal response	Oriented	5	Coos and babbles
	Confused speech	4	Irritable, cries
	Inappropriate words	3	Cries to pain
	Non-specific sounds	2	Moans to pain
	None	1	None
Best motor response	Follows commands	6	Normal spontaneous movements
	Localizes pain	5	Withdraws to touch
	Withdraws to pain	4	Withdraws to pain
	Flexes to pain	3	Abnormal flexion
	Extends to pain	2	Abnormal extension
	None	1	None

Toxic Causes

Poisoning

Neoplastic Causes

Intracerebral tumor

Traumatic Causes

Closed head injury
Subdural or epidural hematoma
Intraparenchymal hemorrhage

Congenital or Vascular Causes

Hemorrhage—secondary to arteriovenous malformation (AVM), aneurysm, coagulopathy
Infarction
Cerebral venous thrombosis
Hypertensive encephalopathy
Hydrocephalus—secondary to ventriculoperitoneal shunt obstruction, obstruction of ventricular outflow from mass or hemorrhage

Metabolic or Genetic Causes

Hypoxic—ischemic encephalopathy (HIE)
Hypoglycemia
Diabetic ketoacidosis
Electrolyte abnormalities
Inborn errors of metabolism
Reye syndrome
Hepatic encephalopathy
Uremic encephalopathy
Hormonal abnormalities—thyroid, adrenal, pituitary
Hypo- or hyperthermia

Miscellaneous Causes

Absence or complex partial status epilepticus
Postictal state

▼ DIFFERENTIAL DIAGNOSIS DISCUSSION

Trauma

Pathogenesis

A closed head injury can result in the loss of consciousness secondary to a hematoma (epidural, subdural, or intraparenchymal), diffuse cerebral swelling, or both. Severe head trauma can also lead to coma by diffuse cerebral swelling and increased intracranial pressure (ICP) without associated hematoma.

Clinical Features

▼ **Epidural hematomas** usually occur following contact injuries, which can be relatively minor (especially in infants).
▼ **Subdural hematomas** are usually associated with more severe head injury and a history of an immediate loss of consciousness. In infants, chronic

subdural hematomas can present with a history of recurrent vomiting, seizures, retinal hemorrhages, and a tense fontanelle and should suggest the possibility of child abuse.

⚡ **HINT** In patients with epidural hematoma, the classic symptom complex of unconsciousness followed by a lucid interval and then deepening coma is rarely seen.

Evaluation

A computed tomography (CT) scan is the test of choice after head injury, but cervical spine radiographs are also essential in all children with significant head injuries. Neck immobilization is critical until a fracture or dislocation has been ruled out.

Treatment

Treatment includes management of cerebral edema, prevention of hypotension, and surgical decompression of large or expanding intracranial hematomas. Phenytoin is indicated to prevent seizures in the immediate posttraumatic period.

Poisoning (See also Part III, "Toxicology")

Poisoning is one of the **most common causes of coma** in children. Information to be elicited in the child's history includes drugs (prescription and nonprescription) and other potentially toxic agents that are accessible in the child's home. Age is an important risk factor for both accidental (toddlers) and intentional (adolescents) ingestions. Clinical features vary depending on the agent ingested (Table 21.2). Toxicology screens of blood and urine are the tests of choice.

Meningitis

Etiology

Meningitis can result from viral, bacterial, mycoplasmal, fungal, and parasitic infections. An initial presentation of coma is most likely from bacterial meningitis. In children, 90% of bacterial meningitis cases are caused by *Haemophilus influenzae, Streptococcus pneumoniae, Neisseria meningitidis, Escherichia coli,* and Group B streptococci. The organism most commonly causing meningitis varies with age group (Table 21.3).

Clinical Features

Signs of meningitis include fever, vomiting, headache, lethargy, irritability, and stiff neck. On examination, there may be lethargy, irritability or coma, fever, bulging fontanelle (infants), nuchal rigidity (children older than 4–6 months), and Kernig or Brudzinski signs (rarely present in children younger than 2 years of age).

Evaluation

The work-up should begin with a **lumbar puncture (LP)** to obtain cerebrospinal fluid (CSF) for analysis. LP should be deferred until a CT scan has been obtained if signs of increased ICP or focal neurologic signs are present. In patients with bacterial meningitis, the CSF typically shows 200–20,000 white blood cells (WBCs) with a polymorphonuclear neutrophil leukocyte

TABLE 21.2. Drugs That Can Cause Delirium or Coma

Drug	Physical Findings
Barbiturates	Small, reactive pupils; hypothermia; flaccidity; doll's eye reflex may be absent
Opiates	Pinpoint, reactive pupils; hypothermia; hypotension; hypoventilation; bradycardia
Psychedelics	Small, reactive pupils; hypertension; hyperventilation; dystonic posturing
Amphetamines	Dilated pupils, hyperthermia, hypertension, tachycardia, arrhythmia
Cocaine	Dilated pupils, hyperthermia, tachycardia
Atropine-scopolamine	Dilated pupils; hyperthermia; flushing; hot, dry skin; supraventricular tachycardia
Glutethimide	Midposition, irregular fixed pupils; hypothermia; flaccidity
Tricyclic antidepressants	Hyperthermia, hypotension, supraventricular tachycardia
Phenothiazines	Hypotension, arrhythmia, dystonia
Methaqualone	Same as with barbiturates; if severe tachycardia, dystonia

Reprinted with permission from Packer RJ, Berman PH: Coma. In *Textbook of Pediatric Emergency Medicine,* 3rd ed. Edited by Fleisher GR, Ludwig S. Baltimore, Williams & Wilkins, 1993, p 126.

(PMN) predominance, an elevated protein level (> 100 mg/dl), and a low glucose level (< 30 mg/dl). **Bacterial culture** with Gram stain and latex agglutination studies are also performed on CSF.

A complete blood cell (CBC) count; prothrombin time (PT); partial thromboplastin time (PTT); serum electrolyte panel; blood urea nitrogen (BUN), creatinine, and glucose levels; and blood cultures also should be obtained.

Treatment

Treatment should begin immediately with appropriate intravenous **antibiotics.** In children older than 3 months, vancomycin plus a third-generation cephalosporin (cefotaxime or ceftriaxone) should be administered initially because of the risk of antibiotic-resistant strains of *S. pneumoniae;* therapy then can be modified once the organism is identified and susceptibility testing is available. The need for empiric therapy with vancomycin (in addition to ampicillin and cefotaxime) in children 1–3 months of age is more controversial. If there is any delay in obtaining the CSF studies, antibiotic therapy should be initiated presumptively. Dexamethasone (0.15 mg/kg, intravenously, every 6 hours for 4 days) should be considered in patients with suspected or confirmed pneumococcal meningitis.

Encephalitis

Etiology

Viruses that can cause encephalitis include:

▼ Herpes simplex virus (HSV)
▼ Arboviruses (California)

TABLE 21.3.   Recommendations for Initial Antimicrobial Treatment of Meningitis in Different Age Groups

	Neonates (<1 month)	Infants (1–3 months)	Children (>3 months)	Older Children, Adults
Most commonly involved organisms	Group B *Streptococcus*; Gram-negative bacilli; *Listeria monocytogenes*	Group B *Streptococcus*; Gram-negative bacteria; *Streptococcus pneumoniae*; *Neisseria meningitidis*; *Haemophilus influenzae*	*S. pneumoniae*; *N. meningitidis*; *H. influenzae*	*S. pneumoniae*
Recommended antibiotic	Ampicillin plus an aminoglycoside	Ampicillin plus an aminoglycoside or third-generation cephalosporin*	Third-generation cephalosporin*	Third-generation cephalosporin*

Reprinted with permission from Virella G: *NMS Microbiology and Infectious Diseases*, 3rd ed. Baltimore, Williams & Wilkins, 1997, p 430.

* Plus additional antibiotics for resistant or tolerant strains of *S. pneumoniae*.

- ▼ Eastern equine encephalitis virus
- ▼ Western equine encephalitis virus
- ▼ St. Louis encephalitis virus
- ▼ Japanese B encephalitis virus
- ▼ Varicella-zoster virus
- ▼ Epstein-Barr virus (EBV)
- ▼ Coxsackie virus
- ▼ Echovirus
- ▼ Poliovirus
- ▼ Rhabdovirus
- ▼ Paramyxovirus
- ▼ West Nile virus

Clinical Features

Evidence of encephalitis in the patient's history includes a viral prodrome of fever, malaise, headache, nausea, and vomiting that progresses to behavioral changes, confusion, seizures, and coma. Focal neurologic deficits (e.g., hemiparesis, cranial neuropathies, visual field loss, aphasia, focal seizures) may be seen and are most common in patients with HSV encephalitis (80% of patients).

Evaluation

Because specific antiviral therapy for HSV encephalitis is available, evidence for the viral cause of the encephalitis should be sought. The following findings on laboratory and imaging studies are suggestive of HSV encephalitis:

- ▼ **CSF analysis.** CSF typically shows a mixed pleocytosis (50–1000 cells/mm^3) with lymphocyte predominance. The presence of red blood cells (RBCs; up to 500 cells/mm^3) in the CSF suggests HSV encephalitis. CSF protein can be normal or mildly elevated; glucose is usually normal. Viral isolation can be helpful but has a low sensitivity. HSV polymerase chain reaction (PCR) is a highly sensitive method for identifying HSV in CSF (approaching 95%) and should be considered in any patient with suspected HSV encephalitis.
- ▼ **CT.** A CT scan may demonstrate focal areas of hemorrhage or hypodensity in one or both temporal lobes.
- ▼ **Magnetic resonance imaging (MRI)** is a more sensitive early indicator than CT. A temporal lobe signal change on MRI suggests HSV encephalitis.
- ▼ **Electroencephalography.** In HSV encephalitis, the electroencephalogram (EEG) typically shows periodic lateralizing epileptiform discharges. In other viral encephalitides, generalized slowing is the most common EEG finding.
- ▼ **Brain biopsy with virus isolation** is the most definitive method of making a diagnosis, but it is not often used.

Treatment

In the presence of a compatible clinical history, presumptive treatment for HSV encephalitis with acyclovir is initiated. The dosage is 1500 mg/m^2/day divided TID, given intravenously, for 14–21 days. The treatment for nonherpes viral encephalitides is supportive.

Hypoxic—Ischemic Encephalopathy (HIE)

Etiology

A decrease in oxygen delivery to the brain is the most common metabolic disturbance that causes coma. There are many possible causes, including:

Respiratory failure
Cardiac arrest or arrhythmia
Congestive heart failure
Hypotension
Severe anemia
Neonatal apnea
Carbon monoxide poisoning
Near-drowning

Evaluation

A **head CT scan** may be normal initially, but evidence of cerebral edema (i.e., decreased density with loss of gray and white matter differentiation) becomes apparent within 24–48 hours of the onset of hypoxia. **MRI** may demonstrate abnormalities earlier than CT. Cerebral edema is usually maximal 48–72 hours following the hypoxia. An **EEG** can be helpful in predicting the prognosis. A burst–suppression pattern or the absence of activity is associated with poor neurologic outcome.

Treatment

Treatment is aimed at reversing the underlying cause of hypoxia–ischemia and managing the cerebral edema.

Hypoglycemia

Etiology

Hypoglycemia, an important and readily treatable cause of coma, often occurs secondary to excessive exogenous insulin. It is less commonly associated with nesidioblastosis, pancreatic adenomas, sepsis, and inborn errors of metabolism.

Clinical Features

The most important part of the history is determining whether **insulin-dependent diabetes mellitus (IDDM)** is present. At blood glucose concentrations of less than 60 mg/dl, dizziness, anxiety, and tremulousness occur. As the glucose level decreases, confusion, delirium, loss of consciousness, and seizures can occur.

Evaluation

Blood glucose measurement is the test of choice.

Treatment

The treatment is immediate intravenous glucose replacement with 25% dextrose (D25, 2–4 ml/kg).

Diabetic Ketoacidosis

Diabetic ketoacidosis is discussed in Chapter 26, "Diabetes."

Reye Syndrome

Etiology

Reye syndrome is a systemic disorder of mitochondrial function that occurs during or after a **viral infection** (e.g., varicella-zoster) and is frequently associated with **salicylate** administration.

Clinical Features

The history includes recurrent vomiting and progressive deterioration of mental status, ranging from lethargy and confusion to coma, over a period of one to several days.

Evaluation

On examination, signs of increased ICP are frequently present, but focal neurologic deficits rarely occur. The head CT scan or MRI shows evidence of diffuse cerebral edema. Elevated ammonia and liver enzymes suggest Reye syndrome, although definitive diagnosis requires liver biopsy. CSF analysis is normal except for increased opening pressure. The EEG shows abnormalities consistent with a diffuse encephalopathy.

Treatment

Treatment is **supportive** with particular attention given to controlling the ICP and treating the hypoglycemia.

Intracerebral Tumor

Etiology

Although chronic symptoms or focal neurologic dysfunction are the most common early findings of a tumor, coma occasionally occurs. The causes of coma from a tumor may be direct compression or infiltration of the brain stem or blockage of the ventricular system that results in hydrocephalus. Often, such an acute presentation is precipitated by hemorrhage into the tumor.

Clinical Features

Signs in the patient's history indicating intracerebral tumor include recurrent headaches, vomiting, or progressive neurologic symptoms (such as gait abnormalities) preceding the onset of coma.

Evaluation

The examination may show evidence of increased ICP with or without focal neurologic signs. The work-up should begin with a head CT scan.

Treatment

Initial therapy focuses on treating the increased ICP. Dexamethasone (0.25 mg/kg every 6 hours) is used to decrease edema around the tumor. Acetazolamide (30 mg/kg/day, intravenously or orally, in 4–6 divided doses) may also be used.

Definitive therapy may include surgery, chemotherapy, radiation therapy, or a combination of modalities, depending on the type and location of the tumor.

Seizure

Seizures are discussed in Chapter 71, "Seizures."

▼ EVALUATION AND TREATMENT OF COMA

Management of a comatose child has two main goals: **preventing further brain damage** and **defining the underlying causes** of the coma. Immediate management is focused on stabilizing the respiratory and hemodynamic status. Endotracheal intubation is often required to ensure airway protection and adequate oxygenation. Large-bore intravenous lines should be placed and isotonic fluid administered as needed to replace intravascular volume and maintain adequate blood pressure.

When the cardiorespiratory status has been stabilized, a focused **neurologic assessment** of the patient's respiratory pattern, pupillary function, oculovestibular function, and motor function should be performed, looking for evidence of increased ICP (Tables 21.4 and 21.5). Signs of increased ICP include the following:

▼ Abnormal respiratory pattern
▼ Unequal or unreactive pupils
▼ Impaired or absent oculocephalic (doll's eye) or oculovestibular (cold water caloric) responses
▼ Systemic hypertension
▼ Bradycardia
▼ Tense fontanelle (infants)
▼ Abnormal body posturing (decerebrate or decorticate) or muscle flaccidity

Patients should be cared for in **pediatric intensive care** units when possible. If there is evidence of increased ICP, hyperventilate the patient immediately to decrease the arterial carbon dioxide tension ($Paco_2$) to 25–30 mm Hg and administer mannitol (0.5–1 g/kg, intravenously). Dexamethasone can also be started with a bolus of 1–2 mg/kg, intravenously. After intravascular volume has been corrected, fluids should be limited to 75% of maintenance, and only isotonic fluids should be given. The head of the bed should be maintained at a 30° angle above horizontal to maximize cerebral venous drainage.

If there is a history or external evidence of head trauma, an **immediate CT head scan** should be obtained. In any unconscious patient with a history of trauma, the neck must be stabilized until cervical spine injury has been ruled out by a cervical spine radiograph or CT scan.

If clinical signs of meningitis or encephalitis (e.g., fever, meningismus) are present, an **LP should be performed immediately** unless there is evidence of a focal neurologic process or increased ICP. In these cases, intravenous antibiotics should be administered, and a CT scan should be performed before the LP to rule out a focal mass lesion or impending herniation.

Initial laboratory tests should include:

▼ A serum electrolyte panel
▼ Serum glucose, BUN, creatinine, calcium, ammonia levels
▼ Arterial blood gases
▼ Liver function tests
▼ A toxicology screen

TABLE 21.4.   Syndrome of Uncal Herniation

Stage	Respiratory Pattern	Pupillary Size and Reactivity	Oculocephalic–Oculovestibular Response	Motor Response to Noxious Stimuli
Early third nerve	Normal	Unilateral,* moderately dilated pupil; dilated pupil reacts sluggishly	Full or dysconjugate†	Appropriate (fends off) or unilateral hemiparesis*
Late third nerve	Central hyperventilation or Cheyne-Stokes	Unilateral,* widely dilated pupil, unreactive	Dysconjugate (absent, late)†	Decorticate or decerebrate (may be asymmetric)
Midbrain, upper pons	Central hyperventilation	Bilateral midposition pupils, unreactive	Impaired or absent	Bilateral, decerebrate

Data from Plum F, Posner JB: *The Diagnosis of Stupor and Coma*, 3rd ed. Philadelphia, FA Davis, 1980. Table reprinted with permission from Packer RJ, Berman PH: Coma. In *Textbook of Pediatric Emergency Medicine*, 3rd ed. Edited by Fleisher GR, Ludwig S. Baltimore, Williams & Wilkins, 1993, p 125.

* Usually ipsilateral to side of lesion.

† Eye with dilated pupil does not move.

TABLE 21.5.   Central Syndrome of Rostrocaudal Deterioration

Stage	Respiratory Pattern	Pupillary Size and Reactivity	Oculocephalic–Oculovestibular Response	Motor Response to Noxious Stimuli
Early diencephalic	Cheyne-Stokes	Small pupils, reactive	Full doll's eye, full ipsilateral* tonic deviation	Appropriate rigidity (fends off stimuli)
Late diencephalic	Cheyne-Stokes	Small pupils, reactive	Full doll's eye (easy to obtain), full ipsilateral* tonic deviation (easy to obtain)	Decorticate posture
Midbrain, upper pons	Central hyperventilation	Midposition, ± irregular pupils, unreactive	Impaired, dysconjugate	Decerebrate posture
Lower pons, upper medulla	Shallow or ataxic	Pinpoint, unreactive	Absent	No response

Data from Plum F, Posner JB: *The Diagnosis of Stupor and Coma,* 3rd ed. Philadelphia, FA Davis, 1980. Table reprinted with permission from Packer RJ, Berman PH: Coma. In *Textbook of Pediatric Emergency Medicine,* 3rd ed. Edited by Fleisher GR, Ludwig S. Baltimore, Williams & Wilkins, 1993, p 124.

* Toward side of ice water irrigation.

TABLE 21.6. Metabolic Alterations That Cause Coma

Acidosis
Metabolic causes (↓ pH, ↓ CO_2, ↓ HCO_3)
  Diabetic ketoacidosis
  Reye syndrome (uncommon)
  Salicylism
  Lactic acidosis (e.g., primary or secondary to anoxia, shock, or seizures)
  Exogenous poisons (ethylene glycol, methyl alcohol, paraldehyde)
  Diarrhea
  Uremia
Respiratory causes (↓ pH, ↑ CO_2, ↑ HCO_3^-)
  Exogenous sedatives
  Chest injury
  Pulmonary dysfunction (intrinsic)
  Brain stem dysfunction
  Neuromuscular disease (e.g., myasthenia gravis, Werdnig-Hoffman syndrome)
Mixed causes (↓ pH, ↑ P_{CO_2}, ↓ HCO_3)
  Salicylism
  Sepsis

Alkalosis
Metabolic causes (↑ pH, ↑ P_{CO_2}, ↑ HCO_3)
  Vomiting
  Bartter syndrome
Respiratory causes (↑ pH, ↓ P_{CO_2}, normal to ↓ HCO_3)
  Reye syndrome (common)
  Salicylism
  Sepsis
  Pneumonia
  Hepatic coma

Reprinted with permission from Packer RJ, Berman PH: Coma. In *Textbook of Pediatric Medicine*, 3rd ed. Edited by Fleisher GR, Ludwig S. Baltimore, Williams & Wilkins, 1993, p 127.

* CO_2 = carbon dioxide; HCO_3 = bicarbonate; P_{CO_2} = partial pressure of carbon dioxide; ↑ = increased; ↓ = decreased.

Arterial blood gases can be particularly helpful for differentiating potential causes of coma (Table 21.6). Once laboratory studies are drawn, 2–4 ml/kg of D25 should be given intravenously. If there is no response, the patient should receive naloxone (0.01 mg/kg, intravenously).

If focal neurologic abnormalities or evidence of increased ICP are present on examination, or if no cause for the coma is apparent after the screening laboratory evaluation, a **noncontrast CT head scan or MRI** should be performed. If there is a history of seizures or if initial evaluation has been unrevealing, an EEG to rule out nonconvulsive status epilepticus may be helpful.

▼ APPROACH TO THE PATIENT (FIGURE 21.1)

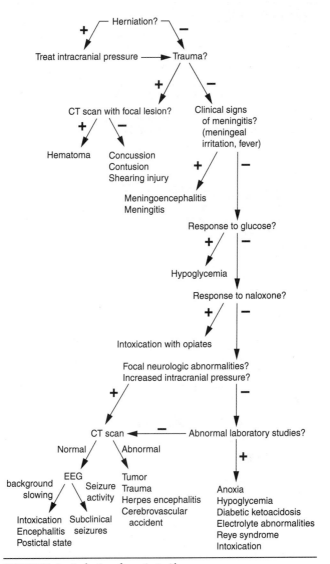

FIGURE 21.1. Evaluation of a patient with coma.
CT = computed tomography; *EEG* = electroencephalogram.

Suggested Readings

American Academy of Pediatrics Committee on Infectious Diseases: Therapy for children with invasive pneumococcal infections. *Pediatrics* 99(2):289–299, 1997.

Durham SR, Clancy RR, Leuthardt E, Sun P, Kamerling S, Dominguez T, Duhaime AC: CHOP Infant Coma Scale ("Infant Face Scale"): a novel coma scale for children less than two years of age. *J Neurotrauma* 17(9):729–737, 2000.

Packer RJ, Berman PH: Coma. In *Textbook of Pediatric Emergency Medicine*, 3rd ed. Edited by Fleisher GR, Ludwig S. Baltimore, Williams & Wilkins, 1993; pp 122–134.

Tasker RC: Neurological critical care. *Curr Opin Pediatr* 12(3): 222–226, 2000.

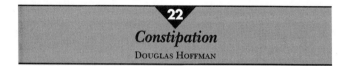

22

Constipation

DOUGLAS HOFFMAN

Constipation is **difficult or delayed passage of stool,** often accompanied by a **decrease in the frequency** of bowel movements. Because **normal stool frequency varies** by age from early in life (Table 22.1), no single definition of constipation fits neatly into pediatric practice. Three to five percent of pediatric primary care visits in the United States are for constipation. This figure reflects the concern among many parents about bowel dysfunction in childhood. In general, constipation is problematic only when stools are hard and dry, but decreased stool frequency can be an **important clue in identifying potentially life-threatening causes** of constipation such as Hirschsprung disease or infantile botulism.

▼ DIFFERENTIAL DIAGNOSIS LIST

Infectious Causes

Chagas disease
Proctitis
Rectal/perirectal abscess
Salmonellosis
Tetanus
Viral ileus

Pharmacological Causes

Aluminum antacids
Amiodarone
Anticholinergics
Antihistamines
Barium
Benzodiazepines
Beta-blockers

TABLE 22.1.   Normal Frequency of Bowel Movements

Age	Bowel Movements Per Week*	Bowel Movements Per Day†
0–3 months old Breast milk	5–40	2.9
Formula	5–28	2.0
6–12 months old	5–28	1.8
1–3 years old	4–21	1.4
>3 years old	3–14	1.0

Acta Paediatr Scand 1989;78:682–684.

* Approximate mean +/− 2 SD.

† Mean.

Reprinted with permission from Baker SS, Liptak GS, Colletti RB, et al: Constipation in infants and children: evaluation and treatment. A medical position statement of the North American Society for Pediatric Gastroenterology and Nutrition. *J Pediatr Gastroenterol Nutr* 29, 1999.

Calcium channel blockers
Calcium supplements
Cholestyramine
Diazoxide
Diuretics
Iron
Laxative, enema, suppository overuse
Mesalamine
Omeprazole
Ondansetron
Opioids
Phenobarbital
Phenothiazines
Phenytoin
Ranitidine
Sucralfate
Tricyclic antidepressants
Ursodiol
Vincristine
Vitamin D intoxication

Toxic Causes

Botulism
Lead

Neoplastic Causes

Pelvic/sacral mass
Polyps
Pregnancy
Spinal cord tumor

Anatomic Causes

Anal atresia
Anal/intestinal stenosis
Anterior displaced anus
Ectopic anus
Gastroschisis
Intestinal bands
Prune belly
Rectal prolapse
Rectal duplication
Rectoperitoneal fistula

Anal Lesions

Fissure
Foreign body
Hemorrhoid
Streptococcal perianal dermatitis

Metabolic Causes

Adrenal insufficiency
Diabetes mellitus (neuropathy)
Diabetes insipidus
Cystic fibrosis (meconium ileus)
Hypothyroidism
Hyperparathyroidism
Hypocalcemia
Hypokalemia
Hypomagnesemia
Hyponatremia
Multiple endocrine neoplasia 2B
Panhypopituitarism
Pheochromocytoma
Porphyria
Renal tubular acidosis

Functional Causes

Anorexia nervosa
Anxiety disorders
Attention deficit disorder
Cognitive deficit/delay
Depression
Excessive cow's milk intake
Genetic predisposition
Insufficient dietary water intake
Introduction to solids
Irritable bowel syndrome
Low fiber intake
Overzealous toilet training
School bathroom avoidance
School entry
Stool withholding

Sexual abuse
Toilet phobia
Underfeeding/malnutrition

Connective Tissue/Autoimmune Disorders

Amyloidosis
Celiac disease
Ehlers-Danlos syndrome
Mixed connective tissue disease
Scleroderma
Systemic lupus erythematosus

Neurogenic/Neuromuscular Causes

Cerebral palsy
Down syndrome
Familial Dysautonomia
Hirschsprung disease
Intestinal neuronal dysplasia
Intestinal pseudoobstruction
Myelomeningocele
Spinal muscular atrophy
Visceral myopathies
Myotonias
Neurofibromatosis
Spina bifida occulta
Spinal cord injury
Static encephalopathy
Tethered cord

Surgical Causes

Appendicitis
Inflammatory bowel disease-induced strictures
Malrotation
Necrotizing enterocolitis
Pyloric stenosis
Volvulus

▼ DIFFERENTIAL DIAGNOSIS DISCUSSION

Like fever or abdominal pain, constipation is a symptom with a broad differential diagnosis. In most cases, constipation is not serious, but one must always consider conditions such as **Hirschsprung disease, neurogenic problems, metabolic disorders,** and **anatomic defects.** Such congenital abnormalities are detected most frequently during infancy, yet the most common presentation of constipation in both infancy and childhood is termed *functional.* The focus here is on functional constipation and Hirschsprung disease.

Functional Constipation

Chronic childhood constipation is functional (idiopathic, nonorganic) without demonstrable underlying disease. The pediatrician can usually identify functional constipation by **thorough history** and **physical examination** alone. Nearly all constipation seen by the general pediatrician and up to 25% seen by pediatric gastroenterologists is functional.

A number of predisposing factors (see differential diagnosis list) appear to be associated with the onset of functional constipation. Whatever the cause, once constipation is triggered, a **positive feedback–type mechanism** ensues. Retained stool in the distal colon begins to lose water across the intestinal wall. As water is resorbed, fecal motility slows, more water is lost, and the feces harden. A **buildup of desiccated stool causes painful defecation** that leads to **ongoing stool retention**. Over time, the **rectum and distal colon expand** to accommodate the growing fecal mass **(acquired megacolon)**, and the **internal anal sphincter,** normally tonically contracted, **loses tone.** Under these conditions, a child's **ability to sense rectal fullness diminishes** and he or she may not appreciate the need to defecate. A classic sign of chronic constipation is the large, infrequent (up to 1 week or more) stool that clogs the household plumbing. **Encopresis, or involuntary fecal soiling,** is for many families a source of tremendous stress. It is a complication of severe functional constipation that occurs when watery stool from the proximal colon leaks around the fecal obstruction, passing involuntarily per rectum. Parents or caretakers often misinterpret encopresis as diarrhea. **Severe constipation** may also **lead to rectal prolapse.**

Evaluation

The medical evaluation of constipation must **differentiate functional from organic or medication-related causes.** In most cases of functional constipation, laboratory tests are unnecessary. Any **predisposing factors** (i.e., low fiber intake, difficult toilet training), **coupled with** telltale signs such as **tenesmus, infrequent/abnormally large stools, stool-withholding behavior** or **soiling,** strongly suggest the **diagnosis. Social stigma** due to excess flatulence and the odor of encopresis is not unusual. Physical examination may reveal **palpable stool** in the abdomen. The **anus** should be checked for **fissures, hemorrhoids** (rare in childhood), surrounding **dermatitis** and **abnormal position. Digital rectal examination** almost always demonstrates abundant stool in the vault. External sphincter tone and anal wink reflex should be intact. A thorough **neurologic examination,** including inspection of the sacral area for sinuses or tufts of hair, is important.

The clinician must **screen for occult blood** in all constipated infants or any child with abdominal pain, failure to thrive, intermittent diarrhea or a family history of either colon cancer or polyps. **Abdominal radiographs** are useful if the diagnosis is in doubt or if rectal examination cannot be performed. Measurement of **abdominal transit time** with **radio-opaque markers** is an option when a patient has infrequent bowel movements but lacks other signs of constipation. In the absence of soiling, a child with normal transit time does not require further evaluation. When there is **soiling with a normal transit time,** treatment relies on **behavioral modification,** sometimes with **psychological evaluation.** Because stool impaction may cause urinary stasis, the need for **urinalysis** and **culture** must be weighed.

Referral to a pediatric **gastroenterologist** is indicated when a constipated child fails therapy or if the physician suspects an organic cause. Tests to consider before referral include serum measurements of thyroid-stimulating hormone, thyroxine, calcium, magnesium, lead, and electrolytes.

Treatment

Management of constipation may be as simple as a **dietary change** for simple constipation, or as complex as a program of **cleanout, bowel "retraining,"** and

family education with close **follow-up. Infants** with simple constipation often do well with **stool softeners** such as **sorbitol-containing juices** (prune, apple, pear), **Karo Syrup,** or **barley malt extract** (Maltsupex). A **glycerin suppository** will usually relieve the acutely constipated infant.

HINT Enemas, mineral oil, and stimulant laxatives are contraindicated in infants.

In **severely constipated children, disimpaction** precedes maintenance therapy. Available agents include **phosphate, saline,** or **mineral oil enemas** and **polyethylene glycol** for **oral lavage.** Cleanout is initiated with a **mineral oil enema** to soften the fecal mass and lubricate the rectal canal. A **hypertonic phosphate enema** is administered **30 minutes later.** A **daily phosphate enema** may be given for up to 5 days to induce evacuation. Tap water, herbal, and soap suds enemas should not be used since they are associated with water intoxication, bowel perforation, and bowel necrosis. Failure to achieve disimpaction at home may require **hospitalization** for polyethylene glycol oral lavage.

Following disimpaction, **maintenance therapy** lasting months and sometimes years is begun. Children should **decrease cow's milk-intake** and consume a **balanced diet** including whole grains, fruits, and vegetables. The most common maintenance agent is **mineral oil,** a lubricant given in doses of 1–3 ml/kg/day. Mineral oil should not be used when there is risk for aspiration (infants, swallowing dysfunction). **Fat-soluble vitamins** in the form of a multivitamin supplement may be given daily at a time when mineral oil is not taken. Occasionally, **stimulant laxatives** such as milk of magnesia or lactulose are used for **short-term "rescue" therapy** to avoid recurrent impaction.

Behavioral modification involves **unhurried toilet sitting** for 10 minutes, two to three times a day after meals. A footstool is often helpful in maximizing Valsalva maneuver. Parents should understand the basic pathophysiology of constipation and be taught to provide **consistent positive reinforcement.** Praise for successful toileting and encouragement after soiling is essential. A **simple reward system** such as stickers on a calendar can be effective and provides a useful record for the physician at follow-up. There is some evidence that biofeedback may be a valid short-term mode of therapy in chronic constipation.

HINT Be aware of pseudoconstipation: Some healthy breast-fed infants may normally only produce a bowel movement two or three times a week. Grunting baby syndrome includes infants without evidence of fecal impaction who strain while passing soft stools. It is thought to result from immature coordination between forced evacuation (Valsalva maneuver) and voluntary relaxation of the external anal sphincter.

HINT Three events in early childhood tend to coincide with the onset of functional constipation: the introduction of solid food in infancy, toilet training, and school entry.

Hirschsprung Disease (Congenital Aganglionic Megacolon)

Hirschsprung disease, the **most common cause of lower intestinal obstruction in newborns, blocks the wave of peristalsis** in aganglionic bowel segments. In many patients the result is **failure to pass stool,** or at best ribbon-like stools, leading to **severe bowel obstruction if undiagnosed.** The incidence is approximately 1 in 5000 live births. The male-to-female ratio is 4 to 1. Hirschsprung disease is unusual beyond infancy, but the diagnosis should always be **considered in any constipated toddler or school-aged child** since the mortality of resulting enterocolitis is high. In addition to several rare genetic disorders, there is an association with **Down syndrome, congenital cardiac anomalies,** and **neuroblastoma** in less than 5% of patients.

Etiology

Hirschsprung disease **originates** sometime during weeks five through twelve of **gestation** when primitive neural crest cells fail to migrate fully caudad. Neural crest cells normally participate in the formation of submucosal and myenteric parasympathetic ganglia; thus, **incomplete migration** gives rise to **aganglionic intestine** having sustained sympathetic contraction. The aganglionic segment always extends proximally from the internal anal sphincter. Eighty percent of cases are limited to some portion of the **rectosigmoid region.** Much less frequently, aganglionosis of the entire colon with or without some small bowel involvement occurs.

Clinical Features

Infants with Hirschsprung disease often have **delayed passage of meconium.** Ninety-four percent of normal-term newborns will pass meconium within 24 hours of birth compared with 6% of infants with Hirschsprung disease. The degree of bowel involvement correlates with the timing of diagnosis. Patients with short-segment disease may not be identified until childhood (or rarely, go undetected into adulthood), whereas those with **more extensive involvement** will **present in infancy** with **bilious vomiting, abdominal distension, failure to thrive,** and **refusal to feed.** On examination, the **abdomen** is often **distended** and anal **sphincter tone** is usually **increased.** The **rectum** is typically **empty** and as the examining digit is withdrawn there may be a forceful gush of liquid stool. **Enterocolitis** is a **life-threatening complication** with acute clinical onset. Increased intraluminal pressure from bowel obstruction is thought to mechanically diminish mucosal blood flow—in turn compromising mucosal integrity—allowing **bacteria and fecal toxins into the bloodstream.** Progression is rapid and septic patients are **febrile** with **abrupt onset** of foul-smelling **bloody diarrhea, abdominal distention,** and **bilious emesis.** The mortality rate in advanced enterocolitis approaches 30%.

Laboratory Evaluation

Several diagnostic methods are available but vary in reliability. Absent rectal air on a prone **abdominal radiograph** suggests Hirschsprung disease. An unprepped **barium enema** demonstrates a narrow distal colonic segment that abruptly transitions to dilated bowel. Because it may take several weeks for a neonate's unaffected proximal bowel segment to dilate with stool, a normal barium study can be misleading. Retention of barium for 24 hours or more is an abnormal finding. A **negative barium study requires further investigation. Anorectal manometry** assesses the internal anal sphincter's response to artificial balloon distention. A normal sphincter relaxes under pressure—an aganglionic sphincter either remains contracted or increases its tone. Normal sphincter relaxation obviates the need for biopsy. When manometry results are abnormal, **rectal biopsy samples** obtained and interpreted by experienced practitioners provide definitive diagnosis.

Management

The treatment of Hirschsprung disease is **surgical resection** of aganglionic bowel with temporary placement of a **diverting ostomy** proximal to the affected segment. The sensitive anoderm is left intact to ensure future continence. Anastomotic stricture occurs in 5% of patients. More than 90% of patients will ultimately have normal bowel function. Before surgery, management of enterocolitis in the intensive-care setting includes **nasogastric decompression, antibiotics,** and **correction of fluid and electrolyte imbalances.**

Table 22.2 compares functional constipation and Hirschsprung disease.

TABLE 22.2. Comparison of Functional Constipation and Hirschsprung Disease

	Functional Constipation	Hirschsprung Disease
Symptoms as a newborn	Rare	Almost always
Late onset (after 3 years)	Common	Rare
Difficult bowel training	Common	Rare
Stool size	Large	Small, ribbonlike
Urge to defecate	Rare	Common
Obstructive symptoms	Rare	Common
Enterocolitis	Rare	Sometimes
Failure to thrive	Rare	Common
Abdominal distention	Rare	Common
Stool in rectal ampulla	Common	None
Barium enema	Copious stool No transition zone	Delayed evacuation Transition zone
Rectal biopsy	Normal	No ganglion cells Increased anticholinesterase staining
Anorectal manometry	Distention of rectum causes relaxation of the internal sphincter	No sphincter relaxation

> ⚡ **HINT** In patients with Hirschsprung disease, the rectum is typically empty on digital exam. However, like functional constipation, patients with short-segment aganglionosis may accumulate stool in the vault. Therefore, patients who do not respond to conventional therapy should be referred to a pediatric gastroenterologist.

Neurogenic Bowel Dysfunction

Neurogenic bowel dysfunction occurs in children when diseases such as **myelomeningocele, tethered cord, lipomeningocele,** or **lumbosacral spinal cord tumors** interfere with the normal neurologic control of defecation. Typical findings include a history of spinal cord trauma, weakness or dysesthesia of the lower extremities, fecal incontinence after successful toilet training, or urinary incontinence. Myelomeningocele-spinal dysraphism in the lumbosacral region can cause constipation and megarectum, but these problems more often manifest as **urinary and fecal incontinence.** Spina bifida occulta (failed fusion of the vertebral arches) is a common finding that usually does not interrupt rectal innervation. **Sacral cysts or fistulae** should be **identified in the newborn** nursery and evaluated by **ultrasound.** Management of patients with neurogenic bowel dysfunction depends on the type, severity, and location of the lesion. Children with moderate-to-severe impairment benefit from interdisciplinary collaboration between physicians, occupational therapists, and behavioral or mental health specialists.

Suggested Readings

Abi-Hanna A, Lake A: Constipation and encopresis in childhood. *Pediatr Rev* 19:23–30, 1998.

Abrahamian FP, Lloyd-Still JD: Chronic constipation in children: longitudinal study of 186 patients. *J Pediatr Gastroenterol Nutr* 3:460–467, 1984.

Baker SS, Liptak GS, Colletti RB, et al: Constipation in infants and children: evaluation and treatment. A medical position statement of the North American Society for Pediatric Gastroenterology and Nutrition. *J Pediatr Gastroenterol Nutr* 29:612–626, 1999.

Davidson M, Jugler MM, Bauer CH: Diagnosis and management in children with severe and protracted constipation and obstipation. *J Pediatr* 62:261–275, 1963.

de Vries M, de Vries M: Cultural relativity of toilet training readiness: a perspective from East Africa. *Pediatrics* 60:170–177, 1977.

Felt B, Wise CG, Olson A, et al: Guideline for the management of pediatric idiopathic constipation and soiling. Multidisciplinary team from the University of Michigan Medical Center in Ann Arbor. *Arch Pediatr Adolesc Med* 153:380–385, 1999.

Goyal R, Hirano I: The enteric nervous system. *N Engl J Med* 334:1106–1115, 1996.

Loening-Baucke V: Encopresis and soiling. *Pediatr Clin North Am* 43:279–298, 1996.

McClung HJ, Boyne L, Heitlinger L: Constipation and dietary fiber intake in children. *Pediatrics* 96:999–1001, 1995.

Rudolph C, Benaroch L: Hirschsprung disease. *Pediatr Rev* 16:5–11, 1995.

Taubman, B: Toilet training and toileting refusal for stool only: a prospective study. *Pediatrics* 99:54–58, 1997.

23
Cough
RICHARD M. KRAVITZ

▼ INTRODUCTION

Cough is one of the most common presenting symptoms in children. The duration of the symptoms determines the level of concern and degree of work-up that is warranted. An **acute cough,** lasting less than 3 weeks, is frequently related to an infectious illness and is often self-limited. This chapter is concerned with **chronic cough**—a cough that persists for longer than 3 weeks and suggests a potentially more serious underlying cause.

A cough has three components. First, there is an **inspiratory phase,** when the patient takes a deep breath. The inspiratory phase is followed by **closure of the glottis and contraction of the expiratory muscles.** During this phase, the intrathoracic pressure increases. Finally, the **glottis opens,** allowing the previously inspired air to be expelled at a high velocity (about 60–70 mph). The purpose of coughing is to shake irritants loose from the airway mucosa and move them proximally (if the irritant is located distally) or expel them (if the irritant is located proximally).

▼ DIFFERENTIAL DIAGNOSIS LIST
Infectious Causes
Bacterial Infection

Bacterial pneumonia
Sinusitis
Tuberculosis
Pertussis
Chlamydia infection
Mycoplasma infection

Viral Infection

Upper respiratory tract infection
Viral pneumonia
Bronchiolitis—respiratory syncytial virus (RSV) infection, parainfluenza infection
Croup
Influenza

Fungal Infection

Aspergillosis
Allergic bronchopulmonary aspergillosis (ABPA)
Histoplasmosis
Coccidioidomycosis

Toxic (Irritant) Causes

Cigarette smoke
Industrial pollutants

Wood-burning stoves
Cleaning solvents

Neoplastic Causes

Teratoma
Lymphoma
Leukemia
Metastatic malignancy

Congenital Causes

Pulmonary Malformations

Bronchogenic cysts
Cystic adenomatoid malformation
Congenital lobar emphysema
Pulmonary sequestration

Vascular Malformations

Aberrant innominate artery
Double aortic arch
Airway hemangiomas

Gastrointestinal Malformations

Esophageal duplications
Tracheoesophageal fistula

Genetic Causes

Cystic fibrosis
Immotile cilia syndrome

Inflammatory Causes

Asthma
Allergies
Sarcoidosis

Psychosocial Causes

Psychogenic (habitual) cough
Paradoxical vocal cord dysfunction

Miscellaneous Causes

Pulmonary Disorders

Bronchopulmonary dysplasia
Laryngotracheobronchomalacia
Foreign body in airway
Bronchiectasis

Ears, Nose, and Throat Disorders

Foreign body in the nose or ear canal
Postnasal drip
Middle ear effusion

Cardiovascular Disorders

Congestive heart failure
Pulmonary edema

Gastrointestinal Disorders

Gastroesophageal reflux disease (GRD)
Diaphragmatic or subdiaphragmatic mass
Foreign body in the esophagus

Immunologic Disorders

Congenital immunodeficiency

▼ DIFFERENTIAL DIAGNOSIS DISCUSSION
Asthma

Asthma, the **most common chronic illness in children,** affects 5%–10% of children in the United States.

Etiology

The underlying cause of asthma is unknown, although airway inflammation is known to be a major component. The triad of **airway inflammation, smooth muscle hyperreactivity,** and **reversible airway obstruction** is characteristic for patients with asthma.

Numerous triggers can precipitate an asthma flare-up, including upper respiratory tract infections, sinus infections, exercise, exposure to cold air, weather changes, exposure to aeroallergens (e.g., dust, cockroaches, animal dander, pollen, grass), exposure to strong odors (e.g., cigarette smoke, strong chemicals), and emotional states (e.g., fear, laughing, crying).

Clinical Features

Asthma symptoms are secondary to airway obstruction and increased airway resistance. **Wheezing** is the classic presentation of asthma, but other symptoms include chronic coughing (cough-variant asthma), shortness of breath, and chest pain or tightness.

Evaluation

A detailed history and physical are key to making the diagnosis of asthma. Wheezing, rhonchi, coarse or decreased breath sounds, or a prolonged expiratory phase may be noted on pulmonary examination. Lung sounds can also be entirely normal at the time of examination, even in a patient with a significant history.

Spirometry with bronchodilator response is used to assess for asthma. In patients with asthma, an obstructive pattern with postbronchodilator normalization is seen. If spirometry is not available, a hand-held peak-flow meter can be substituted.

HINT Pulmonary function testing can be normal in many patients with cough-variant asthma. If asthma is strongly suspected in spite of normal results on pulmonary function testing, provocational testing (e.g., exercise testing, methacholine challenge) is indicated to help elicit airway hyperreactivity. Exercise testing is specific in patients with exercise-induced asthma, whereas the more sensitive methacholine challenge can detect more subtle degrees of airway hyperreactivity.

Treatment

Proper treatment of asthma entails both pharmacologic and nonpharmacologic modalities. For most patients with asthma, ideal therapy includes the use of a daily anti-inflammatory medication with a bronchodilator as required to treat breakthrough symptoms. Short bursts of oral steroids are helpful for treating acute flare-ups of asthma, although the side effects of long-term use preclude the use of oral steroids as a chronic maintenance medication, except in severe cases.

▼ **Anti-inflammatory medications** include mast cell stabilizers (e.g., cromolyn sodium, nedocromil calcium), inhaled steroids (e.g., beclomethasone, triamcinolone, fluticasone, budesonide), and leukotriene inhibitors (e.g., zileuton, zafirlukast, montelukast).

▼ **Bronchodilators.** β_2 Agonists (e.g., albuterol, terbutaline, pirbuterol) are the most effective bronchodilators. Methylxanthine derivatives (e.g., theophylline) and parasympathetic antagonists (e.g., atropine, ipratropium) also may be used.

▼ **Nonpharmacologic management** entails patient education (to improve self-management), environmental control and prevention skills (to decrease the likelihood of developing an asthma attack), and home monitoring with a peak flow monitor (to objectively assess pulmonary status so that interventions can be instituted and the effects measured).

Cystic Fibrosis

Etiology

An autosomal recessive disorder, cystic fibrosis is the **most common genetic disease affecting Caucasians.** The gene is located on chromosome number 7 and codes for a transmembrane protein (cystic fibrosis transmembrane conductance regulator protein-CFTR) that functions as a chloride channel. The most common abnormality is an amino acid defect consisting of the deletion of a phenylalanine.

The disease is characterized by **multi-organ involvement.** Chronic sinopulmonary infections (facilitated by excess altered mucus production in the respiratory tract), pancreatic insufficiency, and abnormalities of the exocrine glands and reproductive tract are major manifestations. In the lungs, dry, thickened secretions hinder clearance of pulmonary secretions. Impaired clearance, in combination with abnormal colonization with organisms (e.g., *Staphylococcus aureus, Pseudomonas aeruginosa*), leads to the development of bronchiectasis and permanent lung damage.

Clinical Features

Major symptoms include a chronic productive cough, yellow-green sputum, hemoptysis, chest congestion, steatorrhea, poor weight gain, failure to thrive, and meconium ileus or meconium ileus equivalent (intestinal obstruction).

Evaluation

A detailed family history should be obtained as well as growth patterns and stool characteristics.

Cardinal features noted on physical examination may include tachypnea, bronchial breath sounds, wheezes, crackles, a prolonged expiratory phase, nasal polyps, upper airway congestion, digital clubbing, reduced height and weight, rectal prolapse, and hepato- and splenomegaly.

The following laboratory studies are indicated:

▼ **Chloride sweat test.** Pilocarpine is used to stimulate sweat collection. The sweat chloride level is considered to be elevated if it exceeds 60 mEq/L.

▼ **Sputum culture.** *P. aeruginosa* and *S. aureus* are the bacterial pathogens most often responsible for the chronic sinopulmonary infections. Other organisms, such as *Burkholderia cepacia, Stenotrophomas maltophilia,* and *Alcaligenes xylosoxidans,* are found less commonly but are more resistant to therapy.

▼ **Complete blood cell (CBC) count.** A CBC should be obtained to rule out anemia and hypersplenism (evidenced by leukopenia and thrombocytopenia).

▼ **Liver function tests** are ordered to assess for hepatobiliary disease and obstruction.

▼ **Prothrombin time (PT).** A PT should be obtained to assess vitamin K sufficiency.

▼ **Vitamin A, E,** and **D** levels should be measured to assess for possible deficiency.

▼ **Fecal fat analysis.** A 72-hour stool collection should be obtained for fecal fat analysis.

▼ A **bentiromide test** may be done to test for protein malabsorption.

▼ **Oxygen saturation analysis** and **pulmonary function tests** should be performed to assess the degree of pulmonary involvement (arterial blood gas analysis is not necessary in most cases).

▼ **Genetic testing** is indicated. More than 70% of patients have the delta F508 mutation.

⚄ HINT All children with recurrent sinopulmonary infections, steatorrhea, growth failure, or asthma who do not respond to appropriate therapy for these conditions should be tested for cystic fibrosis.

⚄ HINT All siblings of patients with cystic fibrosis should be tested for cystic fibrosis using the chloride sweat test. They should also undergo genetic analysis because they have a 2 in 3 chance of being a carrier.

Treatment

Therapy is directed toward maintaining optimal pulmonary function and nutritional status.

▼ **Vigorous daily pulmonary toilet** with chest physiotherapy, breathing exercises, and nebulized bronchodilators are indicated. The efficacy of mucolytic agents such as Mucomyst has been questioned; however, Pulmozyme has been demonstrated to improve lung function in clinical studies.

▼ **Pancreatic insufficiency** is treated with the administration of supplemental pancreatic enzymes and multivitamins. Vitamin K administration is frequently required, especially if the patient takes antibiotics chronically or if the PT is increased (vitamin K should be given intramuscularly if the PT is seriously elevated or if the patient is actively bleeding).

▼ **Hemoptysis** indicates exacerbation of underlying infection. Broad-spectrum oral antibiotics should be used if the infection is mild and the patient is stable. Intravenous administration of antibiotics should be considered if the infection is severe or does not respond to oral antibiotics. It may be necessary to withhold chest physiotherapy until the bleeding subsides (12–24 hours). Most episodes of hemoptysis manifest as blood streaks and respond to a treatment course of antibiotics. Massive hemoptysis, although rare, is a medical emergency that usually results from erosion of an underlying bronchial vessel into a bronchus,

   ▼ **Massive hemoptysis** can be life-threatening, has a high recurrence rate, and carries a poor prognosis.

   ▼ **Locating the bleeding site is urgent** and usually requires an invasive procedure, such as a bronchoscopy and/or catheterization with embolization.

▼ **Other major emergencies** in patients with cystic fibrosis include acute intestinal obstruction, massive hemorrhage from esophageal varices, liver failure, pulmonary hypertension, cor pulmonale with cardiac failure, pneumothorax, and chronic hypoxemia.

Sinusitis

Sinusitis, which is characterized by inflammation and infection of the mucosal lining of the sinuses, is a common cause of chronic cough.

Etiology

In an otherwise healthy host, sinus infections are usually a **complication of upper respiratory tract infections** (i.e., bacterial superinfection following a viral infection). The usual bacterial pathogens include *Streptococcus pneumoniae, Haemophilus influenzae,* and *Moraxella catarrhalis.*

Clinical Features

Sinusitis can present in a variety of ways. Common features include persistent symptoms of an upper respiratory tract infection, chronic cough, a mucopurulent nasal discharge, headaches, and malodorous breath.

Evaluation

The diagnosis can be made clinically, based on the history and physical examination. Physical examination findings may include tenderness over the affected sinus and erythema of the nasal mucosa, with or without a mucopurulent nasal discharge, or the physical examination may be normal.

Radiographic studies that can aid in the diagnosis include **sinus films** and **computed tomography (CT)** of the sinuses. Opacification of the sinuses, mucosal thickening, or the presence of an air–fluid level are typical findings.

Treatment

The usual treatment for sinusitis is a prolonged course of **antibiotics,** usually lasting 14–21 days. Therapy should be directed toward the usual bacterial pathogens. The concomitant use of topical **decongestants** is only recommended for 4–7 days. **Surgical drainage** of the sinus is sometimes used in refractory cases.

Bronchiectasis

Bronchiectasis is a condition in which the bronchi are damaged, leading to the development of bronchial dilatation with the loss of underlying airway support structures (e.g., cartilage and elastic tissue). Acute or chronic inflammation and recurrent infections are also associated with bronchiectasis. Bronchiectasis is the end result of numerous insults to the lung and can be **reversible** (e.g., cylindrical bronchiectasis) or **permanent** (e.g., saccular bronchiectasis).

Etiology

Some of the more common causes of bronchiectasis include **infection** (e.g., following severe pneumonia caused by *S. aureus, S. pneumoniae,* adenovirus, or influenza virus), **genetic conditions** (e.g., cystic fibrosis, immotile cilia syndrome), **recurrent aspiration events,** or a **retained foreign body.**

Clinical Features

Chronic coughing with excessive sputum production is a cardinal sign of bronchiectasis. In severe cases, hemoptysis and recurrent fevers can be seen.

Evaluation

▼ **Physical findings** are related to the extent of the disease. Although the pulmonary examination can be normal early in the course of disease, one is apt to find coarse breath sounds, rhonchi and rales, and expiratory wheezes as the disease progresses. Digital clubbing is also seen in advanced disease.

▼ **Chest radiographs** typically show thickened bronchial walls in the peripheral lung, although early in the course of disease the films may be normal. Other findings include recurrent atelectasis and localized hyperinflation.

▼ **Chest CT scans** are more sensitive than radiographs for defining the extent of the disease, especially in patients with milder cases. Typical findings include bronchial wall thickening extending to the periphery, cystic changes in the bronchi, and air–fluid levels in the damaged bronchi.

▼ **Other studies** may prove useful in the evaluation of the patient with bronchiectasis. These studies depend on the past medical history and can include a sweat test (if cystic fibrosis is to be considered); bronchoscopy (if a foreign body is suspected or if respiratory cultures are desired); an immunologic evaluation (if recurrent pneumonia has occurred); or a pH probe or milk scan (if GRD is suspected).

Treatment

Treatment should be directed toward the underlying cause of the bronchiectasis, if one can be identified.

▼ **Pulmonary toilet.** Maintenance of good pulmonary toilet is important, regardless of the cause of the bronchiectasis. Aiding in the removal of excessive secretions and preventing superinfection can help prevent further bronchial damage. Aerosolized bronchodilators, chest physiotherapy, and postural drainage promote the removal of excess mucus.

▼ **Antibiotics.** Oral or intravenous antibiotics may be indicated for patients with acute exacerbations of bronchiectasis exacerbated by a bacterial infection. Chronic prophylactic antibiotic use to prevent exacerbations is controversial and should be determined on a case-by-case basis.

▼ **Surgery.** In certain patients with well-localized bronchiectasis, surgical removal of the affected lung can be curative. Surgery, however, should only be performed when medical management has failed and the likelihood of disease progression after surgery is minimal.

Immotile Cilia Syndrome

Etiology

Immotile cilia syndrome is an autosomal recessive disease characterized by abnormal function of the cilia. Histologic defects in the cilia may include abnormalities in the dynein arms, defects in the radial spokes connecting the microtubules that form the cilia, and defects in the microtubules themselves.

Clinical Features

Patients with immotile cilia syndrome typically present with recurrent episodes of **otitis media, sinusitis, chronic cough,** and **pulmonary infections.**

Physical findings include recurrent otitis media, chronic sinus drainage, nasal polyps, pulmonary findings suggestive of bronchiectasis, and, in more severe cases, digital clubbing (secondary to the bronchiectasis). **Situs inversus** is seen in 50% of cases.

HINT The triad of sinusitis, bronchiectasis, and situs inversus is referred to as Kartagener syndrome.

HINT Male infertility secondary to abnormally functioning sperm is common.

Evaluation

Frequently the diagnosis is made by clinical history and by ruling out other causes because it is difficult to definitively diagnose the condition. Approaches include **microscopic evaluation** of the cilia, examination of the **ciliary beat frequency or wave form,** and the **saccharin test** (a drop of saccharin is placed in the nose and the length of time it takes the patient to taste the sweetness is measured).

Radiographic findings (chest radiograph or CT scan) are those of cystic fibrosis and bronchiectasis. Sinus films typically show pansinusitis.

Treatment

Treatment is the **same as for bronchiectasis.** Maintaining adequate pulmonary drainage is key to minimizing lung damage. Recurrent otitis media is treated with the placement of myringotomy tubes. Chronic use of antibiotics is controversial.

Gastroesophageal Reflux Disease (GRD)

Gastroesophageal reflux disease is discussed in Chapter 83, "Vomiting."

▼ EVALUATION OF COUGH
Patient History
Present Illness
The present illness should be defined:

▼ What is the duration of the cough?
▼ How frequent is the cough?
▼ When does the cough occur (e.g., upon awakening, later in the evening)?
▼ What does the cough sound like (Table 23.1)?
▼ Is the cough productive or nonproductive for sputum?

✄ HINT   Children frequently swallow rather than expectorate sputum, making assessment of sputum productivity difficult. If the child is too young to expectorate sputum, examination of any emesis can indirectly assess for sputum production.

▼ Were there any precipitating events (e.g., infection, choking episode, allergies)?
▼ Are there any triggers for the cough (Table 23.2)?
▼ Are there accompanying symptoms (e.g., rhinorrhea, watery eyes, headaches, fever, poor weight gain or weight loss, symptoms of food malabsorption, wheezing)?
▼ How many school days have been missed?
▼ Is the cough improving or getting worse?
▼ What medications is the child currently taking? Angiotensin-converting enzyme (ACE) inhibitors can cause a chronic cough and β_2 antagonists can precipitate bronchospasm in patients with asthma.
▼ What is the patient's travel history?
▼ Are other family members ill?

Past Medical History
Important information to be gathered includes:

▼ The patient's birth history
▼ Information regarding any previous illness or surgery
▼ Information regarding allergies
▼ The patient's immunization status

TABLE 23.1. Types of Cough	
Quality	**Likely Diagnosis**
Staccato	Pertussis or parapertussis infection
Bark-like (seal-like) or brassy	Croup
Throat clearing	Postnasal drip, possibly secondary to sinusitis or allergies
Foghorn-like and occurring only when awake	Pathognomonic for a psychogenic (habitual) cough

TABLE 23.2. Triggers for Coughing	
Trigger	**Associations**
Cold air, exercise, or upper respiratory tract infections	Asthma
Supine position	Postnasal drip, GRD
Eating	GRD, tracheoesophageal fistula

GRD = gastroesophageal reflux disease

Family History

The patient's parents should be queried about a family history of any of the following disorders:

▼ Asthma
▼ Allergies
▼ Cystic fibrosis
▼ Emphysema
▼ Tuberculosis
▼ Sarcoidosis

Environmental History

An environmental history can sometimes prove useful in identifying the exacerbating factors in patients with a chronic cough, especially if the underlying cause is asthma or allergies. The following are important factors:

▼ **Home heating system.** Forced-air heating systems that use a duct network can carry dust through the house. Radiator and baseboard heating are much less likely to cause a problem for children with allergies.
▼ **Wood-burning stoves.** Older stoves often do not burn wood efficiently. The incompletely burned wood releases hydrocarbons that can be a potent, noxious irritant for patients with asthma.
▼ **Location of the home.** In rural and suburban settings, patients are exposed to numerous aeroallergens, whereas in urban environments, patients are exposed to industrial irritants.
▼ **Condition of the home.** Dusty homes can aggravate allergies. If the basement is cool and damp, the possibility of mold exposure exists. Older homes, especially in overcrowded, urban areas, can have cockroaches, which have been recognized as potent allergens and can lead to poorly controlled allergies and asthma. Construction within the home can expose the child to various noxious irritants, ranging from dust to paint and chemical odors. Mold spores can also be released into the air. For patients with severe dust allergies, removing the carpeting, drapes, blinds, and stuffed animals from the patient's room and encasing the mattress and pillow in plastic may help minimize exposure to dust mites.
▼ **Cigarette exposure.** Smoking in the home can be a potent trigger for coughing, particularly in children with asthma. Children exposed to cigarette smoke have a higher incidence of asthma, upper respiratory tract infections, and recurrent sinusitis or otitis media.
▼ **Pets.** Exposure to pets can be a problem for children with allergies and asthma.

▼ **Day care.** Recurrent exposure to other children increases the likelihood of the child developing recurrent upper respiratory tract infections.

Physical Examination

The following should be noted on physical examination:

▼ **General appearance**—height and weight, degree of distress
▼ **Skin**—eczema, rashes
▼ **Head, ears, eyes, nose, and throat**—watery eyes, cerumen in the ear, sinus tenderness, nasal discharge, pale or boggy nasal turbinates, postnasal drip, pharyngeal cobblestoning (i.e., a cobblestone-like appearance to the mucosa that is seen in patients with allergic disease)
▼ **Lungs**—respiratory rate, chest appearance, breath sounds (rhonchi, rales, wheezes) and their symmetry
▼ **Heart**—murmur
▼ **Extremities**—cyanosis, clubbing

✍ HINT The presence of digital clubbing raises the possibility of a more severe underlying pulmonary problem, such as cystic fibrosis, bronchiectasis, or chronic hypoxia. Clubbing makes asthma a much less likely etiology for the cough.

Laboratory Studies

Selection of laboratory studies is based on a thorough history and physical examination.

Suspected Allergy

▼ **Diagnostic skin testing** is the most accurate test for determining atopy; skin testing is best done in patients older than 2 years.
▼ **CBC with differential.** Eosinophilia suggests an allergic component.
▼ **IgE level.** Elevation suggests an allergic component.
▼ **Radioallergosorbent testing (RAST).** RAST is used in the evaluation of allergy but is not as clinically sensitive as skin testing.

Suspected Infection

▼ **Purified protein derivative (PPD)** is used to rule out tuberculosis (TB). Tine testing is no longer recommended as a screening test. The usual dose of PPD for the Mantoux tuberculin skin test is 5 units given as an intradermal injection.
▼ **Sputum culture with Gram stain** is indicated for patients who have a productive cough. Acid-fast staining should be done if TB is suspected.

Suspected Immunologic Disorder

A CBC with differential; quantitative IgG, IgA, and IgM levels; functional antibody levels (to assess B lymphocyte function); an anergy panel (to assess T lymphocyte function); and an HIV test are indicated.

Other Disorders

▼ α_1**-Antitrypsin (α_1-AT) level**. An α_1-AT level with genetic variants should be obtained in patients with emphysema to rule out α_1-AT deficiency.
▼ **ACE level.** The ACE level may be elevated in patients with sarcoidosis.

Diagnostic Modalities

▼ **Radiographic studies.** Radiographs or CT scans of the chest or sinuses may be indicated. A barium swallow, milk scan, or pH probe should be considered for most infants with chronic coughing to rule out GRD, tracheoesophageal fistula, or vascular ring or sling.

▼ **Bronchoscopy (with or without lavage)** is useful for inspecting airway anatomy and dynamics, detecting a foreign body, and sampling lung material for culture.

▼ TREATMENT OF COUGH

To properly treat a chronic cough, its underlying cause must be determined. Symptomatic relief should be offered when the cough causes discomfort or interferes with the patient's ability to sleep or perform well in school. Symptomatic cough medications fall into three classes: expectorants, antitussives, and mucolytic agents.

▼ **Expectorants** help to moisturize secretions, making it easier for the patient to cough up sputum. The most effective expectorant is water; patients should be advised to drink plenty of fluids. Another effective expectorant is guaifenesin, which is found in numerous over-the-counter cough and cold preparations.

▼ **Antitussive agents** fall into two classes: peripherally acting and centrally acting medications. Peripherally acting agents (e.g., diphenhydramine) work by decreasing the sensitivity of the cough receptors in the lung. Centrally acting agents (e.g., codeine, dextromethorphan) act on the cough center located in the medulla. They abate coughing by decreasing the stimulus to cough. Dextromethorphan is as effective as codeine but is not a narcotic and thus is not habit-forming. Dextromethorphan is available in several over-the-counter cough preparations, usually in combination with antihistamines, expectorants, or both. Codeine is available only with a prescription and can be obtained as a single agent or mixed with other cough and cold preparations. Antitussive agents are not indicated when the child is otherwise well and not bothered by the cough.

▼ **Mucolytic agents** (e.g., Mucomyst, Pulmozyme) help patients who have thick, tenacious sputum (e.g., patients with cystic fibrosis). These agents help break up the mucus and, with the aid of chest physiotherapy, allow the patient to more easily expectorate sputum.

Suggested Readings

Black P: Evaluation of chronic or recurrent cough. In *Pediatric Respiratory Disease: Diagnosis and Treatment.* Philadelphia, WB Saunders, 1993, pp 143–154.

Chang AB: Cough, cough receptors, and asthma in children. *Pediatr Pulmonol* 28:59–70, 1999.

Chang AB, Asher MI: A review of cough in children. *J Asthma* 38(4):299–309, 2001.

Corrao WM: Chronic persistent cough: diagnosis and treatment update. *Pediatr Ann* 25:162–168, 1996.

Ewig JM: Chronic cough. *Pediatr Rev* 16(2):72–73, 1995.

Harding SM, Richter JE: The role of gastroesophageal reflux in chronic cough and asthma. *Chest* 111:1389–1402, 1997.

Irwin RS, Boulet LP, Cloutier MM, et al.: Managing cough as a defense mechanism and as a symptom. A consensus panel report of the American College of Chest Physicians. *Chest* 114:133S–181S, 1999.

Irwin RS, Curley FJ: The treatment of cough: a comprehensive review. *Chest* 99:1477–1484, 1991.

Katcher ML: Cold, cough and allergy medications: uses and abuses. *Pediatr Rev* 17:12–17, 1996.

Lalloo UG, Barnes PJ, Chung KF: Pathophysiology and clinical presentations of cough. *J Allergy Clin Immunol* 1996;98:S91-97.

Patrick H, Patrick F: Chronic cough. *Med Clin North Am* 79:361–372, 1995.

Schidlow DV: Cough in children. *J Asthma* 33:81–87, 1996.

Wilmott RW: Cough. In *Pediatric Primary Care: A Problem-Oriented Approach.* Edited by Schwartz MW. St. Louis, Mosby, 1997; 216–224.

24

Cyanosis

CLAUDIO RAMACIOTTI

▼ INTRODUCTION

Cyanosis is a **blue discoloration of the skin and mucous membranes** caused by the presence of **deoxygenated hemoglobin** or **abnormal hemoglobin pigments** in the blood. Cyanosis is produced by clinical conditions associated with one or more of the following abnormalities: alveolar hypoventilation, right-to-left shunting, ventilation–perfusion inequality, impairment of oxygen diffusion, or decreased affinity of hemoglobin for oxygen.

▼ **Central cyanosis** implies decreased arterial oxygen saturation.

▼ **Peripheral cyanosis** is caused by a decreased rate of peripheral blood flow. The decreased rate of peripheral blood flow increases the arteriovenous gradient and the absolute amount of desaturated hemoglobin. The most common cause of peripheral cyanosis is generalized vasoconstriction resulting from exposure to cold air or water. Peripheral cyanosis can also be related to severe congestive heart failure, shock, or venous or arterial obstruction.

▓ **HINT** Cyanosis is apparent at a mean capillary concentration of 4 g/dl of reduced hemoglobin (or 0.5 g/dl of methemoglobin). Because it is the absolute quantity of reduced hemoglobin that is responsible for cyanosis, the higher the total hemoglobin content, the greater the tendency toward cyanosis. Polycythemic patients are cyanotic at higher levels of hemoglobin saturation, whereas anemic patients may not become cyanotic even in the presence of marked arterial desaturation.

▼ DIFFERENTIAL DIAGNOSIS LIST
Cardiovascular Disease

Congenital heart defect (Table 24.1)
Eisenmenger syndrome
Arteriovenous fistula—pulmonary or systemic
Primary pulmonary hypertension
Low-output state—e.g., congestive heart failure

Respiratory Disease

Nasal obstruction
Croup syndrome
Foreign body aspiration
Tracheal compression
Tracheobronchomalacia
Bronchiolitis
Reactive airway disease
Respiratory distress syndrome (RDS)
Meconium aspiration
Pneumonia
Pneumothorax
Pleural effusion
Bronchopulmonary dysplasia
Diaphragmatic hernia
Lung hypoplasia
Respiratory muscle dysfunction—e.g., botulism, muscular dystrophy, myasthenia gravis, Werdnig-Hoffmann disease

---

TABLE 24.1.   Structural Defects Associated with Cyanosis

Ventricular septal defect
Unobstructed total anomalous pulmonary venous return
Atrioventricular canal malformation
Patent ductus arteriosus in a term infant
Aorticopulmonary window
Truncus arteriosus
Transposition of the great arteries
Double-outlet right ventricle
Single ventricle
Tricuspid atresia
Pulmonary atresia with an intact ventricular septum
Severe pulmonary stenosis
Tetralogy of Fallot
Ebstein anomaly
Complex malformations with severe pulmonary stenosis or atresia
Obstructed total anomalous pulmonary venous return
Hypoplastic left heart syndrome and a closed interatrial communication
Coarctation of the aorta
Interrupted aortic arch
Hypoplastic left heart syndrome
Severe aortic stenosis
Complex malformations that cause severe subaortic, aortic, or arch obstruction

---

Persistent fetal circulation
Cystic fibrosis

Metabolic Disease

Hypoglycemia
Methemoglobinemia

Neurologic Disease

Seizures
Cerebral edema
Central nervous system (CNS) hemorrhage
CNS infection
CNS depression—e.g., drugs, asphyxia

Miscellaneous Causes

Hypothermia
Crying
Respiratory depressants—e.g., morphine, benzodiazepines
Breath holding
Polycythemia
Sepsis

▼ DIFFERENTIAL DIAGNOSIS DISCUSSION
Heart Failure (Myocardial Dysfunction)
Etiology

Heart failure in infants that occurs in the absence of structural congenital heart disease is commonly caused by **myocarditis, dilated cardiomyopathy, arrhythmia** (e.g., congenital heart block, supraventricular tachycardia), **patent ductus arteriosus** (PDA; in preterm infants), **glycogen storage disease,** or **perinatal asphyxia.**

Heart failure and cyanosis can also be caused by congenital heart defects.

▼ **Poor mixing between the systemic and pulmonary circulations** can result from ventricular septal defect, unobstructed total anomalous pulmonary venous return, atrioventricular canal malformations, PDA (in a term infant), aorticopulmonary window, and truncus arteriosus. Symptoms usually appear 2 weeks after birth. As the pulmonary vascular resistance drops below 25% of the systemic rate, the infant develops signs of pulmonary overcirculation.

▼ **Decreased pulmonary blood flow** in the presence of normal peripheral perfusion can be seen in tricuspid atresia, pulmonary atresia with an intact ventricular septum, critical pulmonary stenosis, tetralogy of Fallot, Ebstein anomaly, and complex manifestations with severe pulmonary stenosis or atresia. Patients typically present with **cyanosis;** the arterial oxygen tension (Pao_2) is typically 20–35 mm Hg. The amount of pulmonary blood flow (and, consequently, the Pao_2 value) depends on the pulmonary vascular resistance as well as the severity of the obstruction between the heart and the pulmonary artery and the size of the ductus arteriosus. No murmurs or a continuous murmur may be heard. An **ejection murmur** is present **with less severe obstruction,** such as occurs in tetralogy of Fallot. The second heart sound (S_2) is often single. On a chest radiograph, a **right aortic arch** is commonly seen in patients with **tetralogy of Fallot,** in addition to signs of decreased pulmonary blood flow. In patients with **tricuspid atresia, left axis deviation on an electrocardiogram is characteristic.**

▼ **Increased pulmonary venous pressure.** Defects leading to increased pulmonary venous pressure include total anomalous venous return (obstructed type) and hypoplastic left heart syndrome accompanied by a closed (or nearly closed) interatrial communication. Increased pulmonary venous pressure leads to pulmonary edema and poor gas exchange. Patients present with severe respiratory distress and cyanosis. The Pao_2 is 15–25 mm Hg.

▼ **Decreased systemic perfusion** can be caused by coarctation of the aorta, interrupted aortic arch, hypoplastic left heart syndrome, critical aortic stenosis, or any complex anomaly that causes severe subaortic, aortic, or arch obstruction. Infants with defects that cause decreased systemic perfusion tend to not be extremely cyanotic—the Pao_2 is 35–50 mm Hg. These infants frequently present with **metabolic acidosis** and other signs of decreased peripheral perfusion. The clinical picture can be similar to that seen in neonatal sepsis.

Clinical Features

Patients present with **respiratory distress** and **cyanosis.** They may have a history of **poor feeding, growth retardation,** or **excessive sweating.**

Evaluation

Tachycardia, tachypnea, and **hepatomegaly** may be noted on physical examination. Peripheral pulses and blood pressure should be evaluated in all four extremities. A **discrepancy between** the **pulses** noted **in the upper extremities and** those measured in the **lower extremities** can be the first clue to the diagnosis of coarctation of the aorta. Severe heart failure can be associated with a **decreased pulse rate;** bradycardia suggests congenital heart block.

The radiographic finding of a small heart contradicts the diagnosis of heart failure. An **echocardiogram** should be obtained.

Treatment

Supportive therapy is **dictated by the defect** (e.g., prostaglandins to prevent closure of the ductus arteriosus, inotropic support for myocardial failure, inhaled nitrogen to decrease pulmonary blood flow in infants with hypoplastic left heart syndrome).

Methemoglobinemia

Etiology

Methemoglobinemia may be toxic or hereditary in origin:

▼ **Toxic causes** include aniline dyes, nitrobenzene, azo compounds, and nitrites.

▼ **Hereditary causes.** There are four described types of hereditary methemoglobinemia.

Clinical Features

Patients with methemoglobinemia present with **cyanosis** in spite of an **increased Pao_2** value. There is no respiratory distress.

Evaluation

Bedside diagnosis of methemoglobinemia entails placing a **drop of the patient's blood on a piece of filter paper.** After 30 seconds of exposure to air, normal blood turns red, while blood taken from a patient with methemoglobinemia remains **chocolate brown.** The physician should also check for the **presence of oxidant drugs.**

Treatment

Methylene blue is administered intravenously.

Pulmonary Disorders

Cyanosis in older children may be a sign of **reactive airway disease (asthma)** or **cystic fibrosis.** Both of these entities are discussed in Chapter 23, "Cough."

Cyanotic Spells

Etiology

Patients with tetralogy of Fallot may have **attacks of paroxysmal hyperpnea** and **increased cyanosis** that occur **spontaneously** or **after early morning feedings, prolonged crying,** or **defecation.** These attacks ("cyanotic spells") occur most commonly in infants 3–18 months of age and constitute a **medical emergency.** Relative **iron deficiency anemia,** which can also precipitate these spells, **must be ruled out.**

Clinical Features

The attacks can be **mild** and last only a few moments (and may erroneously be labeled "colic"); they may be **more prolonged** and followed by **limpness and deep sleep;** or, rarely, they may result in **unconsciousness, convulsions,** or **death.** During an attack, the systolic ejection murmur characteristic of tetralogy of Fallot often disappears.

Treatment

Treatment involves placement of the patient in the **knee–chest position, administration of oxygen,** and the **intravenous administration of phenylephrine, morphine sulfate, and propranolol.** More prolonged attacks should be treated with **sodium bicarbonate** administration. Cyanotic spells are an indication for **surgical intervention.**

▼ EVALUATION OF CYANOSIS

Neonates

Patient History

Important information to obtain from the history includes the following:

▼ Is there a history of maternal infection?
▼ When did the mother's membranes rupture? Early rupture of the membranes predisposes the neonate to infection or sepsis.
▼ Is there a history of asphyxia?
▼ What was the baby's gestational age?
▼ How old was the baby when the first episode of cyanosis occurred?
▼ Has the baby shown signs of feeding intolerance? Does the infant sweat during feedings?

Physical Examination

During the physical examination, the physician should check for signs of impending respiratory failure or circulatory failure, and be prepared to give ventilatory support.

▼ **Vital signs.** The infant's body temperature should be noted. If the baby is hypothermic, examination should take place after measures have been taken to warm the patient.

▼ **Skin color.** Skin color has an impact on the diagnosis; in light skinned patients, cyanosis is usually noted with an arterial oxygen saturation of less than 85%, while in dark-skinned patients, the arterial oxygen saturation must be even lower. Differential cyanosis is present when the degree of cyanosis observed in the hands is different from the degree of cyanosis noted in the feet. In the neonatal period, differential cyanosis is observed in patients with left-sided obstructive heart lesions or arch obstruction and right-to-left ductal shunting, and in those with persistent pulmonary hypertension (PPH) and significant right-to-left ductal shunting. In older patients, differential cyanosis is seen in association with PDA and pulmonary vascular obstructive disease. Pre- and postductal oxygen saturations are useful in documenting differential cyanosis.

▼ **Respiratory examination.** An increased respiratory rate, increased heart rate, grunting, nasal flaring, and retractions are signs of respiratory distress. Breath sounds should be documented. Hyperpnea with cyanosis but without signs of respiratory distress is frequently observed in patients with congenital cardiac defects. Apnea is commonly related to prematurity, intracerebral problems, or medication usage. Tachypnea with nasal flaring, grunting, and intercostal and subcostal retractions often reflects an upper or lower airway disturbance. A high respiratory rate (greater than 80 breaths/min) is unusual with cardiac lesions that are associated with restricted pulmonary blood flow.

▼ **Cardiovascular examination.** Absence of a heart murmur does not rule out congenital heart disease; severe cyanosis without a heart murmur suggests transposition of the great arteries. The pulses and blood pressure should be documented in all four extremities.

Laboratory Studies

A **complete blood count (CBC)** with differential, **blood cultures,** and **urine cultures** should be obtained. If infection is strongly suspected, a **lumbar puncture (LP)** may be indicated. A **serum glucose** level may be appropriate.

The **change in the Pao_2 in response to administration of 100% supplemental oxygen** for 5–10 minutes is useful for differentiating intracardiac shunting from intrapulmonary shunting. If the Pao_2 value increases while the arterial carbon dioxide tension value decreases, PPH of the newborn is a possibility. A **Pao_2 greater than 250 mm Hg excludes a cardiac cause,** whereas a **Pao_2 greater than 160 mm Hg** makes a cardiac cause **less likely. Little or no change** makes the diagnosis of congenital heart disease **highly probable.** Ideally, sampling of the arterial blood should be from the **right temporal or radial arteries** to avoid contamination of blood shunting through a PDA.

The **transcutaneous measurement of oxygen saturation** in patients with good peripheral perfusion can also be helpful. However, one must remember that in the **neonatal period,** the high proportion of fetal hemoglobin in the blood and reduced levels of 2,3-diphosphoglycerate result in a **shift in the** oxygen dissociation curve to the left, so that full saturation can be achieved at lower Pao$_2$ levels than in an older child. Accordingly, in some neonates, 95% saturation may be reached with a Pao$_2$ of 45–50 mm Hg, and a Pao$_2$ of greater than 80 mm Hg causes little change in the oxygen saturation. The equipment currently available for measuring transcutaneous oxygen saturation has been designed (and is more accurate) for the high saturation range. The examiner must always make sure that the heart rate shown corresponds to the actual rate, so that the oxygen saturation rate displayed is reliable.

Older Children

Patient History
▼ What is the onset, duration, and frequency of episodes?
▼ Is there associated coughing, wheezing, or stridor?
▼ Were there any precipitating factors?
▼ Have there been previous episodes?
▼ What is the child's medication history?
▼ Have the child's growth and development been normal?
▼ Has the child had any contact with anyone with an infectious disease?
▼ What is the child's family history?

Physical Examination
As with infants, the physician should check for signs of impending respiratory or circulatory failure, and should be prepared to give ventilatory support.

▼ **Vital signs** should be documented.
▼ **Respiratory examination.** Rhinorrhea should be noted, and the patient should be examined for signs of otitis media, pharyngitis, and sinusitis. Hoarseness, drooling, stridor, and breath sounds (e.g., rales, wheezing) should be noted. If epiglottitis is suspected, the pharynx should not be examined.
▼ **Cardiovascular examination.** The pulse rate and blood pressure in all four extremities should be documented.

⚔ HINT Clubbing refers to selective bullous enlargement of the distal segments (particularly of the dorsal surface) of the fingers and toes. This enlargement is caused by proliferation of connective tissue. Clubbing may be hereditary, idiopathic, or associated with a variety of disorders, including congenital heart disease, infective endocarditis, pulmonary conditions, and gastrointestinal diseases (e.g., regional enteritis, chronic ulcerative colitis, hepatic cirrhosis). It is usually seen only after the first few months of life. Patients with abnormal hemoglobins that cause cyanosis usually do not have clubbing of the fingers and toes.

Laboratory Studies and Diagnostic Modalities
Appropriate studies may include:

▼ A CBC with differential and a blood culture
▼ Arterial blood gas analysis (if the cyanosis is severe)
▼ Pulmonary function tests
▼ A chest radiograph

Suggested Readings

Driscoll, DJ: Evaluation of the cyanotic newborn. *Pediatr Clin North Am* 37: 1–23, 1990.

Grifka RG: Cyanotic congenital heart disease with increased pulmonary blood flow. *Pediatr Clin North Am* 46(2):405–425, 1999.

Grylack LJ, Williams AD: Apparent life-threatening events in presumed healthy neonates during the first three days of life. *Pediatrics* 97(3):349–351, 1996.

Schmitt HJ, Schuetz WH, Proeschel PA, et al: Accuracy of pulse oximetry in children with congenital heart disease. *J Cardiothorac Vasc Anesth* 7:61–65, 1993.

Waldman JD, Wernly JA: Cyanotic congenital heart disease with decreased pulmonary blood flow in children. *Pediatr Clin North Am* 46(2):385–404, 1999.

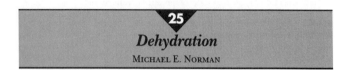

25

Dehydration

Michael E. Norman

▼ DIFFERENTIAL DIAGNOSIS LIST

Hypovolemic Dehydration

Diarrhea
Vomiting
Excessive insensible salt and water loss—e.g., cystic fibrosis
Excessive urinary losses

Hemorrhagic Dehydration

Trauma
Coagulation disorders
Thrombocytopenia
Vascular malformation
Iatrogenic (postsurgical)

Distributive Dehydration

Sepsis
Nephrotic syndrome
Severe liver or pancreatic disorders

▼ DIFFERENTIAL DIAGNOSIS DISCUSSION

Hypovolemic Dehydration

Physiology

In a state of health, **the body regulates fluid volume and tonicity** with precision. This degree of regulation is made possible through the coordinated

TABLE 25.1. Normal Physiologic Losses

Kilograms	Normal Physiologic Loss (ml/100 cal/kg/day)*
1–10	100
10–20	50
20–50	20

* Where 100 calories are expended per kg of weight per day.

efforts of the brain, gastrointestinal tract, and kidneys, as well as through afferent pressure and volume receptors located in the heart and great vessels.

Normally, external fluid balance is maintained because **physiologic fluid losses** through the lungs and skin (i.e., insensible water loss), the stools, and the urine are **matched by oral intake,** particularly in older children who have free access to fluids and an intact thirst center. Water losses through the stool are typically negligible. Insensible water loss (normally two thirds from the skin and one third from the lungs) is a function of metabolic rate, which is ordinarily expressed in caloric expenditure per unit time. **Metabolic rate is highest in early infancy** and varies directly with body size, which parallels surface area in this age group. However, the metabolic rate per unit age/weight slows as the child grows older. The renal osmotic load (i.e., the nonmetabolizable solutes that require renal excretion—sodium and urea in humans) and urinary concentration limits dictate the "physiologic" volume of urine that must be excreted each day to maintain solute balance.

When internal water production is subtracted, normal **physiologic losses** that must be replaced to achieve external water balance are as given in Table 25.1. Thus, a 30-kg child ordinarily would require 1700 ml of fluid per day: 1000 ml for the first 10 kg of weight, 500 ml for the next 10 kg, and 200 ml for the last 10 kg.

Routine electrolyte requirements are given in Table 25.2. The serum concentration of sodium, which is commonly used to classify the type of dehydration, is neither reflective of nor a measure of total body sodium or water. In states of dehydration, the serum sodium concentration may be low, normal, or increased; however, in all cases, the total body sodium value is low because of the net loss of water and sodium. In routine clinical practice, dehydration is isonatremic in 70%–75% of patients (i.e., serum sodium is 135–145 mEq/L); hyponatremic in 15% of patients (i.e., serum sodium is less than 135 mEq/L); and hypernatremic in 10%–15% of patients (i.e., serum sodium is greater than 145 mEq/L).

TABLE 25.2. Routine Electrolyte Requirements

Electrolyte	Requirement (mEq/100 cal/kg/day)
Sodium	2–3
Potassium	1–2
Chloride	3–5

It is important to remember that sodium is predominantly localized in the **extracellular fluid (ECF) compartment,** yet it regulates the free movement of water between the **intracellular fluid (ICF) compartment** and ECF compartment. The **interstitial space,** a potential reservoir for large volumes of fluid and electrolytes in certain pathologic states (e.g., nephrotic syndrome), lies between the ICF and ECF compartments.

Children younger than 1 year of age are especially susceptible to hypovolemic dehydration because of four factors:

▼ They are commonly **infected with a variety of enteric pathogens** that produce diarrhea.

▼ They have a **relatively large body surface area:weight ratio,** resulting in potentially large evaporative losses of fluid.

▼ **Urine is not concentrated as well as it is in older children** and adults. When coupled with a relatively large, fixed urinary solute load (i.e., approximately 20 mOsm/kg/day in bottle-fed infants), the required urine volume needed to avoid solute retention is often greater than in older individuals.

▼ The **percentage of fluid and electrolyte reserves is much less than in older patients** when adjusted for total body weight. Thus, a 10-kg, 1-year-old child becomes symptomatic at a diarrheal (i.e., 90% water and electrolytes) weight loss of 1 kg, or 10%, whereas a 20-kg, 4-year-old child will not become symptomatic with the same illness until he loses twice that amount of fluid and electrolytes.

Clinical Features

Table 25.3 summarizes the clinical features of hypovolemic dehydration. The physical signs of dehydration largely reflect the state of the ECF space. Because water moves freely from the ICF space to the ECF space to restore

TABLE 25.3. Clinical Signs of Dehydration in Children

Parameter	Mild	Moderate	Severe
Activity	Normal	Lethargic	Lethargic to comatose
Color	Pale	Gray	Mottled
Urine output	Decreased (< 2–3 ml/kg/hr)	Oliguric (< 1 ml/kg/hr)	Anuric
Fontanelle	Flat	Depressed	Sunken
Mucous membranes	Dry	Very dry	Cracked
Skin turgor	Slightly decreased	Markedly decreased	Tenting
Pulse	Normal to increased	Increased	Grossly tachycardic
Blood pressure	Normal	Normal	Decreased
Weight loss	5%	10%	15%

Hypernatremic dehydration may be accompanied by moderate clinical signs. Reprinted with permission from Rogers MC: Shock. In *Handbook of Pediatric Intensive Care,* 2nd ed. Edited by Rogers MC, Helfaer MA. Baltimore, Williams & Wilkins, 1994, p 140.

osmotic equilibrium (disequilibrium largely results from the loss or replacement of sodium), **hyponatremic dehydration** presents earlier and with more significant signs of dehydration (water in) than does **hypernatremic dehydration** (water out). In hyponatremic dehydration, net water movement is from the ECF space to the ICF space; in hypernatremic dehydration, the net flow is reversed.

Evaluation

Estimating deficits is critical to designing a successful rehydration program. There are three common approaches to estimating deficits. All take advantage of the clinical observation that most dehydrating illnesses in pediatric patients consist of largely fluid and electrolyte (not solid tissue) losses. In decreasing order of precision, these approaches are:

▼ **Comparison of recent weights.** The patient's basal (pre-illness) weight (obtained at least 4–6 weeks prior to the patient's admission to the hospital) is used as a basis for comparison.
▼ **Average weight for height or length ratio.** For example, if the height or length is at the 50th percentile for the child's chronologic age, then the ratio is 50%, and the patient's "ideal weight" should also be the value at the 50th percentile for that child's chronologic age.
▼ **Bedside assessment of the degree of dehydration.** Bedside assessment is by far the most commonly used assessment tool in routine pediatric practice. The degree of dehydration is usually recorded as "mild, moderate, or severe," or as a percentage signifying weight loss (e.g., 5%, 10%, 15%). The following formula is used to arrive at the predicted "ideal weight:"

$$\frac{X}{\text{current weight}} = \frac{10.0}{100 - (\text{estimated weight loss})}$$

where X is the ideal weight. In this model, mild dehydration is equivalent to a 5% weight loss; moderate dehydration equals a 10% weight loss; severe dehydration equals a 15% weight loss; and shock is usually seen after a weight loss of more than 15%–20%.

Hemorrhagic Dehydration

Clinical Features

Hemorrhage often produces alteration in the level of consciousness as well as skin color changes.

Evaluation

In most patients with hemorrhagic dehydration, the history will yield obvious clues, such as a serious injury, a personal or family history of a bleeding problem, or known vascular abnormalities.

The physical examination typically reveals signs of **hemodynamic instability** that roughly parallel both the amount and the rate of external bleeding. When hemodynamic instability occurs out of proportion to measured losses, internal or concealed hemorrhage must always be considered. Remember that in young children, a high heart rate coupled with an increased basal circulating level of catecholamines makes **hypotension a late and ominous sign** of hemorrhagic hypovolemia; therefore, a normal blood pressure should not be trusted.

When assessing the degree of hemorrhage, remember that it takes several hours for the hemoglobin concentration in plasma to re-equilibrate after acute losses. Internal bleeding may be difficult to ascertain by physical examination, but a high index of suspicion, coupled with serial hemoglobin and hematocrit values, computed tomography, and magnetic resonance imaging, usually yields a prompt and correct diagnosis.

Treatment

The administration of 2 ml/kg of body weight of blood increases the plasma hemoglobin concentration by approximately 1 g/dl. In patients with hemorrhagic hypovolemia, there is no substitute for close clinical and laboratory monitoring of the patient to determine whether the rate of transfusion is keeping pace with the blood loss.

▼ DISTRIBUTIVE DEHYDRATION

In distributive dehydration, there are **no actual net external losses of fluid or electrolytes.** The history and physical findings (lethargy, rapid pulse, poor peripheral perfusion, and poor urine output) often suggest that the ECF volume is diminished, even though the total body water and electrolyte values may be normal.

Etiology

The most common cause of distributive dehydration is the **sepsis syndrome.**

Clinical Features

The history typically reveals the **sudden onset of a high fever,** occurring either de novo or after the onset of an obvious respiratory, gastrointestinal, or urinary tract infection. There is often **listlessness, diminished alertness,** and **age-inappropriate behavior** such as hallucinations or disinterest in the surroundings. Additional history may include vomiting, diarrhea, a nonblanching petechial or hemorrhagic rash, respiratory distress, or oliguria.

Physical findings often include **obvious signs of dehydration** without obvious external losses, meningismus, a petechial or hemorrhagic rash, evidence of septic emboli, and respiratory distress with pulmonary edema. Young children are often obtunded and manifest skin mottling, poor peripheral perfusion, and temperature instability. Frank hypotension for age is a late and often ominous finding.

Evaluation

The laboratory database should be extended to include appropriate **bacterial cultures** plus a **complete blood cell (CBC) count.** Leukopenia or leukocytosis together with elevated bands, thrombocytopenia, evidence of a coagulopathy, liver and pancreatic dysfunction, and a chest radiograph compatible with acute respiratory distress syndrome round out the typical picture of overwhelming sepsis with hypovolemia.

Routine blood chemistry results typically show **metabolic acidosis.** Early on, compensatory respiratory alkalosis with hypocapnia may also be noted. If the respiratory distress syndrome ensues, however, there may be late respiratory acidosis with hypercapnia, aggravating preexisting metabolic acidosis.

Treatment

Treatment consists of maintaining the airway, breathing, and circulation, followed often by the intravenous administration of antibiotics, crystalloids, blood products, and alkali. Therapy, often including intensive support in special care units, is continued until hemodynamic stability (i.e., peripheral perfusion) is achieved.

▼ EVALUATION OF DEHYDRATION

Clinical assessment consists of three elements that must always be addressed (and must be reproducible) in every case of dehydration: patient history, physical examination, and laboratory studies.

Patient History

In taking the history, the following questions should be asked:

▼ **What was the route, duration, and magnitude of the losses?**
▼ **What was given back (and retained) as replacement fluid?** The amount, rate, and composition (which may need to be approximated) must be listed.
▼ **What is the urine output compared with the "norm" for that child when well?** (In infants, how often are diapers changed?)
▼ **What is the course of the child's temperature?**
▼ **What is the child's degree of departure from normal in terms of affect, level of alertness, and sleep–wake cycle?**
▼ **What was the child's weight prior to becoming ill?** (This may not be known.)
▼ **What is the degree of thirst in a child who normally has free access to fluids?**
▼ **What is "going around" in the community at present?** (An epidemiologic search is part of most pediatric histories.)

Physical Examination

The physical examination should include evaluation of the following:

▼ **Comparable weights,** if available; otherwise, "ideal" weight for height or length or bedside estimates of the degree of dehydration
▼ **Skin turgor, color,** and **temperature**
▼ **Peripheral perfusion**
▼ **Presence or absence of tears** in the crying child
▼ **Core temperature and other vital signs,** including blood pressure

---

✔ HINT A dry mouth may reflect mouth breathing.

Laboratory Studies

The following laboratory tests should be ordered to establish a laboratory database:

▼ **Routine serum electrolytes, including sodium, potassium, chloride, and bicarbonate levels.** The serum sodium level is an index of the relative net losses of water and sodium [i.e., (water + sodium gain) − (water + sodium

TABLE 25.4. Normal Values for Fractional Excretion of Sodium (Fe$_{Na}$)

	Prerenal ARF	Intrinsic ARF
Adult or child	< 1.0	> 2.0
Infant (neonate)	< 2.5	> 2.5

ARF = acute renal failure.

loss)], and, when coupled with the history and physical examination, aids in guiding rehydration therapy.

▼ **Serum blood urea nitrogen (BUN) and creatinine levels**
▼ **Urinalysis,** especially specific gravity
▼ **Fractional excretion of sodium (FE$_{Na}$).** Normal values are shown in Table 25.4.

▼ TREATMENT OF REHYDRATION

Generally speaking, rehydration programs in hospitals in the United States call for the **intravenous** (or oral and intravenous) **administration of fluid and electrolytes.** In underdeveloped countries, however, oral rehydration has been widely introduced and successfully practiced. Occasionally it is difficult to obtain intravenous access in a patient presenting with hypovolemic shock; these patients are often given the initial fluid boluses via the interosseous route.

Designing a Rehydration Program

Questions Pertaining to Development of a Program

The following questions can be answered on the basis of the laboratory database and a careful history and physical examination:

▼ Is there a volume deficit and if so, what type?
▼ Is there a disturbance in tonicity or osmolarity?
▼ Is there an acid-base disturbance?
▼ Is there a potassium deficit?
▼ What is the current state of renal function?

Questions Pertaining to Implementation of a Program

▼ What kind of solution should be given?
▼ How much solution should be given?
▼ How fast should the solution be given (i.e., how is the rate of repair staged)?

Oral Rehydration

This technique has **proven efficacy,** is vastly **less expensive** than hospitalization for intravenous rehydration, and features a **minimum of side effects** in well-chosen patients. Numerous investigations have documented the rapid and efficient transport of fluid, electrolytes, and glucose across the infant's gastrointestinal tract, even at a very early age.

Commercially available solutions containing 40–90 mEq/L of sodium (Table 25.5) have been found to be quite effective, regardless of the initial type of dehydration. The prevalence of hypernatremic, isonatremic, or

TABLE 25.5. Commercially Available Oral Rehydration Fluids (in mEq/L)

	Na$^+$	K$^+$	Cl$^-$	Base	Glucose
Pedialyte	45	20	35	30	2.5
Lytren	50	25	45	30	2.0
Rehydralyte	75	20	65	30	2.5
WHO formula	90	20	80	30	2.0

hyponatremic dehydration in a given geographic area determines in part which oral rehydration solutions are commonly available. The choice of commercially available solutions varies in accordance with the nature of the dehydration (osmotic versus secretory diarrhea) and the local epidemiology of disease.

Small, frequent oral feedings are preferred, using lactose-free, high-carbohydrate, low-fat solutions. If milk is introduced early, one must watch for either underlying or secondary cow's milk intolerance by checking stool water for blood, reducing substances, and leukocytes. Generally, it is initially useful in patients with a "typical case" of diarrheal dehydration to "piggyback" oral rehydration and the administration of intravenous solutions, which should run at a reduced rate if the patient is taking fluids well orally. Intravenous solutions should not be summarily discontinued; doing so can cause clinical setbacks in a patient who manifests longer-than-usual gastrointestinal intolerance to oral fluids.

Contraindications to oral rehydration include:

▼ An **inability to take fluids by mouth**
▼ **Ongoing stool water losses** of greater than 5 ml/kg/hour for more than 8–12 hours
▼ **Severe metabolic acidemia,** particularly in patients with underlying renal disease

Intravenous Rehydration

Rate of Repair

▼ **Deficits.** The rate of repair of deficits depends in part on the initial state of serum tonicity. For isonatremic or hyponatremic patients, one should plan to repair one half to two thirds of the calculated deficit in the first 8–12 hours, depending on the degree of dehydration, the presence or absence of complicating factors, and parental expectations. Hypernatremic patients always have a coexisting free water deficit; therefore, 2 full days should be allowed for repair (i.e., approximately 25% of the calculated deficit should be administered every 12 hours).
▼ **Physiologic losses.** The replacement of physiologic losses takes place evenly over 24 hours.
▼ **Ongoing losses.** If the cause of the dehydration is gastrointestinal, ongoing losses will be sharply curtailed once therapy has been initiated, particularly if an intravenous line has been started and the patient takes nothing by mouth.

Replacement of Bicarbonate and Potassium Losses

In younger children, particularly those with dehydration as a result of diarrhea, one should anticipate both **stool bicarbonate and potassium losses** (the average diarrheal stool contains 30–40 mEq/L of potassium). A portion of the sodium-containing fluids should be given as bicarbonate if the serum bicarbonate level is 10 mEq/L or less or if the venous pH value is 7.20 or less. In dehydrated children, the "bicarbonate space" is approximately 0.5 times the total body weight. Thus, the amount of bicarbonate to be given over 24 hours can be determined as follows:

$$\text{Bicarbonate (mEq)} = (\text{ideal} - \text{observed serum bicarbonate}) \\ \times \text{the pre-illness body weight} \times 0.5$$

Solutions

In most rehydration programs, the **maintenance and deficit fluids are mixed into a single solution,** which usually approximates one of the commercially available intravenous solutions: 5% dextrose in physiologic, half-physiologic, third-physiologic, or quarter-physiologic saline (i.e., D5/0.9% physiologic saline solution (PSS); D5/0.45% PSS; D5/0.3% PSS; or D5/0.2% PSS). Using a more dilute solution, especially in patients with hypernatremic dehydration, carries the risk of overzealous correction of hypertonicity and central nervous system (CNS) complications.

Special Problems

▼ **Fever.** For every degree of sustained temperature elevation above the upper limit of normal, 10% must be added to the calculation for insensible water loss.

▼ **Hypernatremia.** Of the total calculated deficit, on average, for every mEq of sodium greater than the upper limit of normal (i.e., 145 mEq/L) there is a "free water deficit" of approximately 4 ml/kg. This fraction of the total fluid deficit should be calculated as a percentage of the total deficit. As always, the tonicity of the intravenous fluids should not fall below D5/0.3 PSS. The deficit repair should not be completed in less than 48 hours, and the serum sodium level should not be lowered by more than 10 mEq/L/day. In hypernatremic patients, the serum electrolyte values should be measured every 12 hours, particularly if the starting serum sodium level is greater than 160 mEq/L.

▼ **Impaired renal function.** A history of poor linear growth, hypertension, chronic enuresis, polyuria, or polydipsia (in the absence of glycosuria) should alert one to the possibility of the presence of underlying renal disease, with its attendant failure to respond to conventional therapy. If the BUN and serum creatinine levels are increased in the presence of dehydration, especially in the setting of an abnormally increased FE_{Na} value and an inappropriately low urine-specific gravity or urine output, the urine output must be followed serially during the process of rehydration. Close attention must also be paid to the urinalysis, particularly to the urine sediment, for signs of chronic renal disease.

▼ **Shock.** In a patient with signs and symptoms of shock, vigorous fluid resuscitation using either crystalloid or colloid solutions must be given until hemodynamic stability is regained. The author usually does not include such fluids in the calculation of the estimated deficit. Physiologic concentrations of saline would be included if that solution were chosen, regardless of the initial laboratory database values. When vascular integrity is assumed to be preserved, the author favors 5% albumin in physiologic saline over physiologic saline or lactated Ringer's solution because approximately two thirds of the crystalloid solution rapidly moves into the ICF space. In the case of Ringer's solution, the lower chloride concentration (which theoretically reduces the acid stress) is more than offset by the need for the liver to convert acetate to bicarbonate rapidly and fully. The ability of the liver to convert acetate to bicarbonate may not be counted on, however, in cases of hypovolemic shock.

Sample Case

A 1-year-old previously well girl presents with a **3-day history of afebrile diarrheal dehydration.** Her pre-illness weight (obtained 1 week ago) was 10.0 kg; her weight on admission is 9.0 kg. The mother says the child has been somewhat lethargic and that previously she had a fever. Her urine output has decreased. When queried, the mother reports that the child has retained "some" Pedialyte, given orally. Physical examination reveals mild tenting of the skin, dry mucous membranes, lethargy, and decreased tears but preserved skin color, temperature, and perfusion. **Laboratory test results** are as follows:

Serum Na^+ = 140 mEq/L
Serum Cl^- = 100 mEq/L
Serum K^+ = 4 mEq/L
Serum HCO_3^- = 15 mEq/L
BUN = 20 mEq/L
Creatinine = 0.8 mEq/L
Urinalysis negative
Urine dipstick negative
Urine-specific gravity = 1.030
FE_{Na} = 0.9%

This patient has 10% diarrheal dehydration with isonatremia, mild metabolic acidosis not requiring bicarbonate therapy, slight azotemia (the BUN and creatinine values top normal for age, especially in the absence of recent protein intake), an appropriately concentrated urine for age and circumstance, and preservation of glomerulotubular balance (i.e., a normal FE_{Na} value) in the face of an appropriate stimulus to concentrate the urine and maximally reabsorb filtered sodium. Potassium losses are assumed because of diarrhea, despite a normal serum potassium value, owing to the acidosis (which caused a transcellular shift of potassium from the ICF to the ECF).

A **worksheet** is a useful and convenient tool for calculating how much fluid to give, how fast to give it, and its tonicity. It also allows the attending physician to supervise and educate the physician-in-training who is writing the rehydration orders. In this patient, a completed worksheet delineating the plan for rehydration would look like Table 25.6.

The resultant fluid for replacement/maintenance might consist of approximately 64 mEq of sodium and half the calculated deficit of potassium per

TABLE 25.6. Rehydration Plan for Sample Case

	Component			
	Water (ml)	Sodium (mEq)	Potassium (mEq)	Chloride (mEq)
Deficit	1000	70*	34–40†	100–110
+ Maintenance	1000	20–30	10–20	30–50
+ Ongoing loss	...	...	...	...
SUBTOTALS	2000	90–100	44–60	130–160
− Initial therapy‡	200	31	0	31
Remaining balance	1800	59–69	44–60	99–121

* In an average case of diarrheal dehydration, occurring over 3 days, approximately half of the electrolytes are lost from the extracellular fluid (ECF). Assuming a 1000-ml fluid loss at an average sodium concentration of 140 mEq/L, half that loss would be approximately 70 mEq in 500 ml of fluid. In acute losses, one should assume a 20% loss from the intracellular fluid (ICF) and an 80% loss from the ECF; in chronic losses, one should assume a 40%:60% loss ratio.

† The average diarrhea stool is more than 90% fluid and contains 30–40 mEq/L of potassium.

‡ The typical fluid bolus given initially to dehydrated patients is 20 ml/kg of physiologic saline at a sodium chloride concentration of 154 mEq/L for each electrolyte.

day (to be administered over 2 days). Chloride is a convenient vehicle (e.g., salt) for replacement of the sodium and potassium. The patient would be given 1800 ml in the first 24 hours (maintenance plus deficit) as D5/0.2% PSS (e.g., approximately 34 mEq/L of sodium chloride with 20 mEq/L of potassium at a rate of approximately 75 ml/hr). At the end of the first day, this should result in the administration of 1800 ml of water, approximately 61 mEq of sodium, 36 mEq of potassium, and 97 mEq of chloride, if potassium chloride is used as a source of potassium replacement. What is most important, however, is not the accuracy of these calculations but the close clinical and laboratory follow-up of the patient. The following items should always be included in the follow-up plan:

▼ **Daily weights plus intake and output**
▼ **Clinical assessments** by the physician, the primary nurse, and, most importantly, the regular caretakers
▼ **Urine volume and specific gravity**
▼ Follow-up values for **serum electrolytes, BUN, creatinine** (if initially abnormal), and **FE_{Na}**

⚡ HINT It is usually not necessary to repeat the serum electrolyte value determination more than once every 24 hours unless the initial presentation was unusually severe, the hospital course is unusual or unanticipated, or the patient has a significant preexisting disease.

▼ APPROACH TO THE PATIENT (FIGURE 25.1)

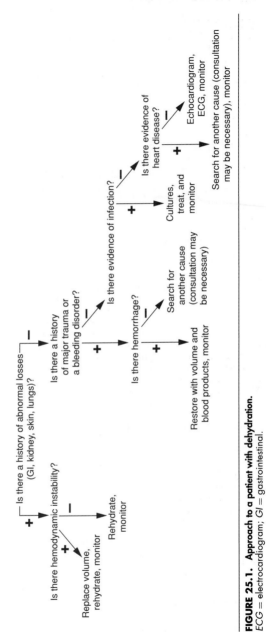

FIGURE 25.1.   Approach to a patient with dehydration.
ECG = electrocardiogram; *GI* = gastrointestinal.

Suggested Readings

Casteel HB, Fiedorek SC: Oral rehydration therapy. *Pediatr Clin North Am* 37:295, 1990.

Espinel CH: The FE$_{Na}$ test. *JAMA* 236:579, 1976.

Mathew OP, Jones AS, James E, et al.: Neonatal renal failure: usefulness of diagnostic indices. *Pediatrics* 65:57, 1980.

Miller TR, Anderson JR, Linas SL, et al.: Urinary diagnostic indices in acute failure: a prospective study. *Ann Intern Med* 89:47, 1978.

26

▼ Diabetes

STUART ALAN WEINZIMER

▼ INTRODUCTION

Diabetes mellitus is a disorder of glucose metabolism characterized by **hyperglycemia** due to insulin deficiency. Diabetes actually encompasses several clinical syndromes. **Type I [insulin-dependent diabetes mellitus (IDDM)]**, formerly called juvenile-onset diabetes mellitus, is characterized by rapid onset, a tendency toward ketoacidosis, and absolute insulin deficiency. **Type II diabetes,** formerly called non-IDDM, is associated with obesity, a lesser likelihood of ketoacidosis, insulin resistance, and nonabsolute dependence on insulin for survival. Both types of diabetes are associated with the same long-term complications. The primary focus of this discussion is type I diabetes, which affects 1 in 350 children younger than 18 years of age.

▼ DIFFERENTIAL DIAGNOSIS LIST

Infectious Disorders

Urinary tract infection (UTI)
Gastroenteritis
Pneumonia
Sepsis

Toxic Disorders

Salicylate ingestion
Steroid use
Diuretic use

Endocrine and Metabolic Disorders

Hypercalcemia
Diabetes insipidus
Inborn error of metabolism

Miscellaneous Disorders

Renal glycosuria
Stress hyperglycemia

Psychosocial Disorders

Psychogenic polydipsia
Enuresis

▼ EVALUATION OF DIABETES

Patient History

- ▼ **Polyuria, polydipsia,** and **polyphagia** are the classic symptoms.
- ▼ **Weight loss** and **poor growth** are the earliest signs and may go undetected.
- ▼ **Nausea, vomiting,** and **lethargy** occur as the child's illness progresses.
- ▼ **A precipitating event** (intercurrent illness or stress) often prompts medical attention.

Physical Examination

Physical examination is usually normal early in the course of the disease. Later findings can include:

- ▼ **Signs of dehydration** (e.g., tachycardia, poor skin perfusion, hypotension)
- ▼ **Hyperpnea (Kussmaul respirations),** a sign of metabolic acidosis
- ▼ **Fruity odor to the breath,** a sign of ketosis

Laboratory Studies

- ▼ A **fasting blood glucose level** greater than 126 mg/dl or **random blood glucose level** greater than 200 mg/dl confirms the diagnosis of diabetes.
- ▼ **Urinalysis** may reveal glycosuria and ketonuria.
- ▼ A **serum electrolyte panel** may reveal hyponatremia (a sodium level of less than 136 mEq/L from hyperglycemia and hypertriglyceridemia; hypokalemia or hyperkalemia (a potassium level of less than 4.0 mEq/L or more than 6.0 mEq/L, respectively); or a metabolic acidosis (bicarbonate level less than 15 mEq/L).
- ▼ **Arterial blood gases** may reveal a low pH (less than 7.3) and a partial pressure of carbon dioxide (pco_2) of less than 35 mm Hg.
- ▼ A **complete blood cell (CBC) count** may reveal elevated white blood cell (WBC) count even in the absence of infection.
- ▼ **Glycosylated hemoglobin** will be elevated.

Differential Diagnosis

The following conditions must be ruled out:

- ▼ **UTI** and **nocturnal enuresis.** The early signs of diabetes (i.e., polyuria and nocturia) may be mistaken for UTI or nocturnal enuresis. Urinalysis, however, reveals the presence of glucose and ketones, which indicate diabetes.
- ▼ **Renal glycosuria** (a condition of abnormal glucose losses in the urine) may be mistaken for diabetes, but the presence of an elevated blood glucose level rules out renal glycosuria.
- ▼ **Other metabolic disorders** may present with acidosis and dehydration, but a history of polyuria, polyphagia, and weight loss with an elevated blood glucose is characteristic of diabetes.
- ▼ **Gastroenteritis and surgical abdomen.** The abdominal pain and vomiting of diabetic ketoacidosis (DKA) may be mistaken for gastroenteritis or a surgical abdomen, but DKA may be differentiated not only from these

disorders but also from other metabolic diseases by the distinct history of polyuria, polydipsia, and characteristic fruity odor to the breath.

▼ **Administration of glucocorticoids** for inflammatory conditions may precipitate hyperglycemia and glycosuria. These conditions must be differentiated from true diabetes. In patients who do not have diabetes, discontinuation of the medications should result in normalization of the blood sugar. Occasionally, a latent case of true diabetes may be discovered. In these cases, the presence of anti-islet cell antibodies or an elevated hemoglobin A_{1c} value indicates true diabetes.

▼ **Asthma or pneumonia.** The Kussmaul respirations that occur with progressive acidosis may resemble asthma or pneumonia, but auscultation and radiography will reveal clear lung fields.

▼ TREATMENT OF DIABETES

Optimal care requires the efforts of the child, the family, and a team of physicians, nurses, dietitians, and counselors specializing in the treatment of children with diabetes. The physician's primary responsibilities are the **prompt recognition of symptoms** leading to a definitive diagnosis, **referral** to a pediatric diabetes center, and **continued supervision** of the child's medical care. Children with diabetes should schedule an appointment every 3–6 months at a pediatric diabetes center.

Treatment goals are to maintain blood glucose level at near-normal range, the use of insulin, and to assure the child's normal growth and development. To accomplish these goals, the child must monitor his own blood sugar several times during the day, exercise, and adhere to a diet with a consistent amount of carbohydrates and without excessive fats. Family members must be trained to monitor blood sugars, give insulin, and recognize and treat low blood sugar reactions. **Psychosocial factors are critical** in the management of children with diabetes, and potential problems should be addressed by experienced behavioral or family therapists.

Insulin

The **target blood glucose level** for a child with diabetes is **80–180 mg/dl.** In patients with persistent hyperglycemia, the insulin dose must be adjusted carefully to avoid overcompensation.

The most commonly used insulin preparations are shown in Table 26.1. **Insulin dosage must be individualized** based on previous response, anticipated food intake, and activity level. Most children require approximately

TABLE 26.1. Pharmacokinetics of Common Insulin Preparations

Insulin	Onset (hr)	Peak	Duration of Action
Rapid-acting (Lispro, Aspart)	0.25	0.5–1	2–3
Short-acting (Regular, Semilente)	0.5–1.0	2–4	4–8
Long-acting (NPH, Lente)	2–4	4–12	12–18
Very-long acting (Ultralente, Glargine)	4–8	n/a	24 +

0.5–0.8 units/kg/day of insulin (less during the "honeymoon period," which may last from a few months to a year or more; often more during adolescence).

Mixtures of short- and long-acting insulin are given two or three times a day (or four times, if necessary) to provide basal levels and peaks of insulin during meals. **Blood sugars are routinely monitored before each meal,** before the insulin is given. Insulin is administered as a subcutaneous injection using a small-gauge needle. Injection sites are rotated among the arms, legs, and stomach to avoid lipoatrophy or lipohypertrophy. Insulin is typically initiated at the following dosages:

▼ 2/3 daily dose before breakfast—1/3 as short-acting, 2/3 as long-acting
▼ 1/3 daily dose before dinner or split before dinner and before bedtime—1/2 as short-acting, 1/2 as long-acting

Timing and doses of insulin must, however, be individualized based on diet, activity, and schedule.

Complications of Insulin Therapy

Hypoglycemia is the most common acute complication of diabetes management. Typical symptoms include hunger, headache, lethargy, dizziness, irritability, confusion, sweating, and tachycardia. Mild symptoms are easily treated with oral glucose (e.g., glucose tablets, orange juice). **Severe hypoglycemia** may lead to seizures and coma. These are treated with glucagon, 1 mg, given intramuscularly. All children with diabetes should carry oral glucose tablets with them at all times and keep glucagon at home. **Recurrent hypoglycemia** should be corrected aggressively. Table 26.2 gives recommended insulin adjustments.

Intercurrent Illness and DKA

Intercurrent illnesses may be managed with more frequent blood glucose monitoring and supplementary insulin. If ketones are present in the urine, give 10%–20% additional short-acting insulin with each dose until ketones have cleared. If the child is vomiting, frequent small doses of short-acting insulin are given, and long-acting insulin is temporarily discontinued. Management of ketosis and DKA is described in Table 26.3.

TABLE 26.2. Insulin Adjustments for Persistent Abnormalities of Blood Glucose

Blood Glucose	Time	Recommended Action
High	Pre-breakfast	Increase evening long/very-long-acting insulin
Low	Pre-breakfast	Decrease evening long/very-long-acting insulin
High	Pre-lunch	Increase morning rapid/short-acting insulin
Low	Pre-lunch	Decrease morning rapid/short-acting insulin
High	Pre-dinner	Increase morning long/very-long-acting insulin
Low	Pre-dinner	Decrease morning long/very-long-acting insulin
High	Bedtime	Increase evening rapid/short-acting insulin
Low	Bedtime	Decrease evening rapid/short-acting insulin

TABLE 26.3.   Guidelines to Treatment of Ketosis

Mild ketosis

Insulin	Usual dose plus 20% morning dose every 2 hours as long as hyperglycemia and ketosis persist
Fluids	Increase oral fluid intake to make up for increased urinary losses and to help clear ketones

Ketoacidosis (DKA)

Ketonemia/ketonuria	Glucose > 200 mg/dL
IV fluids	Serum arterial pH < 7.3 or bicarbonate < 15 mEq/L
	10–20 cc/kg 0.9% saline bolus to restore intravascular volume, repeat if necessary
	Replace deficit slowly over 48 hours using isotonic fluids (0.9% saline)
Sodium	Deficit 10 mEq/kg—replaced with normal saline in rehydration fluid
Potassium	Deficit 5–10 mEq/L–start after patient urinates
	if K > 4.0 add 40 mEq/L
	if K < 4.0 add 60 mEq/L
	Give potassium as 1 : 1 potassium chloride: potassium phosphate
Insulin	0.1 unit/kg/hr (the amount of glucose in the IV fluids and the rate of the insulin infusion should be titrated to lower the blood sugar 50–100 mg/dL/hr
Bicarbonate	Consider use if pH < 7.0–7.1 or if patient shows inadequate respiratory compensation
	Give 2 mEq/L or calculate dose = weight (kg) × 0.3 × (15 − [HCO_3]). Give slowly as intravenous infusion, not rapid bolus.

Monitoring

The goals of **blood glucose monitoring** are to gauge the effectiveness of the current insulin regimen and minimize episodes of hypoglycemia. The availability of accurate, easy-to-use glucometers has facilitated home monitoring of blood sugars and adjustment of therapy. The blood glucose should be monitored before each meal and before the bedtime snack, with more frequent monitoring when the child is sick, vomiting, or having symptoms of hypoglycemia. When blood sugar is out of the target range, prompt modifications should be made to the insulin regimen (see Table 26.2). **Urine should also be monitored** for ketones during periods of intercurrent illness, vomiting, or when the blood sugar exceeds 240 mg/dl.

Diet

The diabetic child's caloric requirements are the same as those for nondiabetic children (approximately 1000 calories plus 100 calories per year of age per day). However, **consistent distribution of these calories** is important —20% of daily calories should be consumed at breakfast, 30% at lunch, 30% at dinner, and 10% at each snack. Snacks are usually in the mid-afternoon and before bedtime, and younger children may also need a mid-morning snack. It is also important to maintain consistency in the amount of carbohydrate, fat, and protein ingested at each meal (carbohydrate counting)— 55% of total energy intake as carbohydrates (complex carbohydrates preferred), 30% or less as fat (10% or less of total diet saturated fat), and 15% as protein.

Exercise

A regular exercise program is important for optimal health and blood sugar control in the diabetic child. Exercise lowers blood sugar and insulin requirements and improves insulin sensitivity. It is also a useful tool to lower the blood sugar level. Vigorous exercise should be avoided in the presence of ketosis.

Psychosocial Factors

Because the safe management of a child with diabetes requires responsible care on the part of the child and family, the physician should assess parenting skills, coping strategies, and any behavior problems in the child. Referral to a behavioral or family therapist is necessary when problems are identified.

Suggested Readings

Diabetes Control and Complications Trial Research Group: The effect of intensive treatment of diabetes on the development and progression of long-term complications in insulin-dependent diabetes mellitus. *N Engl J Med* 329(14):977–986, 1993.
Sperling M: Diabetes mellitus. In *Clinical Pediatric Endocrinology*. Edited by Sperling M. Philadelphia, WB Saunders, 1996, pp 229–263.
Tamborlane WV, Ahern J: Implications and results of the Diabetes Control and Complications Trial. *Pediatr Clin North Am* 44(2):285–300, 1997.

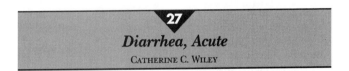

27
Diarrhea, Acute
CATHERINE C. WILEY

▼ INTRODUCTION

Acute diarrhea is defined as stools with **increased water content** that occur at **increased frequency** for a period of less **than 5–7 days.** Most cases of acute diarrhea are of infectious (predominantly viral) origin and are self-limited. Approximately 5% of children with acute diarrhea require medical evaluation.

▼ DIFFERENTIAL DIAGNOSIS LIST
Infectious Causes

Viruses
  Rotavirus
  Norwalk-like viruses
  Adenoviruses
  Enteroviruses
  Astroviruses
  Calciviruses

Bacteria

Salmonella
Shigella
Campylobacter
Yersinia
Pathogenic *Escherichia coli*
Aeromonas
Clostridium difficile
Vibrio

Parasites

Giardia lamblia
Cryptosporidium
Entamoeba histolytica

Parenteral

Otitis media
Urinary tract infection (UTI)
Hepatitis
Sepsis

Toxic Causes

Food-borne illness
Pharmacologic agents—iron, laxatives, antibiotics
Plant or mushroom toxicity
Household cleaners or soap
Serotonin syndrome
Neonatal drug withdrawal

Metabolic or Genetic Causes

Adrenal insufficiency
Congenital adrenal hyperplasia (CAH)
Hyperthyroidism

Inflammatory Causes

Appendicitis
Inflammatory Bowel Disease

Anatomic Causes

Intussusception
Partial obstruction

Miscellaneous Causes

Dietary factors—malnutrition, specific food intolerance, overfeeding, sorbitol
Systemic illness—hemolytic-uremic syndrome, Henoch-Schönlein purpura, immunodeficiency

▼ DIFFERENTIAL DIAGNOSIS DISCUSSION
Infectious Diarrhea

Etiology

As noted previously, infectious diarrhea can be **viral, bacterial,** or **parasitic** in origin. Transmission is usually by the fecal-oral route. Adolescents may have diarrhea or proctitis following the sexual transmission *of Neisseria gonorrhoeae, Treponema pallidum, Chlamydia trachomatis,* or herpes simplex virus (HSV).

Clinical Features

Infectious diarrhea most often affects young children, especially those in daycare. Children commonly present with crampy abdominal pain, vomiting, and 6–10 watery bowel movements per day. Associated symptoms (e.g., fever, vomiting, abdominal pain, rash, joint pain) often support an infectious cause. On examination, the abdomen is usually nondistended and soft, with diffuse tenderness. Bowel sounds may be hyperactive.

Although the clinical syndrome is rarely specific for a particular pathogen, diagnostic clues do exist (Table 27.1). The history may also provide clues regarding the cause:

▼ There is a **seasonal predilection** for many pathogens; viral infections are more common during the winter and bacterial infections occur more frequently in the summer.

TABLE 27.1.   Common Causes of Infectious Diarrhea

Causative Agent	Peak Age	Season	Incubation Period	Fever	Character of Stools
Rotavirus	4 months–3 years	Winter	1–3 days	Variable	Watery, foul-smelling
Norwalk-like viruses	School-age	Winter	12–96 hours	Rare	Loose to watery
Salmonella	1 month–2 years	Summer	8–48 hours	Common	Green, slimy, "rotten egg" odor, occasionally bloody
Shigella	1–5 years	Summer	1–7 days	Common	Watery, bloody, odorless
Campylobacter	1–5 yrs	Summer	1–7 days	Common	Watery, may be bloody
Yersinia	1 month–2 years	Winter	1–14 days	Common	Mucoid, may be bloody
Giardia lamblia	School age	All year	1–4 weeks	Rare	Loose, greasy, pale, and of protracted duration
Entamoeba histolytica	All ages	All year	1–4 weeks	Variable	May be mucoid, bloody

▼ The abrupt onset of diarrhea characterized by the passage of more than four stools per day and no vomiting prior to the onset of diarrhea suggests **bacterial enteritis.**

▼ Bloody diarrhea and fever are seen most commonly in **bacterial enteritis,** although **parasitic** (*Cryptosporidium*) infection should be considered in children with these symptoms who attend daycare.

▼ A **history of contact** with other ill individuals, **daycare attendance, travel,** or certain exposures may provide clues regarding the specific causative agent. For example, G. *lamblia* infection is more common in children who drink well water, and *Campylobacter* and *G. lamblia* can both be transmitted through contact with pets.

▼ *C. difficile* infection occurs predominantly in children who have received **antibiotics** during the preceding 3 weeks.

▼ **Antacid therapy with H$_2$ blockers** increases susceptibility to bacterial pathogens.

Evaluation

In most patients with infectious diarrhea, laboratory studies are not required. However, the following studies may be indicated:

▼ **Serum electrolyte panel.** In children with moderate to severe dehydration (see Chapter 25, "Dehydration," Table 25.3), a serum electrolyte panel may reveal hyponatremia or hypernatremia and significant acidosis, especially if the diarrhea is prolonged. Serum electrolytes may be normal despite significant dehydration.

▼ A **complete blood cell (CBC) count** may show hemoconcentration.

▼ **Stool culture** is generally recommended for hospitalized patients, patients with severe or bloody diarrhea, patients who appear toxic, patients who have been exposed to bacterial enteritis, patients with persistent diarrhea on dietary therapy, patients in daycare or institutional settings, and patients with underlying chronic conditions. Some laboratories test for *Campylobacter, Yersinia,* and pathogenic *E. coli* only by special request. *C. difficile* culture and toxin analysis may be helpful in children with antibiotic exposure. (Of note, the asymptomatic carrier rate for *C. difficile* is 30%–50% in neonates and 3% after 12 months of age.)

▼ **Serology.** Rotazyme, an enzyme-linked immunoassay for rotavirus, is useful in hospitalized patients, in patients with prolonged illness, and for epidemiologic purposes (e.g., during outbreaks). Identification of *Cryptosporidium* requires use of a modified auramine-acid–fast stain or serologic testing.

▼ **Ova & parasites (O&P).** A stool examination for the presence of O& P should be considered for children who attend daycare or who have traveled outside of the country, particularly if the diarrhea is protracted.

Treatment

Antimicrobial agents are not necessary for many patients despite bacterial enteritis. **Antibiotics are contraindicated in some settings.** For example, antibiotic administration may prolong intestinal carriage of salmonella and may increase the risk of hemolytic-uremic syndrome in *E. coli* 0157:H7 infection.

▼ *Campylobacter jejuni.* Erythromycin (10 mg/kg/dose, to a maximum of 500–750 mg/dose) is administered orally every 6 hours for 5–7 days to reduce fecal shedding, shorten illness, and prevent relapse. In severely ill children, consider intravenous administration of erythromycin, chloramphenicol, cefotaxime, or an aminoglycoside. Tetracycline is an alternative for children 8 years and older.

▼ *Shigella.* Trimethoprim-sulfamethoxazole (TMP-SMX) is the drug of choice. The dose is 5 mg TMP/kg/dose (to a maximum of 160 mg/dose), administered orally or intravenously every 12 hours for 5 days. If the organism is sensitive, ampicillin can be used instead: 12.5–18.75 mg/kg/dose administered orally, or 37.5–75 mg/kg/dose administered intravenously or intramuscularly every 6 hours for 5 days. The maximum dose of ampicillin is 500 mg/dose. Because of the increasing incidence of resistance, antimicrobial susceptibility testing should be performed on all isolates.

▼ *Salmonella.* Enterocolitis should only be treated in those patients at risk for developing invasive disease, such as infants younger than 3 months, children with hemoglobinopathies [including sickle cell disease (SCD)], children with malignancies, immunocompromised children (e.g., those with AIDS, those undergoing therapy with immunosuppressive agents, and those with splenic dysfunction), children with cardiac disease at risk for endocarditis, children with *Salmonella typhi* infection, and children with *Salmonella* bacteremia or enteric fever. Antimicrobial susceptibility testing should be performed on all isolates because of the increasing incidence of resistance. If the organism is sensitive to ampicillin or TMP-SMX, one of these agents can be used. The dose is the same as that described for the treatment of *Shigella,* with treatment lasting 7–14 days. Alternatives are chloramphenicol (18.75 mg/kg/dose to a maximum of 1 g/dose, orally or intravenously every 6 hours for 5–7 days), ceftriaxone (25–50 mg/kg/dose to a maximum of 2 g/dose, intravenously every 12 hours for 7–14 days), or cefotaxime (25 mg/kg/dose to a maximum of 3 g/dose, intravenously every 6 hours for 7–14 days). Neonates and patients with meningitis may require different doses, and patients with osteomyelitis need extended treatment (e.g., for 4–6 weeks).

▼ *Clostridium difficile.* Metronidazole (7–11.5 mg/kg/dose to a maximum of 1 g/dose) should be administered orally every 8 hours for 7–10 days after discontinuing administration of other systemic antimicrobials if possible. Vancomycin (5–10 mg/kg/dose to a maximum of 500 mg/dose) can be administered orally every 6 hours for 7–10 days for seriously ill patients or for those in whom treatment has failed.

▼ *Vibrio cholera.* Tetracycline is the treatment of choice in children 8 years of age or older. The dose is 10–12.5 mg/kg/dose to a maximum of 250 mg/dose, administered orally every 6 hours for 3–5 days. TMP-SMX (in the same dosage as that described for the treatment of *Shigella,* for 2–3 days), erythromycin, and furazolidone are alternative therapies.

▼ Enterotoxigenic *E. coli.* Treatment is not usually necessary, but TMP-SMX (in the same dose as that described for *Shigella,* for 3 days) may be administered.

▼ Enteroinvasive *E. coli.* TMP-SMX (in the same dose as that described for *Shigella)* or ampicillin (if the organism is sensitive) may be used. The dose of ampicillin is 12.5–18.75 mg/kg/dose (to a maximum of 500 mg/dose) every 6 hours for 5 days.

▼ *Giardia lamblia.* Metronidazole (5 mg/kg/dose to a maximum of 250 mg/dose, orally every 8 hours for 5–7 days) is the drug of choice.

Furazolidone (1.5–2 mg/kg/dose to a maximum of 100 mg/dose, orally every 6 hours for 7–10 days) is an alternative therapy.

▼ **Cryptosporidium.** Paromomycin (10 mg/kg/dose, every 6 hours) is the agent of choice. This drug has limited efficacy in HIV-infected patients.

▼ **Entamoeba histolytica.** Metronidazole (12–16 mg/kg/dose to a maximum of 750 mg/dose, orally every 8 hours or 15 mg/kg administered as an intravenous bolus, followed by 7.5 mg/kg/dose intravenously every 6 hours) for 10 days is administered to patients with symptomatic colitis or extraintestinal disease. Either method of metronidazole treatment must be followed by iodoquinol (10–13 mg/kg/dose to a maximum of 650 mg/dose, administered orally every 8 hours for 20 days). Additional agents may be needed in the case of severe or invasive disease. If the patient is asymptomatic, iodoquinol alone is used for 20 days. Alternative treatments for asymptomatic infection are also available.

▼ **Cyclospora.** TMP-SMX (in the same dose as for the treatment of *Shigella*) is administered for 7 days.

Food-borne Illness

Etiology

Food-borne diarrhea may occur secondary to ingestion of an infectious agent or ingestion of a preformed toxin. A number of pathogens may be transmitted in contaminated water or food, or via food handlers. Common sources of food-borne diarrhea are listed in Table 27.2.

TABLE 27.2. Common Sources of Food-Borne Gastroenteritis

Source	Infectious Agent or Toxin
Meat	*Staphylococcus aureus* toxins *Clostridium perfringens* toxin Pathogenic *Escherichia coli*
Poultry	*Salmonella* *Shigella* *Campylobacter jejuni*
Eggs	*Salmonella*
Shellfish	*Salmonella* *Vibrio cholerae* *Vibrio parahaemolyticus* Norwalk-like viruses Caliciviruses
Fish	Ciguatera Scombroid
Raw milk	*Salmonella* *Campylobacter jejuni* *Yersinia enterocolitica*
Rice, dried fruit, powdered milk, pork	*Bacillus cereus*
Mushrooms	Mushroom toxin
Pork chitterlings	*Yersinia enterocolitica*

Clinical Features

The **simultaneous, acute onset of gastroenteritis** among individuals who have shared a meal is typical of food-borne illness. These illnesses generally last **less than 24 hours.** Vomiting is prominent in most food poisonings and usually has its onset prior to diarrhea. The severe vomiting of *S. aureus* toxin illness begins 1–6 hours after ingestion of contaminated meat products. Symptoms of *C. perfringens* toxin illness are seen 12 hours after ingestion and typically include secretory diarrhea without vomiting.

⚉ HINT The onset of symptoms the same day as the ingestion suggests that a preformed toxin is the causative agent. Symptoms that begin 24 hours to several days after ingestion suggest enteric pathogens as the cause.

Evaluation

Food poisoning is mainly a clinical diagnosis. Stool cultures may be obtained for detection of enteric pathogens. *C. perfringens* infection may be confirmed by culture of the contaminated food source.

Treatment

Generally, only supportive care is required. Antimicrobial administration is recommended for some enteric pathogens.

Intussusception

Intussusception is discussed in Chapter 9, "Abdominal Pain, Acute."

Hemolytic-Uremic Syndrome

Hemolytic-uremic syndrome is discussed in Chapter 18, "Bleeding and Purpura."

▼ EVALUATION OF ACUTE DIARRHEA

Patient History

The initial patient history aims both to establish **hydration** status and to uncover the **cause of the diarrhea.** The adequacy and type of fluid and solid intake and the urine output should be carefully assessed. In addition, note the size, frequency, and character of the stools (e.g., watery, mucoid, bloody, or foul-smelling) and any associated symptoms. For example, the presence of ear pain or dysuria suggests a diagnosis of parenteral diarrhea.

⚉ HINT *Shigella* emits a neurotoxin and seizures may precede the gastrointestinal symptoms.

Physical Examination

▼ **Vital signs, fontanelles,** and **mucous membranes.** Note signs of dehydration (see Chapter 25, "Dehydration," Table 25.3).

▼ **Skin.** Note maculopapular rash (seen in viral gastroenteritis, typhoid, and *Shigella* infection), pallor, petechiae, or purpura.

▼ **Abdomen.** Auscultate for the presence and quality of bowel sounds, then percuss and palpate for tenderness, organomegaly, or masses.

▼ **Rectum.** Note focal tenderness; stool can be examined and tested for occult blood.

Laboratory Studies

Laboratory studies are unnecessary for most outpatients with acute diarrhea.

If there is a concern about dehydration, testing of **urine specific gravity** may be helpful. In addition, **serum electrolyte analysis** may suggest inadequate fluid replacement (hypernatremic dehydration) or hypotonic fluid replacement (hyponatremic dehydration).

Methylene blue staining of the stool can be used to screen outpatients requiring a bacterial stool culture and may occasionally identify *G. lamblia*. The presence of sheets of polymorphonuclear leukocytes suggests bacterial enteritis and the need for bacterial stool culture. A jar specimen provides a better yield than does a diaper or swab specimen.

Blood cultures should be obtained if there is suspicion of bacteremia or sepsis.

▼ TREATMENT OF ACUTE DIARRHEA

✂ HINT Children with diarrhea and no dehydration should continue to be fed age-appropriate diets.

Oral rehydration therapy is the first line of treatment for all children with mild to moderate dehydration (see also Chapter 25, "Dehydration"). Glucose-electrolyte rehydration solutions contain 75–90 mEq/L of sodium, and maintenance solutions contain 40–60 mEq/L of sodium. Rehydration with oral rehydration solutions should be performed over 4–6 hours. Preliminary research suggests that reduced osmolarity oral rehydration solutions significantly reduce stool volume. **Oral maintenance fluids** can be administered after rehydration, but **age-appropriate foods** should be reintroduced within 24 hours. The "BRAT" diet (bananas, rice, applesauce, and toast) is not recommended. This restricted diet contains inadequate calories and protein to meet nutritional requirements and its use is associated with greater weight loss than age-appropriate diet. The use of lactose-free formulas is not of clear benefit except in the small minority of patients with clinically significant secondary lactase deficiency.

Antidiarrheal medications are not efficacious and are potentially dangerous. They may enhance bacterial proliferation and toxin absorption by promoting reduced gut motility. In addition, they may mask intraluminal fluid loss.

Some studies suggest that bismuth subsalicylate and probiotic agents (*Lactobacillus GG*) may reduce the duration and severity of diarrhea, but confirmation of these findings is needed and they are not currently recommended.

▼ APPROACH TO THE PATIENT (FIGURE 27.1)

▼ **Test a stool sample for the presence of gross or microscopic blood.** The presence of blood should be confirmed using a guaiac reagent test, which

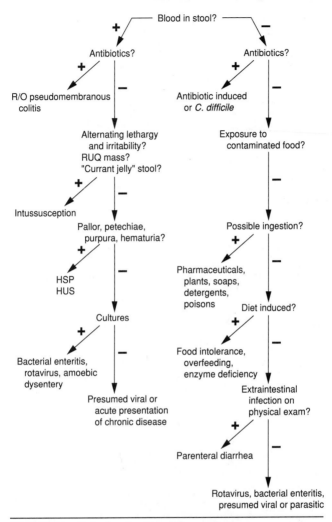

FIGURE 27.1. Evaluation of a patient with acute diarrhea.
HSP = Henoch-Schönlein purpura; *HUS* = hemolytic-uremic syndrome; *R/O* = rule out; *RUQ* = right upper quadrant.

excludes dyes, medications, and vegetable matter as the source of red stools. Broken skin must also be excluded as a source of blood.

▼ **Determine whether the child has recently had antibiotic therapy.** Recent antibiotic therapy in a child with bloody diarrhea suggests the presence of pseudomembranous colitis. Recent antibiotic therapy in a child with nonbloody diarrhea suggests the presence of antibiotic-induced gastroenteritis or *C. difficile* infection without colitis.

▼ **In an afebrile child with bloody diarrhea,** it is particularly important to rule out intussusception (suggested by lethargy, irritability, an abdominal mass, or currant-jelly stools), hemolytic-uremic syndrome (suggested by pallor, petechiae, and oliguria), and Henoch-Schönlein purpura (suggested by purpura, especially of the buttocks and lower extremities).

▼ Most patients are diagnosed as having **presumed viral gastroenteritis.**

Suggested Readings

2000 Red Book: Report of the Committee on Infectious Diseases, 25th ed. Elk Grove Village, IL, American Academy of Pediatrics, 2000.

Brown KH, Peerson JM, Fontaine O: Use of nonhuman milks in the dietary management of young children with acute diarrhea: A meta-analysis of clinical trials. *Pediatrics* 93:17–27, 1994.

Davidson GP: Probiotics in pediatric gastrointestinal disorders. *Curr Opin Pediatr* 12:477–481, 2000.

Guerrant RL, Lohr JA, Williams EK: Acute infectious diarrhea. *Pediatr Infect Dis J* 5:353–359, 1986.

Lifshitz F (ed): Management of acute diarrheal disease. *J Pediatr* 118:S25–138, 1991.

Northrup RS, Flanigan TP: Gastroenteritis. *Pediatr Rev* 15:461–472, 1994.

Provisional Committee on Quality Improvement, Subcommittee on Acute Gastroenteritis: Practice parameter: the management of acute gastroenteritis in young children. *Pediatrics* 97:424–436, 1996.

Sarker SA, et al.: Reduced osmolarity oral rehydration solution for persistent diarrhea in infants: A randomized controlled clinical trial. *J Pediatr* 138:532–538, 2001.

Wong CS, et al.: The risk of the hemolytic-uremic syndrome after antibiotic treatment of *E. coli* 0157:H7 infections. *New Eng J Med* 342:1930–1936, 2000.

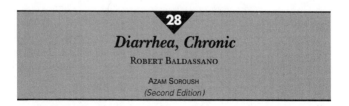

28

Diarrhea, Chronic

ROBERT BALDASSANO

AZAM SOROUSH
(Second Edition)

▼ INTRODUCTION

Stool output of **more than 10 g/kg/day (in infants)** or **200 g/day in children** is defined as diarrhea. Chronic diarrhea is the **persistence of loose, frequent stools for more than 2–3 weeks.**

Diarrhea can be classified as **secretory, osmotic, inflammatory, or motility related.** Presence of an unabsorbable compound in the lumen of the intestine creates an osmolar load that results in osmotic diarrhea. Secretory diarrhea is caused by an imbalance of water and electrolyte absorption and secretion in the intestine.

⚒ HINT If diarrhea stops when the patient is put on NPO status, the patient has osmotic diarrhea.

▼ DIFFERENTIAL DIAGNOSIS LIST

Infectious Causes

Bacterial, parasitic, or viral infection
HIV enteropathy
Bacterial overgrowth
Postinfectious enteritis
Necrotizing enterocolitis
Intra-abdominal abscess
Parenteral diarrhea

Toxic Causes

Antibiotics
Laxatives
Mannitol
Motility agents
Chemotherapeutic agents

Neoplastic Causes

Neuroblastoma
VIPoma
Gastrinoma
Lymphoma
Polyposis
Mastocytosis

Metabolic or Genetic Causes

Carbohydrate malabsorption—lactose intolerance, glucose–galactose transporter defect, sucrose isomaltase deficiency
Fat malabsorption—congenital lipase deficiency, pancreatic disease (cystic fibrosis, chronic pancreatitis, Shwachman syndrome), chronic liver disease, congenital bile salt malabsorption, Wolman disease
Protein-losing enteropathy (PLE)—intestinal lymphangiectasia
Celiac disease
Congenital villous atrophy
Congenital chloride diarrhea
Congenital sodium diarrhea
Acrodermatitis enteropathica
Hyperthyroidism
Hypoparathyroidism
Congenital adrenal hyperplasia (CAH)
Diabetes
Lipoprotein disorders

Anatomic Causes

Malrotation
Partial small bowel obstruction
Short bowel syndrome
Blind loop syndrome
Fistula
Pyloroplasty
Hirschsprung disease with enterocolitis

Dietary Causes

Overfeeding (food or liquid)
Food, milk, or soy-protein allergy
Eosinophilic gastroenteritis
Malnutrition
Fructose
Fiber
Sorbitol

Inflammatory Causes

Inflammatory bowel disease
Severe combined immunodeficiency
Immunoglobulin A (IgA) deficiency
Autoimmune enteropathy
Hemolytic–uremic syndrome

Psychosocial Causes

Irritable bowel syndrome
Munchausen by proxy syndrome

Miscellaneous Causes

Chronic nonspecific diarrhea of infancy
Hepatobiliary disorders—hepatitis, cholestasis, cholecystectomy
Encopresis
Radiation enteritis
Neonatal drug withdrawal syndrome

▼ DIFFERENTIAL DIAGNOSIS DISCUSSION

Chronic Nonspecific Diarrhea of Infancy

Chronic nonspecific diarrhea of infancy (also known as **toddler's diarrhea** or **irritable colon syndrome of childhood**) is the most common cause of diarrhea in children between the ages of **6 months and 3 years.**

Etiology

The cause is unclear. The disorder may be related to **increased bowel motility** or **low intake of fat and fiber,** or it may follow a bout of **infectious gastroenteritis.**

Clinical Features

Patients pass **3–10 loose stools per day,** usually diminishing in frequency in the evening. The child has a good appetite and appropriate weight gain, although undigested food particles are visible in the stool.

Evaluation

The diagnosis is **by exclusion** of other causes. Work-ups for infection and malabsorption are negative. A stool heme work-up is also negative. Clinically, a history of **excessive intake of juices** and a **diet low in fat and fiber** in a child who is thriving supports the diagnosis.

Treatment

The child's consumption of fruit juice and **excessive fluids should be restricted,** and consumption of **dietary fat and fiber** should be **increased.** Reassure parents that the problem will resolve by the time the child is 2–3 years of age.

⚠ HINT   Remember the **four Fs:** fruit juice, fluids, fat, and fiber.

Infectious Enteritis

Infectious enteritis is the **most common cause** of **chronic diarrhea.** Gastrointestinal infections are **usually acute** and resolve in approximately **2 weeks,** but sometimes they can persist for as long as **2 months.** Viral gastroenteritis in an infant can be prolonged as a result of the slow healing of the intestinal mucosa. In addition, infections tend to last longer than usual in immunocompromised patients.

Etiology

Common **bacterial causes** of chronic diarrhea include *Salmonella, Shigella, Yersinia enterocolitica, Campylobacter,* enteroadherent *Escherichia coli, Aeromonas, Clostridium difficile,* and *Plesiomonas.* **Parasitic causes** include *Giardia lamblia, Cryptosporidium, Entamoeba histolytica,* and *Isospora.* Rotavirus, adenovirus, and cytomegalovirus (CMV) are common **viral causes.**

⚠ HINT   Herpes virus, *Mycobacterium avium-intracellulare,* *Blastocystis hominis,* Microsporidia, and fungi can cause chronic diarrhea in immunocompromised patients. Immunocompromised patients usually present with recurrent or prolonged infections.

Clinical Features

▼ *Y. enterocolitica* **infection** involves the terminal ileum a   l can mimic inflammatory bowel disease or appendicitis. It is more common in patients whose normal bowel flora has been changed secondary to antibiotic therapy.

▼ *E. histolytica* **infection** can cause colitis. Blood, mucus, or both are seen in the stool, and patients have a fever.

▼ *Giardia lamblia* **infection** is usually asymptomatic but may manifest with bloating, abdominal pain, anorexia, chronic diarrhea, and failure to thrive (see Chapter 10, "Abdominal Pain, Chronic").

Evaluation

A **stool sample** should be obtained for **bacterial and viral culture.** The laboratory should be instructed to culture for all of the most commonly implicated bacteria and viruses. Stool samples for **Rotazyme** (an enzyme-linked immunoassay for rotavirus) and assays for *C. difficile* **toxins A and B** should also be obtained. **Three stool specimens** should be submitted for **ova and parasites (O&P) analysis.**

Treatment

If the cause is **bacterial,** treatment is with the appropriate **antibiotic** (see Chapter 27, "Diarrhea, Acute"). **Giardiasis** is treated with **furazolidone, metronidazole,** or **quinacrine** (see Chapter 10, "Abdominal Pain, Chronic"). Nutritional supplementation may be required for patients with **viral** diarrhea and **immunocompromised patients.**

C. difficile Colitis (pseudomembranous colitis, antibiotic-induced colitis)

C. difficile colitis is discussed in Chapter 34, "Gastrointestinal Bleeding, Lower."

Parenteral Diarrhea

Etiology

Extraintestinal infection [e.g., upper respiratory tract infection, urinary tract infection (UTI), otitis media, mastoiditis, sinusitis, pneumonia] may be associated with diarrhea. Diarrhea may also be one of the symptoms **associated with other systemic infections** (e.g., toxic shock syndrome, Rocky Mountain spotted fever). The pathogenesis of the diarrhea is unknown.

Clinical Features

The patient may be **otherwise asymptomatic** (e.g., in the case of UTI), or he may have a **range of symptoms** related to the primary illness.

Evaluation

The diagnosis is based on **clinical suspicion.** An appropriate work-up for the suspected primary illness should be performed. In an otherwise asymptomatic child, a **urine culture** is necessary.

Treatment

Treatment of the **primary illness** results in resolution of the diarrhea.

Postinfectious Enteritis

Etiology

In **children,** infectious gastroenteritis is usually **uncomplicated;** however, in **infants** (especially those with a borderline nutritional status), **severe mucosal damage** may follow an infectious gastroenteritis. The mucosal damage results in **disaccharidase deficiency** (most commonly lactase deficiency). Rarely, more **global malabsorption** results.

Clinical Features

Long after the infectious process has been resolved, the patient experiences **intractable watery diarrhea and nutritional compromise,** manifested as **failure to thrive.** Rarely, evidence of vitamin and mineral deficiency is seen.

Evaluation

The diagnosis is made on the basis of **clinical suspicion.** In some patients, a **lactose breath test** may be appropriate.

Treatment

Temporary **avoidance of dairy products** and introduction of a **lactose-free formula or an elemental formula** are needed to allow the brush borders of the small intestine to heal.

Celiac Disease (Gluten-Sensitive Enteropathy)

Etiology

Gluten-sensitive enteropathy is a **hereditary type of malabsorption** that is caused by a **permanent inability to tolerate gluten,** which is present in **wheat, oat, barley, and rye. Gliadin,** the offending protein, **causes severe atrophy of the small intestinal mucosa.** This disease has a **high incidence in Ireland.**

Clinical Features

Symptoms usually start approximately 1 month after gluten is introduced to the diet. Common manifestations include **apathy and irritability, anorexia, vomiting, chronic diarrhea, steatorrhea, abdominal distention, clubbing of the fingers,** and **malnutrition** with symptoms and signs related to nutrient deficiency.

Evaluation

The patient should be **screened for IgA antiendomysial antibodies and IgA anti-transglutaminase antibodies.** However, IgA deficiency must be excluded. IgA antigliadin antibodies result in a very high false-positive rate, and this screening test is no longer used for celiac disease.

Treatment

Removal of gluten from the diet and replacement with corn, rice, or potato starch results in resolution of the symptoms. Complete recovery of the intestinal mucosa is expected in 1–2 years.

Encopresis

Etiology

Patients with **chronic constipation and impaction** may present with chronic diarrhea as a result of **continuous leakage of loose stool around the hard stool.** In patients with **Hirschsprung disease,** diarrhea is usually **secondary to enterocolitis.**

Clinical Features

The patient has a **history of constipation.** On **abdominal examination,** hard stool may be **palpated,** and on **rectal examination,** the **vault is dilated** and **filled with hard stool.**

Evaluation

An **abdominal radiograph** confirms the diagnosis, which is based on clinical suspicion.

Treatment

Treatment entails **evacuation of the bowel** with **multiple enemas. Stool softeners** should be prescribed for **several months,** and **diet** and **behavioral modification** should take place. Patients with **Hirschsprung disease** require **antibiotics** and **surgery** for definitive treatment.

Fat Malabsorption

Etiology

Fat digestion and absorption is a complex process. **Lipase** (a pancreatic enzyme), **bile acid secretion** (to help with micellar solubilization), an intact **intestinal brush border** (to facilitate micelle absorption), intact β **lipoprotein metabolism,** and an intact **transport mechanism** (to carry the chylomicron to the lymphatics) all play a role. A **defect in any of these steps** may result in fat malabsorption.

Clinical Features

Fat malabsorption is manifested with **diarrhea (bulky, greasy stools), failure to thrive,** and signs and symptoms related to **fat-soluble vitamin deficiency** (e.g., rickets, night blindness, neurologic signs, bleeding tendency).

Evaluation

A **stool smear** that stains positive using Sudan III is evidence of fat malabsorption. Definitive diagnosis is with measurement of fat in a **72-hour stool collection.** The work-up for the cause of malabsorption is extensive, and referral to a **gastroenterologist** is recommended.

Treatment

The **underlying cause** must be identified and treated if possible. All patients with fat malabsorption require **additional calorie intake** to compensate for the excessive fat loss. **Medium-chain triglyceride (MCT)–based formulas** are often preferred. Because MCTs have a smaller molecular weight and higher water solubility than do long-chain triglycerides (LCTs), they are absorbed directly into the portal blood (i.e., they bypass the complex absorptive process that is needed for long-chain fatty acids). Patients with fat malabsorption also require **fat-soluble vitamin supplementation.**

Carbohydrate Malabsorption

Etiology

The absorption of carbohydrates involves **amylase** (a pancreatic enzyme); **lactase, isomaltase,** and **sucrase** (intestinal brush border enzymes); and an intact **transport system.** The most common type of carbohydrate malabsorption is **lactase deficiency** (see Chapter 10, "Abdominal Pain, Chronic"). Congenital carbohydrate malabsorption is rare, but it has to be considered in the differential diagnosis of diarrhea in a young infant.

Clinical Features

In general, carbohydrate malabsorption syndromes are manifested with **failure to thrive, osmotic-type diarrhea** (which may be watery), **abdominal cramps, increased flatulence, and borborygmi.**

Evaluation

A positive stool test for reducing substances or a **stool pH lower than 5.0** is indicative of carbohydrate malabsorption. Definitive diagnosis is by a specific **hydrogen breath test** or **mucosal biopsy.**

Treatment

Symptoms usually resolve with complete **removal of the offending carbohydrate** from the diet. **Supplying the deficient enzyme** may be helpful (e.g., lactase for lactose intolerance).

Protein Malabsorption

Diseases that involve the gastrointestinal mucosa or obstruct lymphatic drainage of the gastrointestinal tract can cause **protein-losing entropy (PLE).** **Primary intestinal lymphangiectasia** is a congenital disorder associated with abnormally dilated lymphatics that results in chronic loss of albumin, immunoglobulins, and other proteins. It is also associated with loss of lymphocytes through the gastrointestinal tract.

Clinical Features

Patients may present with signs and symptoms that reflect the **underlying cause, chronic diarrhea, failure to thrive, edema, recurrent infection,** or signs and symptoms related to **loss of proteins.**

Evaluation

Patients have **hypoalbuminemia, hypoproteinemia, abnormal immunoglobulins,** and **lymphocytopenia. Hypocalcemia** and **decreased serum iron and copper levels** occur secondary to the loss of binding proteins. Before making the diagnosis of PLE, **urinary loss of albumin must be ruled out. Increased stool α_1-antitrypsin (α_1-AT)** is the **definitive** means of diagnosing PLE.

Treatment

The **primary cause** of the PLE should be identified. Patients require a **diet that is rich in protein and MCT oil.**

Allergic Enteropathy

Allergic enteropathy is discussed in Chapter 34, "Gastrointestinal Bleeding, Lower."

Inflammatory Bowel Disease

Inflammatory bowel disease is discussed in Chapter 34, "Gastrointestinal Bleeding, Lower."

▼ EVALUATION OF CHRONIC DIARRHEA

A detailed **history** and **physical examination** can obviate the need for laboratory evaluation in some cases.

Patient History

The following details should be sought:

▼ The onset and duration of the diarrhea
▼ The stool pattern and aggravating or alleviating factors
▼ Quality of stool—color; odor; consistency; volume; presence of blood, mucus, or undigested food
▼ The presence of fever and associated symptoms
▼ A history of gastroenteritis, constipation, or recurrent pneumonia before the onset of chronic diarrhea
▼ Dietary history (4 "Fs"—fiber, fluid, fat, fruit juice)

▼ Recent travel or exposure to infections
▼ Medication history
▼ Pertinent family history

Physical Examination

The following should be noted on examination:

▼ **General appearance**—hydration status, weight and height, growth chart
▼ **Skin**—edema, jaundice, pallor, eczematous rash, bruising, clubbing
▼ **Lungs**—wheezing, rales
▼ **Abdomen**—tenderness, mass (stool, abscess, tumor, enlarged organs)
▼ **Rectum**—evidence of perianal disease, rectal prolapse, Hirschsprung disease, constipation

Laboratory Studies

Initial screening studies include:

▼ A serum electrolyte panel
▼ Serum albumin and protein levels
▼ Liver function tests
▼ Complete blood count (CBC) with differential and erythrocyte sedimentation rate (ESR)
▼ Stool sample for white blood cell (WBC) count, occult blood, and eosinophil count
▼ Stool samples for culture, *C. difficile* toxin A and B assay, and O&P
▼ Urinalysis and urine culture
▼ Stool electrolytes, anion gap, magnesium content, osmolarity

Depending on the suspected diagnosis, additional studies may be indicated:

▼ **Carbohydrate malabsorption**—stool pH (< 5.0), reducing substance (positive)
▼ **Fat malabsorption**—Sudan III smear of stool (positive); sweat chloride test; prothrombin time (PT, prolonged); beta carotene, vitamin E, and vitamin D levels (may be decreased)
▼ **PLE**—stool α_1-AT (increased), hypoalbuminemia, lymphopenia, hypogammaglobulinemia
▼ **Small bowel disease**—D-xylose test (abnormal)

▼ TREATMENT OF CHRONIC DIARRHEA

The underlying cause of the diarrhea must be identified and treated.

▼ Consultation with a nutritionist is advisable for patients with disorders such as malabsorption, celiac disease, or allergic enteropathy.
▼ For patients who are not vomiting, an oral glucose electrolyte solution can be given to correct fluid, electrolyte, and acid–base imbalances. Patients may be started on a lactose-free or an elemental formula later, depending on the cause and severity of the diarrhea.
▼ Unstable or malnourished patients should be admitted for stabilization and nutritional rehabilitation. Reinitiation of feeding in a malnourished patient may result in refeeding syndrome, which is manifested by an acute drop in serum potassium, phosphate, magnesium, and calcium levels secondary to the sudden intracellular shift of these elements. If these

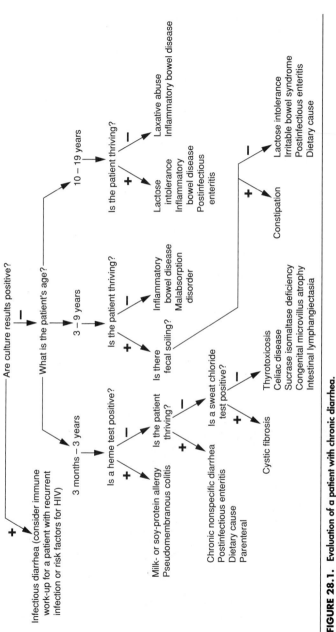

FIGURE 28.1. Evaluation of a patient with chronic diarrhea.
Most patients are diagnosed as having presumed viral gastroenteritis.

electrolyte abnormalities are not corrected in a timely manner, cardiopulmonary compromise and death may result. All electrolyte imbalances must
be corrected before initiation of feeding to prevent refeeding syndrome. A
continuous drip of a diluted formula is started and gradually the rate and
concentration are increased while monitoring the patient's electrolytes
and calcium, phosphate, and magnesium levels.

▼ Total parenteral nutrition may be required for those with severe malnutrition who cannot tolerate feeding.

▼ Additional nutritional supplementation (e.g., zinc, iron, vitamins) may be
required.

▼ APPROACH TO THE PATIENT (FIGURE 28.1)

Suggested Readings

Baldassano RN, Liacouras CA: Chronic diarrhea, a practical approach for the
pediatrician. *Pediatr Clin North Am* 38(3):667–686, 1991.

Guerrant RL, Bobak DA: Bacterial and protozoal gastroenteritis. *New Engl J
Med* 325:327–340, 1991.

Hanauer SB: Inflammatory bowel disease. *N Engl J Med* 334:841–848, 1996.

Heitlinger LA, Lebenthal EB: Disorders of carbohydrate digestion and absorption. *Pediatr Clin North Am* 35:239–255, 1988.

Hyams JS, Stafford RJ, Grand RJ, et al: Correlation of the lactose breath
test, intestinal morphology and lactase activity in young children. *J Pediatr*
97:609–612, 1980.

Picarelli A, Sabbatella L, Di Tola M, et al: Celiac disease diagnosis in misdiagnosed children. *Pediatr Res* 48(5):590–592, 2000.

Smith MM, Lifshitz F: Excess fruit juice consumption as a contributing factor
in nonorganic failure to thrive. *Pediatrics* 93(3):438–443, 1994.

Vanderhoof JA: Chronic diarrhea. *Pediatr Rev* 19(12):418–422, 1998.

Walker-Smith JA, Guandalini S, Schmitz J, et al: Revised criteria for the diagnosis of celiac disease. *Arch Dis Child* 65:909–911, 1990.

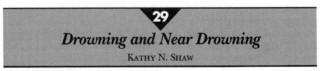

29

Drowning and Near Drowning

KATHY N. SHAW

▼ INTRODUCTION

Terminology

Near drowning is defined as survival, at least temporarily, of suffocation
caused by submersion in water. **"Wet drowning"** is a near drowning or drowning characterized by the **aspiration of a small amount of water** (usually less
than 22 ml/kg). When there is **laryngospasm without aspiration of water**
(approximately 10% of cases), the near drowning or drowning is termed a
"dry drowning." Water temperature at the time of drowning or near drowning is classified as **warm** (20°C), cold (6°C–19°C), or **very cold** ($\leq$ 5°C) and
is **important in determining the prognosis for the hypothermic victim.** The
type of water (e.g., fresh or salt) makes little difference in management of
the patient.

Epidemiology

Nationally, near drowning is **second only to motor vehicle accidents** as the most common cause of death due to nonintentional injury in children younger than 19 years. The **highest rate** of drowning is seen in **children 1–4 years** of age. In California, Arizona, and Florida, drowning is the leading cause of death in this age group. The vast majority of deaths in this age group occur in **residential swimming pools.** **Infants** are most likely to drown in **bathtubs.** A second peak in drowning deaths occurs in the **teen and young adult** age groups in bodies of **fresh water,** with the highest rate in black males.

Near drowning usually results in either **severe permanent brain damage or prompt complete recovery.** There are an estimated 1400 deaths, 7100 hospitalizations and more than 28,000 emergency department visits related to near drowning annually. The annual direct care cost for childhood near drowning exceeds $200 million per year.

Most near drownings are **preventable.** Passage of legislation that requires pool fencing, limits alcohol access at public pools and beaches, and demands pool owners to be proficient in cardiopulmonary resuscitation (CPR) could significantly reduce morbidity and mortality rates. Preventive counseling for parents should also be provided.

Pathophysiology

▼ **Pulmonary injury** results from a lack of surfactant, which is caused by either denaturation (fresh water) or washout (salt water) of surfactant from the alveoli. Alveolar injury and pulmonary edema lead to hypoxemia as a result of an altered ventilation–perfusion ratio and intrapulmonary shunting. Hypercapnia occurs as a result of apnea or hypoventilation but is usually readily corrected with the use of ventilation during resuscitation. The persistent hypoxemia and the effects of anoxic–ischemic cell injury (i.e., cytotoxic edema, cellular disruption) are the primary management issues.

▼ **Central nervous system injury,** including cerebral edema and increased intracranial pressure, is a secondary result of global anoxic–ischemic injury. It is not reversible. Hypothermia may actually protect the brain by causing a decrease in metabolic demand, but this is true only if the hypothermia occurred at the time of the near drowning in cold water.

▼ **Acidosis** may cause dysrhythmias. Shock is usually attributable to intravascular depletion, which develops secondary to the increased capillary permeability caused by anoxia and the loss of protein in the pulmonary edema fluid. Electrolyte imbalances are uncommon but can occur if a large volume of fresh water is absorbed from the gastrointestinal tract.

▼ EVALUATION OF DROWNING AND NEAR DROWNING

Patient History

The **duration of submersion, temperature of the water,** presence of **cyanosis or apnea at the scene, performance of CPR** at the recovery scene, and **amount of time that elapsed until CPR** was initiated are all important historical points that influence prognosis and management (Table 29.1). One should also inquire about the possibility of a **diving injury, alcohol use,** or a past history of a **seizure disorder.**

TABLE 29.1. Prognostic Indicators of Poor Neurologic Outcome in Near-Drowning Victims*

> **At the scene**
> Submersion time > 4–10 minutes
> Delay in beginning CPR
> Resuscitation > 25 minutes
> **In the emergency department**
> Necessity for CPR
> Fixed, dilated pupils
> pH < 7.0
> GCS score < 5
> **After initial resuscitation**
> Persistent GCS score < 5
> Persistent apnea

* Applies to victims of warm water near drownings only. Hypothermic victims of cold water near drownings may have a better prognosis.

CPR = cardiopulmonary resuscitation; GCS = Glasgow coma score.

Physical Examination

During the physical examination, particular attention should be paid to **assessment of vital signs** (including the temperature) and to the neurologic and respiratory examinations. Performing **neurologic and respiratory examinations at periodic intervals** is an **extremely important** component of managing near-drowning victims.

Pupillary response and the **Glasgow coma score (GCS)** (see Chapter 21, "Coma," Table 21.1) should be **assessed serially** to determine the **extent of anoxic–ischemic injury** and the **patient's response to resuscitation** attempts. The child who presents in asystole with fixed, dilated pupils and a GCS score of less than 5 generally has a poor prognosis unless he responds fairly rapidly to resuscitation efforts or he has a core temperature of less than 32°C following a cold-water near drowning. In children with a **GCS score of more than 5** at presentation, the **outcome is generally good.** Unfortunately, **neurologic damage** as a result of near drowning **cannot be reversed.**

Careful attention is paid to the respiratory examination, even in an alert, active child without obvious respiratory distress. **Close monitoring for signs of respiratory involvement** (in the form of serial examinations) **is crucial, even for the initially asymptomatic child.** Signs of lower respiratory involvement (e.g., the use of accessory muscles, tachypnea, cough, wheezing, rales, nasal flaring) **may be delayed** for minutes to hours, and the **injury is usually progressive.**

Laboratory Studies

▼ **Serial pulse oximetry** should be used to detect early signs of pulmonary involvement that are not clinically detectable (e.g., oxygen desaturation of less than 95%).

▼ **Electrolyte values** are rarely abnormal. Respiratory or metabolic acidosis may be present and should be corrected.

▼ **Electrocardiographic monitoring** is indicated for the severely affected patient or for a patient in whom a cardiac electrophysiologic conduction delay (e.g., a prolonged QT interval) may have precipitated unconsciousness, leading to the near-drowning episode.

▼ **Toxicology screens,** including an ethyl alcohol level measurement, may be indicated.

▼ **Chest radiography** is indicated following intubation or if there are signs of lower airway involvement.

▼ APPROACH TO THE PATIENT
Resuscitation

A **brief, well-executed resuscitation effort** with initiation of **advanced cardiopulmonary life support** measures, if necessary, should be made as information is gathered regarding the accident, the patient's core temperature, and the response to therapy. Resuscitation should be initiated **in all apneic and pulseless victims,** but it should only be **continued for prolonged periods in victims of a cold water near drowning** and then only until the **patient's core temperature exceeds 32°C.** The goal of therapy is to prevent further anoxic–ischemic injury.

Airway (Figure 29.1)

The **gag reflex** should be assessed to determine whether the child can protect his or her own airway. In diving accidents, the possibility of a **neck injury** should be considered, and the neck should be **immobilized.** The **airway** should be **suctioned** and properly positioned to ensure air entry.

⚡ HINT The **Heimlich maneuver** (with the victim's head turned sideways) should be used **only if foreign matter** is **obstructing** the airway and it should **never** be used **if cervical trauma** is suspected.

Intubation is required if the child is apneic; if she is in severe respiratory distress; if the administration of more than 50% oxygen is required to maintain an arterial oxygen tension of greater than 60 mm Hg; or if the protective reflexes are missing owing to obtundation. The **stomach** should be **emptied of water** by means of a nasogastric tube once the airway is protected.

Breathing (see Figure 29.1)

Assisted ventilation (e.g., bag-valve-mask ventilation) is initiated if necessary. Use of the **Sellick maneuver** during initial ventilation is an effective means of preventing aspiration. With this technique, an assistant applies anteroposterior pressure to the cricoid cartilage to compress the esophagus against the cervical vertebrae. In children with severe hypoxemia, the most effective treatment is **continuous positive airway pressure,** which helps to improve ventilation–perfusion matching in the lungs.

Children who show signs of **lower respiratory involvement** should be admitted and closely **monitored** for the development of **progressive respiratory failure.** Children **without any symptoms** at presentation to the emergency department, but **with a significant history of submersion or resuscitation** at the scene, should be **observed and monitored** for these signs for a minimum of **4 hours** before discharge.

Circulation

The victim should be assessed for **adequacy of circulation.** If a pulse cannot be felt, chest compressions should be started (but not if the patient is still in the water). An intravenous line should be started and **normal saline**

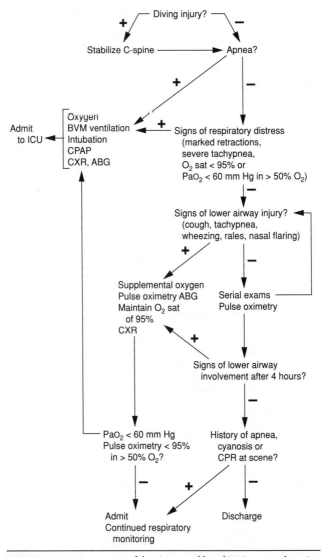

FIGURE 29.1. Management of the airway and breathing in a near-drowning victim.
ABG = arterial blood gases; *BVM* = bag-valve-mask; *CPAP* = continuous positive airway pressure; *CPR* = cardiopulmonary resuscitation; *C-spine* = cervical spine; *CXR* = chest radiograph; *ICU* = intensive care unit; O_2 = oxygen; O_2 sat = oxygen saturation; PaO_2 = arterial oxygen tension.

given in 20-ml/kg aliquots if there are signs of poor perfusion. Poor perfusion usually occurs only in children with severe ischemic injury or pulmonary edema and in those who require mechanical ventilation. Children with **respiratory distress** should receive intravenous fluids at **1.5 times** the maintenance requirement.

Restoration of Core Temperature

In a child who has experienced cold water near drowning, it may be necessary to use a **low-reading thermometer** to obtain the core temperature. The child's **wet clothing** should be **removed** immediately, and the child should be dried and warmed. If the child's core temperature is **32°C–35°C, active external warming** should be started using a heating blanket or radiant warmer. A patient with a core temperature of **less than 32°C** requires **internal warming,** which entails gastric lavage with warm fluid and the administration of heated aerosolized oxygen. In severe cases, **peritoneal dialysis or hemodialysis, mediastinal irrigation,** or **cardiac bypass** may be used if the technique is available.

▨ HINT The popular saying, "A near drowning victim is not dead until he is warm and dead" applies only to hypothermia patients who were immersed in cold water, not to those who are hypothermic because they have been asystolic for an extended period of time following a warm-water drowning.

Suggested Readings

Brenner RA, Trumble AC, Smith GS, et al: Where children drown, United States, 1995. *Pediatrics* 108:85–89, 2001.

Jacinto SJ, Gieron-Korthals M, Ferreira JA: Predicting outcome in hypoxic-ischemic brain injury. *Pediatr Clin North Am* 48(3):647–660, 2001.

Lavelle JM, Shaw KS: Near-drowning: is emergency department cardiopulmonary resuscitation or intensive care unit cerebral resuscitation indicated? *Crit Care Med* 21:368–373, 1993.

Modell JH: Drowning. *N Engl J Med* 328:253–256, 1993.

Quan L, Kinder D: Pediatric submersions: prehospital predictors of outcome. *Pediatrics* 90(6):909–913, 1992.

Shaw KN, Briede CA: Submersion injuries: drowning and near-drowning. *Emerg Med Clin North Am* 7:355–370, 1989.

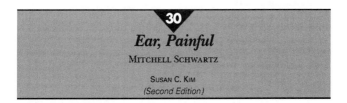

30

Ear, Painful

MITCHELL SCHWARTZ

SUSAN C. KIM
(Second Edition)

▼ INTRODUCTION

Diseases that produce ear pain are some of the most common maladies of childhood. Most cases of otalgia are caused by **acute otitis media. Otitis externa** is also commonly seen, especially during the summer months.

▼ DIFFERENTIAL DIAGNOSIS LIST

External Ear Pain

Infectious Causes

Otitis externa (swimmer's ear)
Infected preauricular sinus
Herpes simplex virus infection
Herpes zoster
Auricular cellulitis
External canal abscess

Neoplastic Causes

Neoplasms of the external auditory canal

Traumatic Causes

Frostbite, burns, lacerations
Hematoma or seroma

Miscellaneous Causes

Foreign body, cerumen impaction

Middle and Inner Ear Pain

Infectious Causes

Acute otitis media
Myringitis
Mastoiditis

Neoplastic Causes

Rhabdomyosarcoma, lymphoma
Histiocytosis X

Traumatic Causes

Traumatic perforation
Barotrauma

Inflammatory Causes

Otitis media with effusion

Miscellaneous Causes

Eustachian tube dysfunction
Cholesteatoma

Referred Pain

Infectious Causes

Dental abscess
Stomatitis, aphthous ulcer
Sinusitis
Cervical lymphadenitis
Pharyngitis or tonsillitis
Retropharyngeal abscess
Peritonsillar abscess
Infected branchial cyst

Parotitis
Meningitis

Neoplastic Causes

Neoplasms of the jaw, oropharynx, nasopharynx, larynx, facial nerve, or central nervous system

Traumatic Causes

Oral cavity, pharyngeal, laryngeal, or esophageal trauma or foreign body

Miscellaneous Causes

Erupting teeth
Impacted teeth
Migraine
Temporomandibular joint dysfunction or arthritis
Bell palsy

▼ DIFFERENTIAL DIAGNOSIS DISCUSSION
Acute Otitis Media

Etiology

Table 30-1 lists risk factors associated with acute otitis media. Acute otitis media occurs **secondary to obstruction of the eustachian tube,** which can result from **infection, allergy, enlarged adenoids, decreased eustachian tube stiffness,** or **inefficient tube opening.** Eustachian tube **obstruction causes a middle ear effusion,** and **contamination** of the effusion (from nasopharyngeal secretions) **causes acute otitis media.** The most common pathogens are *Streptococcus pneumoniae,* nontypeable *Haemophilus influenzae,* and *Moraxella catarrhalis.*

Clinical Features

Symptoms of acute otitis media include **otalgia, fever, irritability, vomiting, diarrhea, hearing loss, anorexia,** and **otorrhea.**

Evaluation

To facilitate examination of the tympanic membrane, the clinician should **properly position the child's ear** (i.e., pull the pinna posteriorly and superiorly and push the tragus forward by applying traction to the skin in front of the ear). **Remove cerumen** with a curette or by irrigation with water (except

TABLE 30.1. Risk Factors for Recurrent Acute Otitis Media
Day care attendance
Passive cigarette smoke exposure
Bottle propping
Formula-fed (as opposed to breast-fed)
Male
Winter season
First episode of acute otitis media before 6 months of age
Siblings in the home
Sibling with recurrent acute otitis media

when a **perforated tympanic membrane** is suspected; in this situation, **irrigation is contraindicated**).

Tympanic membrane mobility should be assessed using **pneumatic otoscopy or tympanometry.** To perform pneumatic otoscopy, use the largest speculum that will fit comfortably in the auditory meatus, fit the speculum tightly to the ear canal, and apply positive and negative pressure to the tympanic membrane with either a rubber bulb or by blowing air into a tube connected to the head of the otoscope. In **acute otitis media,** the tympanic membrane is **red, bulging, opaque,** and has **decreased mobility.**

✄ HINT Tympanic membrane erythema alone is not a reliable indicator of acute otitis media. A red tympanic membrane can also be caused by a viral upper respiratory tract infection, by crying, or by efforts to remove cerumen.

Laboratory evaluation is usually not necessary. Some clinicians do recommend that **febrile infants** with acute otitis media who are **younger than 12 weeks** undergo a full **sepsis evaluation.**

Treatment

Since many patients who have physical findings consistent with diagnosis of otitis media may recover without treatment, **some experts recommend withholding treatment** for 48–72 days before starting antibiotics.

First-line Therapy

▼ **Amoxicillin** (45 mg/kg/day divided three times a day) is still the drug of choice for most episodes of acute otitis media. Reasons for this choice include cost, safety profile, and activity against the common organisms causing otitis media. Recent Food and Drug Administration approval allows for twice a day dosing, which should improve adherence.

▼ Using **higher doses of amoxicillin** (80–90 mg/kg/day) will cover many of the moderately resistant strains of *S. pneumoniae*. Increasing the dose of amoxicillin should be considered when the risk of resistant *S. pneumoniae* is increased, as in the following circumstances:
  ▼ Children less than 2 years of age
  ▼ Recent beta-lactam use
  ▼ Exposure to day care
  ▼ Communities with a high incidence of resistant organisms

▼ A **5-day course** may be sufficient for children over 2 years of age.

▼ **Azithromycin** may be used in patients who are allergic to penicillin.

With appropriate antimicrobial therapy, most children experience **symptomatic improvement within 48–72 hours.** If a patient does not respond fully to amoxicillin, the cause of the otitis may be viral or there may be bacterial resistance.

Second-line Therapy

The choice of a second-line antibiotic depends on the suspected mechanism of resistance. *H. influenzae* and *M. catarrhalis* produce beta lactamase.*S. pneumoniae* alters penicillin binding-proteins. In cases in which resistant *S. pneumoniae* is likely, treatment with **higher doses of amoxicillin** (80–90 mg/kg/day) is recommended if not done initially. **Amoxicillin-clavulanate, cefuroxime axetil**, and **intramuscular ceftriaxone** are also effective against resistant strains. The macrolides, cephalosporins, and trimethoprim-sulfa do not provide reliable coverage for resistant *S. pneumoniae.* **Amoxicillin-clavulanate** or a **second-generation cephalosporin** may be used if *H. influenzae* or *M. catarrhalis* are suspected.

Intramuscular ceftriaxone is not recommended for routine treatment of otitis media. It may be considered **when oral therapy is impossible** or when appropriate **first- and second-line therapy** for *S. pneumoniae* **has already failed.** When used for treatment of resistant organisms, ceftriaxone 50 mg/kg should be given every 1–3 days for three doses.

⚡ HINT With increased use of immunizations against *H. influenzae,* there are fewer cases of otitis caused by *H. influenzae.* Immunization against **S. pneumoniae** has decreased the cases of otitis media caused by that organism, but unfortunately other organisms have caused additional cases of otitis. Recent information shows a net decrease of otitis by about 6%.

⚡ HINT The tympanic membrane does not return to normal appearance for 6–12 weeks. Many times when the ear is examined shortly after an episode of otitis media, the tympanic membrane may appear dull and pink when it is in the healing phase and is not infected.

Infants younger than 4 weeks who present with fever or irritability and acute otitis media should be **hospitalized** for **intravenous antibiotic administration,** pending cultures of the blood, urine, and cerebrospinal fluid. **Well-appearing, afebrile infants younger than 4 weeks** may be treated as **outpatients** with first-line antimicrobials and **careful follow-up.**

Prevention

There is some **controversy** surrounding the administration of **preventive antibiotics** because of the risk of accelerated bacterial resistance and the marginal benefit of prophylaxis found in some clinical trials.

Children who have **repeated cases of otitis media** should be **evaluated for myringotomy.** Although quite popular as a treatment, many critics are questioning the value of this procedure.

Otitis Media with Effusion

Etiology

Otitis media with effusion (i.e., a **middle ear effusion without** the **clinical manifestations** of acute otitis media) is usually either an **extension** of an **upper respiratory tract infection** or a **sequela** to an episode of acute otitis media. The effusion used to be considered sterile; however, recent studies have demonstrated the ability to culture bacterial pathogens (most commonly *H. influenzae, M. catarrhalis, S. pneumoniae,* and *Staphylococcus aureus* from a substantial number of these effusions.

⚡ HINT When otitis media with effusion follows properly treated acute otitis media, it usually represents the beginning of resolution of the infection (as opposed to persistent infection).

Clinical Features

Most children are **asymptomatic,** although some complain of fullness in the ear, hearing loss and, less commonly, tinnitus and vertigo.

Evaluation

Otoscopy often reveals a retracted tympanic membrane with **decreased mobility.** Laboratory evaluation is not necessary.

Treatment

Most cases of otitis media with effusion **clear spontaneously** without active treatment. The management of otitis media with effusion is undergoing re-evaluation. Studies from Europe and the United States show little long-term effect from **insertion of ventilation tubes.** There is some improvement in speech for 6 months in the group treated with ventilation tubes. This effect is no longer present at 1 year. Likewise, treatment with **antibiotics** has some short-term beneficial effects but the effect does not last when compared with patients not treated with antibiotics. Each case has to be individualized, but the main strategy continues to be **patient observation** for infection and speech difficulties.

⚝ HINT Decongestants and antihistamines have not been proven effective in the treatment of acute otitis media or otitis media with effusion.

Otitis Externa (Swimmer's Ear)

Etiology

Otitis externa, **an infection of the ear canal** and **external surface of the tympanic membrane,** results from a loss of cerumen and **chronic irritation** as a result of **excessive moisture** in the ear canal. **Trauma** or **foreign bodies** in the ear canal can also precipitate otitis externa.

Localized abscesses in the ear canal are usually caused by *S. aureus.* Diffuse otitis externa is most commonly caused by *Pseudomonas aeruginosa, Enterobacter aerogenes, Proteus mirabilis, Klebsiella pneumoniae,* streptococci, and *Staphylococcus epidermidis.* Fungi and herpes virus can also cause acute otitis externa.

Clinical Features

The initial symptom of otitis externa is **pruritus** of the auditory canal leading to **ear pain.** The pain **worsens with touching or movement** of the ear and **during chewing.**

Evaluation

Patients may report **purulent drainage,** and **pus** is often noted in the ear canal on examination. The canal appears **erythematous** and **edematous.**

Treatment

Initial management consists of **removing the debris** from the affected ear—usually, wiping the ear canal with a dry cotton swab will suffice, but occasionally gentle suction is needed. A **2% acetic acid otic solution** or a combination **antibiotic–corticosteroid otic preparation** should be instilled in the affected ear four times daily for 10 days, unless a perforated tympanic membrane is suspected. In this case, suspensions (not solutions) should be used. If the canal is particularly edematous, a wick of cotton or gauze should be inserted

10–12 ml into the canal to facilitate medication entry. Patients should be advised that **swimming is to be avoided** during treatment. Failure to respond to **two courses of treatment** or the presence of **severe inflammation** should prompt referral to an **otolaryngologist.**

Adjacent cellulitis or adenitis requires systemic antistaphylococcal coverage.

Prevention

In susceptible patients, prevention of otitis externa entails **abstaining from swimming** or placing **2% acetic acid solution in each ear canal after swimming** or bathing.

Foreign Bodies

Etiology

Foreign bodies rank **second to inflammatory and infectious disorders** of the ear as causes of otalgia. Solid, nonorganic objects are most commonly seen, although live insects can also enter the ear canal.

Treatment

Most foreign bodies can be **gently removed** with an ear curette or otologic forceps. **Insects should be killed** before attempting removal (e.g., with mineral oil, microscope immersion oil, or alcohol). If the object cannot be removed with an ear curette or otologic forceps, **irrigation** of the ear canal with **water at body temperature** is often effective. The stream of water should be directed toward the edge of the foreign body in an attempt to push it toward the external meatus. **Inability to remove the foreign body** necessitates referral to an **otolaryngologist** for removal.

✄ HINT If the foreign body is vegetable matter, irrigation should not be attempted because the vegetable matter can swell and occlude the ear canal.

Acute Mastoiditis

Etiology

Acute mastoiditis is one of the **most serious complications of acute otitis media.** Infection of the mastoid poses a risk because the mastoid is contiguous with the posterior and middle cranial fossae, the sigmoid and lateral sinuses, the facial nerve, the semicircular canals, and the temporal bone. Although all cases of acute otitis media are characterized by concomitant inflammation of the mucosal lining of the mastoid air cells, clinically significant mastoiditis occurs only when the **passageway from the middle ear to the mastoid becomes obstructed.** Acute mastoiditis may be caused by *S. pneumoniae, H. influenzae, Streptococcus pyogenes, S. aureus,* and *M. catarrhalis.*

Clinical Features

Patients with acute mastoiditis present with **persistent otalgia** and **fever.**

Evaluation

Otoscopy usually reveals a **bulging, red, poorly mobile tympanic membrane,** and **purulent drainage** (through a perforation in the membrane) may be visible. **Edema** and **erythema** can be seen **over the mastoid bone,** obliterating the postauricular crease and **causing the characteristic downward and forward displacement of the pinna.** The **mastoid region** is **tender to palpation.**

A **computed tomography (CT) scan** of the temporal bone reveals **inflammation and destruction of the mastoid.** If the tympanic membrane is perforated, the canal should be cleaned of debris and fresh pus should be obtained for culture.

Treatment

Intravenous antimicrobial therapy should be guided by culture results, but **cefuroxime** is often used initially. Placement of **ventilating tubes** may be appropriate to ensure continued drainage. **Mastoidectomy** may be necessary if there **is evidence of osteitis or persistent drainage.** An **otolaryngologist** should be consulted.

Trauma

Etiology

▼ **External ear injuries** can be caused by athletic injuries, falls, direct blows to the ear, earrings that tear through the lobe, burns, or frostbite.

▼ **Middle and inner ear injuries.** The ear canal can be injured by objects used to scratch the ear or to remove cerumen. Traumatic perforation of the tympanic membrane is most commonly caused by poking an object into the ear canal, but trauma to the head and barotrauma can also cause tympanic membrane perforation. Barotrauma occurs when the eustachian tube is obstructed and changes in ambient pressure cannot be transmitted to the middle ear cavity. The increased ambient pressure is transmitted to the vessels of the middle ear mucosa, creating mucosal edema. The pressure differential between the mucosa and the middle ear cavity causes rupture of the mucosal vessels, bleeding into the middle ear, and possibly perforation.

Evaluation

A history of ear trauma may be elicited. The **external ear** should be **examined for hematomas or seromas,** which appear as smooth, blue masses on the lateral auricle and obscure its natural contour. **Microscopic examination** of the tympanic membrane is necessary in patients with suspected traumatic tympanic membrane perforations to ensure that the edges of the perforation do not enter the middle ear cavity. Cholesteatoma formation can occur if the edges of the ruptured tympanic membrane protrude into the middle ear.

Treatment

External ear injuries. Immediate evacuation of hematomas and seromas of the auricle is necessary to prevent cartilage damage. Use of epinephrine should be avoided when lacerations of the pinna are sutured, because epinephrine causes vasoconstriction and may lead to tissue necrosis.

Perforated tympanic membrane. Clean perforations of the tympanic membrane (i.e., those in which the edges do not enter the middle ear cavity) usually heal spontaneously within 2–3 weeks. The perforation should be kept clean and dry. A patient with a traumatic perforation that does not heal in 3 weeks, or one who experiences vertigo, sensorineural hearing loss, or facial nerve paralysis must be referred to an otolaryngologist.

Barotrauma should be treated with antibiotics to prevent infection of the middle ear hemorrhagic effusion. Patients with barotrauma and acute sensorineural hearing loss or vertigo and those with barotrauma injuries that do not heal require prompt referral to an otolaryngologist.

▼ EVALUATION OF A PAINFUL EAR

Patient History

Questions to ask include:

▼ Are any of the risk factors for recurrent acute otitis media present (see Table 30.1)?

▼ What is the season? (Acute otitis media is more prevalent during the winter months, and otitis externa is more common during the summer months.)

▼ Has the patient been swimming recently?

▼ Is there any history of trauma (self-inflicted or barotrauma)?

Physical Examination

Otoscopic examination should provide the diagnosis in most cases. A red, bulging tympanic membrane with poor mobility suggests acute otitis media. If there is concomitant tenderness over the mastoid and obscuring of the postauricular crease, then mastoiditis should be confirmed by **CT scan.** Pain with movement of the pinna and pus or excoriation of the canal suggest otitis externa.

▼ TREATMENT OF A PAINFUL EAR

Until the cause of the ear pain is identified, the patient should be **treated symptomatically. Acetaminophen or ibuprofen** (for children older than 6 months) provides adequate pain control for most patients. **Anesthetic otic drops** are available but should be **avoided** if a **perforation** is suspected.

Suggested Readings

Butler CC, MacMillan H: Does early detection of otitis media with effusion prevent delayed language development? *Arch Dis Child* 85(2):96–103, 2001.

Chan LS, Takata GS, Shekelle P, et al: Evidence assessment of management of acute otitis media: II. Research gaps and priorities for future research. *Pediatrics* 108(2):248–254, 2001.

Dowell SF, Butler JC, Giebink GS, et al: Acute otitis media: management and surveillance in an era of pneumococcal resistance—a report from the Drug-resistant *Streptococcus pneumoniae* Therapeutic Working Group [erratum appears in *Pediatr Infect Dis J* 1999 18(4):341]. *Pediatr Infect Dis J* 18(1):1–9, 1999.

Flynn CA, Griffin G, Tudiver F: Decongestants and antihistamines for acute otitis media in children. *Cochrane Database Syst Rev* (2): CD001727, 2001.

Glasziou PP, Del Mar CB, Hayem M, et al: Antibiotics for acute otitis media in children [update of *Cochrane Database Syst Rev* (2):CD000219; 10796513, 2000]. *Cochrane Database Syst Rev* (4):CD000219, 2000.

Hartman M, Rovers MM, Ingels K, et al: Economic evaluation of ventilation tubes in otitis media with effusion. *Arch Otolaryngol Head Neck Surg* 127(12):1471–1476, 2001.

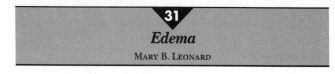

Edema
Mary B. Leonard

▼ INTRODUCTION

Edema is the presence of **abnormally large amounts of fluid in the extracellular tissue spaces** of the body; the term is usually applied to the demonstrable accumulation of excessive fluid in the **interstitial space.** The balance of Starling forces between plasma and the interstitium normally favors the net filtration of fluid from the capillary lumen into the interstitial space. This fluid is then returned to the circulation via the thoracic duct. Edema occurs **when the rate of filtration of fluid from the capillaries increases beyond the capacity of the lymphatics to remove it or when lymphatic function is impaired.** An increase in the hydrostatic pressure gradient or a decrease in the oncotic pressure gradient across the capillary wall favors the formation of edema. Edema may be **localized or generalized.**

Localized edema is found in diseases of the lymphatic system, in diseases associated with venous obstruction, and in conditions associated with increased permeability of the capillary wall (e.g., infection, burns, trauma, allergic reactions). **Allergic reaction** is the **most common cause** of localized edema **in childhood.**

Generalized edema usually develops secondary to increased protein losses, heart failure, or decreased protein production. **Minimal-change nephrotic syndrome (MCNS),** although uncommon (with an incidence of 2 in 100,000 children per year), **accounts for most cases** of generalized edema.

▼ DIFFERENTIAL DIAGNOSIS LIST

Many diseases cause localized or generalized edema; they may be classified according to pathophysiologic mechanism.

Increased Capillary Permeability

Allergic Causes

Insect bites
Contact dermatitis
Drug or food allergy

Infectious Causes

Cellulitis
Scarlet fever
Epstein-Barr virus infection
Roseola

Vasculitic or Rheumatologic Causes

Serum sickness
Henoch-Schönlein purpura
Systemic lupus erythematosus (SLE)

Mucocutaneous lymph node syndrome
Rheumatoid arthritis

Miscellaneous Causes

Hereditary angioneurotic edema
Vitamin E deficiency in premature infants
Sickle cell anemia hand-foot syndrome
Hypothyroidism
Angioedema secondary to use of medications—e.g., enalapril

Decreased Oncotic Pressure (Hypoproteinemia)

Renal Causes

Nephrotic syndrome
Nephrotic syndrome with nephritis

Hepatic Causes

Cirrhosis
Hepatitis
Congenital fibrosis
Metabolic disorders—e.g., galactosemia

Gastrointestinal Causes

Protein-losing enteropathy (PLE)
Cystic fibrosis
Celiac disease
Enteritis with malabsorption

Miscellaneous Causes

Protein-calorie malnutrition (kwashiorkor)
Severe iron-deficiency anemia

Increased Hydrostatic Pressure

Venous Hypertension

Congestive heart failure
Venous thrombosis
Pericardial effusion and tamponade

Increased Vascular Fluid

Excessive iatrogenic intravenous fluid
Salt-retaining steroid therapy
End-stage renal disease
Glomerulonephritis
Medications—e.g., nonsteroidal anti-inflammatory drugs, minoxidil, diazoxide

Impaired Lymphatic Drainage

Hereditary disorders—e.g., Milroy disease
Congenital disorders—e.g., Turner syndrome
Protozoal infections—e.g., filariasis
Trauma
Neoplasia—obstruction secondary to primary or metastatic disease, surgical lymph node resection

▼ DIFFERENTIAL DIAGNOSIS DISCUSSION

This differential diagnosis discussion is limited to **causes of generalized edema.**

Nephrotic Syndrome

Etiology

The nephrotic syndrome, characterized by the **onset of edema with massive proteinuria, hypoalbuminemia,** and **hypercholesterolemia,** may be a manifestation of **numerous clinical entities.** The edema forms **secondary to decreased oncotic pressure** (hypoalbuminemia) **and increased salt and water reabsorption by the kidneys. In primary nephrotic syndrome,** the disease is confined to the **kidney,** whereas **secondary nephrotic syndrome** occurs during the course of a **systemic illness.**

▼ **Causes of primary nephrotic syndrome** in children include MCNS, congenital nephrotic syndrome, focal and segmental glomerulosclerosis, membranoproliferative glomerulonephritis, membranous glomerulonephritis, and crescenteric glomerulonephritis.

▼ **Secondary nephrotic syndrome** may occur in association with vasculitides (e.g., Henoch-Schönlein purpura), SLE, malignant lymphomas (e.g., Hodgkin disease), or infectious diseases (e.g., quartan malaria, hepatitis B, HIV). Nephrotic syndrome during infancy requires special consideration; it may be congenital or caused by congenital syphilis.

Clinical Features

MCNS accounts for more than **75% of cases** of nephrotic syndrome in children. It is **twice as common in boys** as in girls, and onset most commonly occurs between the ages of **2 and 7 years.** Patients usually present with **edema, lethargy, anorexia,** and **decreased urine volume.** The blood pressure is usually normal or decreased; however, in 5%–10% of patients, it is increased. **Hematuria,** present in a minority of patients, is usually microscopic.

The **onset of edema** associated with nephrotic syndrome is usually **insidious;** the fluid characteristically appears in the dependent portions of the extremities or in distensible tissues (e.g., the eyelids, scrotum, or labia). Frequently, the patient's parents notice weight gain, chubbiness, clothes fitting more tightly, or the need for a larger belt during the weeks preceding the patient's presentation for medical attention.

✄ HINT The early symptoms of nephrotic syndrome may be erroneously attributed to an allergic reaction.

Evaluation

Acceptable clinical criteria for confirmation of significant proteinuria include urinary protein losses at a rate of **40 mg/m^2/hour** or a **urine protein-to-urine creatinine ratio** (U$_{PR}$:U$_{CR}$) that **exceeds 1.0** in a randomly collected specimen. A ratio of less than 0.15 is normal; a ratio of greater than 1.0 suggests nephrotic-range proteinuria; and a ratio of more than 2.5 is diagnostic of nephrotic syndrome.

Children usually develop edema when the serum albumin level falls below 2.7 g/dl. The **hemoglobin level may be increased** secondary to hemoconcentration, and the **erythrocyte sedimentation rate** (ESR) is **increased. Mild prerenal azotemia** may be present secondary to reduced intravascular volume. Unless severe hypovolemia is present, the glomerular filtration rate is normal in patients with MCNS. **Hypercholesterolemia** occurs secondary to increased lipoprotein synthesis (stimulated by hypoalbuminemia) and decreased clearance of lipids from the circulation.

Children with nephrotic-range proteinuria, hypoalbuminemia, edema, and hypercholesterolemia have nephrotic syndrome. Their evaluation should include investigation of **possible infectious or systemic causes** based on the history and physical examination. **Syphilis** should be **ruled out** in **patients younger than 6 months** of age.

Treatment

Corticosteroids are the first-line treatment. MCNS is characterized by responsiveness to corticosteroid therapy—treatment with glucocorticoids and a low-salt diet usually results in remission of the renal disease with prompt diuresis and resolution of the edema.

▓ **HINT** Patients with nephrotic syndrome who fail to respond to steroid therapy require a renal biopsy to rule out focal glomerulosclerosis, membranous glomerulopathy, and membranoproliferative glomerulonephritis, which demonstrate a more variable response to therapy and may progress to renal failure.

▼ **Salt restriction** helps minimize the edema.
▼ **Albumin infusions and diuretic administration** may be necessary for patients with severe edema.
▼ **Alkylating agents.** Further immunosuppression with an alkylating agent (e.g., cyclophosphamide, chlorambucil) may be necessary in patients who do not respond to glucocorticoids, or who become glucocorticoid dependent.

Acute Postinfectious Glomerulonephritis

Acute poststreptococcal glomerulonephritis is discussed in Chapter 39, "Hematuria."

Congestive Heart Failure

Etiology

Increased venous pressure is a prerequisite for the development of **cardiac edema,** because the venous back-pressure is critical in the alteration of the transcapillary filtration pressure. Congestive heart failure may occur **secondary to congenital heart disease, myocarditis,** or **cardiomyopathy.**

Clinical Features

In children, the signs and symptoms of congestive heart failure are similar to those seen in adults; however, **edema is a mild finding** and is most often seen in severely decompensated patients. The edema is first noted on the backs of the hands or feet or in dependent areas.

Children may present for medical treatment with fatigue, effort intolerance, anorexia, abdominal pain, or cough. More specific and worrisome signs are **dyspnea, orthopnea, basilar rales, hepatomegaly, cyanosis,** and

cardiomegaly. In **infants,** symptoms of congestive heart failure include **feeding difficulties, tachypnea, diaphoresis,** and **labored respiration;** edema is frequently not detected clinically.

Evaluation

Evaluation is directed toward **identifying the underlying cardiac disease.** The **auscultatory findings** (e.g., gallop rhythm, murmur) are produced by the basic lesion and may help identify the underlying cause. **Echocardiography** delineates structural abnormalities and assesses myocardial function.

Treatment

Therapy is primarily aimed at management of the underlying heart disease. Supportive management strategies may include **diuretics** (to decrease the excessive salt and water load) and **cardiotropic medications** to improve the contractile performance of the heart.

Cirrhosis

Cirrhosis is discussed in Chapter 16, "Ascites."

Protein–Calorie Malnutrition (Kwashiorkor)

Etiology

Kwashiorkor, the most **prevalent form of malnutrition** in the world, is a clinical syndrome that results from **severely deficient protein and calorie intake.** The resultant **hypoalbuminemia** reduces the colloid osmotic pressure, leading to edema.

Clinical Features

Initial signs (e.g., lethargy, irritability) are nonspecific. Patients with advanced cases demonstrate **edema, poor growth, poor stamina, decreased muscle mass, dermatitis,** and **increased susceptibility to infection.** Failure to gain weight may be masked by edema, which is often present in internal organs before it can be identified in the hands or face.

Evaluation

A **decrease in the serum albumin level** is the most **characteristic** laboratory finding. The **hemoglobin level** and **hematocrit** are usually **low.** Height may be normal or retarded, depending on the chronicity of the illness.

Treatment

Restoration of nutritional status can be achieved by **frequent feedings with high-protein, high-energy formulas.** The initial treatment should provide average energy and protein requirements, followed by a **gradual increase to 1.5 times the energy and 3–4 times the protein requirements.** The resolution of the edema may initially result in no change in weight or in weight loss.

▼ EVALUATION OF EDEMA
Patient History

The following information should be sought:

▼ Was the onset of the edema acute or insidious?
▼ What are the associated symptoms (e.g., dark urine, suggestive of nephritis;

respiratory distress, suggestive of congestive heart failure; diarrhea, suggestive of a gastrointestinal disorder)?
▼ Is there a history of a sore throat or cutaneous rash?
▼ Is there a history of recurrent localized edema associated with abdominal pain (suggestive of hereditary angioneurotic edema)?

Physical Examination

When examining a child who presents with edema, the first determination to make is whether the edema is **localized or generalized.** Findings in patients with **localized edema** may include **pruritus** or **urticaria** (associated with an allergic reaction); **tenderness, erythema,** or **fever** (associated with cellulitis); or **localized pronounced swelling** (associated with insect bites, especially those near the eyelids). If the patient has **fixed localized edema** (especially of an **extremity**), **lymphatic obstruction** should be considered (Figure 31.1).

Generalized edema is frequently associated with a **significant underlying disease.** The initial physical examination should include careful attention to the **cardiovascular system,** the **abdomen,** and the **skin.**

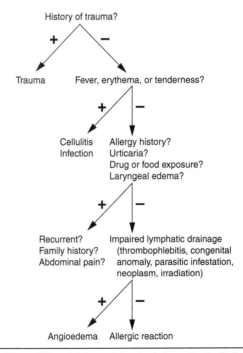

FIGURE 31.1. Differential diagnosis for physical examination findings in a patient with localized edema.

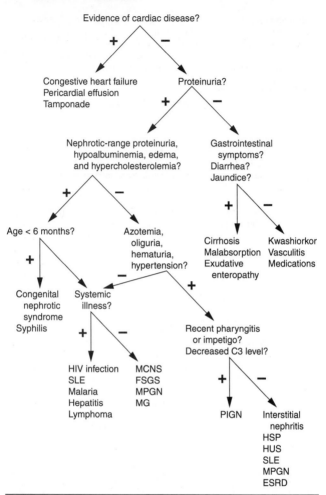

FIGURE 31.2. Approach to the patient with generalized edema.
C3 = complement; *ESRD* = end-stage renal disease; *FSGS* = focal segmental glomerulosclerosis; *HSP* = Henoch-Schönlein purpura; *HUS* = hemolytic-uremic syndrome; *MCNS* = minimal-change nephrotic syndrome; *MG* = membranous glomerulonephritis; *MPGN* = membranoproliferative glomerulonephritis; *PIGN* = postinfectious glomerulonephritis; *SLE* = systemic lupus erythematosus.

Laboratory Studies

The following studies may be indicated for the evaluation of generalized edema:

▼ Urinalysis
▼ Serum albumin level
▼ Blood work (e.g., CBC, hemoglobin level, ESR, PT)
▼ Specific serologic tests (guided by clinical findings)
▼ Serum creatinine level
▼ Serum cholesterol level

HINT The critical step in the laboratory evaluation of edema is to test the urine for evidence of significant proteinuria (i.e., urinary protein losses that exceed 40 mg/m²/hour or a Upr:Ucr ratio that exceeds 1.0).

▼ TREATMENT OF EDEMA

In patients with generalized edema, **treatment of the primary disease** usually results in **resolution of** the edema. The mainstay of edema therapy consists of **salt restriction** and **diuretics,** although in patients with **MCNS** (the most common cause of generalized edema) diuretic therapy is **rarely necessary.** It is often **not necessary to treat the edema before** establishing the **diagnosis.**

▼ APPROACH TO THE PATIENT (FIGURE 31.2)

Suggested Readings

Andreucci M, Federico S, Andreucci VE: Edema and acute renal failure. *Semin Nephrol* 21(3):251–256, 2001.
Fisher DA: Obscure and unusual edema. *Pediatrics* 7:506–528, 1966.
Kelsch RC, Sedman AB: Nephrotic syndrome. *Pediatr Rev* 14:30–38, 1993.
Martin P-Y, Schrier RW: Renal sodium excretion and edematous disorders. *Endocrinol Metab Clin North Am* 24:459–479, 1995.
Powell AA, Armstrong MA: Peripheral edema. *Am Fam Physician* 55: 1721–1726, 1997.
Rosen FS: Urticaria, angioedema, anaphylaxis. 13:387–390, 1992.

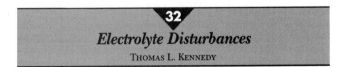

32

Electrolyte Disturbances

THOMAS L. KENNEDY

▼ DIFFERENTIAL DIAGNOSIS LIST

Sodium imbalance
Potassium imbalance
Calcium imbalance
Magnesium imbalance
Phosphate imbalance
Metabolic acidosis
Metabolic alkalosis

▼ DIFFERENTIAL DIAGNOSIS DISCUSSION
Hypernatremia
Etiology

Hypernatremia is a serum sodium level that exceeds 150 mEq/L. The causes of hypernatremia fall into four major categories:

▼ **Water loss** is by far the most common cause of hypernatremia. Usually sodium loss is involved as well, but the water loss exceeds the sodium loss. Major causes of water loss include diarrhea, vomiting, or both with inadequate fluid intake; diabetes insipidus (see Chapter 62, "Polyuria and Urinary Frequency"); increased evaporative water loss (e.g., from radiant warmers or fever); and renal disease with urinary concentrating defect.

▼ **Excess sodium intake** is frequently iatrogenic and results from orally or intravenously administered sodium chloride or sodium bicarbonate.

▼ **Inadequate water intake** can result from an impaired thirst mechanism, an inability to swallow, or a lack of access to water.

▼ **Essential hypernatremia** is rare in childhood and results from defective osmoreceptors.

Clinical Features

The signs and symptoms of hypernatremia vary among individuals and partially depend on the magnitude of the sodium concentration and the rate of change. Signs and symptoms are **nonspecific** and include irritability, lethargy, a harsh "cerebral" cry, increased deep tendon reflexes, seizures, and, occasionally, focal neurologic signs.

Evaluation

Hypernatremic states, especially when associated with water loss, involve significant shifts of fluid from the intracellular space, with relative sparing of the extracellular fluid (ECF). Nevertheless, the physical examination should **focus on ECF volume assessment.** The adequacy of the intravascular compartment can be determined by evaluating the peripheral pulses, perfusion, temperature, and capillary refill time. The adequacy of the interstitial compartment can be ascertained by evaluating the skin turgor, tears, and mucous membranes.

Helpful laboratory studies include serum electrolytes; serum glucose, calcium, blood urea nitrogen (BUN), and creatinine levels; and urinalysis (to evaluate urine sodium, specific gravity, and creatinine).

Findings suggestive of the various underlying mechanisms of hypernatremia are summarized in Table 32.1.

Treatment

Significant **intravascular volume compromise or shock** should be **treated promptly** and independently of the serum sodium concentration by administering normal saline in amounts adequate to restore pulses and perfusion. Initially, a bolus of 20 ml/kg should be administered rapidly (over 20–30 minutes). The child should be reassessed, and additional fluid given as needed.

After the patient has been stabilized, an attempt should be made to **reduce the serum sodium level slowly,** generally at a rate of approximately

TABLE 32.1. Assessment of Hypernatremia

Underlying Cause	ECF Volume	Urine Output	Urine Sodium	Specific Gravity
Sodium excess	Increased	Normal or increased	Increased	High
Water loss (DI)	Decreased	Increased	Decreased	High
Sodium and water loss (water > sodium)	Normal or decreased	Decreased	Increased	Low

DI = diabetes insipidus; ECF = extracellular fluid.

0.5 mEq/L/hr. Administering intravenous fluids consisting of one-third normal saline and spreading the administration of maintenance and deficit fluids evenly over 48 hours is usually adequate, although calculated sodium needs are usually less (i.e., one-eighth to one-fourth normal saline). The use of very hypotonic fluids, especially when given rapidly, can lead to intracellular water shift, cell swelling, and cerebral edema.

In **dehydrated patients** (i.e., those that have experienced sodium and water loss), the sodium deficit should not be overlooked, although it is generally modest (approximately 2 mEq/kg).

In patients with **severe sodium excess,** judicious use of fluids, with or without furosemide administration, dialysis, or both, is recommended (under the guidance of a nephrologist).

Hyponatremia

Etiology

Hyponatremia is defined as a serum sodium level of less than 130 mEq/L. All causes of hyponatremia can be considered to be dilutional, depletional, or both (Table 32.2).

▼ **Dilutional hyponatremia.** The total body water is generally expanded and is increased relative to total body sodium.
▼ **Depletional hyponatremia.** There is a decreased (or normal) amount of total body water and a sodium deficit, in which the sodium loss exceeds the water loss.
▼ **Pseudohyponatremia.** Sodium is not distributed throughout the serum and its concentration is artificially lowered. Causes of pseudohyponatremia include hyperlipidemia and hyperproteinemia.

Clinical Features

As with hypernatremia, the signs and symptoms are variable, nonspecific, and depend on both the severity of the hyponatremia and the rapidity with which it developed. Findings include lethargy, weakness, encephalopathy, and seizures.

Evaluation

Because depletional hyponatremia is associated with a water shift to the intracellular fluid (ICF) compartment, careful assessment and prompt restoration of the **ECF and intravascular volume** are critical.

TABLE 32.2. Causes of Hyponatremia

Dilutional hyponatremia
  Water intoxication (excess ingestion or iatrogenic administration)
  Edema-associated states
    Congestive heart failure
    Nephrotic syndrome
    Renal failure
    Hepatic failure
    Neuromuscular blockade (e.g., pancuronium-induced)
  Excess antidiuretic hormone (ADH)*
    Exogenous administration
    Syndrome of inappropriate antidiuretic hormone (SIADH)
  Reset osmostat
  Hyperglycemia
Depletional hyponatremia
  Renal sodium wasting (e.g., Fanconi syndrome)
  Adrenal sodium wasting (e.g., adrenal insufficiency)
  CAH (21-hydroxylase deficiency)
  Diuretic therapy
  Osmotic diuresis (e.g., glucosuria)
  Gastrointestinal fluid losses with hypotonic replacement
  Excessive perspiration associated with large sodium loss (e.g., cystic fibrosis)

CAH = congenital adrenal hyperplasia.

* Conditions associated with increased ADH or an ADH-like effect and hyponatremia include pain, vomiting, central nervous system (CNS) disorders (e.g., trauma, infection, neoplasia), intrathoracic conditions (e.g., infection, mechanical ventilation), and some drugs [e.g., narcotics, barbiturates, carbamazepine, nonsteroidal anti-inflammatory agents (NSAIDs), cyclophosphamide, vincristine].

Useful **laboratory studies** include serum electrolytes; glucose, BUN, creatinine, albumin, and cholesterol levels; serum cortisol, with and without ACTH stimulation, and adrenocorticotropic hormone (ACTH) levels (if adrenal insufficiency is suspected); and **urinalysis** to evaluate urine sodium and creatinine. A random urine sample permits calculation of the fractional excretion of sodium (FE_{Na}), which can be useful when the urine sodium concentration is borderline (e.g., 19–21 mEq/L):

$$FE_{Na} = [U_{Na} \times P_{Cr}]/[U_{Cr} \times P_{Na}] \times 100\%$$

Figure 32.1 demonstrates how the differential for the specific cause of the hyponatremia can be narrowed on the basis of urine output and urine sodium excretion.

Therapy

▼ **Compromised intravascular volume.** When indicated, the intravascular volume should be restored promptly with the administration of isotonic saline. A reasonable initial fluid volume is 20 ml/kg, given rapidly intravenously over a period of about 30 minutes. Additional isotonic fluid boluses may be indicated.

▼ **Sodium deficit.** The sodium deficit should be calculated and measures

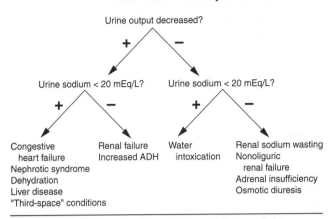

FIGURE 32.1. Narrowing the differential diagnosis for the underlying cause of hyponatremia.
ADH = antidiuretic hormone.

taken to restore the sodium level. The sodium deficit can be calculated as follows:

$$Na^+ \text{ deficit (mEq)} = 0.6 \times wt \text{ (kg)} \times (\text{desired } Na^+ - \text{observed } Na^+)$$

When a rapid increase in the serum sodium level is required (e.g., with hyponatremia-induced seizures), 3% saline (which contains 0.5 mEq/ml of sodium) should be administered. Care should be taken not to over-correct hyponatremia. The goal is to prevent or reverse symptoms. In general, in acute hyponatremia, the sodium level should be corrected to 125 mEq/L or to a level slightly higher than that associated with symptoms. Overzealous correction, especially of chronic hyponatremia, can lead to neurologic deterioration (osmotic demyelinization syndrome or central pontine myelinolysis).

▼ **Severe hyperglycemia.** Hyponatremia may be associated with severe hyperglycemia as a result of transcellular fluid shifts. The fluid shifts are caused by the osmotic effect of the hyperglycemia. The following formula can be used to calculate the sodium concentration after hyperglycemia has been resolved:

$$\text{Final } Na^+ \text{ (mEq/L)} = \text{measured } Na^+ + 0.16 \text{ [glucose (mg/dl)} - 100]$$

▼ **Acute edematous states.** In patients with acute edematous states secondary to hypoalbuminemia it is important not to restrict water intake because intravascular volume may be compromised. It is more important to restrict sodium intake to prevent further edema.
▼ **Adrenal insufficiency.** If adrenal insufficiency is suspected, hydrocortisone (50 mg/m^2) should be given as an initial bolus intravenously, followed by a hydrocortisone drip or doses given every 6 hours.

⚒ HINT Syndrome of inappropriate ADH (SIADH) is an uncommon syndrome in pediatric patients, but it should be considered when hyponatremia occurs in the absence of volume depletion, edema, or renal insufficiency, or in association with certain drugs (Table 32.2). The diagnosis is based on the excretion of urine that is not maximally dilute in the presence of a serum osmolality of less than 280 mOsm/kg. Under most circumstances, a reliable estimate of the serum osmolality can be obtained by doubling the serum sodium level (mEq/L) and adding 10. In patients with hyperglycemia or azotemia, the serum osmolality can be calculated as follows:

$$2 \times Na \ (mEq/L) + glucose/18 + BUN/2.8$$

It is often mistakenly assumed that to diagnose SIADH, the urine osmolality and sodium levels must be very high. The urine osmolality need only be inappropriately increased (i.e., not maximally diluted) in the presence of hypotonic ECF with normovolemia. Treatment consists of restricting fluid intake to slightly less than the total of the estimated insensible water loss plus the urine output, the sum of which approximates two-thirds of maintenance fluids. The condition is usually transient in children, and chronic measures are not required.

Hyperkalemia

Etiology

Hyperkalemia is defined as a serum potassium level that exceeds 5.5 mEq/L. There are four major underlying mechanisms:

▼ **Transcellular potassium shifts** are the most common cause of hyperkalemia in childhood. Shifts of potassium from the ICF to the ECF can be associated with acidosis (especially metabolic acidosis), β-adrenergic blockade, strenuous exercise, insulin deficiency, and hyperkalemic periodic paralysis.

⚒ HINT The presence of acidosis does not always account for the hyperkalemia and may lead to failure to recognize and treat another cause.

▼ **Increased potassium intake** can result from potassium supplements, drugs containing potassium (e.g., potassium penicillins), salt substitute use, blood transfusions (stored blood), and geophagia (some clays are potassium-rich).

▼ **Decreased renal excretion of potassium** can result from renal failure, certain drugs (Table 32.3), type 4 renal tubular acidosis (RTA), mineralocorticoid deficiency, or mineralocorticoid resistance. Types of mineralocorticoid deficiency include adrenal insufficiency, congenital adrenal hyperplasia (CAH), hyporeninemic hypoaldosteronism, and primary mineralocorticoid deficiency. Mineralocorticoid resistance may be a transient condition in the newborn or caused by obstructive nephropathy or pseudohypoaldosteronism.

▼ **Increased endogenous cellular release of potassium** is associated with hypoxic or toxic cell death, burns, intravascular hemolysis, rhabdomyolysis, and acute tumor lysis syndrome.

TABLE 32.3. Drugs Associated with Hyperkalemia

Potassium-sparing diuretics (e.g., spironolactone, triamterene, amiloride)
Potassium supplements (e.g., potassium chloride)
Potassium-containing penicillins
Stored blood
Cyclosporine
Nonsteroidal anti-inflammatory drugs (NSAIDs)
Heparin
Angiotensin-converting enzyme (ACE) inhibitors
β-adrenergic blockers
Chemotherapeutic agents

Clinical Features

Symptoms of hyperkalemia are neither predictably present nor specific. They include muscle weakness, decreased deep tendon reflexes, ileus, anorexia, tingling of the mouth and extremities, malaise, and tetany.

Evaluation

A **serum electrolyte panel** should be obtained. Cardiac changes are usually seen when the potassium level exceeds 6.0 mEq/L and are more likely with a rapidly increasing potassium level. Cardiotoxicity is increased with concomitant hyponatremia or hypocalcemia.

▲ **HINT** Spurious hyperkalemia may be seen with hemolyzed specimens, significant thrombocytosis, or extreme leukocytosis. Because heel-stick samples, which are commonly obtained in infants, frequently result in hemolyzed specimens, increased potassium values are common and need immediate verification (by repeating the test) if treatment is considered. Venipuncture with a 22-gauge needle is preferred.

An **electrocardiogram (ECG)** should be obtained to assess for cardiac changes associated with the hyperkalemia, commonly manifested as tall, "tented" T waves (especially in the precordial leads) and prolonged PR intervals or a widened, prolonged QRS complex. Late ECG changes include flattened P or T waves (or both) with ST segment depression, a sine wave pattern, and tachyarrhythmias or bradyarrhythmias.

Indications for serious concern and instituting treatment include the following:

▼ A potassium value of more than 7.0 mEq/L
▼ A rapidly increasing potassium concentration
▼ A clinical state in which the potassium level is expected to continue to increase (e.g., rhabdomyolysis)
▼ The presence of renal failure
▼ Symptoms of hyperkalemia

Treatment

If the potassium level is high or the hyperkalemia is causing symptoms, emergency measures should be initiated. Options for the management of hyperkalemia are summarized in Table 32.4.

TABLE 32.4.   Treatment of Hyperkalemia

Agent	Indication	Mechanism of Action	Dose	Side Effects/Potential Problems
10% Calcium gluconate	ECG changes	Stabilizes membranes	1 mg/kg IV over 5–10 minutes	Hypercalcemia
Sodium bicarbonate	ECG changes or very high K^+ level	Shifts K^+ to intracellular compartment	1 mg/kg IV over 5–10 minutes	Sodium load
Glucose plus insulin	ECG changes or very high K^+ level	Shifts K^+ to intracellular compartment	0.25–0.5 gm/kg glucose plus 0.3 U insulin/gm glucose over 30–60 minutes	Hyper or hypoglycemia
Kayexalate resin	To remove K^+ from body	K^+ binds to resin in gut	1 gm/kg PO or PR in 50%–70% sorbitol	Constipation
Furosemide	Symptomatic hyperkalemia	Enhances urinary K^+ excretion	1–2 mg/kg IV	May not be enough renal function to be effective
Hemo- or peritoneal dialysis	No renal function	Removes K^+ in dialysate	…	Risks associated with dialysis
Exchange transfusion	ECG changes or very high K^+ level	Donor blood has had most K^+ removed	Double volume	Risks associated with exchange transfusion

ECG = electrocardiogram; IV = intravenous; K^+ = potassium; PO = orally; PR = parenterally.

⚥ HINT Sodium bicarbonate and calcium salts are incompatible in intravenous solutions.

⚥ HINT Increased potassium excretion can be achieved with the use of furosemide, even in children with significant renal impairment.

Hypokalemia

Etiology

Hypokalemia is defined as a serum potassium level of less than 3.5 mEq/L. There are five major underlying mechanisms:

▼ **Severely limited dietary intake**—anorexia nervosa
▼ **Increased gastrointestinal losses**—vomiting, diarrhea, cathartic abuse, geophagia (certain clays bind potassium)
▼ **Increased skin losses**—excessive perspiration
▼ **Increased renal losses**—Fanconi syndrome, RTA, Bartter syndrome, diuretic therapy, osmotic diuresis (e.g., glucosuria), hyperaldosteronism, CAH, 11-β-hydroxysteroid dehydrogenase deficiency (or inhibition with natural licorice ingestion), Liddle syndrome, Gitelman syndrome (magnesium-losing tubulopathy), excess adrenocorticotropic hormone (ACTH), drugs (Table 32.5), magnesium depletion, and chloride depletion
▼ **Transcellular potassium shifts**—alkalosis (metabolic and respiratory), excess insulin, hypokalemic periodic paralysis, and certain drugs (Table 32.5)

⚥ HINT The administration of intravenous glucose, especially in high concentrations, may worsen hypokalemia by stimulating insulin release, which increases cellular uptake of potassium.

Clinical Features

Signs and symptoms of hypokalemia, as in other electrolyte disturbances, are multiple, variable, and nonspecific.

TABLE 32.5. Drugs Associated with Hypokalemia
Drugs associated with increased renal loss
Aminoglycoside toxicity
Amphotericin B
Cisplatin
Penicillins in high doses
Corticosteroids
Diuretics (except for potassium-sparing ones)
Drugs associated with increased cellular uptake of potassium
Terbutaline
Epinephrine
β-adrenergic agents (e.g., albuterol)
Theophylline toxicity
Barium toxicity
Insulin

▼ **Neuromuscular signs** include weakness, paralysis, tetany, ileus, ureteral aperistalsis, lethargy, confusion, autonomically mediated hypotension, and rhabdomyolysis.

▼ **Cardiovascular signs** include brady- and tachyarrhythmias.

▼ **Renal and metabolic abnormalities** include impaired renal concentrating capacity and polyuria, chronic nephrotoxicity, and impaired insulin secretion.

Evaluation

Laboratory studies should include a serum electrolyte panel; serum calcium, magnesium, and glucose levels; and urinalysis to evaluate urine potassium and creatinine (to calculate the fractional excretion of potassium, FE_K). Hyperglycemia may be seen. Other tests (e.g., aldosterone assessment) should be ordered if a specific disorder is suspected on the basis of the history and physical examination.

An **ECG** should also be obtained. ECG changes are seen with severe potassium deficit (i.e., less than 2.5–3.0 mEq/L). In addition, hypokalemia increases susceptibility to digitalis toxicity. Potential changes include T-wave flattening, U waves [which give the appearance of a long corrected QT interval (QTc)], ST segment depression, and prolonged PR intervals (Fig. 32.2).

Therapy

Potassium deficits frequently occur with other abnormalities (e.g., calcium, magnesium, and chloride depletion) and cannot be completely corrected until the accompanying deficits are repaired.

Potassium replacement for hypokalemia should be via the oral route whenever possible, although **oral potassium supplements** may cause gastric irritation or vomiting and may be nonpalatable to a young child. Table 32.6 summarizes available oral preparations. A normal diet usually provides potassium in excess of maintenance requirements (2–3 mEq/kg). Foods rich in potassium include dried fruits, bananas (1.5 mEq/inch), tomatoes, and most other fruits. Prune juice and orange juice provide 16 mEq and 12 mEq of potassium per 8 ounces, respectively.

Patients with severe or symptomatic hypokalemia should receive **potassium intravenously** at a rate of no greater than 0.3–0.5 mEq/kg/hr. Because most of the body's potassium is not in the ECF, the serum potassium concentration may not reflect (and does not permit calculation of) the total potassium deficit. Serum potassium level and acid-base status must be followed closely when repairing deficits. Potassium should not be administered intravenously until it is certain that the patient is not anuric.

⚡ HINT In the intravenous administration of potassium, concentrations of 40 mEq/L or more are irritating to small peripheral veins and often result in pain or loss of access site. Administration of high concentrations (more than 60 mEq/L) through a central line does not cause pain but is potentially dangerous, and benefits must be weighed against the risk of development of fatal arrhythmias. Children should be carefully and continuously monitored.

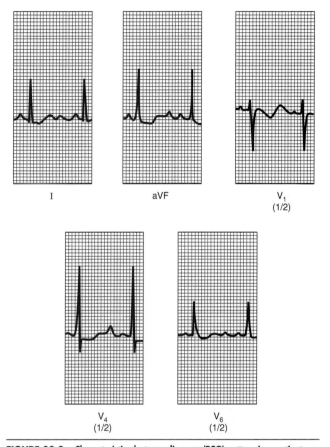

FIGURE 32.2. Characteristic electrocardiogram (ECG) pattern in a patient with hypokalemia.
These tracings are from a 4-year-old with nephrotic syndrome. Note the prominent U waves in all leads with ST segment depression and T wave inversion in leads I, aVF, V_4, and V_6. (Reprinted with permission from Garson A, Jr: Electrocardiography. In *The Science and Practice of Pediatric Cardiology*, 2nd ed. Edited by Garson A, Jr, Bricker JT, Fisher D, et al. Baltimore, Williams & Wilkins, 1998, p 772.)

HINT In acute metabolic acidosis, the serum potassium level may be increased owing to extracellular shift, while the total body potassium level is diminished. A rule of thumb is that a 0.1 decrease in pH acutely results in an increase in potassium level of 0.7 mEq/L.

TABLE 32.6. Oral Potassium Supplements

Preparation	Formulation	Potassium Supplied
Potassium phosphate	Tablet	1.1, 2.3, or 3.7 mEq
Potassium chloride	Extentabs	10 mEq
	Powder packet	20 mEq
	Effervescent tablets	20 mEq
	Liquid	20 mEq
Potassium citrate	Tablets, crystals, or syrup	1 mEq/ml (Polycitra) or 2 mEq/ml (Polycitra-K)
Potassium gluconate	Liquid	20 mEq/15 ml

Hypercalcemia

Etiology

Hypercalcemia is defined as a serum calcium level that exceeds 11 mg/dl or an ionized calcium level that exceeds 5.0 mg/dl. Hypercalcemia reduces renal blood flow [and as a result, decreases the glomerular filtration rate (GFR)]; increases sodium, potassium, and magnesium excretion; decreases renal concentrating capacity; and leads to metabolic acidosis. Causes of hypercalcemia include:

▼ **Enhanced vitamin D activity**—excess vitamin D administration, increased endogenous vitamin D sensitivity or activity (such as occurs in idiopathic infantile hypercalcemia, sarcoidosis, certain malignancies, and neonatal fat necrosis)
▼ **Skeletal disorders of calcium deposition or mobilization**—hyperparathyroidism, immobilization hypercalcemia, hypophosphatasia, vitamin A intoxication, skeletal dysplasias, and metastatic bone disease
▼ **Renal disorders**—hypocalciuric hypercalcemia, thiazide diuretic therapy, rhabdomyolysis with acute myoglobinuric renal failure
▼ **Miscellaneous causes**—milk-alkali syndrome, severe hypophosphatemia, blue diaper syndrome (tryptophan transport defect), excessive intravenous calcium administration, hypo- or hyperthyroidism

Clinical Features

The onset and severity of symptoms vary among individuals, but generally symptoms are more severe the higher the serum calcium level. Symptoms are uncommon at levels of less than 12 mg/dl. Levels of more than 16 mg/dl are life-threatening and should be treated as an emergency.

Hypercalcemia that is renal in origin is characterized by polyuria, polydipsia, and signs of renal insufficiency, nephrocalcinosis, and nephrolithiasis.

Nonrenal hypercalcemia can cause a variety of symptoms:

▼ **General**—fatigue, weakness, anorexia
▼ **Gastrointestinal**—nausea, vomiting, constipation, xerostomia, symptoms of pancreatitis
▼ **Central nervous system (CNS)**—headache, drowsiness, apathy, apnea (infancy)
▼ **Skin and mucous membranes**—pruritus, conjunctivitis

▼ **Musculoskeletal**—myalgias, arthralgias, bone pain, hypotonia
▼ **Cardiovascular**—hypertension, short QT interval, arrhythmias, heart block

Evaluation

Laboratory studies should include total and ionized calcium levels; a serum electrolyte panel; serum phosphorus, alkaline phosphatase, magnesium, urea, creatinine, total protein, and albumin levels; and an intact or aminoterminal assay for parathyroid hormone (PTH). **Other studies,** such as vitamin D levels, should be chosen based on clinical suspicion.

Calcium excretion can be assessed using a 24-hour collection (normal is < 4 mg/kg/day) or, more quickly, by determining the calcium:creatinine ratio from a random sample (normal is < 0.2).

Therapy

Dehydration should be corrected, **hydration status** should be closely monitored, and **intravascular volume** should be maintained. If possible, the underlying cause of the hypercalcemia should be identified and removed. Calcium excretion should be maximized via saline diuresis and the use of loop diuretics.

Other therapies (e.g., steroids, calcitonin, mithramycin, bisphosphonates, chelators) may be indicated, depending on the specific disorder that is responsible for the hypercalcemia. These therapies should be used under the direction of a nephrologist or endocrinologist.

Hypocalcemia

Etiology

Hypocalcemia is defined as a serum calcium level of less than 9.0 mg/dl (7.0 mg/dl in newborns) or an ionized calcium level of less than 4.8 mg/dl (4.0 mg/dl in newborns). Causes include:

▼ Hypoalbuminemia (total calcium is decreased, but ionized calcium usually remains normal)
▼ Hyperphosphatemia
▼ Renal failure
▼ Hypocalcemia of the newborn, early (within 72 hours of birth) or late (5–7 days after birth)
▼ Hypoparathyroidism
▼ Pseudohypoparathyroidism
▼ Exchange transfusion
▼ Vitamin D–deficient rickets
▼ Vitamin D–dependent rickets
▼ Pancreatitis
▼ Hypomagnesemia

Clinical Features

The following signs and symptoms may be seen, especially with a reduced ionized calcium level:

▼ Muscle weakness, fasciculations, or both
▼ Numbness and tingling in extremities
▼ Cramps
▼ Hyperreflexia

▼ Positive Chvostek and Trousseau signs
▼ Tetany
▼ Seizures

Evaluation

Laboratory studies should include those recommended for the evaluation of hypercalcemia.

Ionized calcium level determinations may be useful in assessing a child with hypocalcemia; unfortunately, this test is frequently unavailable in hospital laboratories, and it can be unreliable.

A prolonged QTc interval may be seen on ECG (Figure 32.3).

Treatment

The decision to treat is based on the presence of symptoms, the calcium concentration, and the cause of hypocalcemia. Commonly used calcium preparations are summarized in Table 32.7.

Oral therapy is indicated only for correction of **chronic and mildly symptomatic states.** Maintenance calcium needs are not precisely known but are generally considered to be 20–50 mg/kg/day of elemental calcium. In patients with hyperphosphatemia, therapy includes the use of phosphate binders (either calcium- or aluminum-containing salts). When indicated, vitamin D therapy increases absorption of calcium from the gastrointestinal tract and increases phosphaturia.

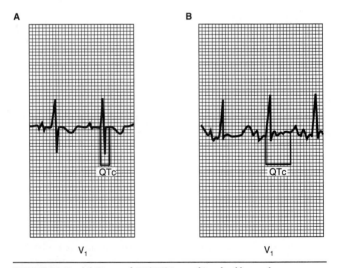

FIGURE 32.3. (A) Corrected QT (*QTc*) interval in a healthy newborn.
(B) Prolonged QTc interval in a patient with hypocalcemia.
(Reprinted with permission from Garson A, Jr: Electrocardiography. In *The Science and Practice of Pediatric Cardiology*, 2nd ed. Edited by Garson A, Jr, Bricker JT, Fisher D, et al. Baltimore, Williams & Wilkins, 1998, p 746.)

TABLE 32.7. Commonly Used Calcium Preparations

Preparation	Elemental Calcium Content	Route
Calcium gluconate (10%)	1 ml = 9 mg = 0.45 mEq	Intravenous
Calcium chloride (10%)	1 ml = 27 mg = 1.36 mEq	Intravenous
Calcium glubionate	1 ml = 23 mg = 1.12 mEq	Oral

Patients with **severe symptoms** (e.g., seizures) require 10–20 mg/kg elemental **calcium administered intravenously and slowly.** The child must be monitored for bradyarrhythmias. Extravasation of calcium into the subcutaneous tissues may cause serious skin sloughs. Treatment with hyaluronidase should be considered for these patients.

✄ HINT Hypomagnesemia frequently accompanies hypocalcemia, so the magnesium level should always be measured. If it is low in a child with apparent symptoms of hypocalcemia, the magnesium level should be corrected.

Hypermagnesemia

Etiology

Hypermagnesemia is defined as a serum magnesium level that exceeds 2.5 mEq/L. Mechanisms include excess intake (almost always accompanied by significant renal insufficiency) and decreased renal excretion (seen with a GFR of less than 10 ml/min, hypothyroidism, and familial hypocalciuric hypercalcemia). Sources of excess magnesium intake include magnesium-containing antacids, laxatives, or enemas; high-dose intravenous magnesium administration; and, in newborns, prepartum administration of large amounts of magnesium sulfate to the mother.

Clinical Features

Signs and symptoms, including decreased deep tendon reflexes, weakness, confusion, lethargy, and hypotension, relate to adverse effects on neuromuscular transmission and usually first appear when the magnesium level exceeds 7 mEq/L.

Evaluation

It is important to assess the GFR (to assess the level of renal function) and the calcium concentration because hypocalcemia worsens the signs and symptoms of hypermagnesemia.

Therapy

The source of the increased magnesium level must be discovered and removed. **Continuous heart rate and blood pressure monitoring** are indicated for patients with magnesium levels that exceed 5 mEq/L. If the patient has symptoms, or if the magnesium level is greater than 7 mEq/L, **intravenous administration of calcium** is indicated to temporarily decrease the serum magnesium level. In patients with severe hypermagnesemia and renal insufficiency, **peritoneal dialysis or hemodialysis** may be required.

TABLE 32.8.   Causes of Hypomagnesemia
Increased gastrointestinal losses
Small bowel disease or inflammation
Fat malabsorption (including cystic fibrosis)
Laxative abuse
Protein-calorie malnutrition
Gluten sensitivity
Gastroenteritis or chronic diarrhea
Increased renal losses
Primary renal tubular magnesium wasting (Gitelman syndrome)
Postobstructive diuresis
Recovery phase of acute renal failure
Diuretic therapy
Hypokalemic states
Hyperaldosteronism
Drugs (aminoglycosides, amphotericin, cyclosporine)
Hypo- or hyperparathyroidism
Renal tubular acidosis
Hyperthyroidism
Redistribution
Refeeding, total parenteral nutrition
Pancreatitis
"Hungry bone" syndrome

Hypomagnesemia

Etiology

Hypomagnesemia is defined as a serum magnesium level of less than 1.5 mEq/L and is frequently seen in association with hypocalcemia and hypokalemia. Rarely, hypomagnesemia is caused by dietary insufficiency. More common causes include increased gastrointestinal losses, increased renal excretion, and redistribution (Table 32.8).

▓ HINT   The association of hypomagnesemia with hypocalcemia and hypokalemia is common but confusing. In some situations, a cause-and-effect relationship may be in place. For example, hypomagnesemia leads to hypocalcemia as a result of diminished PTH secretion or decreased responsiveness of bone to PTH. Likewise, hypomagnesemia increases renal potassium loss. In other situations, a shared cause (e.g., aminoglycoside toxicity) accounts for the overlap. Attempts to treat one of these deficiencies without recognizing the presence of another will not be successful.

Clinical Features

The signs and symptoms of hypomagnesemia are sometimes difficult to separate from those associated with concomitant electrolyte disturbances. Clinical features of hypomagnesemia include weakness, tremors, anorexia, lassitude, and, rarely, seizures.

Evaluation

Laboratory studies should include a serum electrolyte panel and serum calcium, phosphorus, alkaline phosphatase, and PTH levels.

An ECG may reveal associated cardiovascular problems, such as tachycardia (sinus or nodal), premature beats (supraventricular or ventricular), and changes similar to those seen in hypokalemia (i.e., flat, broad T waves; prolonged PR and QT intervals). Patients with hypomagnesemia also have increased susceptibility to digitalis toxicity.

Treatment

Therapy of symptomatic hypomagnesemia entails the administration of **magnesium sulfate** (25–50 mg/kg intravenously via a slow drip, or every 4–6 hours intramuscularly). The patient must be monitored for hypotension.

Prevention involves ensuring an adequate supply of magnesium in the diet or in parenteral fluids. Normal requirements are approximately 4 mg/kg/day (0.3 mEq/kg/day). Oral magnesium supplements frequently produce diarrhea and should be used with caution in children with renal insufficiency.

Hyperphosphatemia

Etiology

The normal phosphorus values vary according to age (Table 32.9). Causes of hyperphosphatemia include:

- **Renal failure** (defined as a GFR of less than 20% of normal)
- **Increased renal tubular reabsorption**—hypoparathyroidism, pseudohypoparathyroidism
- **Increased phosphate intake**—cow's milk in infants, phosphate-containing enemas
- **Increased endogenous phosphate release**—tumor lysis syndrome
- **Most hypocalcemic states**

Clinical Features

Hyperphosphatemia is almost always accompanied by hypocalcemia, and signs and symptoms are related to the latter.

HINT A serious complication of hyperphosphatemia is metastatic or ectopic calcification in vessel walls and tissues. The risk is greatly increased when the calcium and phosphorus product exceeds 70.

Evaluation

Appropriate laboratory studies include those for the assessment of calcium disorders as well as those that allow determination of renal function and

TABLE 32.9. Normal Phosphorus Values

Age	Normal Phosphorus Value (mg/dl)
Newborn	4.8–8.2
1–3 years	3.8–6.5
4–11 years	3.7–5.6
12–15 years	2.9–5.4
15 +	2.7–4.7

assessment of the urine creatinine and phosphate level. Assessment of the urine creatinine and phosphate level allows determination of tubular reabsorption of phosphate (TRP):

$$\text{TRP} = 1 - (\text{U}_{\text{Phos}}/\text{P}_{\text{Phos}})/(\text{U}_{\text{Cr}}/\text{P}_{\text{Cr}}) \times 100\%$$

Normal is a TRP that exceeds 80%.

Treatment

Phosphate intake must be restricted and an **oral phosphate binder** (e.g., calcium carbonate, aluminum-containing salts) should be administered. Calcium carbonate is the preferred agent; a reasonable starting dose is 1 g with each meal, titrated thereafter as indicated.

Phosphate excretion should be maximized by **saline diuresis** if renal function is normal. In patients with severe renal insufficiency, both **peritoneal dialysis and hemodialysis** may be effective.

Hypocalcemia should be corrected, if possible.

Hypophosphatemia

Etiology

Normal phosphate values are given in Table 32.9. Hypophosphatemia can result from hypercalcemic states, decreased phosphate intake, binding of phosphate in the gastrointestinal tract (e.g., antacid abuse), or increased renal phosphate loss (e.g., hyperparathyroidism, Fanconi syndrome, hypophosphatemic rickets).

Clinical Features

Symptoms and signs generally do not occur until the phosphorus level is less than 1.5 mg/dl. Clinical features include muscle weakness, rhabdomyolysis, bone pain, arthralgias, hemolytic anemia, anorexia, nausea, and vomiting.

Evaluation

Appropriate laboratory studies include those for the assessment of calcium disorders as well as those that allow determination of renal function and assessment of the urine creatinine and phosphate level.

Treatment

The underlying condition should be treated or removed. If possible, the **accompanying hypercalcemia** should be treated. Often, treatment of the hypercalcemia resolves the hypophosphatemia.

If necessary, **phosphate** should be administered to increase the serum phosphorus level to 2.0 mg/dl. Phosphate should be given at a rate of 15–20 mg/kg/day, either orally or intravenously. It is important to ensure that the patient's renal function is normal before administering phosphate. The intravenous administration of phosphate is **contraindicated in the presence of hypercalcemia** because it may lead to the development of metastatic calcifications.

Metabolic Acidosis

Etiology

Metabolic acidosis is defined as any state that reduces the serum bicarbonate concentration to less than the normal range of 24–26 mmol/L.

TABLE 32.10. Causes of Metabolic Acidosis

Normal anion gap
  Gastrointestinal loss of bicarbonate
    Diarrhea
    Drainage of intestinal fluid (e.g., ileostomy, nasojejunal tube drainage)
  Administration of acid
    Total parenteral nutrition (e.g., amino acids)
  Acute extracellular fluid expansion (e.g., following the rapid administration of
    intravenous fluids)
  Renal loss of bicarbonate or failure to secrete net acid
    Renal tubular acidosis
    Therapy with carbonic anhydrase inhibitors (e.g., acetazolamide)
Wide anion gap
  Renal failure
  Ketoacidosis
    Diabetes mellitus
    Starvation
  Lactic acidosis
  Other organic acidosis (e.g., methylmalonic acidemia)
  Intoxications (e.g., methanol, salicylates, ethylene glycol)

Metabolic acidosis may be accompanied by either a normal anion gap (hyperchloremic metabolic acidosis) or a wide anion gap. Causes of metabolic acidosis are summarized in Table 32.10.

Renal tubular acidosis (RTA) is a group of disorders in which hyperchloremic metabolic acidosis occurs because of excess renal tubular loss of bicarbonate, failure to excrete dietary net acid, or both. There are many causes of RTA (Table 32.11), which can be categorized according to the type of RTA: **type 1** (distal or classic) RTA, **type 2** (proximal) RTA, or **type 4** (hyperkalemic) RTA. Characteristics of each of these types of RTA are summarized in Table 32.12.

Clinical Features

Signs and symptoms of metabolic acidosis are nonspecific, variable, and generally overshadowed by the illness or disorder leading to the acidosis. Isolated metabolic acidosis (e.g., RTA) is occasionally associated with anorexia and vomiting. Hyperventilation, an almost immediate compensatory response to metabolic acidosis, is often, but not always, apparent.

Evaluation

The serum bicarbonate concentration is virtually equivalent to the total carbon dioxide value reported with serum electrolytes. The first step in the evaluation of a low bicarbonate level is to **calculate the anion gap:**

$$\text{Anion gap} = (Na^+) - [(Cl^-) + (HCO_3^-)]$$

The normal gap is 12, with a range of 8–16.

▼ If the **anion gap is normal,** a history of diarrhea or other gastrointestinal losses should be sought. If there is none, an accurate (meter) pH determination using a freshly voided urine sample transported in an airtight container should be obtained, and evaluation for RTA should be undertaken.

TABLE 32.11.   Selected Causes of Renal Tubular Acidosis (RTA)

Type 1 (distal or classic) RTA
  Idiopathic
    Sporadic
    Inherited (autosomal dominant or recessive)
  Associated with renal disease
    Obstructive nephropathy
    Reflux nephropathy
    Postrenal transplant
  Associated with disorders causing nephrocalcinosis
    Medullary sponge kidney
    Hyperparathyroidism
    Hypervitaminosis D
  Associated with systemic disease
    Sickle cell disease (SCD)
    Marfan syndrome
    Ehlers-Danlos syndrome
    Hereditary elliptocytosis (HE)
    Wilson disease
  Associated with autoimmune disorders
    Systemic lupus erythematosus (SLE)
    Sjögren syndrome
    Polyarteritis nodosa
    Hypergammaglobulinemia
  Associated with drug toxicity
    Amphotericin B
    Lithium
Type 2 (proximal) RTA
  Idiopathic or isolated
    Sporadic
    Inherited (autosomal dominant)
  Associated with Fanconi syndrome*
  Associated with systemic disease
    Cystinosis
    Lowe (oculocerebrorenal) syndrome
    Galactosemia
    Glycogen storage disease
    Hereditary fructose intolerance
    Tyrosinemia
    SLE and other autoimmune disorders
  Associated with toxins
    Drugs (e.g., aminoglycosides, chemotherapeutic agents)
    Heavy metals
  Associated with renal disorders
    Nephrotic syndrome
    Medullary cystic disease
    Renal venous thrombosis
    Renal transplant rejection
  Associated with carbonic anhydrase deficiency
    Congenital (sporadic or familial)
    Drug-induced (acetazolamide)
Type 4 (hyperkalemic) RTA
  Associated with renal disease
    Diabetic nephropathy
    Obstructive nephropathy
    Hyporeninemic hypoaldosteronism†

Continued

TABLE 32.11. Selected Causes of Renal Tubular Acidosis (RTA) (continued)

Associated with aldosterone deficiency
  Addison disease
  Chronic adrenal suppression
  Congenital adrenal hyperplasia (21-hydroxylase defect)
Associated with aldosterone resistance
  Pseudohypoaldosteronism
  Transient resistance (in newborns)
Associated with drugs
  Spironolactone
  Triamterene
  Amiloride
Chloride shunt (excess reabsorption of chloride)

* Fanconi syndrome is characterized by generalized proximal tubular dysfunction.

† Type 4 RTA may be found with any chronic tubulointerstitial nephritis.

▼ If the **anion gap is greater than 16,** the source of the unexplained anion should be considered. For example, the possibility of lactic acidosis or diabetic ketoacidosis (DKA) must be excluded. Although the history is helpful, several laboratory studies may be useful as well. A blood gas analysis should be obtained to assess the pH and arterial carbon dioxide tension ($PaCO_2$) to determine the degree of compensation or the presence of a mixed acid-base disturbance. A blood ammonia level and evaluation of urine for organic acids may be helpful.

HINT Not all low serum bicarbonate levels indicate metabolic acidosis. Finger-stick carbon dioxide levels are often spuriously low because of prolonged exposure of the blood to air. Decreased bicarbonate concentrations may occur as compensation for chronic respiratory alkalosis.

TABLE 32.12. Characteristics of Renal Tubular Acidosis

	Type 1	Type 2	Type 4
Renal function?	Normal	Normal	Normal or decreased
Failure to thrive?	Yes	Yes	Yes
Polyuria or polydipsia?	Yes	Yes	No
Potassium level?	Normal or low	Normal or low	Elevated
Bicarbonate leak?	Usually	Significant	Small
Urine maximally acid?	No (pH > 6)	Yes	Yes
Nephrocalcinosis or nephrolithiasis?	Yes	No	No
Fanconi syndrome?	No	Often	No
Osteomalacia or rickets?	Rarely	If Fanconi syndrome is present	No

---

▓ HINT Metabolic acidosis may occur with a normal bicarbonate value in children with mixed metabolic acid-base disturbances. For example, an infant with bronchopulmonary dysplasia who is receiving furosemide chronically (metabolic alkalosis) may develop severe diarrhea (metabolic acidosis) and have a normal bicarbonate concentration.

▓ HINT A change in the bicarbonate concentration of 10 mmol/L is expected to lead to a change in pH of 0.15 in the same direction.

Therapy

Treatment should be directed at correcting or removing the cause of the acidosis (e.g., insulin administration in a patient with DKA). Because the lungs permit the removal of volatile acid as carbon dioxide, it is important to ensure **adequate ventilation.**

Alkali therapy is controversial and usually is not indicated in the treatment of acute acidosis. In chronic acidosis, **alkali therapy** may help to prevent both growth failure and the use of the skeleton as a buffer, which can lead to calcium loss. **Bicarbonate therapy** may be started at 2 mEq/kg/day and may be increased as needed to normalize the bicarbonate level. (The normal serum bicarbonate level is 22–24 mmol/L.) In patients with renal bicarbonate loss, up to 20 mEq/kg/day of bicarbonate may be required. Commonly used oral alkalinizing agents in children include:

▼ **Polycitra syrup,** which provides 2 mEq/ml of bicarbonate, 1 mEq/ml of sodium, and 1 mEq/ml of potassium
▼ **BICITRA solution,** which provides 1 mEq/ml of bicarbonate and 1 mEq/ml of sodium
▼ **Shohl solution (citric acid and sodium citrate),** which supplies 1 mEq/ml bicarbonate
▼ **Sodium bicarbonate tablets,** which supply 650 mg of bicarbonate (8 mEq/tablet)

Metabolic Alkalosis

Etiology

Metabolic alkalosis is defined as any state that increases the serum bicarbonate concentration to greater than the normal level of 24–26 mmol/L.

Metabolic alkalosis is either **chloride-sensitive** or **chloride-resistant** (Table 32.13). Chloride-sensitive metabolic alkalosis is associated with a decreased extracellular fluid volume and the urinary chloride level is less than 10 mEq/L. Chloride-resistant metabolic alkalosis is associated with a urinary chloride level that exceeds 20 mEq/L.

Clinical Features

As with metabolic acidosis, signs and symptoms are generally those of the underlying disorder. Sudden, severe metabolic alkalosis may result in diminished ionic calcium levels, leading to hypocalcemic cramps or tetany.

Evaluation

The physical examination should focus on assessment of the ECF volume status.

TABLE 32.13. Causes of Metabolic Alkalosis

Chloride-sensitive
Vomiting or nasogastric suction
Chronic diuretic therapy
Chloride-deficient diet
Cystic fibrosis (increased skin loss of chloride)
Congenital chloride diarrhea (autosomal recessive)
Chloride-resistant
Alkali administration (e.g., antacid therapy)
Acute diuretic therapy
Hypokalemic state
Mineralocorticoid excess
Compensation for respiratory acidosis
Bartter syndrome
Liddle syndrome

Laboratory studies should include a serum electrolyte panel; serum urea and creatinine levels; and urine electrolyte levels, including chloride. In some children, a sweat chloride determination is indicated.

▼ **HINT** There may be mixed metabolic acidosis and alkalosis occurring together, and the measured bicarbonate concentration may be normal.

▼ **HINT** Metabolic alkalosis and frank alkalemia may occur if long-standing respiratory acidosis is corrected suddenly (e.g., with mechanical ventilation). This condition is called "posthypercapneic alkalosis."

Treatment

If there is volume contraction, **hydration status** should be restored with normal saline. If present, **hypokalemia** should be corrected. Diuretic therapy should be discontinued, if possible, or given intermittently. Alkali therapy should be discontinued.

Suggested Readings

Adrogue HJ, Modios NE: Hypernatremia. *New Engl J Med* 342(20):1493–1499, 2000.

Chon JC, Scheinmann JI, Roth KS: Renal tubular acidosis. *Pediatr Rev* 22(8):277–286, 2001.

Hanna JD, Scheinman JI, Chan JC: The kidney in acid-base balance. *Pediatr Clin North Am* 42(6):1365–1395, 1995.

Marks KH, Kilav R, Naveh-Many T, et al.: Calcium, phosphate, vitamin D, and the parathyroid. *Pediatr Nephrol* 10(3):364–367, 1996.

Rodriguez-Soriano J: Potassium homeostasis and its disturbances in children. *Pediatr Nephrol* 9(3):364–374, 1995.

Trachtman H: Sodium and water homeostasis. *Pediatr Clin North Am* 42(6):1343–1363, 1995.

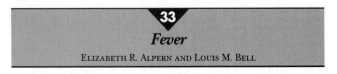

33
Fever
ELIZABETH R. ALPERN AND LOUIS M. BELL

▼ INTRODUCTION

Fever is the abnormal elevation of body temperature. It is a **nonspecific sign** of disease. The significance of fever lies in its indication of disease processes. Fever is defined as a core body temperature ≥ 38.0°C. However, the clinically relevant defined cut-point of an abnormally elevated temperature is based on a particular child's risk for infection. Fever in neonates or in immunocompromised patients is defined as ≥ 38.0°C (100.4°C) and in older children at 38.5°–39.0°C.

Body temperature is usually measured by **rectal thermometry** in infants and young children and by **sublingual thermometry** in older children and adolescents. Because temperature may vary in different areas of the body, tympanic, temporal artery, and pacifier thermometers may not correlate with rectal measurements in young children.

Because fever is an indication of disease, the most important management and therapeutic measures are to determine the underlying cause of the fever (e.g., infection, inflammation, neoplasm). When the underlying disease is treated appropriately, the fever can be managed with antipyretics as needed to make the child comfortable.

▼ DIFFERENTIAL DIAGNOSIS LIST
Infectious Causes

Systemic

Sepsis
Occult bacteremia
Viral syndrome
Tick-borne infections (Lyme disease, Rocky Mountain spotted fever)

CNS

Meningitis
Encephalitis

Respiratory Tract

Upper respiratory tract infection
Pharyngitis/tonsillitis
Retropharyngeal abscess
Otitis media
Croup
Sinusitis
Pneumonia
Bronchiolitis

Abdominal/Pelvic

Gastroenteritis
Appendicitis

Genitourinary
Urinary tract disease
Pelvic inflammatory disease
Tubo-ovarian abscess

Musculoskeletal
Osteomyelitis
Septic arthritis

Cutaneous
Cellulitis

Miscellaneous
Abscess
Adenitis
Orbital cellulitis
Fever of unknown origin

Toxicologic Causes
Salicylates
Cocaine
Amphetamine
Anticholinergics
Malignant hyperthermia

Neoplastic Causes
Leukemia
Lymphoma

Inflammatory Causes
Acute rheumatic fever
Systemic lupus erythematosus
Juvenile rheumatoid arthritis
Kawasaki disease
Inflammatory bowel disease
Serum sickness
Drug and immunization reactions

Miscellaneous Causes
Heat stroke
Thyrotoxicosis
Dehydration
Prolonged seizures
Factitious

▼ EVALUATION OF COMMON PRESENTATIONS
Infant Less Than 2 Months of Age

Well-appearing infants (0–60 days of age) with a fever ($\geq$ 38.0°C) but without an identifiable source of infection are at risk for **occult serious bacterial**

infections. These young infants may have only vague or nonspecific signs and symptoms of illness that do not indicate the severity of potential infection.

History
▼ **High risk**—prematurity, perinatal complication, immunocompromised state (sickle cell disease, HIV), exposure to recent antibiotics, steroids, surgery
▼ **Low risk**—full-term gestation, uncomplicated prenatal course

Physical Examination
Physical examination should concentrate on identifying infections that are more common in neonates, such as meningitis, HSV encephalitis, omphalitis, pneumonia, and pyelonephritis.

Screening Tests
Low-risk criteria for three published screening protocols are presented in Table 33.1.

Management
The management of febrile infants is determined by age, history, and screening tests. The management options are presented in Figure 33.1.

Children 2 Months to 24 Months of Age

Occult bacteremia is the presence of pathogenic bacteria in the blood of a well-appearing febrile child (usually defined as $\geq 39.0°C$) who lacks a focal bacterial source of infection. The risk of occult bacteremia is approximately 2%. This risk increases with increasing temperature or a white blood cell count greater than 15,000/mm^3. Occult bacteremia carries a risk of **progression to focal infection, meningitis, or sepsis.** The degree of this risk is dependent on the etiology of the bacteremia. In a population immunized with the *Haemophilus influenzae* B vaccine, the risk of serious adverse outcome is extremely low. In this population, the most common bacterial isolate causing occult bacteremia is *Streptococcus pneumoniae*, which usually resolves spontaneously.

History

An **immunocompromised state** (e.g., long-term steroid use, oncologic processes, acquired or inborn immunodeficiencies, sickle cell anemia, congenital heart disease) or the presence of an **indwelling medical device** (e.g., ventriculoperitoneal shunts, indwelling catheters) will put a child at increased risk of invasive bacterial infection. The child's **immunization history** is also important. The newly licensed pneumococcal conjugate vaccine may significantly decrease the risk of bacteremia. Prior antibiotic use may mask presenting signs or symptoms of focal bacterial infections and should be noted.

Physical Examination

Any sign of focal **bacterial infection** (e.g., pneumonia, abscess, urinary tract infection) or **pathognomonic viral illness** (e.g., varicella, stomatitis) will guide diagnosis and treatment plans appropriate for that particular infection. However, the well-appearing child without focal infection should be evaluated for

TABLE 33.1. Low-Risk Screening Criteria

	Philadelphia Protocol	Boston Protocol	Rochester Criteria
History/Physical Exam	Normal	Normal	Normal
WBC Count	5,000–15,000/mm³	< 20,000/mm³	5,000–15,000/mm³
Differential	Band:Neutrophil ratio <0.2		Absolute band count ≤ 1500/mm³
Urinalysis	<10 WBC/hpf	<10 WBC/hpf	<10 WBC/hpf
CSF	<8 WBC/hpf	<10 WBC/hpf	
CXR	Normal	Normal	
Stool	If symptoms: negative blood and few WBC on smear		If symptoms: <5 WBC/hpf
Social	Readily available transportation and phone	Readily available transportation and phone	Readily available transportation and phone
Negative Predictive Value (for SBI) of Screen	100%	94.6%	98.9%
Treatment option if low risk	Home without antibiotics and follow-up in 24 hours	Home with Ceftriaxone IM and follow-up in 24 hours	Home without antibiotics and follow-up in 24 hours

WBC = white blood cell count; CSF = cerebral spinal fluid; CXR = chest x-ray; SBI = serious bacterial infection; IM = intramuscular.

occult bacteremia. Children with **nonspecific viral syndromes** and **otitis media** are also at risk for occult bacteremia.

Screening Tests

▼ **Blood culture** is the gold standard for diagnosing occult bacteremia. The white blood cell count has been advocated by some authorities for use as a risk stratification measure when considering expectant antibiotic therapy for the child at risk for occult bacteremia. Unfortunately, because of the low incidence of occult bacteremia, there are significant limitations to this screening test. A WBC count ≥ 15,000 mm³ has a positive predictive value of only approximately 5%.

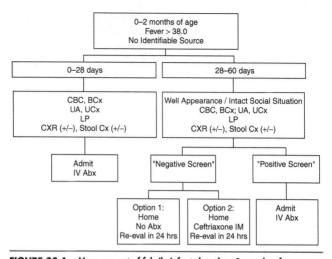

FIGURE 33.1. Management of febrile infants less than 2 months of age. *CBC* = complete blood cell count; *BCx* = blood culture; *UA* = urinalysis; *UCx* = urine culture; *CSF* = cerebral spinal fluid; *LP* = lumbar puncture; *CXR* = chest x-ray; *IV Abx* = intravenous antibiotics.

▼ **Chest radiographs** are indicated in children with significant respiratory symptoms or persistent tachypnea.

▼ **Urinalysis and culture** are helpful for those children with dysuria, foul-smelling urine, prior history of urinary tract infection, urinary tract abnormality, or other risk factors for occult urinary tract infections (UTI). See Table 33.2 for risk factors associated with occult UTIs in young children.

Management

Reevaluation in 24–48 hours is imperative if the diagnosis of occult bacteremia is suspected. Controversy exists regarding whether presumptive therapy for children at risk for the development of occult bacteremia is indicated.

TABLE 33.2. Risk Factors for Urinary Tract Infections

Girls	Boys
Temperature ≥ 39°C	Age ≤ 6 months
Fever ≥ 2 days	Uncircumcised penis
Caucasian	Lack of other focal source of infection
Age ≤ 1 year	
Lack of other focal source of infection	

Two meta-analyses have failed to show a significant difference in risk of meningitis in children with occult bacteremia who are treated with antibiotics.

Suggested Readings

Alpern ER, Henretig FM: "Fever" in *Textbook of Pediatric Emergency Medicine*, 4th ed. Editors Fleisher GR, Ludwig S. Lippincott, Williams & Wilkins, Philadelphia, 2000.

Alpern ER, Alessandrini EA, Bell LM, Shaw KN, McGowan KL: Occult bacteremia from a pediatric emergency department: Current prevalence, time to detection, and outcome. *Pediatr* 106:505–511, 2000.

Bulloch B, Craig WR, Klassen TP: The use of antibiotics to prevent serious sequelae in children at risk for occult bacteremia: A meta-analysis. *Acad Emerg Med* 4:679–683, 1997.

Gorelick MH, Shaw KN: Clinical decision rule to identify febrile young girls at risk for urinary tract infection. *Arch Pediatr Adolesc Med* 154:386–390, 2000.

Jaskiewicz JA, McCarthy CA, Richardson AC, et al.: Febrile infants at low risk for serious bacterial infection—An appraisal of the Rochester criteria and implications for management. *Pediatrics* 94:390–396, 1994.

Lee GM, Harper MB: Risk of bacteremia for febrile young children in the post-*Haemophilus influenzae* type b era. *Arch Pediatr Adolesc Med* 152(5):624–628, 1998.

Rothrock SG, Harper MB, Green SM, et al.: Do oral antibiotics prevent meningitis and serious bacterial infections in children with *Streptococcus pneumoniae* occult bacteremia? A meta-analysis. *Pediatrics* 99(3):438–444, 1997.

Shaw KN, Gorelick MH: Urinary tract infection in the pediatric patient. *Pediatr Clinic North Am* 46(6):1111–1124, 1999.

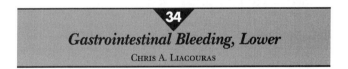

34

Gastrointestinal Bleeding, Lower

Chris A. Liacouras

▼ INTRODUCTION

The presence of **blood in the gastrointestinal tract is always abnormal.** Blood in the stool can occur in several forms: **hematochezia** (bright red blood on the stool), **"currant jelly" stools** (thickened, brick-red blood on the stool), **melena** (dark or black stools), or **occult bleeding** (normal-appearing stools that test positive by Hemoccult or guaiac testing).

Blood acts as a cathartic that decreases intestinal transit time. Therefore, hematochezia usually signifies colonic disease (i.e., bleeding from a site between the distal colon and the terminal ileum), but it may be the result of profuse proximal gastrointestinal tract bleeding. Melena usually signifies profuse upper intestinal bleeding (proximal to the terminal ileum), whereas "currant jelly" stools commonly occur as a result of an active Meckel diverticulum or intussusception. Normal-appearing stools that test positive for blood suggest slow gastrointestinal tract bleeding. Table 34.1 lists causes of bloody stools by site.

TABLE 34.1. Causes of Bloody Stools by Site

Site	Cause
Nasopharynx	Epistaxis, gum disease, oral or nasal trauma, tonsillectomy, adenoidectomy
Esophagus	Esophageal stricture, esophagitis, ulcer, varices, eosinophilic enteritis, graft-versus-host disease (GVHD)
Stomach	Gastritis, ulcer, foreign body, vascular anomaly, tumor, duplication, polyp, infection
Duodenum	Ulcer, celiac disease, malrotation, vascular anomaly, postviral enteritis, parasitic infection
Small bowel	Inflammatory bowel disease, celiac disease, volvulus, malrotation, necrotizing enterocolitis, infection, Henoch-Schönlein purpura, duplication, Meckel diverticulum, vascular anomaly, tumor, eosinophilic enteritis
Colon	Polyp, inflammatory bowel disease, infection, Hirschsprung disease, trauma, sexual abuse, hemorrhoid, tumor, hemolytic-uremic syndrome, Henoch-Schönlein purpura, milk- or soy-protein allergy, varices, intussusception, volvulus, fissure, solitary rectal ulcer, foreign body, vascular anomaly, GVHD

✂ HINT   Rapid upper gastrointestinal tract bleeding should always be considered in any child with first-time bloody stools, and a nasogastric tube should be passed.

▼ DIFFERENTIAL DIAGNOSIS LIST

The following are common causes of hematochezia and melena.

Infectious Causes

Bacterial Infection

Salmonella
Shigella
Campylobacter
Yersinia
Enterohemorrhagic *Escherichia coli*
Aeromonas
Plesiomonas
Clostridium difficile

Parasitic Infection

Entamoeba histolytica
Balantidium coli
Necator americanus (hookworm)
Strongyloides stercoralis
Ascaris lumbricoides

Viral Infection

Adenovirus
Rotavirus

Cytomegalovirus (CMV)
HIV

Neoplastic Causes

Leiomyoma
Lymphoma
Adenocarcinoma
Carcinoid

Traumatic Causes

Anal fissure
Foreign body
Sexual abuse

Congenital or Vascular Causes

Meckel diverticulum
Enteric duplication
Arteriovenous malformation (AVM)
Hemangioma
Hemorrhoids
Rectal varices
Esophageal varices (rapid flow)
Hirschsprung enterocolitis

Inflammatory Causes

Juvenile polyps
Polyposis syndromes
Inflammatory bowel disease
Lymphonodular hyperplasia
Necrotizing enterocolitis
Milk- or soy-protein allergy
Eosinophilic gastroenteritis
Graft-versus-host disease
Vasculitis [systemic lupus erythematosus (SLE)]

Miscellaneous Causes

Rapid upper gastrointestinal bleeding
Intussusception
Volvulus
Solitary rectal ulcer
Coagulopathy
Thrombocytopenia
Anticoagulant drug therapy
Henoch-Schönlein purpura
Hemolytic–uremic syndrome

💥 HINT Certain foods, drugs, and occurrences (e.g., factitious menstrual bleeding, hematuria, swallowed maternal blood) can mimic blood in the stool and must be ruled out (Table 34.2).

TABLE 34.2. Foods and Drugs Mimicking Blood in the Stool		
False Hematochezia	**False Melena**	**False Heme-Positive Stools**
Foods that contain red dye	Spinach	Red meat
Juice	Blueberries	Cherries
Candy	Licorice	Tomato skin
Kool-Aid	Purple grapes	Iron supplements
Jell-O	Chocolate	
Tomatoes	Grape juice	
Beets	Bismuth subsalicylate	
Cranberries	Iron supplements	

▼ DIFFERENTIAL DIAGNOSIS DISCUSSION

✂ HINT Lower gastrointestinal tract bleeding in children is most often caused by infection. Bacterial infections often present with acute abdominal pain, fever, and bloody diarrhea.

C. difficile Colitis (Pseudomembranous Colitis, Antibiotic-Induced Colitis)

Etiology

The toxins produced by *C. difficile* have **cytotoxic effects** on the colonic mucosa. Although *C. difficile* colitis is usually associated with an imbalance of the gastrointestinal flora **following the administration of broad-spectrum antibiotics** (e.g., clindamycin, amoxicillin, cephalosporin), it can develop in patients with **underlying intestinal disorders** (e.g., inflammatory bowel disease) and those who have undergone **recent abdominal surgery.** *C. difficile* can also cause disease in **young infants** (secondary to an increase in intestinal colonization), **institutionalized patients** (as a result of cross-infection), and sporadically, in otherwise healthy patients.

✂ HINT Antibiotic-induced colitis commonly occurs within 2 weeks of introducing the drug.

Clinical Features

C. difficile is associated with a **wide variety of clinical symptoms.** Patients may be **asymptomatic,** or they may experience **frequent, painful, bloody diarrhea, a sign of severe, life-threatening colitis.** Typically, children present with abdominal pain and bloody, mucus-streaked, foul-smelling, watery stools that occur at frequent intervals. Some patients may be **dehydrated.**

Evaluation

C. difficile-induced colitis should be suspected whenever a patient presents with bloody diarrhea. **Fresh stool specimens** (transported on ice or frozen) should be collected and evaluated for the presence of *C. difficile* toxins A and B. In patients with persistent bloody diarrhea and a negative microbiologic evaluation, **colonoscopy** should be performed. Colonoscopy often reveals the classic mucosal pseudomembrane formation (raised, yellow plaques).

Treatment

Therapy varies depending on the severity of symptoms. Mild cases may be self-limited and usually respond to the **discontinuation of the inciting antibiotic.** Patients with features of more severe colitis are treated with either **oral metronidazole or vancomycin** (see Chapter 27, "Diarrhea, Acute"); symptoms usually resolve within 3–5 days. Dehydrated patients require **intravenous fluids** and the short-term introduction of clear liquids.

Recurrent episodes may occur following cessation of therapy; in this situation, repeat treatment and further evaluation for other underlying systemic disorders (e.g., inflammatory bowel disease) are indicated.

Meckel Diverticulum

Etiology

Meckel diverticulum, the **most common** of all **congenital gastrointestinal anomalies,** occurs in 1%–3% of all infants. The diverticulum is derived from a congenital remnant of the embryonic yolk sac that originates from the antimesenteric border of the intestine. This abnormality is typically located within 2 feet (60 cm) of the ileocecal valve. The diverticulum commonly contains ectopic gastric tissue, which can cause **peptic ulceration** (manifested as painless, bright red or "currant jelly" rectal bleeding).

⚟ HINT Enteric duplications (intestinal cysts) originate from the mesenteric border of the bowel and, like a Meckel diverticulum, can also contain ectopic gastric tissue and manifest with hematochezia or "currant jelly" bleeding.

Clinical Features

Intermittent, painless rectal bleeding in a 2-year-old child is the most common presentation. A small percentage of patients may present with massive life-threatening rectal bleeding.

Bowel obstruction (secondary to internal herniation or intussusception of the enteric diverticulum) can lead to abdominal pain and bilious vomiting.

Evaluation

The diagnosis is made either via a **Meckel scan,** a specific nuclear medicine test that uses a radioisotope to identify gastric mucosa, or by a **nonspecific tagged red blood cell (RBC) scan** that identifies sites of rapid gastrointestinal bleeding. Routine abdominal radiographs and contrast studies are almost never useful for making the diagnosis of a Meckel diverticulum.

Treatment

Surgical excision is performed in all cases of documented Meckel diverticulum.

Colonic Polyps

Etiology

Most juvenile polyps are **inflammatory** in origin. **Polyposis syndromes,** which may involve a few polyps or hundreds of polyps, are typically **genetic** in origin and include inflammatory, hamartomatous, and adenomatous changes. The presence of **five or more polyps** usually carries an **increased risk of cancer.**

Clinical Features

Painless hematochezia in a child between the ages of 2 and 10 years is the typical presentation. (Juvenile polyps are the most common cause of painless hematochezia in children who have no evidence of perianal or rectal trauma.) Other common presentations include **tenesmus, mucus-streaked stools, and rectal (or polyp) prolapse** through the rectum. Rarely, intussusception occurs secondary to a lead point (e.g., a colonic polyp or Meckel diverticulum).

Juvenile polyps are usually palpable on rectal examination.

As many as 30% of children may develop an **iron-deficiency anemia.**

Evaluation

In the past, barium enemas were used to diagnose colonic polyps; however, because stool retention secondary to improper bowel preparation may "hide" polyps, and because the present treatment of choice is polypectomy, **colonoscopy** is now the preferred diagnostic tool. In addition to allowing visualization of the entire colon (thus identifying the exact cause and all possible polyps), colonoscopy allows the endoscopist to treat the problem by performing a polypectomy.

Treatment

In the past, conservative therapy consisted of observation with the hope that the polyp would auto-amputate. However, currently, **colonoscopy with polypectomy** is recommended to eliminate the source of bleeding, to identify the presence of other polyps, and to identify the type of polyp so that future management of the patient can be determined.

Inflammatory Bowel Disease

Etiology

Inflammatory bowel disease is an **idiopathic, multifactorial inflammatory condition** of the alimentary tract.

▼ **Crohn disease** may occur in both the upper and lower gastrointestinal tract and results in chronic intestinal inflammation associated with severe mucosal damage, transmural wall thickening, serosal induration, granuloma formation, fistula and abscess formation, intestinal strictures, and perforation. The terminal ileum is the most common site of involvement, although the disease may "skip" to noncontiguous areas.

▼ **Ulcerative colitis** is confined to the colon and rectum and typically causes severe mucosal destruction without transmural involvement. Unlike Crohn disease, ulcerative colitis is continuous along the lower gastrointestinal tract, although the rectum may be spared.

✂ HINT Toxic megacolon, a potential complication of ulcerative colitis, is a true surgical emergency and should be ruled out promptly.

Clinical Features

Children with inflammatory bowel disease usually present with **fever, bloody diarrhea, weight loss, and crampy abdominal pain.** Associated systemic abnormalities in inflammatory bowel disease include growth failure, arthralgias, arthritis, skin lesions (pyoderma gangrenosum, erythema nodosum), perianal disease (rectal abscess, skin tags, or fistula formation), ophthalmologic abnormalities (episcleritis and uveitis), mouth sores, and hepatobiliary disease. Many children with Crohn disease develop an **iron-deficiency anemia** and a **secondary lactase deficiency.**

⚔ HINT Profuse rectal bleeding, hypogastric pain, tenesmus, and frequent diarrhea usually suggest ulcerative colitis, whereas right lower quadrant pain, weight loss, failure to thrive, and perianal disease typify Crohn disease.

Evaluation

▼ The **physical examination** may reveal abdominal tenderness that is usually focal in the lower quadrants and signs of systemic involvement (e.g., mouth sores, joint involvement, erythema nodosum, pyoderma gangrenosum, perianal disease).
▼ **Laboratory studies** such as a complete blood count (CBC), erythrocyte sedimentation rate (ESR), chemistry panel, and lactose breath test are useful for determining the biochemical abnormalities associated with inflammatory bowel disease. Patients with inflammatory bowel disease usually have an elevated ESR, hypoalbuminemia, and an elevated white blood cell (WBC) count.
▼ **Colonoscopy with biopsy** is the test of choice for diagnosing ulcerative colitis and Crohn disease. The diagnosis may be made by visual inspection of the intestinal mucosa (aphthous ulcers and mucosal damage) or by biopsy (granulomas, crypt abscesses, and mucosal inflammation).
▼ **Upper gastrointestinal small bowel follow-through contrast studies** are useful for assessing small bowel (terminal ileal) disease.

Treatment

The prognosis depends on aggressive treatment of exacerbations, but aggressive intervention with nutritional support is equally important.

▼ **Corticosteroids** are the first line of therapy for patients with moderate to severe disease. The recommended dosage (1–2 mg/kg/day) is tapered over 4–8 weeks, depending on the clinical response. Immunosuppressive agents (e.g., 6-mercaptopurine, azathioprine, cyclosporin A) have been used in children who have an increased risk for complications from steroid treatment, who require prolonged steroid use, or who are refractory to other treatment regimens.
▼ **Oral salicylate derivatives,** which help to heal the intestinal mucosa, are the mainstay of treatment. In the past, sulfasalazine (50–100 mg/kg/day) was used for patients with mild to moderate exacerbations. Folic acid (1 mg/day) was administered concurrently, because sulfasalazine competitively inhibits folate absorption. 5-Aminosalicylic acid (5-ASA), the active component, is minimally absorbed and thus acts directly on the mucosa as an anti-inflammatory agent. Recently, mesalamine, which does not require coliform bacteria to metabolize itself to 5-ASA, has been used. The dose is 30–70 g/kg/day.
▼ **Antibiotics** have been shown to be effective for patients with perianal disease and mucosal inflammation. Metronidazole, used when evidence of bacterial overgrowth, fistulae, or perianal disease exists, has been effective against anaerobes but also has anti-inflammatory properties.

▼ **Surgical intervention,** such as resection with colectomy and eventual endorectal pull-through, is useful in patients with ulcerative colitis. Surgery should be avoided, however, in children with Crohn disease unless abscess, fistula, toxic megacolon, perforation, acute obstruction, or uncontrolled bleeding exist.

As an adjunct to therapy, **nutritional support** is paramount to achieve optimal growth. Special issues, such as deficiencies in trace elements (e.g., zinc, magnesium, calcium), protein-losing enteropathy (PLE), and fat malabsorption resulting in vitamin A, D, E, and K deficiency, must be addressed. An oral elemental diet, total parenteral nutrition, or both are the primary modes of nutritional support for these patients. The goal is to provide at least 125%–140% of the recommended daily allowance for calories and protein.

Because of the chronicity of this disease, **psychological support** is vital. It is important to teach adaptive responses to the illness, rather than enabling maladaptive responses to progress.

Hirschsprung Enterocolitis

Etiology

Hirschsprung disease is caused by a **congenital absence of ganglion cells** (see Chapter 22, "Constipation"). An associated enterocolitis occurs secondary to poor colonic motility, stagnation of fecal material in the rectum, and breakdown of the mucosal barrier.

Clinical Features

Although Hirschsprung enterocolitis is **uncommon,** the possibility should be considered in any infant with **rectal bleeding** who has **abdominal distention, foul-smelling diarrhea, a history of delayed meconium passage, constipation, fever, and sepsis.** There may also be evidence of intestinal obstruction.

Evaluation

A **barium enema** (unprepped—to prevent dilatation of the colonic transition zone) may suggest the diagnosis. Often, a submucosal or full-thickness **rectal biopsy** (demonstrating absence of ganglion cells and hypertrophied nerve bundles) is required to confirm the diagnosis.

Treatment

Infants with suspected Hirschsprung enterocolitis should be placed **"NPO"** and administered **fluids and broad-spectrum antibiotics intravenously. A nasogastric tube** should be inserted to decompress the proximal bowel. **Surgical correction** is required to remove the aganglionic bowel segment and to relieve the intestinal obstruction.

Milk- or Soy-Protein Allergy

Etiology

Milk- or soy-protein allergy is the **most common immunologic cause of gastrointestinal bleeding** in infants. The most common explanation for milk-protein allergy is that it is caused by an antigen-induced, IgE-mediated reaction with subsequent mast cell activation and eosinophilic infiltration of the intestinal mucosa.

Clinical Features

Many children have a history of rhinitis, bronchospasm, and coughing.

There are several clinical manifestations, including an **immediate hypersensitivity reaction,** a **delayed systemic reaction** (characterized by a rash and headache), and a **gastrointestinal reaction** that occurs several days later. Infants most commonly present with bloody, mucus-streaked **diarrhea, abdominal pain, weight loss, and vomiting.** Patients may also have signs of **anaphylaxis** (e.g., urticaria, bronchospasm, hypotension).

Peripheral eosinophilia is often present.

HINT Approximately 20% of infants with milk-protein allergy are also allergic to soy and 1% may also be allergic to most simple foods.

Evaluation

The diagnosis is usually made on the basis of the **clinical history.** Although a strict placebo-controlled **food challenge test** is the only way to make a definitive diagnosis, food elimination can often strongly suggest the offending agent. Helpful diagnostic tests include a **Wright stain of the stool** (to reveal stool eosinophils) **or endoscopy,** which may demonstrate eosinophilic infiltration of the intestinal mucosa.

Treatment

Treatment consists of **removing the offending antigen** from the diet. In infants, this disorder typically resolves by 2 years of age. Older children who develop food allergies often require a lifetime of avoidance.

Eosinophilic Enteritis

Etiology

Idiopathic eosinophilic gastroenteritis is a rare disorder caused by eosinophilic tissue infiltration and mast cell activation without known antigenic stimulation. Three forms exist: **mucosal infiltration** (vomiting, diarrhea, PLE), **muscular infiltration** (gastric outlet obstruction), and **serosal infiltration** (ascites without other intestinal symptoms). Common sites of involvement include the gastric antrum, esophagus, and colon. Eosinophilic enteritis can produce **severe esophagitis, gastritis, duodenitis, or all three.**

Clinical Features

Patients present with **nausea, vomiting, abdominal pain, and upper or lower gastrointestinal bleeding. Hematemesis** results from mucosal infiltration, which promotes an inflammatory response. Other clinical findings include **diarrhea, weight loss, failure to thrive, ascites, and peripheral edema.**

Laboratory findings include **peripheral eosinophilia, iron-deficiency anemia, elevated serum IgE levels, and hypoalbuminemia** (secondary to PLE).

Evaluation

Initial evaluation includes searching for evidence of mucosal malabsorption using the **D-xylose absorption test** and performing **radiographic contrast**

studies, which may show small bowel edema and ulceration. Definitive diagnosis can be made by **endoscopy with biopsy.**

Treatment

Treatment involves **supportive care, dietary manipulation,** and the administration of **corticosteroids** (in severe cases) and **oral cromolyn sodium.** Long-term care should be coordinated by a pediatric gastroenterologist.

Intussusception

Intussusception is discussed in Chapter 9, "Abdominal Pain, Acute."

▼ EVALUATION OF LOWER GASTROINTESTINAL BLEEDING

Patient History

▼ **Travel history.** The travel history may suggest an infectious cause.
▼ **Events suggesting upper gastrointestinal tract trauma.** A recent history of epistaxis, nasogastric or gastrostomy tube placement, retching (suggestive of a Mallory-Weiss tear), surgery (e.g., tonsillectomy, adenoidectomy), or caustic ingestion may explain melena or heme-positive stools.
▼ **Medication history.** Melanotic stools can be caused by drug-induced gastritis [e.g., from nonsteroidal anti-inflammatory agents (NSAIDs) or salicylates]. In addition, certain drugs can mimic blood in the stool (see Table 34.2).

Physical Examination

▼ **Perianal and digital rectal examinations** should always be performed in children with hematochezia to look for anal fissure, hemorrhoids, rectal trauma, foreign bodies in the rectum, and signs of sexual abuse (e.g., cutaneous bruising, anal tears, labial or penile irritation).
▼ **Abdominal palpation** may reveal hepatosplenomegaly, which suggests portal hypertension and possible varices.
▼ **Cutaneous examination** may reveal hemangiomas (suggestive of an alimentary AVM), purpura on the buttocks and lower extremities (consistent with Henoch-Schönlein purpura), or erythema nodosum and pyoderma gangrenosum (seen in children with inflammatory bowel disease).

Laboratory Studies

Stool culture and **testing for WBCs** is always indicated for a child who presents with bloody diarrhea.

Diagnostic Modalities

Upper gastrointestinal endoscopy and colonoscopy are the most important tests for the diagnosis of gastrointestinal bleeding and may be therapeutic. Other diagnostic modalities and their indications are summarized in Table 34.3.

▼ TREATMENT OF LOWER GASTROINTESTINAL BLEEDING

Lower gastrointestinal bleeding can be life threatening. Patients with persistent, rapid bleeding or associated dizziness, fatigue, or severe abdominal

TABLE 34.3. Useful Diagnostic Tests for Evaluation of Gastrointestinal Bleeding

Test	Indication
Meckel scan	Identification a Meckel diverticulum or intestinal duplication
Tagged red blood cell (RBC) scan	Identification of a site of rapid intestinal bleeding
Colonoscopy	Evaluation of hematochezia or colonic disease
Upper endoscopy	Evaluation of causes of upper gastrointestinal bleeding proximal to the ligament of Treitz
Angiography	Identification of vascular causes of gastrointestinal bleeding
Barium enema	Identification of anatomic abnormalities of the colon (Hirschsprung disease, intussusception, stricture, mass)
Upper gastrointestinal series	Identification of anatomic and inflammatory abnormalities of the esophagus, stomach, and small intestine
Enteroclysis	Used when enhancement of the mucosal detail of the small intestine is required
Abdominal radiograph	Identification of foreign body, intestinal obstruction, mucosal edema (thumbprinting)

pain require immediate evaluation and stabilization:

▼ Orthostatic vital signs and a CBC should be obtained as soon as possible.
▼ Patients with hypotension or anemia should receive intravenous fluids and blood products (when necessary).
▼ A plain abdominal radiograph is useful for revealing intestinal obstruction or perforation.
▼ In patients with significant lower gastrointestinal bleeding, a nasogastric tube should be placed to decompress the bowel and to determine the severity and origin of the bleeding (e.g., from the stomach or esophagus).
▼ The patient should be admitted under the care of a pediatric gastroenterologist.

Suggested Readings

Brown RL, Azizkhan RG: Gastrointestinal bleeding in infants and children: Meckel's diverticulum and intestinal duplication. *Semin Pediatr Surg* 8(4):202–209, 1999.

Fox VL: Gastrointestinal bleeding in infancy and childhood. *Gastroenterol Clin North Am* 29(1):37–66, v, 2000.

Hoffenberg EJ, Sauaia A, Maltzman T, et al: Symptomatic colonic polyps in childhood: not so benign. *J Pediatr Gastroenterol Nutr* 28(2):175–181, 1999.

Lee KH, Yeung CK, Tam YH, et al: Laparoscopy for definitive diagnosis and treatment of gastrointestinal bleeding of obscure origin in children. *J Pediatr Surg* 35(9):1291–1293, 2000.

Saulsbury FT: Henoch-Schönlein purpura in children. Report of 100 patients and review of the literature. *Medicine* 78(6):395–409, 1999.

Silverman A, Roy CC: *Pediatric Clinical Gastroenterology*, 3rd ed. St. Louis, Mosby, 1983.

Sleisenger MH, Fordtran JS: *Gastrointestinal Disease*, 4th ed. Philadelphia, WB Saunders, 1989.

Treem WR: Gastrointestinal bleeding in children. *Gastrointest Endosc* 4:75, 1994.

Walker WA, Durie PR, Hamilton JR, et al: *Pediatric Gastrointestinal Disease*, 2nd ed. Philadelphia, BC Decker, 1996.

Wyllie R, Hyams JS: *Pediatric Gastrointestinal Disease*. Philadelphia, WB Saunders, 1993.

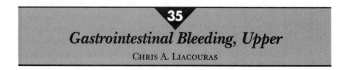

35
Gastrointestinal Bleeding, Upper
CHRIS A. LIACOURAS

▼ INTRODUCTION

The presence of hematemesis usually suggests that the site of bleeding is proximal to the ligament of Treitz. Common sites of upper gastrointestinal tract bleeding are summarized in Table 35.1.

▼ DIFFERENTIAL DIAGNOSIS LIST

Infectious Causes

Bacterial gastritis—*Helicobacter pylori* infection
Viral infection—cytomegalovirus, varicella, herpes, adenovirus
Fungal esophagitis or gastritis

TABLE 35.1. Causes of Hematemesis by Site

Site	Cause
Oropharynx	Epistaxis
	Mouth-/nose-/throat-surgery trauma
	Foreign body
Esophagus	Esophagitis
	Esophageal stricture
	Mallory-Weiss tear
	Infection
	Foreign body
	Esophageal varices
Stomach	Ulcer
	Gastritis (drug, infection, caustic ingestion)
	Eosinophilic enteritis
	Graft-versus-host disease (GVHD)
	Vascular abnormality
	Varices duplication
	Tumor
	Gastric polyps
Duodenum	Ulcer
	Eosinophilic enteritis
	Hemobilia

Toxic Causes

Drugs—nonsteroidal anti-inflammatory drugs (NSAIDs), aspirin, steroids
Caustic substances
Alcohol gastritis

Neoplastic Causes

Zollinger-Ellison syndrome
Leiomyoma
Leiomyosarcoma

Traumatic Causes

Mallory-Weiss tear
Epistaxis
Oropharyngeal trauma—e.g., postsurgical trauma
Nasogastric or gastric tube trauma
Foreign body

Congenital or Vascular Causes

Enteric duplication
Dieulafoy ulcer
Arteriovenous malformation (AVM)
Esophageal or gastric varices

Inflammatory Causes

Gastric or duodenal ulcer
Esophagitis (reflux or chemical)
Gastritis (caustic or chemical)
Duodenitis
Eosinophilic gastritis

Miscellaneous Causes

Hemobilia
Graft-versus-host disease
Swallowed maternal blood
Pulmonary disease (hemoptysis)
Factitious bleeding (Munchausen by proxy syndrome)

▼ DIFFERENTIAL DIAGNOSIS DISCUSSION

Mallory-Weiss Tear

Etiology

A Mallory-Weiss tear is a **linear mucosal tear of the distal esophagus** that occurs as a result of **forceful vomiting or retching.**

Clinical Features

Bloody streaks are seen in the vomitus.

Evaluation

Mallory-Weiss tears, which are not visible on radiographs, are diagnosed using **upper endoscopy.** Initially, the tear appears as a **vertical, linear red streak;** after healing, it is seen as a **white streak** with surrounding erythema.

Treatment

Most patients can be managed in the outpatient setting because Mallory-Weiss tears usually **resolve spontaneously.** In severe cases, hospital observation is indicated. Rarely, blood transfusion, vasopressin therapy, or balloon tamponade may be necessary.

Esophagitis

Etiology

Esophagitis **(inflammation of the esophageal mucosa)** can be caused by acid or bile reflux, viral or *H. pylori* infection, inflammation, allergy, or caustic ingestions. Esophagitis may cause vomiting, or it may result from disorders that promote delayed gastric emptying and vomiting.

Clinical Features

Typically, patients with esophagitis experience **heartburn, chest pain, water brash** (sour taste in the mouth), or **vomiting and regurgitation. Blood-streaked emesis** occurs in patients with severe or untreated esophagitis.

In infants with reflux esophagitis, parents may notice **pooled bloody secretions on the infant's bedding.** In **older children** with esophagitis, **bloody emesis** is usually **associated with epigastric or chest pain** and a **history of frequent regurgitation** and a **"sour taste"** in the mouth.

Evaluation

Upper endoscopy, the test of choice when esophagitis is suspected, allows inspection of the esophageal mucosa and biopsy of the esophagus to determine the cause of the inflammation and the degree of histologic involvement.

Contrast radiography is often useful for determining the anatomic configuration of the upper gastrointestinal tract. This study is most valuable for ruling out other causes of upper gastrointestinal bleeding (e.g., gastric or duodenal ulcer disease, esophageal strictures, esophageal or gastric varices).

Treatment

The treatment of esophagitis depends on its cause.

▼ **Acid reflux esophagitis** is treated with a combination of prokinetic agents (e.g., metoclopramide, cisapride) and gastric acid blockers.
▼ **Inflammatory esophagitis** requires the use of protective agents, such as sucralfate, and treatment of the underlying inflammatory process (e.g., Crohn disease, allergic esophagitis) with corticosteroids or food elimination.
▼ **Strictures** necessitate dilatation.
▼ **Infectious esophagitis** is treated with antimicrobials.

Gastritis
Etiology

Gastritis **(inflammation of the gastric mucosa)** can be classified as primary or secondary:

▼ **Primary gastritis** results when acid or bile causes direct mucosal damage.
▼ **Secondary gastritis** is either a complication of another disease process (e.g., severe burns, systemic illness, Henoch-Schönlein purpura)

or is caused by an offending agent (e.g., ingested drugs or corrosives, infections).

Clinical Features

Epigastric pain and vomiting are the most common symptoms of gastritis in children. The pain often occurs during, or just after, meals and the patient often complains of **nausea and early satiety.** Small amounts of **fresh blood or "coffee ground" material** may be seen **in the vomitus.**

Evaluation

In children, radiographic contrast studies often do not have the sensitivity necessary to show gastritis. **Upper endoscopy** is a more valuable tool; the gastric mucosa can be directly visualized and biopsies can be obtained to determine the cause of the gastritis.

Treatment

Although it is important to identify and treat the specific cause of the gastritis, a generalized treatment approach is usually necessary initially. **Acid-blocking medications** (e.g., antacids, H_2 blockers) are required to raise the gastric pH above 4.0. **Drugs** (e.g., aspirin, NSAIDs) **should be eliminated.** Patients with major hemorrhage require **fluid resuscitation and transfusion.**

Gastric or Duodenal Ulcer

Etiology

Gastric or duodenal ulcers may result from **infection** (*H. pylori*), increases in **hormones** (Zollinger-Ellison syndrome), **increased gastric acidity,** or **direct injury** (drugs, caustic ingestion, foreign body). In addition, the development of ulcers has been associated with several **systemic diseases,** including sickle cell disease, cystic fibrosis, and asthma.

HINT Gastric ulcers are more common in children younger than 6 years, whereas duodenal ulcers occur more frequently in older children.

Clinical Features

Major symptoms include **upper gastrointestinal bleeding, abdominal pain, vomiting, anorexia, syncope or dizziness** (secondary to anemia), **weight loss or failure to thrive,** and **heartburn.** The pain can awaken the child at night or in the early morning and usually occurs after meals. Symptoms of ulcer disease have often been present for as long as 2 years prior to diagnosis.

Evaluation

Although an upper gastrointestinal contrast study can confirm the diagnosis in up to 50% of patients, **upper endoscopy** remains the most efficacious test. Upper endoscopy allows identification of the ulcer, determination of the cause (via a biopsy), and, in some cases, treatment (e.g., cauterization in the case of acute bleeding).

HINT When the ulcers are multiple or recurrent, disorders such as Zollinger-Ellison syndrome or antral G cell hyperplasia should be considered.

Treatment

Routine medical therapy consists of **gastric acid suppression** (with antacids, H_2 blockers, and proton pump inhibitors) and **mucosal protection** (with sucralfate). **Infectious causes and systemic diseases should be treated** to prevent recurrences.

Profuse bleeding may require endoscopy with **electrocautery; surgery** is indicated in the rare case of intractable bleeding or perforation.

Esophageal or Gastric Varices

Etiology

Varices occur **secondary to portal hypertension caused by chronic liver disease, vascular obstruction** (Budd-Chiari syndrome), **or portal vein obstruction** (cavernous transformation, thrombosis). The portal hypertension and subsequent vascular shunting cause the development of varices (esophageal, gastric, and rectal) and an abdominal caput medusae. Increased vascular pressure results in elevated wall tension, thinning of the blood vessel wall, and eventually, vascular rupture.

Clinical Features

Painless, profuse vomiting of bright-red blood is often the first sign of bleeding varices. Approximately 25% of children with varices have had no prior diagnosis and present with hematemesis.

Patients may have **signs of liver disease** (e.g., jaundice, palmar erythema, spider angiomas). Almost all patients with varices have palpable **splenomegaly.**

Evaluation

An **abdominal examination** is revealing, because most children with varices have evidence of either hepatomegaly or splenomegaly.

There may be **laboratory evidence of liver disease** (e.g., elevated transaminases).

Although radiographic studies may provide some additional information—for example, a contrast study can show the outline of the varices and an abdominal ultrasound can detect associated liver disease and the direction of blood flow in the portal system—**upper gastrointestinal endoscopy** is the most accurate method of diagnosing varices.

Treatment

Bleeding varices are an **absolute medical emergency.** The patient must be admitted to a **pediatric intensive care facility** and placed in the care of a **pediatric gastroenterologist.** Upper gastrointestinal endoscopy is indicated for diagnosis and treatment **(sclerotherapy).**

▼ EVALUATION OF UPPER GASTROINTESTINAL BLEEDING

Patient History

▼ Is there a history of prolonged retching or recent stress?
▼ Could the child be swallowing blood as a result of epistaxis, tonsillectomy or adenoidectomy, trauma to the teeth or gums, or trauma from foreign objects or nasogastric tube insertion?
▼ Has the child eaten any food that may resemble blood in the vomitus?

▼ Does the child's medication history include NSAIDs or aspirin (which can cause gastritis) or steroids (which can cause gastric ulcers)?

Physical Examination

▼ **The nares, mouth, and throat of any child who presents with hematemesis should be carefully examined.**

▼ **The child's fingernails should be inspected for evidence of dried blood** because digital manipulation of the nose is the most common cause of nosebleeds in children. A negative rectal examination for occult blood should alert the physician to the possibility that epistaxis is responsible for the blood in the vomitus.

▼ **Hepatosplenomegaly or isolated splenomegaly** almost always occurs in conjunction with portal hypertension and varices.

▼ **Freckles over the lips and under the axilla** may suggest Peutz-Jeghers syndrome with gastric polyps.

Diagnostic Modalities

Upper gastrointestinal endoscopy and contrast studies are useful for discovering the cause of hematemesis. Although an upper gastrointestinal contrast study occasionally shows pathognomonic esophageal findings, **upper endoscopy with biopsy and culture** is the study of choice.

For children who have recurrent bleeding episodes and for whom endoscopy or contrast studies have been negative, **nuclear medicine bleeding scans** may be useful. The patient must be actively bleeding at the time of the test.

▼ TREATMENT OF UPPER GASTROINTESTINAL BLEEDING

The first step in the management of a patient with upper gastrointestinal tract bleeding is to provide supportive care:

1. Obtain vital signs and manage the airway, breathing, and circulation.
2. Place a large-bore intravenous line.
3. Obtain a complete blood cell count (CBC), type and cross-match, serum electrolyte panel, and blood urea nitrogen (BUN) and creatinine levels.
4. Administer crystalloid (normal saline) or a blood transfusion (if necessary).
5. Place a nasogastric tube to irrigate the stomach.
6. Place a deep venous line for central venous pressure measurement (if indicated).
7. Obtain the patient's history and evaluate for prior bleeding episodes or chronic disease.
8. Consult a pediatric gastroenterologist.

In addition to supportive care, acute medical management entails the **intravenous administration of vasopressin** to promote vasoconstriction of bleeding blood vessels. Vasopressin is extremely useful in children with active esophageal or gastric varices and ulcers. Patients given vasopressin should be monitored in an **intensive care setting** and should be in the care of a **pediatric gastroenterologist.**

Other medical treatments include **endoscopy with sclerotherapy or electrocautery** and **balloon tamponade. Surgery** is indicated for patients with uncontrolled bleeding in whom medical treatment has failed.

▼ APPROACH TO THE PATIENT

The **first episode** of upper gastrointestinal tract bleeding in children should always be **treated as a medical emergency.** Once the patient is stabilized, a careful history and physical examination should be performed to determine the cause of the bleeding.

Suggested Readings

Polin RA, Ditmar MF: *Pediatric Secrets,* 2nd ed. Philadelphia, Hanley & Belfus, 1997.

Silverman A, Roy CC: *Pediatric Clinical Gastroenterology,* 3rd ed. St. Louis, Mosby, 1983.

Sleisenger MH, Fordtran JS: *Gastrointestinal Disease,* 5th ed. Philadelphia, WB Saunders, 1993.

Treem WR: Gastrointestinal bleeding in children. *Gastrointest Endosc* 4:75, 1994.

Walker WA, Durie PR, Hamilton JR, et al: *Pediatric Gastrointestinal Disease,* 2nd ed. Philadelphia, BC Decker, 1996.

Wyllie R, Hyams JS: *Pediatric Gastrointestinal Disease.* Philadelphia, WB Saunders, 1993.

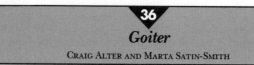

36
Goiter
CRAIG ALTER AND MARTA SATIN-SMITH

▼ INTRODUCTION

Goiter (**enlargement of the thyroid gland**) arises under a variety of clinical circumstances. Morbidity from enlarged thyroid ranges from that associated with carcinoma to simple cosmetic effects.

▼ DIFFERENTIAL DIAGNOSIS LIST

Infectious Causes

Acute suppurative thyroiditis
Subacute thyroiditis

Toxic Causes

Environmental goitrogens
Lithium carbonate
Amiodarone
Iodide-containing drugs

Neoplastic Causes

Thyroid-stimulating hormone (TSH)-secreting adenoma
Thyroid adenoma
Papillary carcinoma
Follicular carcinoma
Medullary carcinoma
Anaplastic carcinoma
Nonthyroid carcinomas—lymphoma, teratoma, hygroma

Congenital Causes

Ectopic gland
Unilateral agenesis
Dyshormonogenesis
Thyroxine (T$_4$) resistance

Metabolic Causes

Iodine deficiency

Inflammatory Causes

Chronic lymphocytic thyroiditis (CLT, Hashimoto thyroiditis)
Graves disease (acquired and neonatal)

Miscellaneous Causes

Simple colloid goiter (adolescent goiter)
Multinodular colloid goiter
Thyroglossal duct cyst

▼ DIFFERENTIAL DIAGNOSIS DISCUSSION

Chronic Lymphocytic Thyroiditis (CLT, Hashimoto Thyroiditis)

Etiology

CLT, an autoimmune condition, is the **most common cause of goiter** in the pediatric population. Its incidence is **highest in adolescent girls,** with a female:male ratio of 2:1.

Clinical Features

Some patients with CLT present for medical examination with symptoms of **hypothyroidism** (Table 36.1). Most have enlargement of the gland without systemic complaints. Rarely, patients with CLT show symptoms of

TABLE 36.1. Signs and Symptoms of Hypothyroidism and Hyperthyroidism

Hypothyroidism	Hyperthyroidism
Goiter in some patients	Goiter, bruit over thyroid
Lethargy, slow speech	Nervousness, restless sleep
Cold skin, decreased sweating	Sweating, heat intolerance
Bradycardia	Palpitation, tachycardia
Weakness	Fatigue, weakness
Anorexia	Increased appetite
Weight gain	Weight loss
Constipation	Increased stool frequency
Stiff, aching muscles	Tremor of hands and tongue
Edema of face and eyelids	Exophthalmos, lid lag
Dry, coarse skin	Increased skin pigmentation
Hair loss with increased coarseness	Fine hair
Poor growth	Accelerated growth
Delayed puberty and tooth eruption	Poor school performance
	Moodiness or irritability

hyperthyroidism. These children **progress toward hypothyroidism** over a period of months. The **thyroid gland** itself **is diffusely enlarged** (though possibly with **asymmetry**), **mobile, nontender,** and **firm.** It usually has a granular or pebbly texture but can be smooth. However, in the most severe cases of hypothyroidism and CLT, the thyroid is often so **degenerated** that it is not easily palpable. Enlargement may be due to lymphocytic infiltration or due to stimulation by the increased TSH.

There is a **family history** of thyroid disease in 30%–40% of patients with CLT. Histologic findings include infiltration of the gland with plasma cells and lymphocytes, parenchymal atrophy, and eosinophilic degeneration of acini.

Evaluation

Laboratory studies should include assessment of T_4, **TSH,** and **antithyroglobulin and antithyroperoxidase antibodies.** Normal values of thyroid function studies are shown in Table 36.2. In children with CLT, thyroid function tests indicate either a **euthyroid state** (no abnormalities), **compensated hypothyroidism** (normal level of T_4 with increased TSH) or **hypothyroidism** (low level of T_4 with increased TSH). **One or both of the antithyroid antibodies is present** in 90%–95% of patients with CLT. These antibodies represent the immunologic response to the presence of elements of thyroid tissue in the bloodstream and are not the cause of the thyroiditis.

Treatment

Thyroid hormone replacement is indicated for the treatment of overt hypothyroidism and occasionally for compensated hypothyroidism accompanied by a significantly enlarged gland. Initial doses of **sodium L-thyroxine** at $100 \mu g/m^2$ of body surface area or 2–5 $\mu g/kg/day$ should be **adjusted after 1 month** of therapy to keep T_4 and TSH levels in the normal range. Shrinkage of the goiter may not occur if the inflammation is long-standing and the fibrosis is extensive. Once an appropriate dose of sodium L-thyroxine has been established, **biannual follow-up** is necessary to ensure compliance and appropriate growth. Some may require more frequent laboratory studies.

Spontaneous remission occurs in up to 30% of adolescents. It is acceptable to discontinue hormone replacement therapy when growth is completed to ascertain whether spontaneous remission has occurred. If the child is euthyroid at presentation and again at 6 months, yearly monitoring of T_4 and TSH is indicated.

TABLE 36.2. Normal Thyroid Hormone Levels

Parameter	Normal Finding
T_4	
Total	7.0–15.0 uU/dl
Free	0.8–2.3 ng/dl
T_3	80–250 ng/dl
TSH	0.5–5.0 uU/ml

T_3 = triiodothyronine; T_4 = thyroxine; TSH = thyroid-stimulating hormone.

Simple Colloid Goiter

Etiology

Simple colloid goiter **(adolescent goiter)** is the **second most common** cause of nontoxic thyroid enlargement in the pediatric population. Its cause is uncertain. There is often a **family history** of goiter.

Clinical Features

There is **diffuse enlargement** of the thyroid gland in **asymptomatic adolescents.** The gland is enlarged and is usually softer than in chronic lymphocytic thyroiditis. **Nodularity** may develop after several years, even in those patients in whom regression has occurred.

Evaluation

There are usually **no antithyroid antibodies,** and the T_4 **and TSH levels are normal.** Some patients have an increased level of thyroid growth-stimulating antibodies in their serum, which suggests that this may be a mild form of autoimmune disease.

Treatment

Treatment with sodium L-thyroxine is not required. In many cases, the goiter **resolves with time.**

Graves Disease

Etiology

Graves disease, a **multisystem autoimmune disorder,** is the **most common cause of hyperthyroidism** in the pediatric population. The incidence in males and females is equal in infancy and early childhood, with a female predominance occurring in adolescence. In Graves disease, elaboration of an immunoglobulin G1 antibody stimulates the TSH receptor, resulting in hyperfunctioning follicular cells with **increased production and release of thyroid hormone.** Other antibodies, including thyroid growth-stimulating antibody, may contribute to enlargement of the gland. Exophthalmos in Graves disease may be caused in part by a collagen-stimulating antibody.

Clinical Features

Graves disease presents with signs of **hyperthyroidism** and **thyromegaly. Exophthalmos** is occasionally present, and rarely, dermopathy. Children with hyperthyroidism caused by Graves disease often are brought to medical attention because of **worsening school performance** and a **change in behavior** (emotional lability and irritability). The majority of symptoms of hyperthyroidism (see Table 36.1) are caused by stimulation of the sympathetic nervous system resulting from increased levels of thyroid hormones.

Evaluation

On physical examination, the thyroid gland is symmetrically **enlarged, smooth,** and **nontender.** The texture is soft to firm, and the size is variable. Graves disease is rare in a child without a **goiter.** The child is usually **tachycardic** with a widened pulse pressure and an active precordium. A **vascular bruit** may be heard over the gland. **Proptosis with stare** and **upper lid lag** is noted in many cases; however, the eye disease in children rarely reaches the severity seen in adults. Dermopathy, caused by an accumulation of mucopolysaccharide in the skin and subcutaneous tissue, is uncommon in children.

Laboratory and radiologic studies that support the diagnosis of Graves disease and help to distinguish it from other causes of hyperthyroidism are shown in Table 36.3.

Treatment

There are three main approaches to management of Graves disease: **antithyroid medications, iodine-131 (^{131}I) ablation therapy,** and **subtotal thyroidectomy.** In general, medical management with **medications should be the first intervention,** followed by either ablation with ^{131}I or surgery. The mainstays of long-term medical treatment in children are the **thioamide derivatives,** propylthiouracil (PTU) and methimazole. These medications inhibit the organification of iodide, thus blocking the synthesis (but not the release) of thyroid hormone. *β*-**Blocking agents** are used as adjuvant treatment to control symptoms when long-term therapy is initially introduced; they may be discontinued when the thyroid disease is well controlled. Side effects of the medication include skin rash, pruritus, and rarely, agranulocytosis. If a **child on PTU or methimazole** presents with a **severe sore throat,** a complete blood cell count should be obtained.

Thyroid Storm (Thyroid Crisis)

Etiology

Thyroid storm is a **medical emergency.** A very rare condition, it typically occurs in individuals who have **preexisting hyperthyroidism** and who are **undertreated or noncompliant.** Infection, trauma, and surgical procedures are the most common precipitating events. Pneumococcal sepsis is occasionally

TABLE 36.3. Laboratory Findings in Graves Disease

Parameter	Finding Suggestive of Graves Disease
Total T_4	Levels increased
Free T_4	Levels increased
T_3	Levels increased
TSH	Significantly suppressed and often undetectable
Thyroid-stimulating immunoglobulin	Elevated
Thyroid antibodies	
Antithyroglobulin antibody	May be detectable but rarely increased to the degree seen in CLT; if levels are very high, consider the possibility of CLT
Antithyroperoxidase antibody	May be detectable but rarely increased to the degree seen in CLT; if levels are very high, consider the possibility of CLT
^{123}I uptake study	Increased uptake of the isotope at 6 and 24 hours postadministration is supportive of Graves disease (decreased uptake is seen in CLT and subacute thyroiditis)

CLT = chronic lymphocytic thyroiditis; ^{123}I = iodine-123; T_3 = triiodothyronine; T_4 = thyroxine; TSH = thyroid-stimulating hormone.

found. The release of large amounts of thyroid hormone leads to a **hyper-metabolic state** with **excessive thermogenesis** and **significant fluid losses. Increase in temperature** can be extreme.

Clinical Features

Children with thyroid storm show **fever, rapid tachycardia, tremor, nausea and vomiting, diarrhea, dehydration,** and **delirium or coma.** Occasionally, patients have a true **toxic psychosis.** The markedly increased cardiac workload can lead to **congestive heart failure.**

Treatment

Treatment of thyroid storm includes the **immediate administration of** β**-blocking agents** to suppress the activity of the sympathetic nervous system. Next, **hydration** must be achieved, and appropriate measures must be taken to **lower the body temperature slowly. Propylthiouracil** (6–10 mg/kg/day, divided, every 8 hours) is administered. Subsequently, **iodide treatment** to rapidly terminate the release of thyroxine is administered in the form of Lugol iodide, 5 drops every 8 hours, or sodium iodide, 125–250 mg/day intravenously over 24 hours.

Acute Suppurative Thyroiditis

Etiology

A **fistula tract** may have formed between the **left pyriform sinus of the pharynx** and the **left lobe of the thyroid gland.** Because of high endogenous levels of iodine, the thyroid gland is inherently resistant to bacterial infection. However, **infections** do occur and **must be treated promptly** to prevent abscess formation.

Clinical Features

Patients present with the rapid onset of **anterior neck pain** associated with **dysphagia, pharyngitis, mandibular pain,** and a **hoarse voice; fever;** and signs of **systemic toxicity.** The thyroid itself is **exquisitely tender and nonmobile** and may have areas of fluid. The **pain increases with neck extension.**

Evaluation

Organisms identified by means of needle biopsy include *Streptococcus pyogenes, Staphylococcus aureus, Streptococcus pneumoniae,* anaerobes, fungi, and parasitic organisms. Marked leukocytosis and an increased sedimentation rate are the most consistent laboratory findings. Thyroid function tests usually are normal, but a transient increase in T_4 levels can occur. Nuclear medicine scanning with iodine-123 (^{123}I) demonstrates decreased uptake of the isotope.

Treatment

Antibiotic treatment should be tailored to the suspected organism. Areas of abscess may require **surgical drainage.** β**-Blocking drugs** can be used if signs of transient thyrotoxicosis develop. Recovery without residual thyroid disease is the natural course.

Subacute Thyroiditis

Etiology

Subacute thyroiditis is a **self-limited inflammation** of the thyroid gland that most often is associated with, or follows, a **viral illness.** Viral agents implicated include mumps virus, adenovirus, coxsackievirus, influenza virus, Epstein-Barr virus, and enteric cytopathic human orphan virus. The incidence is the same in boys and girls.

Clinical Features

It can be **difficult to distinguish between subacute and acute** suppurative thyroiditis. Patients present for treatment with **fever** and **anterior neck pain.** The **area over the thyroid** may be **warm and erythematous.** The thyroid is usually tender and **enlarged.** Signs and symptoms of **hyperthyroidism** develop because of the release of stored hormone from the inflamed gland. These symptoms can persist for 1–4 weeks and can be followed by a 2- to 9-month period of hypothyroidism.

Evaluation

T_4 **and triiodothyronine (T_3) levels** are increased in the majority of patients with subacute thyroiditis for a period of **several weeks.** Most patients do not develop antithyroid antibodies. As in acute suppurative thyroiditis, an ^{123}I scan will demonstrate decreased **uptake of isotope.**

Treatment

Treatment includes the administration of **nonsteroidal anti-inflammatory drugs** and **propranolol.** In severe cases, the use of **corticosteroids** may be indicated. Typically, full recovery of thyroid function occurs. If **hypothyroidism** develops, it is usually transient, but it **should be treated.**

Congenital Goiter

Etiology

Most cases of newborn goiter are caused by **inborn defects of thyroid hormone metabolism** (dyshormonogenesis). Most of these defects are inherited as autosomal recessive traits. These defects include:

▼ Abnormal iodide trapping or organification
▼ Iodotyrosine deiodinase defect
▼ Defects in thyroglobulin synthesis, transport, or processing

A second cause of congenital goiter is the **maternal ingestion of goitrogenic agents** during pregnancy, leading to a transient congenital hypothyroidism in the infant. Treatment of maternal hyperthyroidism with PTU or methimazole usually does not cause congenital hypothyroidism unless extremely high doses are used (more than 150 mg/day of PTU).

Evaluation

In dyshormonogenesis, T_4 **levels may be normal or low** while the **TSH is elevated.** ^{123}I scanning usually reveals an **enlarged gland** with **abnormal isotope uptake.**

Treatment

As with other causes of congenital hypothyroidism, infants with dyshormono-genesis need treatment with **sodium L-thyroxine** (10 μ/kg/day) to ensure the normal T$_4$ levels needed for central nervous system development.

Infants with **presumed transient hypothyroidism** can be **followed closely** without treatment for **2 weeks.** If the T$_4$ level remains low and the TSH level is elevated, then treatment should be started and continued for 3–6 months.

▼ EVALUATION OF GOITER

Patient History

The major goals during the initial history are to determine if a child has signs or symptoms of **hypothyroidism or hyperthyroidism** (see Table 36.1). The **rapidity of enlargement** of the gland may allow one to focus on an **acute process** (e.g., suppurative thyroiditis) as opposed to a **chronic problem** (e.g., CLT). In the case of a **solitary nodule or unilateral enlargement,** exposure to **radiation** either for treatment of a medical condition or accidental **exposure should be determined.**

HINT The incidence of thyroid carcinoma in Belarus has increased dramatically following the Chernobyl nuclear accident. Children adopted from this area need to be carefully screened.

Physical Examination

- ▼ **Vital signs.** Heart rate and blood pressure findings are important in both hypothyroid and hyperthyroid states.
- ▼ **Growth.** Poor overall growth may be the first sign of hypothyroidism associated with CLT. Obesity with normal linear growth argues against hypothyroidism as the cause of the increased weight. Accelerated growth is common in hyperthyroidism.
- ▼ **Neurologic examination.** Restlessness, tremor, exophthalmos, and hyper-reflexia are common features of hyperthyroidism. In contrast, decreased energy and delayed relaxation phase of deep tendon reflexes are common findings in hypothyroidism.
- ▼ **Thyroid examination.** Careful palpation and measurement of the gland is performed with the examiner standing behind a seated or standing patient. The size and texture of the gland, symmetry of enlargement, associated lymphadenopathy, and any tenderness should be noted.

Laboratory Studies

Laboratory studies are guided by the history and physical examination findings. They commonly include **evaluation of T$_4$, TSH,** and **thyroid antibodies** (thyroglobulin and peroxidase). In cases of suspected hyperthyroidism, **T$_3$** should also be measured since children occasionally manifest predominantly T$_3$ toxicosis. Elevations in total T$_4$ are seen in states of increased binding such as in pregnancy and use of oral birth control pills with an associated increase in thyroid-binding globulin. Free T$_4$ assays may be affected by certain medications.

Suggested Readings

Alter CA, Moshang T: Diagnostic dilemma: the goiter. *Pediatr Clin North Am* 88:567–578, 1991.

Foley TP: Thyroid disease. *Pediatr Ann* 21:13–57, 1992.

Hopwood N, Kelch RP: Thyroid masses: approach to diagnosis and management in childhood and adolescence. *Pediatr Rev* 14:481–487, 1993.

Jaruratanasirikul S, Leethanaporn K, Khuntigij P, et al: The clinical course of Hashimoto's thyroiditis in children and adolescents: 6 years longitudinal follow-up. *J Pediatr Endocrinol Metab* 14:177–184, 2001.

Jaruratanasirikul S, Leethanaporn K, Suchat K: The natural clinical course of children with an initial diagnosis of simple goiter: a 5-year longitudinal follow-up. *J Pediatr Endocrinol Metab* 13:1109–1113, 2000.

Mahoney CP: Differential diagnosis of goiter. *Pediatr Clin North Am* 34:891–905, 1987.

Thyroid Internet Textbook, http://www.thyroidmanager.org/thyroidbook.htm

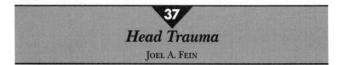

37

Head Trauma

JOEL A. FEIN

▼ INTRODUCTION

Head injury in children accounts for more than 600,000 emergency department visits, 95,000 hospitalizations, and 7,000 deaths per year. Fatal or irreversible injury is usually a sequela of neuronal cell death and vascular disruption during the first few milliseconds of impact. Another irreversible cause of morbidity is the shearing of the white matter tracts as a result of an acceleration–deceleration injury. **The only injuries that are reversible with therapy are those with secondary effects on the brain and blood vessels.**

▼ DIFFERENTIAL DIAGNOSIS LIST

Focal Injuries

Scalp lacerations
Hematoma
Cerebral contusion
Fractures

Diffuse Injuries

Concussion syndrome
Diffuse axonal injury
Increased intracranial pressure (ICP)

▼ DIFFERENTIAL DIAGNOSIS DISCUSSION

Scalp Lacerations

Scalp lacerations are common findings in patients with head injuries. Blood loss can be extensive, especially in infants and young children. The physician should carefully assess the depth of the wound and evaluate it for **retained**

foreign bodies. In addition, the **integrity of the galea aponeurotica** (a tendinous sheath located just above the periosteum) should be evaluated; some clinicians suture this layer separately to control bleeding. Finally, the physician should search for **skull fractures or "step-offs" (dents).**

Hematoma

Hematoma caused by head injury may exist outside of the confines of the skull (e.g., cephalohematoma, subgaleal hematoma), or inside the skull (e.g., epidural or subdural hematoma). **Intracranial lesions** may require **neurosurgical intervention,** whereas **extracranial lesions** rarely require any treatment other than **supportive care.**

Cephalohematoma

Newborn infants commonly incur a cephalohematoma, in which blood collects between the periosteum and the table of the skull and is therefore prevented from spreading past the midline. This type of injury is common in traumatic deliveries.

Subgaleal Hematoma

A posttraumatic, well-circumscribed "lump" on an older child's head usually represents a subgaleal hematoma.

Epidural and Subdural Hematomas (Table 37.1)

Epidural hematomas are less often associated with underlying brain injury than are subdural hematomas.

Cerebral Contusions and Lacerations

Cerebral contusions can occur as a **coup injury** (at the contact location) or as a **contrecoup injury** (rebounding, on the opposite side). A cerebral contusion commonly manifests as **posttraumatic epilepsy.**

Cerebral lacerations usually result from **penetrating injury** to the brain or from a **depressed skull fracture.** Clinical manifestations are more often a result of the associated concussion and the underlying brain injury than of the focal lesions themselves. These lesions can be visualized on computed tomography (CT) scans.

Skull Fractures

Linear Skull Fractures

Linear skull fractures comprise 75%–90% of all skull fractures. **Usually no treatment is necessary.** However, if the fracture is located over a vascular structure (e.g., the middle meningeal artery), there is an increased incidence of epidural hemorrhage. Diastatic ("growing") fractures can develop when meninges get caught between the bone edges and continue to separate them.

Basilar Skull Fractures

Basilar skull fractures typically occur in the **petrous portion of the temporal bone.** Potential findings on physical examination of a patient with a basilar skull fracture are:

▼ "Raccoon" eyes (ecchymosis below the eyes)
▼ Battle sign (ecchymosis at the mastoid)
▼ Hemotympanum (blood behind the eardrum)
▼ Cerebrospinal fluid (CSF) otorrhea or rhinorrhea
▼ Cranial nerve dysfunction, especially involving the seventh and eighth cranial nerves

TABLE 37.1. Epidural versus Acute Subdural Hematoma

	Epidural Hematoma	Subdural Hematoma
Common mechanism	Blunt direct trauma, frequently to parietal region	Acceleration–deceleration injury
Etiology	Arterial or venous	Venous (bridging veins below dura)
Incidence	Uncommon	Common
Peak age	Usually > 2 years	Usually < 1 year Peak at 6 months
Location	Unilateral Commonly parietal	75% Bilateral Diffuse, over cerebral hemispheres
Skull fracture	Common	Uncommon
Associated seizures	Uncommon	Common
Retinal hemorrhages	Rare	Common
Decreased level of consciousness	Common	Almost always
Mortality	Rare	Uncommon
Morbidity in survivors	Low	High
Clinical findings	Dilated ipsilateral pupil, contralateral hemiparesis Period of lucidity prior to acute decompensation and rapid progression to herniation	Decreased level of consciousness Irritability, lethargy
Onset	Acute	Acute (within 24 hours), subacute (within 1 day–2 weeks), or chronic (after 2 weeks)
Findings on CT	Convex "lens-shaped" cerebral hemisphere	Concave, diffusely surrounding cerebral hemisphere

CT = computed tomography.

Depressed Skull Fractures

Depressed skull fractures can sometimes be diagnosed clinically, by palpation of the depression of the skull underneath a hematoma, or radiographically, using tangential views of the skull or a CT scan. **Surgical elevation** may be necessary **if the fracture extends past the inner table of the skull.**

Concussion Syndromes

Concussion syndromes are diagnosed when blunt head injury results in a transient impairment in awareness and responsiveness. The **symptoms can last from seconds to hours.** Some patients complain of persistent headaches, dizziness, and subtle differences in memory, anxiety level, and sleep patterns lasting a few weeks after head injury.

Diffuse Axonal Injury

Diffuse axonal injury occurs when nerve fibers are sheared on initial impact. Patients exhibit **persistent functional neurologic deficits** (e.g., a prolonged comatose state) without obvious radiographic abnormalities. Diffuse axonal injury is associated with high morbidity and mortality rates.

Increased Intracranial Pressure (ICP)

Increased ICP **affects the delivery of oxygen and substrate to the brain tissue.** An increase in one component of the intracranial contents (i.e., blood, CSF, or tissue) necessitates a decrease in another component because, under normal conditions, the sum of these compartments in the cranial vault remains constant. Therefore, if the ICP increases to more than the normal limit (15 mm Hg), small changes in the volume of the intracranial contents result in large changes in ICP. The **brain tissue and blood vessels** become **increasingly compressed,** disrupting cerebral blood flow or causing herniation of brain tissue through the dural reflections.

▼ **Herniation of the uncal portion of the temporal lobe** through the tentorium disrupts the parasympathetic fibers of the third cranial nerve, resulting in ipsilateral pupillary dilatation and contralateral motor deficits. In diffuse injury, the uncal herniation and, therefore, the pupillary and motor deficits, can be noted bilaterally.

▼ **Herniation of the brain stem** is frequently a premorbid event. Compression of medullary autonomic structures affects heart rate, respirations, and level of consciousness. "Cushing's triad," resulting from increased ICP and consisting of hypertension, bradycardia, and irregular respirations, is a classic finding. Decerebrate posturing may also be noted. However, serious sequelae can ensue even if the child has not experienced this constellation of findings.

▼ APPROACH TO THE PATIENT
Stabilization

Initial priorities for any severely injured child are **protection of the airway, maintenance of adequate tissue perfusion,** and **rapid assessment of neurologic status.** Although the primary injury to the brain is irreversible, the secondary injury may be minimized in the acute care setting.

Airway

Upper airway obstruction is initially managed with proper **adjustment of the head, neck, and mandible** to clear the soft tissues and tongue away from the airway (Table 37.2). Examination of the cervical spine is considered part of the airway evaluation. Before undertaking radiographic and clinical examination of the cervical spine, a **cervical collar** should be used with side immobilization, or manual immobilization should be provided.

TABLE 37.2. Possible Indications for Endotracheal Intubation

Upper airway obstruction unrelieved by airway repositioning
Abnormal respiratory rate or rhythm
Loss of protective airway reflexes
Concomitant trauma
   Chest wall instability
   Pulmonary contusion
Signs of increased intracranial pressure (ICP)

Breathing

The head trauma victim with a clear upper airway but decreased breath sounds may have one of many injuries:

▼ Pneumothorax
▼ Pulmonary contusion
▼ Flail chest
▼ Central nervous system (CNS) depression

Circulation

Lack of brain perfusion can lead to irreversible neuronal cell damage. **The cerebral perfusion pressure equals the mean arterial pressure minus the ICP.** Therefore, the goal of management is to normalize the mean arterial pressure while minimizing ICP.

Shock should be dealt with aggressively in the trauma patient, regardless of concern about increased ICP. Shock must be addressed as if it were hypovolemic shock until proven otherwise; it cannot be presumed to be secondary to spinal cord injury (neurogenic shock). The administration of crystalloid (e.g., lactated Ringer's solution) or colloid (e.g., whole blood) should be based on the patient's heart rate, skin perfusion, and urinary output.

Assessment of Neurologic Disability

The **Glasgow coma scale (GCS) score** should be obtained (see Chapter 21, "Coma," Table 21.1), and the **pupils** and **gag reflex** should be evaluated relatively early to determine the presence of brain herniation as well as the need for endotracheal intubation. The GCS score is a prognostic tool for patients with head trauma (Table 37.3).

Management of Increased ICP

▼ **Hyperventilation** reduces the "blood" portion of the cerebral vault by constricting the cerebral vessels. The arterial carbon dioxide tension ($Paco_2$) should be maintained at approximately 30 mm Hg. Alternatively, the end-tidal CO_2 ($et\ co_2$) should be maintained at approximately 35 mm Hg.
▼ **Mannitol administration** (0.5–1.0 g/kg intravenously) is thought to reduce the "tissue" portion of the intracranial vault by drawing water out of the brain. The presence of hypotension or hypovolemia is a relative contraindication to the use of mannitol.
▼ **Maintenance of adequate mean arterial pressure** is facilitated by elevating the head 30 degrees and taking measures to stop seizure activity, if present.

TABLE 37.3. Factors Associated with a Poor Outcome

Age < 2 years
Glasgow coma scale (GCS) score of less than 5
Subdural hematoma
Decerebrate or flaccid posture
Coma of more than 24 hours' duration

Further Evaluation

Patient History

A brief history of the **events preceding and subsequent to the traumatic episode** should be obtained, focusing on the timing and mechanism of injury, duration of unconsciousness, presence of amnesia, neurologic assessment at the scene, and any preexisting medical conditions.

Physical Examination

A **secondary survey** should follow soon after the primary survey and should include a close inspection of the head, torso, abdomen, genitalia, and extremities. It is important to examine the head for lacerations, depressions, contusions, or signs of basilar skull fracture.

In the comatose patient, a **normal oculovestibular response** implies that the cranial nerve pathways most proximal to the brain stem (i.e., the third, sixth, and eighth cranial nerves) are intact and that, by association, the neighboring brain stem is functional. Performance of this test can be delayed until after the secondary survey has been completed.

The **oculocephalic ("doll's eye") reflex** should not be evaluated in patients who might have a cervical spine injury.

Diagnostic Modalities

The decision to obtain **skull radiographs** is based on the patient's age, the mechanism of injury, and the need for other radiologic evaluation. Children less than two years old, especially those with a hematoma over the parietal area, may benefit from a skull radiograph as an indicator of whether or not to get a CT scan. When a **CT scan** of the head is required to investigate the possibility of intracranial lesions, it is not necessary to obtain skull radiographs. CT of the head is indicated for patients with:

▼ A persistently diminished level of consciousness
▼ Clinical neurologic deterioration
▼ A persistent focal neurologic deficit
▼ A parietal skull fracture (middle meningeal location)
▼ A significant mechanism of injury
▼ A history of amnesia or loss of consciousness

Management of Complications

Posttraumatic seizures develop in a small percentage of patients who have experienced head trauma. In the acute setting, a **benzodiazepine** should be administered because of its rapid onset of action. **Phenytoin** should be used as a second antiepileptic agent in this setting. Patients with cerebral contusions on CT scan may receive phenytoin initially to prevent rather than treat seizures.

▼ **Early-onset posttraumatic seizures** (occurring within 1 week of injury) often accompany cerebral lacerations and contusions. Twenty percent of these patients experience late seizures, but the condition rarely progresses to epilepsy.
▼ **Late-onset posttraumatic seizures** (developing more than 1 week after injury) are associated with seizures that persist for the next few years in 50% of patients.

▼ TREATMENT OF HEAD TRAUMA

Severe Head Trauma

Treatment consists of **head CT scan** and **management of intracranial pressure** as needed. Patients with "severe" head trauma include those with:

▼ An abnormal neurologic examination
▼ Persistent seizures
▼ A GCS score less than or equal to 14
▼ A depressed or basilar skull fracture

Moderate Head Trauma

Treatment consists of **12–24 hours of observation.** CT of the head may be considered. Patients with "moderate" head trauma include those with a history of amnesia or a brief loss of consciousness, but a normal neurologic examination. Patients with persistent or worsening headache, vomiting, or reported seizure activity are also considered to have moderate head injury.

Mild Head Trauma

For the head trauma to be considered "mild," the patient must have never lost consciousness, and he must have a normal neurologic examination and no reported amnesia. **CT evaluation and a longer observation period** should be considered for the asymptomatic child under 2 years with a significant scalp hematoma, and an infant younger than 2–3 months with a moderate or high-impact mechanism. Other patients can be **observed at home** by a reliable caretaker. This caretaker should be instructed to awaken the patient every 3–4 hours to walk and talk. The caretaker should bring the patient back to the emergency department if any of the following conditions develop:

▼ A headache that worsens or is unrelieved by acetaminophen
▼ Frequent vomiting or vomiting beyond 8 hours postinjury
▼ Change in behavior or gait
▼ Vision problems
▼ Fever or stiff neck
▼ Evidence of clear or bloody fluid draining from the nose or ear
▼ Difficulty in awakening from sleep
▼ Seizures
▼ Bleeding that is unrelieved by the application of pressure for 5 minutes

Suggested Readings

American Academy of Pediatrics Committee on Quality Improvement: The management of closed head injury in children. *Pediatrics* 104:1407–1415, 1999.

Duhaime AC, Alario AJ, Lewander WJ, et al: Head injury in very young children: mechanisms, injury types, and ophthalmologic findings in 100 hospitalized patients younger than two years of age. *Pediatrics* 90:179–185, 1992.

Goldstein B, Powers KS: Head trauma in children. *Pediatr Rev* 15:213–219, 1994.

Raphaely RC, Swedlow DB, Downes JJ, et al: Management of severe pediatric head trauma. *Pediatr Clin North Am* 27:715–727, 1980.

Schutzman SA, Barnes P, Duhaime AC, et al: Evaluation and management of children younger than two years old with apparently minor head trauma: proposed guidelines. *Pediatrics* 107:883–993, 2001.

Schutzman SA, Greenes DS: Pediatric minor head trauma. *Ann Emerg Med* 37:65–74, 2001.

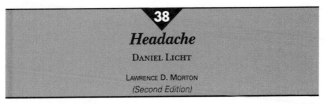

38

Headache

DANIEL LICHT

LAWRENCE D. MORTON
(Second Edition)

▼ INTRODUCTION

Headache, a common complaint in childhood, occurs in up to 10% of children ages 5 to 15 years old, and is a major cause of missed school. Children are usually brought to medical attention for evaluation of a severe, recurrent, or persistent headache in hope of relieving the discomfort and to rule out serious intracranial disease.

For clinical purposes, it is **useful to classify headaches by time course** rather than by pathophysiology. There are four patterns of headache: **acute, acute recurrent, chronic progressive, and chronic nonprogressive.** It is usually possible to determine the nature of the headache from the history and physical examination alone.

🏃 HINT A chronic, progressive headache generally implies a worsening pathological process. Beware of the headache that wakes the child from sleep or is associated with vomiting on waking.

▼ DIFFERENTIAL DIAGNOSIS LIST

Acute Headache

Emergent Causes

Central nervous system infection
Vasculitis
Hemorrhage
Trauma
Mass lesion or tumor
Abscess
Subdural hematoma
Hydrocephalus
Systemic infection with fever
Hypertension
Pseudotumor cerebri

Localized, Acute Headache

Sinusitis
Otitis media

Trauma
Dental or temporomandibular joint dysfunction
First migraine

Generalized, Acute Headache

Systemic infection with fever
Central nervous system (CNS) infection
Hypertension
Vasculitis
Hemorrhage
Postlumbar puncture (LP) headache
Exertional headache
First migraine

Acute, Recurrent Headache

Migraine, with or without aura
Complex migraine
Migraine variant
Cluster headache
Seizure

Chronic, Progressive Headache

Pseudotumor cerebri
Mass lesion
Tumor
Abscess
Subdural hematoma
Hydrocephalus

Chronic, Nonprogressive Headache

Muscle contraction (tension headache)
Postconcussion syndrome
Psychosomatic—depression, conversion disorder, malingering, school
phobia

▼ DIFFERENTIAL DIAGNOSIS DISCUSSION
Localized, Acute Headache

The underlying cause of an acute, generalized headache may be suggested
by the presence of a **fever with meningismus, focal neurologic signs such as
nystagmus, cranial neuropathies, ataxia, papilledema, or an altered level of
consciousness.** There may be a history of **head trauma** or a relationship to
exertion.

If these signs are absent, examination should reveal the cause of the
headache: **sinusitis** (characterized by localized head pain), **otitis media** (characterized by a hyperemic tympanic membrane), or **ocular abnormalities** (refractory errors, evidence of cellulitis, or retrobulbar neuritis, although the
latter are rare). **Localized pain that persists** following head trauma may indicate **neuroma or leptomeningeal cyst formation. Pain in the occiput** may
indicate **cervical disc abnormality** as a result of trauma or a malformation
(e.g., Klippel-Feil sign, Arnold-Chiari malformation, or platybasia).

Generalized, Acute Headache

The underlying cause of an acute, generalized headache may be suggested by the presence of a fever (which may cause cranial artery dilatation), meningismus, focal neurologic signs, papilledema, retinal hemorrhages, or an altered level of consciousness. There may be a history of head trauma or a relationship to exertion.

Migraine Headache

Etiology

Migraine accounts for **75% of headaches** in young children referred for neurologic consultation. Family history is common and reassuring. Common triggers include **anxiety, stress, fatigue, head trauma, exercise, menses, illness, diet** (e.g., caffeine and caffeine withdrawal), and medication (e.g., oral contraceptives, ephedrine, albuterol, theophylline, prednisone).

Clinical Features

▼ **Common migraine.** Migraine without aura is associated with nausea, vomiting, and light and sound sensitivity. The headache is less often well localized than it is in migraine with aura. Migraine with aura (classic migraine) is a biphasic event. The first phase (aura) most commonly includes visual aberrations, sparkling lights or lines, and blind spots. The patient moves into the next phase as the pain commences. The pain is classically pulsating or throbbing and can be unilateral or bilateral. Attacks usually last 2–6 hours and are commonly associated with anorexia, nausea, vomiting, and photophobia. The patient usually wishes to lie in a dark, quiet room; symptoms usually resolve with sleep.

▼ **Complicated migraine.** Symptoms are similar to those listed for common migraine but also involve distal symptoms such as impairment of body image and time ("Alice in Wonderland" migraine), sensory changes, or focal motor deficits (e.g., ophthalmoplegia, hemiplegia).

The distinction of common and complicated migraine has treatment implications.

⚗ HINT Migraine can occur in very young children, who might not be able to verbalize the pain. Instead, the child may experience repeated bouts of vomiting or ataxia followed by behavioral changes (e.g., irritability, lethargy).

Evaluation

The diagnosis can often be made exclusively on the basis of the **history and physical examination.** A child with typical migraine symptoms and a strong family history of migraine may not require imaging studies [e.g., head computed tomography (CT) or magnetic resonance imaging (MRI)]. Generally, electroencephalography is of little diagnostic value, because nonspecific electroencephalogram (EEG) abnormalities have been found in as many as 9% of all migraine patients.

Treatment

Acute attacks may be treated with the administration of **acetaminophen, salicylates, or nonsteroidal anti-inflammatory drugs (NSAIDs),** although sometimes children do just as well with **sleep** and **antiemetics** (occasionally justifying the intramuscular administration of promazine or chlorpromazine). **Serotonin agonists** like sumatriptan succinate (Imitrex), rizatriptan (Maxalt), and zolmitriptan (Zomig) have been established as effective medications, and are available in a variety of formulations (subcutaneous injection, nasal spray, oral wafer, and pill). Alternatively, **dihydroergotamine (DHE)** can be administered intramuscularly, or intravenously as part of an established protocol for the treatment of status migrinosis.

⚡ IMPORTANT: All serotonergics, including DHE, are **contraindicated** in the treatment of complex migraine.

Prophylaxis

Prophylaxis for migraine consists of avoiding activities that trigger headaches. A **"migraine diet"** (elimination of chocolate, caffeine, peanuts, pizza, and hot dogs) benefits some patients. If conservative preventative measures fail, consideration needs to be given to the daily use of medications such as **tricyclic antidepressants** (e.g., amitriptyline), **cyproheptadine,** β-**blockers** (e.g., propranolol), or **calcium channel blockers** (e.g., verapamil). Miscellaneous agents, such as valproate, phenytoin, and lithium, have also been used.

Cluster Headache

Clinical Features

Cluster headache is **uncommon** in children. **Unilateral, retro-orbital pain** is the initial symptom, followed by symptoms of **hemicranial autonomic dysfunction** (e.g., injection of the conjunctiva, tearing of the eye, rhinorrhea, Horner syndrome, and flushing). Patients with cluster headaches are usually ambulatory during the attack and rarely experience nausea and vomiting.

Evaluation

Diagnosis is made on the basis of the **history and physical examination.**

Treatment

Some attacks can be aborted by having the patient breathe **100% oxygen** for 5–10 minutes. **Lithium** is considered by some to be the prophylactic agent of choice.

Brain Tumor

Headaches are a common complaint in children, but brain tumors are a **rare cause.** However, 50%–70% of children with brain tumors may present with headache. **Posterior fossa tumors** (e.g., ependymomas, pontine gliomas, medulloblastomas, and cerebellar astrocytomas) most commonly present with headaches.

Clinical Features

Nausea, vomiting, visual disturbances, and lethargy may be noted. The headache may **worsen with recumbency. Papilledema and sixth cranial nerve palsy** may be seen. Children with brain tumors frequently present with symptoms of **increased intracranial pressure (ICP),** as well as other symptoms that correlate with the location of the tumor (e.g., seizures, focal deficits).

Evaluation

MRI is the imaging study of choice for diagnosing a brain tumor, although **CT** is adequate for most patients.

Treatment

Treatment consists of **surgery, chemotherapy, and radiation therapy,** singly or in combination.

Pseudotumor Cerebri

Etiology

Pseudotumor cerebri is a condition in which there is **increased ICP without a mass lesion or hydrocephalus.** Pseudotumor cerebri has been associated with **obesity, menses, and the use of various medications** (e.g., tetracycline, corticosteroids).

Clinical Features

Headache is the most common symptom, often accompanied by **visual obscuration and diplopia. Decreased visual acuity** with an **expanded blind spot and papilledema** are found on examination.

Evaluation

An **emergent head CT** should be done on **all patients presenting with papilledema.** If the head CT shows **no evidence of obstructive hydrocephalus,** then an LP can be done safely. The LP must be performed in a recumbent position in a relaxed patient to accurately measure pressure. Opening pressure will be greater than 200 mm H_2O and the spinal fluid should show no evidence of infection.

Treatment

The **first LP** should alleviate most symptoms, after which the administration of **acetazolamide** will maintain lower pressures. The patient should be **followed by an ophthalmologist** to monitor visual deficits.

Chronic, Nonprogressive Headache

Etiology

This category encompasses **tension headaches, conversion disorders, depression, and malingering.**

Clinical Features

Pain is usually **diffuse and generalized,** with a **dull, aching quality.** Nonprogressive headache is not associated with neurologic disturbances.

Evaluation and Treatment

Nonprogressive headache is a **diagnosis of exclusion.** Treatment is difficult; administration of **amitriptyline** with use of **biofeedback** can be of benefit. Concomitant **counseling** may be needed as well.

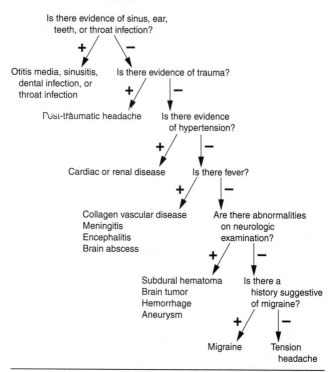

FIGURE 38.1. Approach to the patient with headache.

▼ APPROACH TO THE PATIENT (FIGURE 38.1)

Suggested Readings

Barlow CF: Migraine in the infant and toddler. *J Child Neurol* 9(1):92–94, 1994.

Fenichel GM: *Clinical Pediatric Neurology: A Signs and Symptoms Approach,* 4th ed. Philadelphia, WB Saunders, 2001, pp 77–116.

Hanson RR: Headaches in childhood. *Semin Neurol* 3(1):51–60, 1988.

Rothner AD: Headaches in children and adolescents—classification and recommendations. *Postgrad Med* 81(8):223–230, 1987.

Schulman EA, Silberstein SD: Symptomatic and prophylactic treatment of migraine and tension-type headache. *Headache* 42 (suppl 2):16–21, 1992.

Silberstein S, Lipton R: Overview of diagnosis and treatment of migraine. *Neurology* 44(10):6–16, 1994.

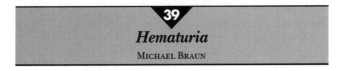

Hematuria
MICHAEL BRAUN

▼ INTRODUCTION

Hematuria, as defined by the presence of greater than 5 red blood cells/(RBCs/HPF) by light microscopy on two or more consecutive samples, is a common pediatric problem. Hematuria can originate as a **primary disorder** from any portion of the urinary system or as a **sign of systemic disease.** The list of potential causes of hematuria is extensive.

▼ DIFFERENTIAL DIAGNOSIS LIST

Infectious

Pyelonephritis
Cystitis
Urethritis

Malignancy

Wilms tumor
Renal cell carcinoma
Angiolipoma

Hematologic

Sickle cell trait/disease
Protein C deficiency
Protein S deficiency

Metabolic

Hypercalcuria

Idiopathic
Vitamin D excess
Distal renal tubular acidosis
Bartter syndrome
Hyperparathyroidism
Immobilization
Tumors

Hyperoxaluria

Primary
Enteric
Short bowel syndrome
Inflammatory bowel disease

Hyperuricosuria

Tumors (leukemia/lymphoma)
Gout
Lesch-Nyhan syndrome

Cystinuria

Glomerular Disorders

Alport syndrome
Benign familial hematuria
Benign hematuria (nonfamilial)

Cystic Disease

Polycystic kidney disease
Simple cysts
Multicystic dysplasia

Glomerulonephritis

Hypocomplementemic

Acute poststreptococcal glomerulonephritis
Lupus nephritis
Membranoproliferative glomerulonephritis

Normocomplementic

IgA nephropathy
Membranous nephropathy
Henoch-Schönlein purpura
Hemolytic uremic syndrome
Focal segmental sclerosis

Miscellaneous

Renal vein thrombosis
Vasculitis
Obstruction of the collecting system
Drugs
Trauma
Exercise
Foreign body
Munchausen syndrome

▼ DIFFERENTIAL DIAGNOSIS DISCUSSION

The most common causes of persistent microscopic hematuria and gross hematuria are listed in Table 39.1.

Urinary Tract Infection (UTI)

Etiology

The frequency of specific bacterial pathogens varies with age. Although *Escherichia coli* and gram-negative bacteria typically predominate, other infectious agents such as group B streptococci, coagulase-negative staphylococci, *Neisseria Gonorrhoeae*, chlamydia, parasites, and viruses (adenovirus) can also be found. Worldwide the most common infectious cause of hematuria is **schistosomiasis.** Individuals with recurrent UTIs have a high frequency of **associated disorders,** including structural abnormalities of the urinary tract, voiding dysfunction, poor hygiene, chronic constipation, and spinal cord abnormalities.

TABLE 39.1.   Common Causes of Hematuria

Gross Hematuria* Microscopic Hematuria	Persistent
UTI (49%)	Hypercalcuria
Perineal irritation (11%) hematuria (non-familial)	Benign
Meatal stenosis with ulceration (7%) familial hematuria	Benign
Unknown (9%) nephropathy	IgA
Trauma (7%)	Alports syndrome
Acute nephritis (3%)	Idiopathic
Coagulopathy (3%)	
Stone (2%)	

UTI = urinary tract infection; IgA = immunoglobulin A.

* From Ingelfinger JR, Davis AE, Grupe WE: Frequency and etiology of gross hematuria in a general pediatric setting. *Pediatrics* 59:557–561, 1977.

Clinical Features

Because UTIs present in young infants and toddlers with fever, vomiting, irritability, and poor feeding, it can be **difficult to differentiate UTIs from other causes of febrile illnesses.** In older children, organ-specific complaints of dysuria, frequency, urgency, or loss of bladder control are clinically useful and more common.

▟ **HINT** Severity of illness may help discriminate lower tract UTIs (cystitis) from upper tract infections (pyelonephritis) in young children. Upper urinary tract infections are more commonly found in older children with complaints of high fever, costovertebral tenderness, and manifestations of systemic illness.

Evaluation

A detailed history of **prior episodes** of UTIs in conjunction with the patient's voiding patterns should be sought. In adolescents risk factors for **sexually transmitted diseases** should be identified. **Physical examination** should include examination of the genitalia, abdomen, back, and neurologic integrity. **Microscopic urinalysis** frequently reveals large amounts of WBCs and bacteria. Confirmation of the diagnosis must be obtained by **urine culture.** Given the frequency of associated anatomic abnormalities, boys over the age of 6 months with an episode of UTI or girls with a second documented UTI should have **radiographic evaluation** of the urinary tract performed (i.e., renal ultrasound, VCUG).

▟ **HINT** Urinalysis by dipstick typically is positive for nitrites (produced by gram-negative bacteria) and leukocyte esterase (an enzyme found in white blood cells), although the risks of false-negative findings reduce the sensitivity of this test.

Treatment

Antibiotic therapy tailored to organism-specific antibiotic sensitivities is the primary therapy for UTIs. Further evaluation and treatment may be required if structural abnormalities or voiding dysfunction are noted during evaluation.

Malignancy

Etiology

Wilms tumor accounts for greater than 90% of childhood malignancies that arise from the urogenital tract. Other tumors include renal cell carcinoma, mesoblastic nephroma, rhabdomyosarcoma, hemangioma, and sarcomas. Up to 80% of patients with **tuberous sclerosis** may develop hematuria associated with hemorrhage from renal angiolipomas.

Clinical Features

Wilms tumor typically presents as an **abdominal mass with or without associated abdominal pain.** Microscopic **hematuria** is found in about 50% of patients at presentation, and gross hematuria is unusual. Hematuria as a sole presenting feature of Wilms tumor is exceedingly rare. Renal cell carcinoma frequently presents with isolated hematuria, particularly in the adult population; however, this tumor is very uncommon in the pediatric population.

Evaluation/Treatment

Wilms tumor and other urologic malignancies are suggested by the finding of a **renal mass** on physical examination or by ultrasound or computed tomography (CT) scan. Further evaluation and treatment should be directed by oncological/surgical referral.

Sickle Cell-Associated Hematuria

Etiology

Hematuria is a **common manifestation** of sickle cell hemoglobinopathy. Affecting patients with either sickle cell disease or sickle cell trait (hemoglobin S heterozygotes), it is thought to be due to sickling and sludging of RBCs in the renal medulla. Typically occurring in **adolescent males,** it can be precipitated by **trauma, exercise, dehydration,** or **infection. Papillary necrosis** is also seen with severe dehydration and renal infarction. When hematuria is associated with significant proteinuria (>50 mg/dl) the possibility of concurrent **focal segmental glomerular sclerosis** should be considered.

Clinical Features

Hematuria can be painless or painful and can range from microscopic to severe gross hematuria.

▲ **HINT** Sickle cell nephropathy frequently is accompanied by a loss of urinary concentrating ability (isosthenuria).

Evaluation

Hematuria with **little to no proteinuria** is typical. Severe gross hematuria associated with pain or significant proteinuria requires **evaluation of renal function** and possibly **renal imaging** (nuclear scan or renal ultrasound). In patients with suspected, but not confirmed, sickle cell disease, **hemoglobin electrophoresis** should be obtained.

Treatment

Treatment is focused on **hydration** and, depending on the severity of symptoms, **alkalinization** of the urine with bicarbonate or loop diuretics. In severe cases, **vasopressin, blood transfusion,** or **surgical intervention** may be required.

Trauma

Traumatic injury to the urogenital tract is frequently seen with blunt force trauma, and may be **life threatening,** depending on the severity of injury.

> **HINT** The presence of hematuria with minimal traumatic injury is highly suggestive of anatomic abnormalities of the kidney or collecting system.

Evaluation

Hematuria associated with renal trauma requires evaluation by **CT scan, renal ultrasound,** or **intravenous pyelography (IVP).** When traumatic injury to the lower urinary tract is suspected, any imaging study involving placement of urethral or bladder catheters should be ordered only with urologic consultation.

Treatment

Treatment is directed on the basis of severity of injury. Most renal contusions or lacerations can be managed **conservatively;** however, significant lacerations of the kidney or injury to the collecting system or lower urinary tract may require **emergent surgical intervention.**

Hypercalciuria

Etiology

Hypercalciuria occurs in states of both **hypercalcemia** and **eucalcemia.** In eucalcemic patients, the most common cause is idiopathic; other causes include vitamin D excess, immobilization, Cushing syndrome, distal renal tubular acidosis, and Bartter syndrome. Disorders associated with hypercalcemia include hyperparathyroidism, vitamin D intoxication, hypophosphatasia, tumors, and immobilization bone resorption.

Clinical Features

Idiopathic hypercalcuria typically presents with **asymptomatic microscopic hematuria.** As with secondary forms of hypercalcuria, these patients can present with gross hematuria, renal colic, and dysuria.

Evaluation

The initial screening test for hypercalcuria is a **urine calcium-to-creatinine ratio** on a spot urine sample; a ratio of greater than 0.2 in older children and adults is highly suggestive of hypercalcuria. Normal values are higher in infants and young children. Confirmation should be obtained by **24-hour urine collection** with an excretion of greater than 4 mg/kg/24 hours. **Serum chemistries,** including calcium, phosphorus, magnesium, urine pH, and renal function, should also be obtained. A detailed **family history** for stone disease, diet history, and evaluation of medications and nutritional supplements should be sought. **Renal ultrasound** for evaluation of urolithiasis or nephrocalcinosis is recommended.

Treatment

Treatment of secondary hypercalcuria is directed toward the underlying disorder. Treatment of patients with idiopathic hyperkaluria is controversial. **Increased fluid intake** is often recommended, as is a trial of **thiazide diuretics** to reduce calcium excretion. These children are at increased risk of kidney stone formation.

Urolithiasis

Etiology

The differential diagnosis of urolithiasis is based on the **mineral content of the renal stone** and includes disorders of calcium, oxalate, cystine, and purine metabolism. The causes of calcium stones are discussed earlier. Disorders of oxalate metabolism result in the excretion of excess oxalate in the urine, precipitating calcium oxalate stone formation. Cystinuria, a genetic deficiency in the dibasic amino acid transporters, results in decreased reabsorption of all dibasic amino acids. As a result of its low solubility, cystine forms crystals in the urine and promotes stone formation. Disorders of purine metabolism induce hyperuricemia and promote uric acid stones. While not common in this country, infectious stones are the most common cause worldwide. Staghorn calculi are frequently associated with chronic *Proteus mirabilis* infections.

Clinical Features

Stone disease typically presents with **grossly bloody urine and renal colic:** severe crampy abdominal or flank pain. Presentation with microscopic hematuria, penile pain, and passage of the stone or gravel may also be seen.

Evaluation

A family history of stone disease is frequently noted, particularly in older patients. **Renal ultrasound, IVP, or spiral CT scan** should be considered. If a stone is suspected, **blood chemistries** including calcium, phosphorus, magnesium, uric acid, and creatinine; **urine pH;** and **24-hour urine collections** for calcium, cystine, oxalate, phosphorus, and uric excretion should be obtained. UTI, either acute or chronic, should be excluded by **urine culture.** Attempts should be made to **recover the stone** or gravel for analysis of mineral content.

⚉ HINT Simple X-rays can detect kidney stones if the stone is radio-opaque (calcium, oxalate, cystine, or struvite). Urate stones are radiolucent and not seen by plain film.

Treatment

Management of these patients is twofold. First, **treat the acute event.** Mineral solubility is increased with hydration and either alkalinization or acidification of the urine. Pain management should be optimized. Surgical intervention or lithotripsy is indicated in cases of urinary obstruction or recurrent stones with superimposed UTIs. Once the cause has been determined, therapy to **prevent stone recurrence** can be implemented; this includes increased fluid intake to ensure dilute hypotonic urine, dietary manipulation, and drug therapy in some cases.

Alport Syndrome

Etiology

Alport syndrome is defined by the presence of **hereditary nephritis** associated with **sensorineural hearing loss.** This disorder occurs in 1 in 1500 live births. Eighty-five percent of cases are transmitted as an X-linked dominant trait [autosomal dominant (AD) and autosomal recessive (AR) transmission has been reported]. The primary genetic defect involves the gene for collagen 4A5; mutations have been described in the A3 and A4 chains in patients with AR and AD forms of Alport's.

Clinical Presentation

Alport syndrome presents as intermittent or persistent **microscopic hematuria,** although gross hematuria and proteinuria may also be seen. In children, both **ocular defects** (anterior lenticonus and macular lesions) and high-frequency **sensorineural hearing loss** can be found. While this syndrome typically has an indolent progression to renal failure, rapid progression to renal failure does occur.

Evaluation

Alport is strongly suggested by a **family history of chronic renal failure associated with hearing loss.** Diagnosis is confirmed by **renal biopsy.** Genetic analysis is available on a research basis, and family screening can be considered.

Therapy

There is **no current therapy** to prevent the progression to renal failure. In families with a history of Alport, progression usually follows a similar pattern. Males typically have a worse prognosis than do affected females.

Benign Familial Hematuria (BFH)

Etiology

Benign familial hematuria is transmitted in an autosomal dominant fashion, although other patterns of transmission have been reported. The **genetic basis** of this disorder is thought to be due to heterozygotic mutations in the genes encoding collagen 4.

Clinical Features

This disorder is defined by the presence of persistent **microscopic hematuria without proteinuria, hearing loss, or progressive renal disease.**

Evaluation

This is a diagnosis primarily of **exclusion** and **family history.** Family history should be positive for microscopic hematuria only. Any finding of renal failure or sensorineural hearing loss in family members excludes this diagnosis and should alert the clinician to the possibility of Alport syndrome. Diagnosis can be confirmed by **renal biopsy.**

Treatment

Because this disorder is nonprogressive, **no treatment** is indicated, although patients should be followed closely.

Glomerulonephritis

Glomerulonephritis can be categorized according to serum complement (C3) levels at presentation. The most common forms of nephritis are **acute poststreptococcal glomerulonephritis (APSGN)** and IgA nephropathy. An unusual form of glomerular disease noted for its acuity at presentation is **rapidly progressive glomerulonephritis (RPGN).**

Clinical Features

Most acute episodes of nephritis present with proteinuria associated with **hematuria** or tea-colored urine. **Decreased urine output** may be noted as well as signs of **peripheral edema.** Signs of **acute renal failure** may be present; these include anuria, marked volume overload with hypertension, congestive heart failure, and hypertensive encephalopathy. APSGN typically presents 10–14 days after an upper respiratory infection with β-hemolytic streptococci or, in some cases, an episode of impetigo. IgA nephropathy is commonly associated with a viral prodrome and the subsequent development of grossly bloody urine. Signs of lethargy, weight loss, and lassitude may antecede MPGN.

Evaluation

All patients with suspected glomerulonephritis should have a complete blood count, ASO or streptozyme, C3, antinuclear antibody (ANA), blood chemistries including renal function studies, and a microscopic urinalysis performed. The presence of **RBC casts in the urine is diagnostic.** Renal biopsy may be indicated in some instances.

⚡ HINT While ASO titres can remain elevated for up to 6 months following an episode of APSGN, C3 levels should return to normal within 6 weeks after presentation; a persistently low C3 level is suggestive of MPGN.

Treatment

The treatment of acute nephritis is largely **supportive.** Careful attention to **fluid and electrolyte balance** is essential. **Urine output** should be optimized and diuretics may be needed. **Blood pressure should be carefully monitored and treated aggressively.** In some instances, **immunosuppressive or dialytic therapy** may be warranted.

Renal Vein Thrombosis (RVT)

Etiology

Renal vein thrombosis is **uncommon.** It can be seen in either **hypercoagulable states** (protein C or protein S deficiency) or with **extreme volume depletion.** It is most frequently seen in patients with **florid nephrotic syndrome.** It is also a common cause of hematuria in neonates, particularly in infants of diabetic mothers.

Clinical Features

Patients typically present with an **abrupt drop in urine output** associated with an **enlarging abdominal mass.**

TABLE 39.2.	Drugs Associated with Hematuria	
Ampicillin	Aspirin
Penicillin	Amitriptyline
Polymyxin	Chlorpromazine
Sulfonamide	Cholchine
Indomethacin	Phenylbutazone
Cyclophosphamide	Gold salts

Evaluation

Patients may have signs of **hypotension or shock.** Complete blood counts show **falling hemoglobin levels** and **low platelet counts.** Renal ultrasound demonstrates an **enlarged kidney** with little to no blood flow by Doppler.

Treatment

Intravascular volume repletion is critical. Depending on the severity and extension of the thrombus, **thrombolytic therapy** may be warranted. On rare occasions **surgical removal** of the clot may be required.

Medications

Etiology

Microscopic hematuria due to drug exposure is not uncommon. While some of these medications are commonly used in pediatrics, most are not (Table 39.2).

Clinical Features

Patients typically present with **isolated microscopic hematuria** without other associated findings on physical examination or biochemical analysis. **Cyclophosphamide** is frequently associated with gross hematuria that can be severe in some cases.

Evaluation

A thorough **drug history** is often all that is needed.

Treatment

The **offending agent should be withdrawn** if possible. Usually no further treatment is indicated; however, in the case of cyclophosphamide, induced hemorrhagic cystitis, urologic evaluation, and treatment may be needed.

▼ EVALUATION OF HEMATURIA (FIGURE 39.1)

Patient History

A **complete and thorough history** is essential to guiding the diagnostic evaluation of hematuria. The following information should be obtained:

▼ Previous episodes of gross hematuria or UTI
▼ Pattern of hematuria (initial, total, terminal)
▼ History of recent upper respiratory tract infections, sore throat, or impetigo
▼ Dysuria, frequency, voiding patterns, fever, weight loss, abdominal or flank pain, skin lesions

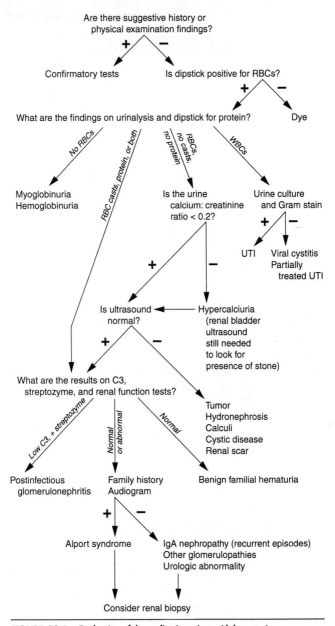

FIGURE 39.1. Evaluation of the pediatric patient with hematuria.
C3 = activated third component of complement; *IgA* = immunoglobulin A;
RBCs = red blood cells; *UTI* = urinary tract infection; *WBCs* = white blood cells.

▼ Trauma or foreign body
▼ Drug, dietary, and vitamin or nutritional supplements
▼ Family history of renal disease, hematuria, urolithiasis, sickle cell disease, coagulation disorders, hearing loss
▼ Travel to developing countries

Physical Examination

The examination of the patient should focus on the following:

▼ Blood pressure
▼ Edema
▼ Rash or purpura
▼ Arthritis
▼ Abdominal mass
▼ Ocular defects
▼ Genito-urinary abnormalities

Laboratory Evaluation

The diagnostic evaluation of hematuria should be guided by findings on history and physical examination and may include:

▼ Fresh urinalysis with microscopic examination of sediment for RBCs, crystals, and casts (Table 39.3 for causes of discolored urine)
▼ Serum electrolytes: BUN, creatinine, calcium, phosphorus, uric acid
▼ Complete blood count with platelets
▼ Complement studies (C3, C4, CH50 or THC)
▼ ASO/Streptozyme
▼ ANA
▼ Urine culture
▼ Urine Ca/Cr ratio or 24-hour urine Ca excretion
▼ Urinary excretion of cystine, oxalate, phosphorus, citrate, and urate
▼ Urine pH

✂ HINT   Hematuria, even gross hematuria, does not cause proteinuria per se. The finding of >50 mg/dl of protein by dipstick strongly suggests a glomerular pathological condition.

Diagnostic Modalities

Radiographic imaging is frequently indicated. **Ultrasound evaluation** of the kidneys and bladder may demonstrate the presence of tumors, urinary obstruction, renal stones, or evidence of renal parenchymal disease. Small stones or abnormalities of the collecting system may be missed by ultrasound.

TABLE 39.3. Causes of Discolored Urine (Hemastix Negative)

Urates
Beets
Blackberries
Rifampin
Phenazopyridine

IVP are useful for delineating the anatomic structure of the collecting systems as well as for defining functional obstructions. CT scans also provide valuable anatomic information, in addition to information about the presence of stones, tumors, or obstructions. Like IVPs, CT scans are more invasive and require the use of a contrast agent. Additional studies such as cystoscopy, angiography, or renal biopsy should be considered in consultation with a sub-specialist.

▼ TREATMENT OF HEMATURIA

The treatment of hematuria is driven by the underlying pathophysiology and is in large part **conservative.** Hematuria with concurrent proteinuria, hypertension, renal failure, trauma, or severe hemorrhage may indicate the need for more **aggressive therapy.**

Suggested Readings

Diven SC, Travis LB: A practical primary care approach to hematuria in children. *Pediatr Nephrol* 14:65–72, 2000.

Feld LG, Meyers KE, Kaplan BS, et al: Limited evaluation of microscopic hematuria in pediatrics. *Pediatrics* 102(4):E42, 1998.

Feld LG, Waz WR, Perez LM, et al: Hematuria: an integrated medical and surgical approach. *Pediatr Clin North Am* 44(5):1191–1210, 1997.

Ingelfinger JR, Davis AE, Grupe WE: Frequency and etiology of gross hematuria in a general pediatric setting. *Pediatrics* 59:557–561, 1977.

Lieu TA, Grasmeder HM III, Kaplan BS: An approach to the evaluation and treatment of microscopic hematuria. *Pediatr Clin of North Am* 38(3):579–592, 1991.

Mahan JD, Turman MA, Menster MI: Evaluation of hematuria, proteinuria, and hypertension in adolescents. *Pediatr Clin North Am* 44(6): 1573–1589, 1997.

Polito C, La Manna A, Cioce F, et al: Clinical presentation and natural course of idiopathic hypercalciuria in children. *Pediatr Nephrol* 15(3–4):211–214, 2000.

Roy S III: Hematuria. *Pediatr Ann* 25(5):284–287, 1996.

40

Hemolysis

KIM SMITH-WHITLEY

▼ INTRODUCTION

Hemolysis is **increased red blood cell (RBC) destruction with compensatory increased RBC production.** The patient with hemolysis usually presents with symptoms of **anemia and hyperbilirubinemia.** Hemolysis may rarely be an incidental finding when a complete blood count (CBC) is obtained for other reasons.

The causes of hemolysis can be classified as intrinsic or extrinsic. **Intrinsic causes** are abnormalities that occur within the RBC (i.e., changes that involve the RBC membrane, enzymes, or hemoglobin). **Extrinsic causes** involve

TABLE 40.1. Intravascular and Extravascular Causes of Hemolysis

Intravascular hemolysis
Disseminated intravascular coagulation (DIC)
Hemolytic-uremic syndrome
Burns
Acute hemolytic transfusion reactions
Organ graft rejection
Prosthetic heart valves
Hemangiomas
March hemoglobinuria
Drugs
Venoms
Infections
Acute G6PD deficiency
Paroxysmal nocturnal hemoglobinuria
Extravascular hemolysis
Alloimmune hemolysis
Autoimmune hemolysis
Red blood cell (RBC) membrane abnormalities
RBC enzyme abnormalities
Hemoglobinopathies
Thalassemia syndromes

G6PD = glucose-6-phosphate dehydrogenase.

damage to normal RBCs by any external process. A second classification system categorizes the causes of hemolysis according to whether **RBC destruction occurs intravascularly or extravascularly** (Table 40.1).

▼ DIFFERENTIAL DIAGNOSIS LIST
RBC Membrane Abnormalities

Hereditary spherocytosis (HS)
Hereditary elliptocytosis (HE)
Hereditary pyropoikilocytosis
Infantile pyknocytosis
Paroxysmal nocturnal hemoglobinuria

Enzyme Defects

Embden-Meyerhof pathway defects—pyruvate kinase deficiency
Nucleotide metabolism defects—pyrimidine-5'-nucleotidase deficiency
Hexose monophosphate shunt defects—glucose-6-phosphate dehydrogenase (G6PD) deficiency

Hemoglobin Disorders

Hemoglobinopathies—hemoglobin S, C, D, E
Thalassemia syndromes—alpha-thalassemia, beta-thalassemia
Unstable hemoglobin syndromes—congenital Heinz-body hemolytic anemia, hemoglobin M disease

Alloimmune Causes

Hemolytic disease of the newborn
Hemolytic transfusion reaction

Autoimmune Causes

Warm-Reactive Antibodies

Idiopathic
Neoplastic causes
Immunodeficiency

Infectious Causes

Viruses—e.g., cytomegalovirus (CMV), hepatitis, influenza, coxsackievirus
Bacteria—e.g., *Streptococcus, Escherichia coli, Salmonella typhi*
Postimmunization—e.g., diphtheria-tetanus-pertussis (DTP), polio, typhoid

Toxic Causes

Antibiotics—penicillin, cephalothin, tetracycline, rifampin, sulfonamides
Phenacetin
5-Aminosalicylic acid
Quinine and quinidine
Insulin
Lead
Chlorpromazine

Collagen Vascular Disease

Systemic lupus erythematosus (SLE)
Scleroderma
Juvenile rheumatoid arthritis (JRA)
Polyarteritis nodosa
Dermatomyositis

Cold-Reactive Antibodies

Infectious Causes

Mycoplasma
Epstein-Barr virus (EBV)

Neoplastic Causes

Lymphoproliferative disease

Nonimmune Causes

Microangiopathic hemolytic anemia
Hypersplenism

Toxic Causes

Drugs—e.g., vitamin K, phenacetin, sulfones, benzenes, phenylhydralazine
Lead
Venoms

Infectious Causes

Viruses—EBV, hepatitis
Bacteria—*Clostridium perfringens, E. coli, Streptococcus*
Parasites—malaria, histoplasmosis

▼ DIFFERENTIAL DIAGNOSIS DISCUSSION
Hereditary Spherocytosis (HS)

Etiology

HS is the most common **inherited RBC membrane defect** and is most often seen in patients of **northern European descent.** RBC skeletal protein abnormalities lead to membrane instability and subsequent **hemolytic anemia** in affected individuals. Although HS is inherited in an autosomal dominant fashion, 10%–25% of all cases are sporadic.

Clinical Features

The clinical severity depends on the severity of the hemolysis, which can be **mild to severe,** and on the degree of compensation by the patient. Half of patients have a history of **neonatal hyperbilirubinemia.** The classic clinical presentation of hemolytic anemia is **jaundice, pallor, and splenomegaly.** Patients may have episodes of increased hemolysis with infections, transient aplastic crises, and splenomegaly.

Evaluation

The **peripheral blood smear** shows an **increased** number of **spherocytes** (i.e., small, round, dark-staining RBCs that lack central pallor). The **osmotic fragility test** demonstrates decreased resistance to osmotic lysis as compared with normal RBCs.

Treatment

Treatment of HS is **supportive.** Although transfusion of RBCs may be necessary for transient aplastic episodes, only a small number of patients depend on **RBC transfusions. Splenectomy** should be considered in children with poor growth or increased RBC transfusion requirements.

Hereditary Elliptocytosis (HE)

Etiology

Like HS, HE is **inherited** in an autosomal dominant pattern, but sporadic mutations are not as common.

Clinical Features

Most children with HE are **asymptomatic** but may present for evaluation with a transient aplastic or a hyperhemolytic episode.

Evaluation

The **peripheral blood smear** will reveal more than 15% elliptocytes (i.e., elongated, cigar-shaped, or oval RBCs). The peripheral blood smear in normal patients may contain up to 15% elliptocytes.
    The differential diagnosis of HE includes **iron-deficiency anemia.**

Treatment

Splenectomy is curative but is not indicated unless anemia is profound.

Glucose-6-Phosphate Dehydrogenase (G6PD) Deficiency

Etiology

G6PD deficiency, **inherited** in an X-linked pattern, is the most common enzyme deficiency of the hexose monophosphate shunt. Affected patients are either heterozygous males or homozygous females. There is an increased incidence of G6PD deficiency in people of **African and Mediterranean descent.** Affected children may have **drug-induced hemolysis** or a **chronic hemolytic process.**

Medications and substances that can induce hemolysis in G6PD-deficient patients include acetanilid, doxorubicin, methylene blue, naphthalene, nitrofurantoin, primaquine, pamaquine, and sulfa drugs.

Clinical Features

Presentation depends on the type of G6PD deficiency variant inherited.

▼ **Patients with the African variant** of G6PD deficiency rarely present for evaluation with neonatal jaundice or chronic hemolytic anemia. They are usually identified when they present for evaluation following drug (or other substance) exposure. Drug-induced hemolysis can be severe, involving the acute onset of pallor, malaise, scleral icterus, dark urine, and abdominal or back pain.

▼ **Patients with the Mediterranean variant** of G6PD deficiency usually have a more severe form of G6PD deficiency and may present for evaluation with signs and symptoms of neonatal hyperbilirubinemia, chronic hemolytic anemia, or drug-induced hemolysis.

Evaluation

If G6PD deficiency is suspected, a **blood sample** should be sent for analysis of G6PD enzyme activity. **"Bite" or "blister" cells** (RBCs with small outpouchings or blisters on the outer rim) may be identified on the **peripheral blood smear.**

Treatment

Drug-induced intravascular hemolysis is **self-limited and reversible** when the offending drug is discontinued. Children with a **chronic hemolytic process** may require **RBC transfusions** for exacerbations of anemia characterized by cardiovascular compromise.

Sickle Cell Disease (SCD)

Etiology

Hemoglobin S (Hb S) is the predominant hemoglobin in the group of **genetic disorders** that encompass SCD. Hb S is an abnormal hemoglobin caused by a single nucleotide base substitution: valine replaces glutamic acid in the sixth position of the β globin chain, resulting in structural changes in the RBC membrane. SCD variants include SCD-SS, SCD-SC, SCD-Sβ-thalassemia, and others.

Clinical Features

Patients with SCD disorders have **hemolytic anemia** and **vaso-occlusive complications** and are at **increased risk for infection.** People with **sickle cell trait** are generally **asymptomatic** but may have occasional hematuria. Currently, most patients are identified through **newborn screening** for hemoglobinopathies. Others, not identified as newborns, present with signs and symptoms of SCD complications:

▼ **Infection.** Children with SCD, especially those younger than 3 years, are at increased risk for the development of bacterial infections as a result of splenic hypofunction and other immunologic abnormalities. *Streptococcus pneumoniae* is the most commonly implicated agent; however, *Haemophilus influenzae*, *E. coli*, *Salmonella* species, and *Staphylococcus aureus* are common pathogens in patients with SCD as well. Pneumococcal sepsis can be rapidly fatal in these patients, despite the use of penicillin prophylaxis and immunization with polyvalent pneumococcal vaccines.

▼ **Osteomyelitis.** Patients with SCD are at increased risk for osteomyelitis; therefore, any child with SCD, bone pain, and fever or soft tissue swelling should be evaluated for the presence of osteomyelitis. The most common organisms causing osteomyelitis in this patient population are *Salmonella* and *S. aureus*. It is difficult to discriminate between osteomyelitis and a vaso-occlusive episode in the child with SCD. Evaluation should include radiographic studies and orthopedic evaluation.

▼ **Stroke.** Children with SCD, particularly types SS and $S\beta^0$-thalassemia, may develop hemorrhagic or infarctive strokes. The clinical presentation includes seizures, hemiplegia, difficulty speaking, or a change in mental status; however, subtle intermittent neurologic symptoms or severe headaches may indicate neurologic complications as well.

▼ **Acute chest syndrome (ACS)** is one of the leading causes of morbidity and mortality in patients with SCD. The cause of ACS may be multifactorial in an individual patient and includes infection, pulmonary vascular damage, infarction, and cytokine release. ACS is classically defined as a new infiltrate on chest radiograph.

▼ **Painful episodes,** the most common complications of SCD, are unpredictable and often progressive. The exact pathophysiology is unknown but may be related to occlusion and damage of the microvasculature, leading to organ ischemia and infarction.

▼ **Splenic sequestration** is one of the leading causes of death in children with SCD. These children develop hypovolemic shock as the result of the loss of large volumes of blood into the spleen. Although the spleen in children with SCD-SS has usually autoinfarcted by the time the patient reaches 8 years of age, children with SCD-SC and SCD-$S\beta^+$ thalassemia can present with splenic sequestration at any age. Acute splenic sequestration episodes are characterized by splenic enlargement with evidence of hemoglobin levels below baseline and increased reticulocyte counts. Mild to moderate thrombocytopenia may also occur. Any child who has had one episode of splenic sequestration is at increased risk for another.

▼ **Priapism** is a prolonged, painful penile erection and can occur in boys and men with SCD at any age. Priapism may be sustained over a long period of time or may be "stuttering" in nature (i.e., characterized by recurrent episodes within short periods of time).

▼ **Transient aplastic episode** [see also Chapter 58, "Pallor (Paleness)"]. Any patient with chronic hemolytic anemia can experience aplastic episode (i.e., a transient arrest in erythropoiesis characterized by the acute onset of pallor, frequently following a viral illness). Parvovirus B19 infection is the most common cause. The anemia is often severe and reticulocyte counts are usually less than 1%.

Evaluation

Important historic information to obtain from patients with SCD includes:

▼ Specific disease phenotype
▼ Baseline hemoglobin and reticulocyte counts
▼ Past disease complications
▼ Dates of last transfusion and related complications

Appropriate laboratory tests in a child suspected of having SCD include a hemoglobin electrophoresis, CBC, and reticulocyte count.

Treatment

▼ **Suspected infection.** Any child with SCD and fever should be considered bacteremic or septic until proven otherwise. Blood cultures should be obtained promptly and parenteral antibiotics strongly considered, particularly in children with severe disease phenotypes (SS, Sβ^0thalassemia).

▼ **Stroke.** Exchange transfusions are recommended for patients with acute strokes to decrease further cerebral damage. In children who have had a stroke, chronic transfusion therapy is strongly recommended to decrease the high risk of recurrent stroke.

▼ **ACS.** Because the underlying cause is often unclear, supportive care should include antibiotics, analgesics, aggressive pulmonary toilet, and supplemental oxygen as needed. Transfusion therapy is controversial in this setting. However, any child who is experiencing hypoxia or significant difficulty in breathing should receive an RBC transfusion, either simple or exchange.

⚡ HINT Any patient who has experienced an episode of ACS is at increased risk for recurrence. This risk may be decreased with chronic transfusion or hydroxyurea therapy.

▼ **Painful episode.** Care is directed at pain control and close monitoring of patients for other disease complications and side effects of medications. Musculoskeletal pain can be managed acutely with analgesics and non-pharmacologic therapies (e.g., heat and relaxation). Dehydration should be avoided; *ACS* may be prevented by ambulation and frequent incentive spirometer use. Hydroxyurea (HU), an antimetabolite medication, has decreased painful episodes in patients with SCD-SS and SCD-Sβ^0thalassemia. However, HU therapy is best prescribed and monitored by a pediatric hematologist.

▼ **Splenic sequestration.** If transfusions are necessary, it is important to acutely transfuse small aliquots of RBCs, because the spleen will release the patient's RBCs as the sequestration episode resolves. Long-term management of these children is controversial; however, splenectomy or a chronic transfusion program should be considered for children who have experienced a life-threatening episode or repeated episodes requiring multiple transfusions.

▼ **Priapism.** If untreated, impotence may result. Initial management includes the use of intravenous hydration and analgesia. A urologist should be consulted, particularly if urinary retention develops or if detumescence does not occur promptly despite medical management.

▼ **Transient aplastic episode.** Because most children have parvovirus infections, hospitalized patients should be admitted to single rooms with contact and respiratory isolation. No pregnant caretakers should be permitted in the room. Children with congestive heart failure require RBC transfusion.

Hemoglobin C (Hb C)

Etiology

Hb C results from a substitution of lysine for glutamic acid in the sixth position of the β-polypeptide chain.

Clinical Features and Evaluation

Patients with **homozygous disease** usually have **mild chronic hemolytic anemia with splenomegaly** and the **peripheral blood smear** shows a marked number of **target cells.** Patients with **Hb C trait** are **asymptomatic.**

Hemoglobin E (Hb E)

Etiology

Hb E is a common hemoglobin variant, particularly in the **Asian population.**

Clinical Features and Evaluation

Patients with **Hb E trait** are **asymptomatic.** Patients with **homozygous Hb E** have **mild hemolytic anemia, target cells and microcytosis on the peripheral blood smear, and a mean corpuscular volume (MCV)** that is usually **less than 70 fl.** Variants of Hb E with α-thalassemia and β-thalassemia exist as well.

Thalassemia

Etiology

The thalassemia syndromes represent a group of **inherited disorders** caused by **decreased or absent** synthesis of the α **or** β **human globin chains.** The thalassemia syndromes occur more frequently in **Mediterranean, Asian, and African populations.** Because of unbalanced globin chain synthesis, unstable hemoglobin complexes are produced. Precipitation of the unpaired globin chains and subsequent RBC membrane damage cause **premature RBC lysis,** which leads to **hemolytic anemia** and a compensatory **increase in RBC production** in affected individuals.

Clinical Features—α-Thalassemia

There are four clinical classifications of the α-thalassemias:

▼ **One α gene mutation.** These patients, the silent carriers of α-thalassemia, have no clinical symptoms, a normal hemoglobin level, and a normal MCV.

▼ **Two α gene mutations.** Patients with α-thalassemia trait, caused by two α gene mutations, have mild microcytic hypochromic anemia. Because the degree of microcytosis is out of proportion to the degree of anemia, the likelihood of iron-deficiency anemia as a possible diagnosis is diminished.

▼ **Three α gene mutations.** Hemoglobin H (Hb H) disease, caused by three α gene mutations, is characterized by moderate to severe microcytic hypochromic anemia. The excess β chains form tetramers, a fast-migrating hemoglobin (seen on hemoglobin electrophoresis) referred to as "Hb H." Hemoglobin Bart's or γ globin chain tetramers can also be present in neonates with Hb H disease or α-thalassemia trait. In Hb H disease, anemia may be severe, with hemoglobin values ranging from 3 to 4 g/dl. Hemolytic episodes may be exacerbated by fever or infection.

▼ **Four α gene mutations.** Hydrops fetalis is caused by mutations of all four α genes. These infants fail to produce α globin in utero. They are severely anemic, develop congestive heart failure, and are usually stillborn.

Clinical Features—β-Thalassemia

The β thalassemia syndromes are categorized according to three levels of clinical severity:

▼ **Thalassemia minor (β-thalassemia trait).** Patients are asymptomatic and have mild hypochromic anemia.

▼ **Thalassemia intermedia.** Patients have mild to moderate hypochromic anemia and are not transfusion dependent.

▼ **Thalassemia major (Cooley anemia).** Patients have severe hypochromic microcytic anemia (characterized by hemoglobin levels of 3–4 g/dl) and usually present for evaluation within the first 2 years of life with pallor, lethargy, and hepatosplenomegaly. Bony expansion, a sign of exuberant intramedullary hematopoiesis, may be found on physical examination.

Evaluation

Patients with **thalassemia major** may be diagnosed by **newborn screening for hemoglobinopathies. Hemoglobin A may be low to absent.** For all patients suspected to have thalassemia, a **CBC** should be obtained from the patient and both parents. If **microcytic anemia** is present in either parent or both parents, then **hemoglobin electrophoresis studies** should be obtained.

α- and β-**Thalassemia trait must be distinguished from iron-deficiency anemia** since all patients with these disorders may have an MCV of less than 75 fl. In patients with β-thalassemia trait, the MCV would be disproportionately low for the mild degree of anemia seen if the anemia were caused by iron deficiency, and the RBC mass would be increased.

▼ The red blood cell distribution width index (RDW) is increased in iron deficiency but normal in thalassemia trait.

▼ Hemoglobin electrophoresis shows an increased amount of Hb A2, Hb F, or both in patients with β-thalassemia trait, but not in those with α-thalassemia trait or iron deficiency.

Iron studies may not suggest the presence of iron deficiency in patients with β-thalassemia; however, iron-deficiency anemia and β-thalassemia trait can coexist and make diagnosis difficult. After treatment for iron deficiency, if the MCV remains low, then diagnostic studies for thalassemia traits should be pursued.

Treatment

Transfusion therapy in thalassemia major is directed at treating the anemia as well as suppressing endogenous RBC production. **Splenectomy** may be indicated in patients with an increasing need for RBC transfusions, in patients with significant growth retardation, or in patients in whom hypersplenism is associated with a worsening of the anemia.

Hemolytic Disease of the Newborn (Isoimmune Hemolytic Anemia)

Etiology

Hemolytic disease of the newborn results from **maternal sensitization to fetal RBC antigens** that differ from her own.

▼ **In Rh hemolytic disease,** the Rh(D)-negative mother (previously exposed to the D antigen through pregnancy or transfusion) may produce anti-D. During each subsequent pregnancy, transplacental passage of maternal antibody may cause fetal hemolysis.

▼ **No previous exposure is necessary for ABO hemolytic disease** because anti-A and anti-B are naturally occurring isohemagglutinins. ABO incompatibility is the most common cause of hemolytic disease of the newborn, but Rh incompatibility is associated with the most severe hemolysis in the fetus or the newborn.

▼ **Hemolytic disease of the newborn can also develop when the mother lacks one of the so-called minor blood group antigens** (C, E, Kell, Duffy, or Kidd) that the fetus has inherited from the father.

Clinical Features

Newborns with hemolytic disease of the newborn present for evaluation with **varying degrees of illness,** depending on the degree of anemia. Clinical manifestations result from the rate of RBC destruction and the degree of compensation. Newborns have **jaundice and anemia,** usually within the first 24 hours of life. Anemia may cause **congestive heart failure,** and, if the anemia is severe in utero, **hydrops fetalis** may develop. Neonates with hydrops fetalis usually die shortly after birth. **Hyperbilirubinemia** can also be severe and can lead to **kernicterus.**

Delayed anemia can occur in neonates who have been recognized as having isoimmune hemolytic anemia during the first few days of life or in those with mild hemolysis that was undetected initially. Hemoglobin levels may fall to 4–6 g/dl within the first 4–6 weeks of life.

Evaluation

If the patient's mother is Rh negative and the father is Rh positive, then the infant is at risk for the development of hemolysis. The **Rh-negative mother** should be **screened routinely for the presence of anti-D** during gestation and should receive **RhoGAM** (anti-D immune globulin) prophylactically at termination of pregnancy or postpartum.

Antibody bound to the surface of the neonate's RBCs can often be demonstrated using a direct **antibody test (DAT),** although a negative DAT does not rule out isoimmune hemolytic disease. The **maternal serum should be tested** for the presence of a specific antibody that may cause the hemolysis.

Treatment

Treatment is directed at reducing severe unconjugated hyperbilirubinemia and correcting severe anemia. **Exchange transfusion** should be considered if the hemoglobin level is less than 12 g/dl and falling within the first 24 hours of life or if the serum bilirubin level is greater than 20 mg/dl within the first 24 hours of life. **Phototherapy** and **hydration** for hyperbilirubinemia may be the only treatments necessary.

Details regarding the management of women at risk for carrying a fetus with Rh disease can be found in standard obstetrics textbooks. Routine immunization of mothers at risk has succeeded in decreasing the incidence of Rh hemolytic disease of the newborn in the United States.

✄ HINT If the neonate has type O blood or is Rh negative, he is not at risk for development of major blood group incompatibility. However, he may still be at risk for development of minor blood group incompatibility.

Acute Hemolytic Transfusion Reactions

Etiology

Acute hemolytic transfusion reactions result when a **recipient with preformed antibodies receives an ABO-incompatible RBC transfusion.** These **life-threatening reactions** are usually caused by the **misidentification** of the donor or recipient of the blood for transfusion and, therefore, are avoidable.

Clinical Features

Patients develop **fever, chills, and tachycardia** commensurate with the volume of blood that has been transfused. Delayed hemolytic transfusion reactions are caused by the presence of preformed antibodies to **minor blood group antigens** in previously transfused patients. These reactions usually include **back pain and dark urine.**

Evaluation

The **urine dipstick test** results may be positive for the **presence of heme** with an **absence of RBCs.** Laboratory findings include a **positive DAT** in both kinds of hemolytic transfusion reactions. **Disseminated intravascular coagulation (DIC) and renal failure** may develop.

Treatment

The first intervention when an acute hemolytic transfusion reaction is suspected is to **stop the blood transfusion.** Treatment should include **aggressive intravenous hydration** and the use of **diuretics** to prevent fluid overload. **Alkalinization** may be considered to prevent renal failure.

Autoimmune Hemolytic Anemia (AIHA)

Etiology

AIHA, which may be **idiopathic or secondary,** can cause **acute, life-threatening anemia** in the pediatric population. The idiopathic diagnosis is the more common in the pediatric population because specific causes are difficult to identify. Secondary AIHA may be caused by warm-reactive or cold-reactive antibodies and may result from infection, malignancy, collagen vascular diseases, drugs, or toxins.

Clinical Features

Children with AIHA may have a **sudden onset of pallor, fever, scleral icterus, and dark urine.** However, a more insidious onset of AIHA may be seen, particularly in children older than 10 years. **Splenomegaly** is usually present on physical examination. The course of the disease varies from a limited single short episode to a more prolonged illness, with relapses associated with infections.

Evaluation

Laboratory findings include **normochromic, normocytic anemia with sphe-rocytes** seen on **peripheral blood smear,** as well as **reticulocytosis. Hyper-bilirubinemia** is present. The **DAT is usually positive;** however, a negative DAT does not eliminate the possibility of AIHA. Childhood AIHA is usually mediated by IgG. The presence of hemolysis with IgM may be associated with *Mycoplasma* or Epstein-Barr virus infection.

Treatment

Treatment is directed at **cardiovascular support** and **decreasing the amount of RBC destruction. Prednisone** (2 mg/kg/day) is given orally if the child is stable, or the equivalent dose in a parenteral form can be given. **Urine output should be maintained** to avoid renal failure.

RBC transfusions should be avoided unless hypoxia or cardiovascular compromise is present, because severe hemolytic transfusion reactions can occur. **If RBC transfusion is necessary,** the "least incompatible" donor unit of blood should be used. The **first 15 ml of blood should be administered under very close observation.** The urine should be checked for the presence of hemoglobin, and the plasma layer of a spun hematocrit should be checked for a pink tinge consistent with hemolysis.

Microangiopathic Hemolytic Anemia

Etiology

Microangiopathic hemolytic anemia is associated with a variety of conditions, including **DIC, prosthetic heart valves, cardiac disease** (e.g., coarctation of the aorta, severe valvular disease, endocarditis), **hemolytic–uremic syndrome, thrombotic thrombocytopenic purpura, severe burns, march hemoglobin-uria, renal transplant rejection, and hemangioma.**

Clinical Features

The degree of anemia is **variable.** Thrombocytopenia may or may not be present, and **reticulocytosis** is usually present. DIC may occur.

Evaluation

The peripheral blood smear shows **prominent RBC fragments,** such as helmet cells and schistocytes.

Treatment

Treatment should be directed at the **underlying cause.**

▼ EVALUATION OF HEMOLYSIS
History and Physical Examination

A well-focused history and physical examination can direct the physician in ordering appropriate tests and making a diagnosis (Table 40.2).

✂ HINT Some patients with congenital hemolytic anemias present for evaluation during transient aplastic episodes without histories suggestive of chronic hemolysis.

TABLE 40.2. Clinical Evaluation of Pediatric Patients with Suspected Hemolytic Anemia

Question	If the Answer is "Yes," Consider . . .
History	
Is the patient a neonate?	Hemolytic disease of the newborn
Has the child had previous episodes of scleral icterus or dark urine, particularly with intercurrent illnesses?	Chronic (versus an acute) hemolytic process
Is the patient currently taking medications or has he received medications recently?	G6PD deficiency or drug-induced hemolysis, depending on the type of medications and the ethnic background of the child
Are there mothball products in the household?	G6PD deficiency
Has the patient participated in very strenuous exercise recently, such as running a marathon?	March hemoglobinuria
Does the patient have cardiac disease or prosthetic heart valves?	Microangiopathic hemolytic anemia
Has the patient had recent severe diarrheal illness or viral prodrome?	HUS and chronic hemolytic anemia
Is the patient an African-American?	G6PD deficiency, thalassemia, SCD
Is the patient of Mediterranean descent?	G6PD deficiency, thalassemia
Has the patient had a blood transfusion recently? Is the patient on a chronic transfusion protocol?	Acute or delayed hemolytic transfusion reaction, particularly if the patient is chronically transfused
Is there a family history of gallstones or splenectomy in early childhood? Is there a family history of anemia?	Chronic hemolytic anemia, inherited
Physical examination	
Is there scleral icterus, jaundice, and splenomegaly?	Hemolytic anemia
Is there evidence of maxillary hyperplasia, towering forehead, or other evidence of bone marrow expansion?	Chronic hemolytic process
Laboratory studies	
Are there prominent spherocytes?	Hereditary spherocytosis, autoimmune hemolytic anemia, hemolytic disease of the newborn
Are there prominent schistocytes?	Microangiopathic hemolytic anemia
Are there prominent target cells?	Hb C disease, SCD-SC type, Hb E, thalassemia, liver disease, LCAT, beta lipoproteinemia
Are there prominent elliptocytes?	Hereditary elliptocytosis, iron-deficiency anemia
Is the DAT positive?	Autoimmune hemolytic anemia, hemolytic disease of the newborn, hemolytic transfusion reaction

DAT = direct antibody test; G6PD = glucose-6-phosphate dehydrogenase; Hb C = hemoglobin C; Hb E = hemoglobin E; HUS = hemolytic-uremic syndrome; LCAT = lecithin cholesterol acyltransferase; SCD = sickle cell disease.

Laboratory Studies

At minimum, the initial laboratory evaluation should include a **CBC** and **reticulocyte count**. **Liver function tests** and **bilirubin levels** may be indicated. A DAT can be revealing: when RBC destruction is caused by antibody production against erythrocytes (e.g., in AIHA or hemolytic disease of the newborn), hemolysis is extravascular, occurring primarily in the spleen and reticuloendothelial system.

▼ The **DAT is positive** without hemoglobinemia or hemoglobinuria and there are spherocytes on the peripheral blood smear.
▼ The **DAT is negative** when RBC destruction is caused by microvascular or mechanical destruction (e.g., in DIC or hemolytic–uremic syndrome), and the resulting intravascular hemolysis is characterized by the release of free hemoglobin, decreasing haptoglobin, and increased schistocytes.

⚡ HINT Three common conditions are frequently mistaken for hemolytic anemia: hemorrhage, recovering bone marrow (e.g., seen after chemotherapy or viral illness), and partially treated nutritional deficiencies. The reticulocyte count is often increased with evidence of anemia; however, this finding is not related to intrinsic or extrinsic causes of hemolysis.

▼ APPROACH TO THE PATIENT (FIGURE 40.1)
▼ TREATMENT OF HEMOLYSIS

Generally, treatment for hemolytic anemia is directed toward **managing cardiovascular compromise** and **treating the underlying cause** in patients with acquired disease.

Splenectomy

Splenectomy should be considered for children with **congenital hemolytic anemia** to reduce RBC transfusion requirements and to manage complications of hypersplenism (e.g., poor growth). All children who have had their spleens removed are at **greater risk for development of an infection,** particularly with *S. pneumoniae, H. influenzae, Neisseria meningitidis,* or *E. coli.* The risk of infection is greater after splenectomy in young children, particularly in those younger than 4 years, and in those who have underlying conditions associated with increased risk of infection. Immunizations against *H. influenzae, S. pneumoniae,* and *N. meningitidis* are recommended before splenectomy. Prophylactic use of oral penicillin has been shown to be effective in reducing the incidence of bacterial sepsis.

Chronic Transfusion

Children with chronic hemolytic anemia, particularly children with β-thalassemia major or SCD with severe complications, often require **frequent transfusions** (i.e., every 3–6 weeks), either to maintain the hemoglobin level above a certain value or to keep the percentage of Hb S below a certain value. **Complications** of frequent blood transfusions include **iron overload, RBC alloimmunization,** and **viral infection.** Iron overload is treated with **chelation therapy,** usually with subcutaneous or intravenous deferoxamine preparations, or **exchange transfusions** in appropriate patients with SCD.

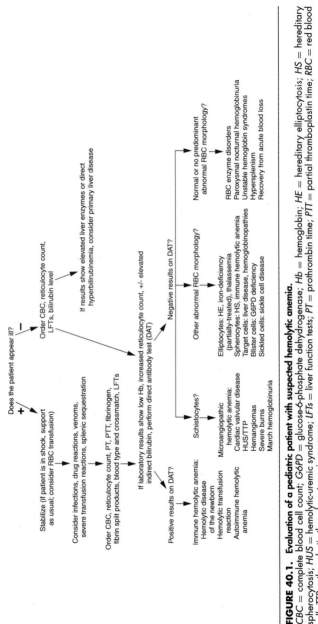

FIGURE 40.1. Evaluation of a pediatric patient with suspected hemolytic anemia.
CBC = complete blood cell count; G6PD = glucose-6-phosphate dehydrogenase; Hb = hemoglobin; HE = hereditary elliptocytosis; HS = hereditary spherocytosis; HUS = hemolytic-uremic syndrome; LFTs = liver function tests; PT = prothrombin time; PTT = partial thromboplastin time; RBC = red blood cell; TTP = thrombotic thrombocytopenic purpura.

Complications of Chronic Hemolytic Anemia

Generally, the complications of chronic hemolytic anemias are related to increased RBC destruction, increased RBC production, and anemia. These complications include **folic acid deficiency** and **gallstones** as a result of increased RBC turnover, **splenomegaly** as a result of increased RBC entrapment and extramedullary hematopoiesis, and **transient aplastic episode.**

Suggested Readings

Cohen AR: Pallor. In *Textbook of Pediatric Emergency Medicine*, 3rd ed. Edited by Fleisher GR, Ludwig S. Baltimore, Williams & Wilkins, 1993, pp 388–396.
Segel GB: Anemia. *Pediatr Rev* 10:77, 1988.
Stewart CL, Tina LU: Hemolytic uremic syndrome. *Pediatr Rev* 14:218, 1993.

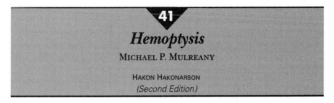

41
Hemoptysis
MICHAEL P. MULREANY

HAKON HAKONARSON
(Second Edition)

▼ INTRODUCTION

Hemoptysis includes the **expectoration of blood-streaked sputum,** as well as **gross bleeding** from the airways and lung. Spitting or coughing up of blood may occur in many bronchopulmonary diseases, the most common being infection. Although bleeding of more than a few ounces is uncommon in children, **massive hemoptysis** (loss of more than 8 ml blood/kg or 300 ml blood/24 hr) is a **life-threatening condition** requiring immediate evaluation and therapy.

✄ HINT Patients with massive hemoptysis most likely have a single focus of bleeding.

▼ DIFFERENTIAL DIAGNOSIS LIST

Infectious Causes

Bacterial Infection

Pneumococcus
Staphylococcus
Meningococcus
Group A *Streptococcus*
Mycoplasma
Bordetella pertussis
Pseudomonas

Viral Infection

Influenza virus
Varicella-zoster virus
Hepatitis B virus

Fungal Infection

Aspergillus
Coccidioides
Blastomyces

Parasitic Infection

Visceral larva migrans
Filariasis
Toxoplasmosis

Arthropod Infestation

Hemorrhagic fevers

Toxic Causes

Cocaine
Penicillamine
Trimellitic anhydride
Radiologic contrast medium

Neoplastic Causes

Benign Chest Masses

Hemangiomas
Angiomas—angiokeratoma diffusum, spider angioma
Bronchogenic cysts
Enteric cysts

Malignant Chest Masses

Bronchial carcinoid tumor
Bronchial adenoma (premalignant)
Sarcoma
Teratoma
Metastatic lesions—sarcoma, Wilms tumor, osteogenic sarcoma

Traumatic Causes

Foreign body
Lung contusion

Congenital or Vascular Causes

Arteriovenous malformation or fistula—Rendu-Osler-Weber syndrome
Systemic vasculitis—periarteritis nodosa, Henoch-Schönlein purpura, hypersensitivity angiitis

Cardiac Causes

Congenital pulmonary vein stenosis—pulmonary veno-occlusive disease
Tetralogy of Fallot with pulmonary atresia and multiple collaterals
Pulmonary arterial stenosis
Mitral stenosis with left atrial hypertension

Metabolic or Genetic Causes

Cystic fibrosis
Immotile cilia syndrome
Congenital bronchiectasis

Inflammatory Causes

Collagen Vascular and Immune-Related Disorders

Goodpasture syndrome—pulmonary renal disease
Wegener granulomatosis
Systemic lupus erythematosus
Immune complex—mediated glomerulonephritis
Cryoglobulinemia
Progressive systemic sclerosis
Behçet syndrome

Psychosocial Causes

Munchausen by proxy syndrome

Miscellaneous Causes

Pulmonary Disorders

Pulmonary hemosiderosis, pulmonary embolism, bronchopulmonary dysplasia

Hematologic Disorders

Consumption coagulopathy
Incompatible blood transfusion
Bleeding disorders—hemophilia A and B, von Willebrand disease
Sickle cell disease
Acute chest syndrome
Pulmonary infarct

Other Disorders

Chronic or recurrent aspirations
Pulmonary compression injury
Pulmonary alveolar proteinosis
Pulmonary sequestration

▼ DIFFERENTIAL DIAGNOSIS DISCUSSION

HINT An inhaled foreign body must always be considered in any child with hemoptysis.

HINT Pneumonia, bronchitis, lung abscess, and laryngotracheitis can be associated with hemoptysis.

Bronchiectasis

Bronchiectasis is discussed in Chapter 23, "Cough."

Cystic Fibrosis

Cystic fibrosis is discussed in Chapter 23, "Cough."

Pulmonary Hemosiderosis

Etiology

Hemosiderosis may be primary or secondary.

▼ **Primary hemosiderosis.** Primary idiopathic hemosiderosis is caused by bleeding into the lungs of unknown cause and is a diagnosis of exclusion. Classification is as follows:

1. Isolated
2. With cardiac or pancreatic involvement
3. With glomerulonephritis (Goodpasture syndrome)
4. With sensitivity to cow's milk and milk protein allergies (Heiner syndrome)

▼ **Secondary hemosiderosis** can result from cardiac disease, collagen vascular disease or systemic vasculitis, bleeding disorders, or granulomatosis.

Clinical Features

Typically, the infant or child appears ill (i.e., **pale, tachypneic, tachycardic, lethargic**) and is usually afebrile. The pallor results from **anemia,** which is caused by recurrent subclinical bleeding. **Sputum is frequently rust colored;** frank hemoptysis is less common as a presentation. **Infiltrates** on a chest radiograph may be **diffuse. Intercostal or substernal retractions** are usually noted on physical examination.

Evaluation

The diagnosis is confirmed by demonstrating **macrophages containing hemosiderin.** A macrophage sample may be obtained via **gastric lavage** (performed three times in the morning before the patient has risen from the supine position) or via **bronchoscopy.**

⚗ HINT Primary idiopathic hemosiderosis is a diagnosis of exclusion and requires a comprehensive work-up, including evaluation for immunologic, infectious, and cardiac causes. Milk protein precipitin values should be obtained for any child with pulmonary hemorrhage of unknown cause.

Treatment

Blood transfusions may be required in the acute phase. Conventional therapy includes prednisone (2 mg/kg/day for 4–6 weeks, tapered over 1–2 months in an attempt to wean the patient completely or to at least achieve an every-other-day regimen). **Azathioprine or cyclophosphamide** is used for patients who do not respond to steroid therapy, or in place of steroids.

Children who test **positive for milk precipitin values** should be placed on a **non–casein-based diet.** Although some children respond, many do not.

Goodpasture Syndrome

A pulmonary–renal immune complex disorder, Goodpasture syndrome is characterized by **deposits of antiglomerular basement membrane (anti-GBM) antibodies in the kidneys and lungs.** Anti-GBM antibodies are also found in the **serum.** Injury caused by viral infections, volatile hydrocarbon exposure, or ingestion of certain drugs (e.g., penicillamine) has been implicated in the pathogenesis of Goodpasture syndrome. The disorder is most common in **young Caucasian boys. Hemoptysis** is common and usually occurs prior to renal disease developing.

Wegener Granulomatosis

Characterized by **angiitis with granuloma formation,** Wegener granulomatosis involves both the **lung and the kidney.** The cause is unknown, but the disorder has been associated with drug ingestion, infections, and chemicals. Wegener granulomatosis is distinguished by necrotizing lesions of the upper and lower respiratory tract and necrotizing glomerulonephritis. The **sinuses, nasal septum, and nasopharynx** are usually involved. The disorder can present with **massive hemoptysis** secondary to **necrotizing pneumonitis** in the lower respiratory tract. **Acute glomerulonephritis** and **renal failure** usually precede the pulmonary manifestations.

▼ EVALUATION OF HEMOPTYSIS
Patient History

A careful history is important to rule out an exogenous agent or an underlying pulmonary disorder. A description of the **color of the blood,** the **duration of the bleeding,** and the **amount of blood** is helpful in defining the severity of the condition and making a specific diagnosis.

HINT It is important to distinguish hemoptysis (coughing of blood) from hematemesis (vomiting of blood). In hematemesis, the blood is often brown and has a low pH as a result of contact with gastric acid. Care must also be taken to differentiate hemoptysis from epistaxis, oral or nasopharyngeal bleeding, and bleeding caused by tonsillitis or gingivitis.

HINT The main features of alveolar hemorrhage, apart from hemoptysis, are shortness of breath, anemia, hypoxemia, and diffuse pulmonary shadowing on a chest radiograph.

Physical Examination

Features of **systemic illnesses** (e.g., collagen vascular diseases, vasculitides, chronic hypoxemia) should be sought, and the patient's **cardiopulmonary status** should be evaluated. The physician should ensure that the patient's **vital signs and hemodynamic status** are stable. Specific findings that may be suggestive of the cause include the following:

▼ **Putrid sputum** suggests the presence of a lung abscess or bronchiectasis.
▼ **Acute pleuritic chest pain** raises the possibility of pulmonary embolism or another pleura-based lesion (e.g., abscess, fungal cavity, vasculitis).
▼ **Localized wheezing** occurs with an intramural lesion (e.g., foreign body, tumor).
▼ **Pleural rub** suggests the presence of pleural disease.
▼ **Clubbing** and **chronic hypoxemia** suggest the presence of a chronic pulmonary or cardiac disorder (e.g., cystic fibrosis, bronchiectasis, cyanotic congenital heart disease).

Laboratory Studies

A **complete blood count with differential, coagulation studies,** and **sputum culture** and **Gram stain** should be obtained in all patients with significant hemoptysis (more than a few teaspoons).

Other laboratory studies are ordered according to clinical suspicion for a particular condition. These studies may include:

▼ **Urinalysis, urine microscopy,** and **serum blood urea nitrogen and creatinine levels** to exclude the existence of a kidney disorder
▼ **Erythrocyte sedimentation rate, complement antinuclear antibodies, rheumatoid factor,** and **cryoglobulin** to exclude the existence of vasculitis and connective tissue disorders
▼ **Serum anti-GBM antibody level** to evaluate suspected Goodpasture syndrome
▼ **Serum antinuclear cytoplasmic antibody** to evaluate suspected Wegener granulomatosis
▼ **Bacterial, viral, fungal,** and **parasitic cultures** and to exclude the presence of an infection
▼ **Purified protein derivative analysis** to exclude the presence of tuberculosis
▼ **Chloride sweat test** to exclude the presence of cystic fibrosis
▼ **Lung biopsy** may be indicated if the work-up is negative (consistent with idiopathic or primary pulmonary hemosiderosis) and suspicion of an underlying condition still exists

Diagnostic Modalities

▼ **Chest radiograph.** A chest radiograph should be obtained for all patients with significant hemoptysis or clinical distress. The radiographic changes are usually diffuse and bilateral, often sparing the apices and costophrenic angles. Unilateral hyperlucency may indicate a radiolucent foreign body; in that case, a lateral decubitus film should be evaluated for paradoxical asymmetry.
▼ **Laryngoscopy** or **bronchoscopy** (or both) can differentiate upper from lower respiratory tract bleeding and focal from diffuse bleeding. These modalities can also localize the bleeding to a particular bronchopulmonary segment. A rigid scope should be used for patients with severe bleeding because the rigid scope enables the physician to ventilate the patient (if necessary), to control the airway, and to provide definitive treatment in some cases. A flexible scope is better suited for diagnostic purposes, lavage, and obtaining samples for culture.
▼ **Cardiac catheterization and angiography** can help to delineate the bronchial and pulmonary vasculature, localize an isolated bleed, define the underlying cause (dilated tortuous bronchial vessels, increased number of vessels, bronchopulmonary anastomosis), and evaluate hemodynamics (in congenital heart disease and suspected pulmonary hypertension). Angiography can include treatment (coiling of collateral vessels) and guide surgical resection in large vessel, diffuse disease.
▼ **High-resolution computed tomography (HRCT) of the chest with contrast** is more sensitive and specific than a chest radiograph for demonstrating the alveolar pattern in an intrapulmonary bleed. HRCT is also helpful in diagnosing sequestration and locating anomalous vessels.

▼ **Magnetic resonance imaging and magnetic resonance angiography** are valuable for detecting neoplasia and anomalous vasculature.

▼ **Echocardiography** may allow exclusion of an underlying cardiac disorder.

▼ **Radionuclide scanning** with technetium 99m–labeled sulfur colloid can detect perfusion defects caused by emboli and may be helpful in detecting a localized bleeding site.

▼ TREATMENT OF HEMOPTYSIS

Stabilization

An **aggressive approach** in an **intensive care setting** is indicated when a massive hemorrhage occurs. An airway must be **established immediately.** (Aspiration of blood and asphyxia are more likely to kill the patient than is exsanguination.) One should be prepared to use **intubation and mechanical ventilation. Catheters with suction and oxygen** must be available at the bedside.

Hypovolemia requires **fluid resuscitation, blood transfusion, or both. Hypoxia** should be treated with **oxygen. Acidosis** requires the administration of **fluids** (e.g., 0.9% normal saline, lactated Ringers solution) and blood.

Infants with intrapulmonary bleeding almost always have concomitant **left-sided heart failure with pulmonary edema** and may require **positive-pressure ventilation** with **positive end-expiratory pressure, pressor administration** (e.g., dopamine, dobutamine, epinephrine), and **fluid restriction** (except for blood transfusion, when necessary).

Termination of Bleeding

Methods of terminating bleeding include the following. The effectiveness of conservative therapy is well established and is the mainstay except for massive hemoptysis.

▼ **Bronchoscopic lavage** of a segment of the lung with iced saline can be successful in some cases but is rarely used.

▼ **Foley catheter placement.** A balloon-tipped catheter is placed in the affected bronchus, inflated, and left in place for 24 hours.

▼ **Selective embolization** of the bronchial or pulmonary vessels with catheter-introduced coils is an effective way of stopping the bleeding.

▼ **Electrocoagulation** is found to be useful by some authors.

▼ **Selective intubation** of a main bronchus with a cuffed tube may be useful in unilateral bleeding.

▼ **Surgical resection** of the focus of bleeding may provide definitive treatment in isolated bleeding segments.

☒ HINT A major pitfall in dealing with hemoptysis is to ascribe recurrent episodes of hemoptysis to a previously established diagnosis, such as chronic bronchiectasis or bronchitis. Failing to search for a new diagnosis may result in missing a serious but potentially treatable condition.

Suggested Readings

Batra PS, Holinger LD: Etiology and management of pediatric hemoptysis. *Arch Otolaryngol Head Neck Surg* 127(4):377–382, 2001.

Corey R, Hla KM: Major and massive hemoptysis: reassessment of conservative management. *Am J Med Sci* 301–309, 1987.

DiLeo MD, Amdee RG, Butcher, RB: Hemoptysis and pseudohemoptysis: the patient expectorating blood. *Ear Nose Throat J* 74:822–824, 1995.

Fabian MC, Smitheringale A: Hemoptysis in children: The Hospital for Sick Children experience. *J Otolaryngol* 25(1):44–45, 1996.

Panitch HB: Hemoptysis. In *A Practical Guide to Pediatric Respiratory Diseases.* Edited by Schidlow DV, Smith DS. 1994, pp 15–18.

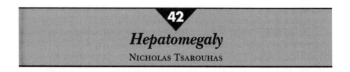

42

Hepatomegaly

NICHOLAS TSAROUHAS

▼ INTRODUCTION

Hepatomegaly, an enlarged liver, is an important clue to a variety of systemic pathological conditions. Alternatively, it may herald disease of the liver itself. **Palpation** is the most common technique used to diagnose hepatomegaly. A palpable liver, however, does not necessarily denote hepatomegaly. In a normal child, the liver edge usually is palpable 1–2 cm below the right costal margin in the right midclavicular line. In an infant, the liver edge may be palpable 2–3 cm below the costal margin. While a liver palpable beyond these parameters suggests hepatomegaly, the **liver span is a more reliable indicator.** The liver span is ascertained by percussing the upper edge, and by palpating or auscultating the lower edge. **Auscultation** is performed by placing the stethoscope below the xiphoid and "scratching" superiorly from the right lower quadrant until the lower edge of the liver causes a change in the transmitted sound. In the neonate, the normal liver span is 4–5 cm, while in older children, the span reaches 7–8 cm in boys and 6–7 cm in girls.

▼ DIFFERENTIAL DIAGNOSIS LIST

Infectious Causes

Viral Infections

Benign infection
Hepatitis (types A–E)
Mononucleosis
Cytomegalovirus (CMV) infection
AIDS

Bacterial Infections

Sepsis
Liver abscess
Cat-scratch disease
Brucellosis
Rocky Mountain spotted fever
Ehrlichiosis

Tuberculosis
Syphilis
Leptospirosis

Other Infections

Malaria
Toxoplasmosis
Babesiosis
Histoplasmosis
Amebiasis
Ascariasis
Toxocariasis
Echinococcosis
Schistosomiasis

Hematologic Causes

Hemolytic anemia (e.g., sickle cell anemia)
Thalassemia
Erythroblastosis fetalis

Neoplastic Causes

Neuroblastoma
Hepatoblastoma
Hepatocellular carcinoma
Leukemia
Lymphoma
Wilms tumor
Adenoma
Hemangioma
Hemangioendothelioma
Hemartoma
Other metastatic disease

Vascular Causes

Congestive heart failure
Constrictive pericarditis
Budd-Chiari syndrome

Anatomic Causes

Extrahepatic

Biliary atresia
Biliary hypoplasia
Bile duct stenosis or stricture
Choledochal cyst
Cholelithiasis
Tumors (hepatic, biliary, pancreatic, duodenal)

Intrahepatic

Alagille syndrome
Intrahepatic biliary duct hypoplasia or paucity

Traumatic Causes

Laceration
Hematoma
Traumatic cyst

Metabolic Causes

Wilson disease (hepatolenticular degeneration)
α_1-Antitrypsin (α_1-AT) deficiency
Hemochromatosis (primary or secondary)
Cystic fibrosis
Diabetes mellitus
Crigler-Najjar syndrome (type I glucuronyl transferase deficiency)
Dubin-Johnson syndrome
Zellweger (cerebrohepatorenal) syndrome
Amino acid metabolism defects
    Tyrosinemia
    Urea cycle disorders
    Methylmalonic acidemia
    Homocystinuria

Carbohydrate metabolism defects
    Galactosemia
    Hereditary fructose intolerance
    Glycogen storage diseases
        Von Gierke disease
        Pompe disease

Lipid metabolism defects
    Fatty acid oxidation disorders
    Hyper- or hypolipoproteinemia
    Mucolipidoses (I-cell disease)
    Lipid storage diseases
        Niemann-Pick disease
        Gaucher disease
        GM_1 and GM_2 gangliosidosis

Mucopolysaccharidoses
    Hurler syndrome
    Hunter syndrome

Nonalcoholic steatohepatitis

Toxic Causes

Drugs
Hypervitaminosis A

Miscellaneous Causes

Obesity
Protein-calorie malnutrition
Chronic intravenous alimentation
Autoimmune chronic active hepatitis
Reye syndrome
Chronic granulomatous disease
Juvenile rheumatoid arthritis (JRA)

Systemic lupus erythematosus (SLE)
Histiocytic disorders
    Langerhans cell histiocytosis
    Hemophagocytic lymphohistiocytosis
    Malignant histiocytic disorders

Amyloidosis
Sarcoidosis
Congenital hepatic fibrosis
Idiopathic neonatal hepatitis

▼ DIFFERENTIAL DIAGNOSIS DISCUSSION
Benign Viral Infection

It is not uncommon for children with viral syndromes to have **mild hepatomegaly**. The liver is nontender, and serum transaminase levels are occasionally slightly high. Only **observation** for resolution of the infection is required.

Liver Abscess
Etiology

Bacterial agents are the usual culprits; occasionally, a **parasitic agent** can cause a liver abscess. The following are risk factors for liver abscess:

▼ Bacteremia
▼ Intra-abdominal infection
▼ Anti-inflammatory drug therapy
▼ Antineoplastic drug therapy
▼ Immunodeficiency
▼ Umbilical vein catheterization

Clinical Features

Patients present with **right upper quadrant pain, fever, anorexia, weight loss,** and, occasionally, **jaundice.**

Evaluation

The patient's liver enzyme levels, white blood cell (WBC) count, and erythrocyte sedimentation rate (ESR) are usually increased. Blood culture results may be positive. **Ultrasound, computed tomography (CT),** and **magnetic resonance imaging (MRI)** are useful diagnostic modalities.

Treatment

Therapy includes the use of **antibiotic agents** in concert with CT- or ultrasound-guided **aspiration or surgical drainage.** Appropriate empiric antibiotic therapy includes a penicillinase-resistant penicillin (e.g., nafcillin, oxacillin) and an aminoglycoside (e.g., gentamicin). Anaerobic coverage is sometimes added as well. Common antimicrobial choices for anaerobic abscesses include clindamycin, cefoxitin, or metronidazole.

Viral Hepatitis

Viral hepatitis is discussed in Chapter 47, "Jaundice."

Infectious Mononucleosis

Infectious mononucleosis is discussed in Chapter 53, "Lymphadenopathy."

Cytomegalovirus (CMV) Infection

CMV infection is discussed in Chapter 76, "Splenomegaly."

AIDS

AIDS is discussed in Chapter 73, "Sexually Transmitted Diseases."

Sepsis

Sepsis is discussed in Chapter 46, "Infections, Newborn."

Neuroblastoma

Neuroblastoma is discussed in Chapter 8, "Abdominal Mass."

Biliary Atresia

Biliary atresia is discussed in Chapter 48, "Jaundice, Newborn."

Wilson Disease (Hepatolenticular Degeneration)

Etiology

Wilson disease is an autosomal recessive disease of **copper metabolism.** Decreased biliary excretion of copper causes copper accumulation in hepatocytes.

Clinical Features

The onset of symptoms, which are usually the result of **hepatic or neurologic involvement,** usually occurs during **late childhood or adolescence.** There may be a family history of undiagnosed hepatic, neurologic, or psychiatric disease.

▼ **Hepatic involvement** is usually characterized by increased transaminase levels and by cholestasis. Patients may also develop a brisk hemolysis that can cause unconjugated hyperbilirubinemia.
▼ **Psychiatric and neurologic manifestations** include subtle problems (e.g., a decline in school performance or behavioral changes) that progress if a diagnosis is not made and therapy initiated. Late symptoms include tremors, slurring of speech, and severe dystonia.

Evaluation

Urine and serum copper levels are increased, and the **serum ceruloplasmin level is decreased.** Slit-lamp examination to detect the presence of Kayser-Fleischer rings should be performed. **Cranial CT and MRI scans** may show central nervous system (CNS) lesions.

Treatment

Dietary intake of copper should be minimized, and **copper chelation therapy** with D-penicillamine is initiated. Some experts advocate **liver transplantation.**

α_1-Antitrypsin (α_1AT) Deficiency

α_1-AT deficiency is discussed in Chapter 47, "Jaundice."

Tyrosinemia

Etiology

Tyrosinemia is an aminoacidopathy characterized by an increased level of **plasma tyrosine.** The liver, the kidneys, and the CNS are primarily affected.

Clinical Features

Symptoms, which include **vomiting and irritability,** develop early in the first year of life. Other manifestations include jaundice, hypoglycemia, failure to thrive, and developmental delay.

Evaluation

Laboratory test results may show **anemia, hyperbilirubinemia,** and an **increase in liver enzyme values.** The α-fetoprotein level may also be high.

Treatment

Treatment includes **dietary management** and **liver transplantation.**

Urea Cycle Disorders

Etiology

Urea cycle disorders involve **defects or deficiencies** in the **enzymes** that detoxify ammonia to urea.

Clinical Features

After a few days of dietary protein intake, neonates develop **vomiting, seizures, lethargy,** and even **coma.** Infants and older children present with vomiting and neurologic symptoms.

Evaluation

Increased levels of ammonia, a **decreased blood urea nitrogen (BUN) level,** and **metabolic acidemia** are present.

Treatment

Treatment entails **dietary protein restriction** and the oral administration of **ammonia-removing compounds** (e.g., sodium benzoate, sodium phenylacetate, arginine, lactulose).

Galactosemia

Etiology

Classic galactosemia is caused by galactose-1-phosphate uridylyltransferase deficiency, which leads to the inability to metabolize **galactose-1-phosphate** and the **accumulation** of this substance in the liver, kidney, and brain.

Clinical Features

Infants and children may present for examination with **irritability, lethargy, vomiting, jaundice, hepatosplenomegaly, failure to thrive, cataracts,** and **hypoglycemia.** It is important to make the diagnosis at birth to prevent permanent brain damage.

TABLE 42.1. Comparison of Glycogen Storage Diseases

	von Gierke Disease	Pompe Disease
Etiology	Hepatorenal glycogenosis	Cardiac glycogenosis
Clinical features	"Doll face" appearance; failure to thrive; hydronephrosis; gout; normal mental status; hypoglycemia with an increase in the amount of lactic acid, lipids, and uric acid; no muscle involvement	Cardiomegaly, hypotonia, normal mental status, muscle involvement
Treatment	Dietary control	No effective therapy
Prognosis	Near-normal life	Death usually results from respiratory muscle failure

Treatment

Treatment entails reduction or **exclusion of dietary galactose.**

Glycogen Storage Diseases

von Gierke disease and Pompe disease are compared in Table 42.1.

Niemann-Pick Disease

Etiology

Classic Niemann-Pick disease is an autosomal recessive disease caused by a sphingomyelinase deficiency, which results in **excess storage of sphingomyelin and cholesterol** in the liver, spleen, brain, and bone marrow ("foam" cells). Classic Niemann-Pick disease ultimately **progresses to mental retardation, neurologic deterioration, and death.**

Clinical Features and Evaluation

Infants present for evaluation with **developmental delay, hearing and vision abnormalities, hypotonia, feeding difficulties,** and **failure to thrive.** Other findings on physical examination include a "wasted" appearance, hepatosplenomegaly, and, in some, a "cherry-red" spot on the macula. The diagnosis is made by means of **enzyme analysis.**

▟ HINT Patients with Tay-Sachs disease, another devastating lipid storage disorder, classically have the "cherry-red" spot on the macula, but notably do not have associated hepatosplenomegaly.

Mucopolysaccharidoses

Hunter syndrome and Hurler syndrome are compared in Table 42.2.

TABLE 42.2. Comparison of Mucopolysaccharidoses

	Hunter Syndrome	Hurler Syndrome
Etiology	X-linked recessive disorder caused by iduronate-2-sulfatase deficiency	Autosomal recessive disorder caused by α-L-iduronidase deficiency
Clinical features	Coarse facial features, short stature, hearing abnormalities, cardiac abnormalities, hepatosplenomegaly, hernias, joint stiffness, skin problems, mental retardation	Developmental delay, macrocephaly, coarse facial features, clouded corneas, nasal discharge, hepatosplenomegaly, hernias, kyphosis
Prognosis	More mild course than that of Hurler syndrome	Joint immobility, skeletal disturbances, developmental regression, and neurologic deterioration progress to death by early adolescence

Drug Toxicity

Drugs that can cause hepatitis and cholestasis through direct hepatotoxicity or fatty infiltration are summarized in Chapter 47, "Jaundice," Table 47.1.

Protein-Calorie Malnutrition

Etiology

Starvation states are commonly associated with **hepatomegaly. Kwashiorkor,** which is characterized by **severe protein deficiency,** is the most prevalent form of malnutrition in the world.

Clinical Features

Children with kwashiorkor have a **severely wasted appearance, growth retardation, apathy, lethargy, dermatitis,** and **edema. Susceptibility to infection** is increased. Severely ill patients may develop stupor and coma.

Evaluation

Laboratory test abnormalities include **anemia, hypoglycemia, hypoalbuminemia,** and **hypoproteinemia. Vitamin and mineral deficiencies are universal.** Urinalysis is notable for the presence of **ketones.** Bone age, measured by radiographic study of the left hand and wrist, shows a **delay in skeletal maturation** with respect to chronologic age.

Treatment

Enteral "refeeding" (with careful monitoring of laboratory nutritional indices and electrolytes) is usually curative.

Chronic Intravenous Alimentation

Etiology

Hyperalimentation hepatitis, or total parenteral nutrition (TPN) hepatitis, is a common complication when parenteral nutrition using crystalline amino acid solutions has been provided on a long-term basis.

Clinical Features

Jaundice usually marks the onset of this complication. **Chronic liver disease** may ensue. Children who tolerate TPN for more than 2.5 years are less likely to have significant chronic liver disease.

Evaluation

Liver enzymes, bilirubin, and **nutritional indicators** (e.g., albumin, protein) should be monitored.

Treatment

When possible, attempts should be made to use **enteral nutrition.**

Autoimmune Chronic Active Hepatitis

Etiology

Autoimmune chronic active hepatitis, which is characterized by the presence of **circulating autoantibodies,** may be caused by an abnormality of suppressor T cells.

Clinical Features

Like most autoimmune diseases, autoimmune chronic hepatitis is **most common in girls.** Symptoms include **fever, fatigue, weakness, abdominal pain,** and **joint pain.** Symptoms of other autoimmune manifestations may also be present (e.g., thyroiditis, autoimmune hemolytic anemia).

Evaluation

Physical examination signs include **hepatosplenomegaly, jaundice, palmar erythema,** and **spider angiomata.** Laboratory results may show **hypergammaglobulinemia;** the presence of specific anti-smooth muscle, anti-liver, or anti-kidney **microsomal antibodies;** and **hemolytic anemia.**

Treatment

Patients often respond to **immunosuppressive therapy** with corticosteroids (e.g., prednisone) or azathioprine, but relapse often occurs when the patient is weaned from the steroids. **Liver transplantation** may be necessary.

Reye Syndrome

Etiology

Reye syndrome is a **rare, reversible, noninflammatory** encephalopathy of unknown etiology, which is characterized by **fatty degeneration of the liver.** There is an **association between Reye syndrome and aspirin use** during varicella infection or an influenza-like illness.

Clinical Features

The initial presentation is the **abrupt onset of vomiting** following prodromal viral (or varicella) symptoms. **Neurologic changes** rapidly develop. The ensuing **progressive encephalopathy** is characterized by quietness, irritability, combativeness, confusion, delirium, stupor, and coma.

Evaluation

Laboratory test abnormalities include increases in liver enzyme levels, the ammonia level, the BUN value, and the prothrombin time. Decreases in the serum glucose level, bicarbonate level, and arterial carbon dioxide tension ($Paco_2$) may also be present. **Liver biopsy** is usually confirmatory.

Treatment

Fluid restriction, hyperventilation, and **mannitol therapy** are commonly used to combat the lethal effects of cerebral edema.

Histiocytic Disorders

Etiology

Reactive disorders associated with the proliferation of the mononuclear phagocytic system are classified into 3 groups:

▼ **Langerhans cell histiocytosis (LCH)**
▼ **Hemophagocytic lymphohistiocytosis (HPLH)**
▼ **Malignant histiocytic disorders**

✄ HINT Langerhans cell histiocytosis (dendritic cell-related disorders) was previously classified as a "histiocytosis X syndrome" and referred to as Hand–Schüller–Christian syndrome, Letterer–Siwe disease, and eosinophilic granuloma.

▼ **LCH is characterized by cells similar to the Langerhans cells of the skin,** causing organ damage to multiple body systems through the production of cytokines and prostaglandins.
▼ **HPLH is a macrophage-related disorder** characterized by a proliferation of erythrophagocytic histiocytes in the bone marrow, spleen, lymph nodes, skin, or CNS.

Both LCH and HPLH have been **linked to underlying immunodeficiencies and viruses.**

Clinical Features

▼ **LCH** may present as a **single system disease,** with isolated bony lesions, or as a **multisystem disease** involving the skin, teeth, liver, bone marrow, lungs, liver, spleen, GI tract, or CNS. **Complications** include pulmonary and hepatic fibrosis, liver and bone marrow failure, and neurologic abnormalities.
▼ **HPLH** patients commonly present with **fever, fatigue, jaundice,** and **hepatosplenomegaly. Complications** include overwhelming infection, bleeding, and progressive CNS disease.

Evaluation

CBC, coagulation studies, liver enzymes, and **chest x-ray** are important initial studies in all the histiocytic disorders. A **skeletal survey** is used in LCH to search for bony lesions. HPLH is usually associated with pancytopenia, hypertriglyceridemia, hepatitis, and hyperferritinemia. **Bone marrow evaluation** is usually confirmatory.

Treatment

Chemotherapy, radiotherapy, immunotherapy (cyclosporin A, antithymocyte globulin), and **bone marrow transplantation** have been used in the histiocytic disorders with variable success.

▼ EVALUATION OF HEPATOMEGALY

Patient History

The following questions may lead to a diagnosis:

▼ **Is there a history of a minor preceding viral illness?** Mild hepatomegaly may be apparent with even benign viral illnesses.

▼ **Did a prodromal illness lead to jaundice?** Hepatitis A infection is a common diagnosis in the setting of a jaundiced child after a mild prodromal illness.

▼ **Is there a history of poor feeding with respiratory distress?** Eating is a "stress test" for infants, so congestive heart failure should be considered in the setting of respiratory distress or ill-appearance.

▼ **Is there a history of trauma?** Moderate abdominal trauma may result in a liver laceration or hematoma.

▼ **Is the patient lethargic or irritable?** When parents describe an irritable or lethargic child, serious consideration should be given to the possibility of sepsis or a metabolic disorder.

▼ **Is there a history of vomiting with developmental delay or behavioral abnormalities?** Metabolic disorders may present with vomiting and non-specific neurodevelopmental abnormalities.

▼ **Is there a family history of early death or neurologic disease?** Metabolic disorders should be considered with vague family histories of infantile deaths of unknown etiology.

▼ **What is the patient's medication history?** Many drugs can cause liver abnormalities and hepatomegaly. Aspirin use is associated with Reye syndrome.

▼ **Is there a maternal history of perinatal illness or poor prenatal care?** Poor prenatal care should lead one to consider infectious etiologies such as AIDS, hepatitis, CMV, and syphilis infections.

▼ **Is there a history of umbilical catheterization?** Hepatic abscess is a known complication of umbilical catheterization (as well as amebiasis).

▼ **Is there a history of foreign travel?** Malaria, as well as other infectious etiologies should be considered if the patient has recently traveled abroad.

▼ **Is there a history of a tick bite?** Rocky Mountain spotted fever, ehrlichiosis, and babesiosis are all concerns after tick bites.

▼ **Is there a history of animal contact?** Cats or kittens are the main culprits in cat scratch disease (via scratches) and toxoplasmosis (commonly from the litter box); contact with cat or dog feces is also a risk factor for toxocariasis; dogs are also occasional carriers of echinococcus, as are coyotes, wolves, and other canines; leptospirosis is usually caused by contact with the urine or waters contaminated by rats, dogs, or cattle; brucellosis should also be considered if there has been contact with cattle (or unpasteurized milk), goats, or swine; inhalation of spores containing the fecal droppings of birds or bats might lead to histoplasmosis.

Physical Examination

▼ **Jaundice** is often the presenting sign in patients with viral hepatitis, hemolytic anemia, anatomic pathologies, and drug hepatotoxicity.

▼ **Fever** supports an infectious or inflammatory diagnosis.

▼ **Exudative pharyngitis** suggests Epstein-Barr virus (EBV) or CMV infection

▼ **Adenopathy** raises suspicion for an infectious or oncologic process.

▼ **An abdominal mass** is a concern for neuroblastoma.

▼ **Splenomegaly** occurs with metabolic, infectious, oncologic, and anatomic (obstructive) disorders.

▼ **Eye findings** may be seen in metabolic (e.g., Wilson disease) or infectious (e.g., CMV) disorders.

▼ **Facial dysmorphism** suggests a metabolic disorder or Alagille syndrome.

Laboratory Studies

Appropriate laboratory studies may include:

▼ **Liver enzymes.** Hepatocellular injury is marked initially by rises in liver enzymes. Alanine aminotransferase (ALT) and aspartate aminotransferase (AST) are the two most common markers. The ALT level is more specific for liver disease, as the AST level also rises with muscle disorders. Alkaline phosphatase (which is also nonspecific) and gamma glutamyl transferase (GGT) levels rise—especially with cholestatic disorders. Lactate dehydrogenase (LDH) is another nonspecific marker of liver injury.

▼ **Bilirubin.** Elevations in conjugated (direct) bilirubin are found in cholestatic disorders, while rises in unconjugated (indirect) bilirubin are seen in hemolytic processes and congenital disorders of bilirubin metabolism.

▼ **Prothrombin time (PT), albumin, and glucose.** The true "liver function tests" are PT, albumin, and glucose. These studies reflect the synthetic function of the liver.

▼ **CBC.** The WBC and platelet counts are useful when certain infections are suspected. The hemoglobin should be closely monitored in hemolytic processes, as well as traumatic hepatic injuries. The overall CBC, of course, is also important when oncologic processes are suspected.

▼ **Reticulocyte count.** The reticulocyte count is diagnostic in hemolytic anemias.

▼ **Routine blood smear.** Evidence of hemolysis can be also seen on the blood smear. Parasitic diseases like malaria and babesiosis often can be identified on blood smears as well.

▼ **Ammonia.** The ammonia level is important in many metabolic disorders as well as in Reye syndrome.

▼ **Viral serologies.** Serologic studies are confirmatory in cases of many viral infections (e.g., hepatitis A-E, EBV, CMV).

▼ **Blood cultures.** Blood cultures should be obtained in cases of sepsis or suspected liver abscess.

▼ **Urinalysis (UA).** Hemoglobinuria is a common finding in hemolytic anemias. Metabolic disorders are sometimes associated with abnormalities on the UA.

▼ **Plasma amino acids and urine organic acids.** Metabolic studies of the plasma and urine are warranted when metabolic disorders are suspected.

Appropriate ancillary studies may include:

▼ **Ultrasound.** Ultrasound is useful to noninvasively visualize the anatomy of the liver and surrounding structures. Intrahepatic and extrahepatic masses are readily identified, and the anatomy of the biliary tree can be evaluated. Doppler studies add important information about hepatic blood flow.

▼ **CT scan and MRI scan.** CT and MRI are useful to detect smaller masses, and may better delineate between tumors, cysts, and abscesses. CT is the most useful study when liver trauma is a possibility.

▼ **Radionuclide scan.** Nuclear scintography is excellent in distinguishing hepatitis (impaired liver uptake) from biliary atresia (impaired intestinal excretion).

▼ **Cholangiography.** Direct visualization of the intrahepatic and extrahepatic biliary tree is possible through cholangiography.

▼ **Liver biopsy.** Biopsy of the liver is indicated in cases of suspected oncologic processes, metabolic disorders, and anatomic pathologies (e.g., atresia).

▼ **Bone marrow biopsy.** Bone marrow biopsy is confirmatory in many oncologic and metabolic (e.g., storage) disorders.

▼ TREATMENT OF HEPATOMEGALY

Most patients with hepatomegaly require **supportive care** only. Most importantly, however, it must be ensured that the **synthetic function of the liver is adequate.** Prolongation of the PT, which is seen earlier than decreases in albumin, is treated with vitamin K and, sometimes, fresh frozen plasma. Albumin infusions are sometimes used for hypoalbuminemia. A "burned out" liver also loses its ability to maintain satisfactory glucose levels, and these patients must be vigorously supported with glucose infusions.

Additionally, the **cause of the hepatomegaly should be treated** if possible (e.g., antibiotics for infections, antineoplastics for oncologic disorders, surgical management for anatomic disorders). Traumatic liver injuries are usually managed conservatively with **observation,** but surgical intervention is occasionally necessary. **Surgical intervention** is also used in cases of biliary atresia, choledochal cysts, and sometimes liver abscesses.

▼ APPROACH TO THE PATIENT (FIGURES 42.1 AND 42.2)

The approach to hepatomegaly is guided by the patient's acuity and age; neonatal management differs from older infants and children.

▼ **Acutely ill neonate. Infection** must be considered first and foremost. If infection is likely, broad-spectrum antibiotics are initiated, and then the distinction of bacterial versus viral should be investigated. **Noninfectious causes** that should be considered in an acutely ill neonate include hemolytic, metabolic, congestive, and anatomic abnormalities. Importantly, **biliary atresia** is an important diagnosis that should be made swiftly, as surgical correction is most likely to be successful in the first few months of life. Clues to this diagnosis include a conjugated hyperbilirubinemia in the absence of splenomegaly.

▼ **Acutely ill older infant or child.** Beyond the neonatal age groups, **oncologic** and **toxic causes** must also be considered.

▼ **Non-acutely ill neonate.** Bacterial sepsis is unlikely, whereas **viral causes** and **syphilis** are more common. Hemolytic anemias and anatomic causes are likely considerations in a non-acutely ill neonate with hepatosplenomegaly but no evidence of infection.

▼ **Non-acutely ill older infant or child.** Viral hepatitis is one of the most common diagnoses, but many other possibilities need to be eliminated first. Toxic, hemolytic and oncologic causes are not uncommon, and nutritional, rheumatologic, and metabolic disorders are also possible.

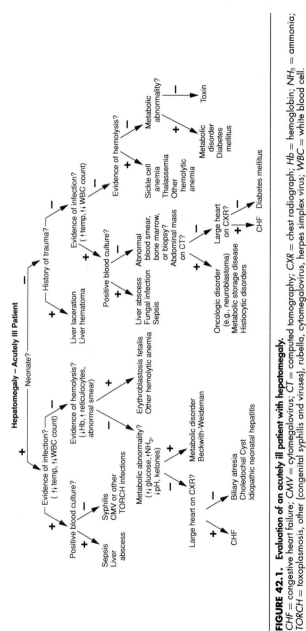

FIGURE 42.1. Evaluation of an acutely ill patient with hepatomegaly.

CHF = congestive heart failure; CMV = cytomegalovirus; CT = computed tomography; CXR = chest radiograph; Hb = hemoglobin; NH_3 = ammonia; $TORCH$ = toxoplasmosis, other (congenital syphilis and viruses), rubella, cytomegalovirus, herpes simplex virus; WBC = white blood cell.

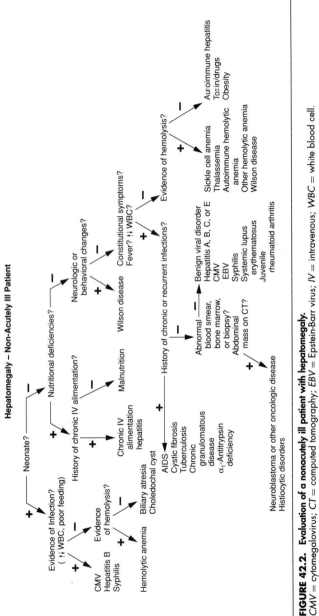

FIGURE 42.2. Evaluation of a nonacutely ill patient with hepatomegaly.
CMV = cytomegalovirus; CT = computed tomography; EBV = Epstein-Barr virus; IV = intravenous; WBC = white blood cell.

Suggested Readings

De Kerguenec C, Hillaire S, Molinie V, et al: Hepatic manifestations of hemophagocytic syndrome. *Am J Gastroenterol* 96:852–857, 2001.

Fitzgerald JF: Cholestatic disorders of infancy. *Pediatr Clin North Am* 35:357–373, 1988.

Krugman S: Viral hepatitis: A, B, C, D, and E. *Pediatr Rev* 13:203–212; 245–247, 1992.

Mews C, Sinatra F: Chronic liver disease in children. *Pediatr Rev* 14:436–444, 1993.

Misra S, Ament ME, Vargas JH, et al: Chronic liver disease in children on long-term parenteral nutrition. *J Gastroenterol Hepatol* 11:S4–S6, 1996.

Wolf AD, Lavine JE: Hepatomegaly in neonates and children. *Pediatr Rev* 21:303–310, 2000.

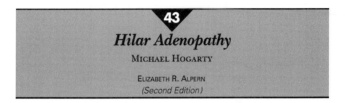

43

Hilar Adenopathy

MICHAEL HOGARTY

ELIZABETH R. ALPERN
(Second Edition)

▼ INTRODUCTION

The pulmonary hilum is the root of the lung where the bronchus, pulmonary blood, and lymphatic vessels, nerves, and bronchopulmonary lymph nodes intersect. Hilar adenopathy is the **nonspecific enlargement of lymph nodes at the hilum.** Signs and symptoms that may lead to evaluation for hilar adenopathy include supraclavicular lymphadenopathy, bronchial obstruction with cough or wheeze, hoarseness, inspiratory stridor, dyspnea, dysphagia, or swelling of the neck and face resulting from compression of the superior vena cava. Most commonly, however, recognition of **hilar adenopathy is an incidental finding** on a chest radiograph. It can be unilateral or bilateral depending on the cause. Hilar adenopathy must be differentiated from other mediastinal masses of nonlymphatic origin.

▼ DIFFERENTIAL DIAGNOSIS LIST

Infectious Causes

Bacterial Infection

Mycobacterium tuberculosis, atypical mycobacterium, *Mycoplasma pneumoniae* infection
Mediastinitis
Lung abscess

Viral Infection

Epstein-Barr virus (EBV)
HIV
Adenovirus
Pertussis

Fungal Infection

Histoplasmosis
Coccidioidomycosis
Blastomycosis

Parasitic Infection

Toxoplasmosis

Neoplastic Causes

Lymphoma
Leukemia
Metastatic solid tumors (less common; neuroblastoma, testicular carcinoma)

Miscellaneous Causes

Langerhans cell histiocytosis
Sinus histiocytosis with massive lymphadenopathy (Rosai-Dorfman disease)
Sarcoidosis
Cystic fibrosis
Castleman disease (benign giant lymph node hyperplasia)
Phenytoin hypersensitivity syndrome

❏ HINT Diseases that mimic hilar adenopathy are listed in Table 43.1.

▼ DIFFERENTIAL DIAGNOSIS DISCUSSION
Lymphomas

Lymphomas are the third most common group of childhood malignancies. **Hodgkin disease** accounts for 40% of childhood lymphomas, and **non-Hodgkin lymphoma (NHL)** accounts for 60%. Both types of lymphoma may

---

TABLE 43.1. Diseases that Mimic Hilar Adenopathy

Vascular diseases
　Engorgement of the pulmonary veins
　Thymic hemangioma
　Total anomalous pulmonary venous return
　Aortic aneurysm
Skeletal diseases
　Vertebral osteophytes
Neoplastic diseases
　Thymic neoplasm
　Germ cell tumor
　Neurofibromatosis
　Teratomas
Cystic diseases
　Cystic hygroma
　Thymic cyst
　Esophageal duplication cyst

be associated with underlying **congenital or acquired immune system dysfunction** (e.g., HIV infection, ataxia–telangiectasia).

Hodgkin disease most commonly presents with **bilateral hilar adenopathy** (with or without an associated mediastinal mass), as well as **cervical or supraclavicular adenopathy.** The hilar adenopathy causes **tracheobronchial compression** in more than 50% of children with Hodgkin disease.

Hodgkin disease and NHL are discussed in detail in Chapter 53, "Lymphadenopathy."

Tuberculosis (TB)

Etiology

Mycobacterium tuberculosis infection (TB) is most often found **in children exposed to adults with high risk** of the disease (Table 43.2). The incidence of this disease has been increasing since 1985. The increase in HIV infection in adults and children has significantly contributed to the increase in the incidence of TB.

Clinical Features

In children, *M. tuberculosis* infection is most commonly **asymptomatic** and represents **primary** (rather than reactivated) **infection.** A **1- to 6-month incubation period** between infection and the development of symptoms is seen in children. Primary infection most often presents with hilar adenopathy, visible on a **chest radiograph** (especially in children younger than 3 years). **Unilateral hilar adenopathy** (usually on the right side) is a more common finding than bilateral hilar adenopathy. Symptoms of **fever, weight loss, night sweats, pneumonia, atelectasis from bronchial compression, miliary TB,** and **extrapulmonary disease,** including **meningitis,** may be present. The **severity of disease is inversely related to the patient's age.**

Evaluation

Sputum, gastric lavage, or bronchoalveolar lavage samples should be evaluated by **Gram stain and culture** for *M. tuberculosis.* However, it is difficult to obtain positive culture proof of infection in children and diagnosis often relies on the **identification of the index adult case,** a **chest radiograph,** and a **positive purified protein derivative (PPD), or Mantoux, tuberculin skin test.** A positive result on the PPD test is indicated by induration at the site caused by the body's hypersensitivity to the tuberculin protein 2–10 **weeks after infection.** Prior to this time, a false-negative result may occur. Anergy owing to other underlying illness may also cause a false-negative skin test.

TABLE 43.2. Groups at High Risk for Tuberculosis

People from endemic areas (Asia, Middle East, Africa, Latin America)
Residents and former residents of correctional facilities
Residents of nursing homes
Homeless people
Users of intravenous drugs
Poor and medically indigent urban dwellers
Health care workers
HIV-infected patients
Children living with high-risk adults

▓ **HINT** Rapid identification techniques [e.g., DNA probes, gas chromatography, immunoassays, and polymerase chain reaction (PCR) assays for M. *tuberculosis* DNA] are becoming available.

Treatment

Reporting of suspected and proven cases of TB is mandated by law. Treatment is determined by the extent of infection. Treatment of active disease is based on eradicating the disease and minimizing the development of resistant organisms. **Directly observed therapy by a trained health care worker** is a standard of treatment in the United States.

▼ **Patients with pulmonary TB** are treated with 2 months of isoniazid, rifampin, and pyrazinamide therapy, followed by 4 months of isoniazid and rifampin therapy. If drug-resistant organisms are suspected, ethambutol or streptomycin is added until susceptibility results are available.

▼ **For patients with severe extrapulmonary TB,** 12 months of therapy are required. Local health officials and TB specialists are helpful in determining optimal treatment regimens.

Histoplasmosis

Etiology

Histoplasma capsulatum, a **fungus** that is endemic to the **Mississippi and Ohio River valleys, Argentina,** and the **Caribbean,** causes histoplasmosis.

Clinical Features

When the spores of *H. capsulatum* are inhaled, an **asymptomatic infection** usually occurs. However, **acute symptomatic pulmonary infections or disseminated infections** may occur (especially in immunocompromised patients) and are associated with **persistent fever, coughing, wheezing, chest pain, and fatigue. Hilar adenopathy** is seen in 75% of patients hospitalized for histoplasmosis. **Pulmonary infiltrates, atelectasis, or effusions** may also be present. **Cardiomegaly** may indicate pericardial involvement.

Evaluation

Culture of *H. capsulatum* **from blood, bone marrow, sputum, or cutaneous lesions** is the basis of diagnosis. **Serologic testing** for complement-fixing antigen or radioimmunoassay for polysaccharide antigen **in urine or serum** may aid diagnosis. Histoplasmin skin testing is not indicated for diagnosis of disease.

Treatment

Histoplasmosis is usually a **self-limiting** disease; however, antifungal agents may be indicated in selected cases. A course of 6 weeks or longer of **amphotericin B** may be used to treat disseminated disease.

Sarcoidosis

Etiology

Sarcoidosis is a **multisystemic disease of noncaseating epithelioid granulomas** involving the **lungs, lymph nodes, eyes, skin, liver, and spleen.** Its cause is unknown.

Clinical Features

Sarcoidosis is **rare in children,** occurring most often in young adults. Adolescents and adults present with involvement of the lung, lymph node, and eye. Younger children usually have skin, joint, and eye involvement. Most patients present with multiple constitutional symptoms, including **fatigue, malaise, fever, weight loss, nonproductive cough, and exertional dyspnea.**

Evaluation

Sarcoidosis is difficult to differentiate from infectious pulmonary diseases (e.g., tuberculosis, histoplasmosis, coccidioidomycosis). Diagnosis depends on **tissue biopsy, clinical and radiographic features, and exclusion** of other possible infectious or malignant diseases.

Most children with sarcoidosis have **bilateral hilar adenopathy.** Other radiographic findings may include **lung parenchymal infiltrates, pleural effusions, or calcifications.** Sarcoidosis is **staged** based on radiographic findings (Table 43.3).

Peripheral lymphadenopathy is common in children with sarcoidosis; these nodes may be **biopsied** for tissue confirmation. The **serum angiotensin-converting enzyme level is usually elevated** in children with sarcoidosis, and **hypercalciuria** and **hypercalcemia** are often present.

Treatment

Corticosteroids are used for the treatment of symptomatic sarcoidosis. **Routine evaluation of all organ systems** that may become involved is necessary in the management of sarcoidosis.

▐▌ HINT Patients with **stage I disease** have a **good chance of resolution** or substantial improvement. Other patients may progress to pulmonary fibrosis.

Virus-Associated Hilar Adenopathy

Viruses that cause lower respiratory infections (e.g., respiratory syncytial virus, parainfluenza virus, influenza virus) rarely cause hilar adenopathy; however, **adenovirus** can cause hilar adenopathy in as many as 57% of infected children. Conditions **associated with HIV and AIDS** that may lead to hilar adenopathy include **TB and *Pneumocystis carinii* pneumonia, lymphomas, and lymphocytic interstitial pneumonitis.**

TABLE 43.3. Stages of Sarcoidosis	
Stage	**Chest Radiograph Findings**
0	Normal radiograph
I	Bilateral hilar lymphadenopathy alone
II	Bilateral hilar lymphadenopathy with pulmonary infiltrates
III	Pulmonary infiltrates without hilar adenopathy
IV	Pulmonary fibrosis and emphysema

▼ **HINT** Other mediastinal masses associated with HIV include thymic enlargement and multiloculated thymic cysts.

Evaluation

▼ **Adenovirus** can be isolated by fluorescent antibody testing or culture from respiratory secretions.
▼ **HIV.** In children older than 18 months, HIV is diagnosed by enzyme-linked immunosorbent assay and Western blot analysis. In younger children, culture and PCR are needed for the diagnosis.

Treatment

▼ **Adenovirus.** Adenovirus infection is self-limited; treatment is supportive.
▼ **HIV.** Management of HIV in children depends on a multidisciplinary team, antiretroviral therapy, and treatment of opportunistic infections.

▼ EVALUATION OF HILAR ADENOPATHY
Patient History

The history should be aimed at gathering the following information:

▼ **Travel and place of residence.** Has the patient been exposed to locations that would place him at risk for infections causing hilar adenopathy (Table 43.4)?
▼ **HIV risk factors**
▼ **Exposure to TB**
▼ **Recurrent pulmonary infections**
▼ **Constitutional symptoms**—weight loss, night sweats, fever, pruritus, myalgias, arthralgias
▼ **Pulmonary symptoms**—orthopnea, dyspnea, wheeze, cough

Physical Examination

The following should be noted on physical examination:

TABLE 43.4. Regions Associated with Certain Infectious Causes of Hilar Adenopathy

Region	Cause
Mississippi and Ohio River valleys Argentina Caribbean	*Histoplasma capsulatum*
American Southwest San Joaquin Valley of California Parts of Mexico	*Coccidioides immitis*
Great Lakes region Southeastern and Central United States Mexico Central and South America Africa Middle East	*Blastomyces dermatitidis*

▼ **Lungs**—wheezing, stridor, rales, or rhonchi
▼ **Head and neck**—swelling (suggestive of superior vena cava syndrome)
▼ **Peripheral lymph nodes**—enlargement, especially of the supraclavicular nodes
▼ **Liver and abdomen**—hepatosplenomegaly or abdominal masses
▼ **Skin**—pallor, petechiae, viral exanthem, or erythema nodosum
▼ **Joints**—arthritis, arthralgias

Laboratory Studies

The following laboratory studies may be appropriate:

Complete blood count (CBC)
Erythrocyte sedimentation rate (ESR)
EBV titers
HIV test
PPD (Mantoux) tuberculin skin test
Sputum, gastric aspirate, or bronchoalveolar lavage cultures

Diagnostic Modalities

The following studies may be appropriate:

▼ **Chest radiography.** Posteroanterior and lateral views should be obtained, and compared with prior films.
▼ **Computed tomography (CT).** An unenhanced CT scan should be followed by a contrast-enhanced CT scan. The unenhanced CT scan allows recognition of calcification in nodes, which is suggestive of granulomatous disease. Abnormal nodes are defined by an unusual location, a diameter greater than 1 cm, or enhancement.
▼ **Magnetic resonance imaging (MRI).** MRI may not identify calcifications within lymph nodes.
▼ **Biopsy** is necessary unless TB or histoplasmosis has been definitively diagnosed by another method. The tissue sample does not necessarily need to be hilar (e.g., enlarged peripheral nodes or the bone marrow can be biopsied).

Suggested Readings

Blackmon GM, Raghu G: Pulmonary sarcoidosis: a mimic of respiratory infection. *Semin Respir Infect* 10(3):176–186, 1995.

Butler JC, Heller R, Wright PF: Histoplasmosis during childhood. *South Med J* 87(4):476–480, 1994.

Hudson MM, Donaldson SS: Hodgkin's disease. *Pediatr Clin North Am* 44(4):891–905, 1997.

Kelly CS, Kelly RE Jr: Lymphadenopathy in children. *Pediatr Clin North Am* 45(4):875–888, 1998.

Marks MJ, Haney PJ, McDermott MP, et al: Thoracic disease in children with AIDS. *Radiographics* 16:1349–1362, 1996.

Sandlund JT, Downing JR, Crist WM: Non-Hodgkin's lymphoma in childhood. *N Engl J Med* 334(19):1238–1248, 1996.

Smith KC: Tuberculosis in children. *Curr Probl Pediatr* 31(1):1–30, 2001.

Wildin SR, Chonmaitree T, Swischuk LE: Roentgenographic features on common pediatric viral respiratory tract infections. *Am J Dis Child* 142(1):43–46, 1988.

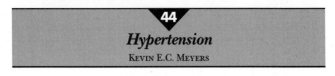

44

Hypertension
KEVIN E.C. MEYERS

▼ INTRODUCTION

▼ **Hypertension** is defined as blood pressure (systolic, diastolic, or both) that is **consistently above the 95th percentile** for the patient's age, height, and sex (see Chapter 87, "Cardiology Laboratory," Figure 87.1). Hypertension and an elevated blood pressure are not synonymous. The most common causes for isolated high blood pressure readings are anxiety and incorrect measurement techniques.

▼ **Labile blood pressure** refers to blood pressure (systolic, diastolic, or both) that is sometimes above and sometimes below the 95th percentile for the patient's age, height, and sex and **does not result in hypertensive damage to organs.** Labile blood pressure is frequently found in teenagers.

▼ **Borderline hypertension** is present when the blood pressure is **between the 90th and 95th percentile** for age, height, and sex.

▼ **Hypertensive urgency** occurs when the an asymptomatic patient has systolic or diastolic blood pressure measurements that **exceed the 95th percentile** for the patient's age, height, and sex by more than 50%.

▼ **Malignant hypertension** is a **rapid increase in blood pressure** with clinical evidence for **end-organ damage** (retinopathy, papilledema, and seizures).

▼ DIFFERENTIAL DIAGNOSIS LIST

Primary
Polygenetic

Familial
Sporadic
Labile

Monogenetic

Gordon syndrome
Liddle syndrome
Syndrome of apparent mineralocorticoid excess (AME)

Renal Causes
Renoparenchymal

Glomerulonephritis—acute and chronic
Hemolytic–uremic syndrome
Focal segmental glomerulosclerosis
Lupus nephritis
Pyelonephritis (acute or chronic) or reflux nephropathy
Polycystic kidney disease—autosomal recessive, autosomal dominant
Wilms tumor

Obstructive uropathy
Trauma

Vascular Causes

Coarctation of the aorta
Narrow aorta (Williams syndrome, Takayasu arteritis)
Renal artery stenosis
Fibromuscular dysplasia
Renal venous thrombosis

Endocrine Causes

Cushing syndrome
Thyrotoxicosis
Pheochromocytoma
Neuroblastoma
Congenital adrenal hyperplasia
Conns syndrome (hyperaldosteronism)

Neurologic Causes

Increased intracranial pressure (ICP)
Dysautonomia
Guillain-Barré (acute) syndrome

Drug-Related Causes

Corticosteroids
Cyclosporine A
Epinephrine
Cocaine
Amphetamines
Sympathomimetics
Oral contraceptives

Miscellaneous Causes

Stress
Pain
Orthopedic traction
Burns
"White coat" hypertension

▼ DIFFERENTIAL DIAGNOSIS DISCUSSION

Eighty percent of **preteen patients** have **renal or renovascular causes** for their hypertension and are **more likely to have an underlying cause** for their hypertension than are adolescents. The **younger the patient** and **higher the blood pressure,** the more likely it is that a **secondary cause** will be found for the hypertension. Endocrine causes, such as pheochromocytoma and thyrotoxicosis, occur much less frequently.

Renal Artery Stenosis (RAS)

Etiology

A patient with renal artery stenosis may have a history of **umbilical artery catheterization** as a neonate. The stenosis may result from **idiopathic**

fibromuscular dysplasia or may be associated with **neurofibromatosis**. A neurofibroma may rarely cause compression of a renal artery. Fibromuscular dysplasia involves hyperplasia of the intimal and medial layers of the renal artery. **Williams syndrome** and **Takayasu arteritis** are also associated with RAS. The cause for the RAS is not always identifiable.

Clinical Features

Preteens with markedly increased hypertension should be evaluated carefully for the existence of **abdominal bruits.** Most patients have an abdominal bruit lateral to the periumbilical area.

Evaluation

The evaluation consists of **renal ultrasonography, magnetic resonance angiography (MRA)**, and **renal angiography.**

Treatment

Patients may be treated with **dilatation** of the narrowed renal artery, **autotransplant** of the kidney, **vascular repair**, and **antihypertensives. Angiotensin-converting enzyme (ACE) inhibitors** are **contraindicated** in patients with bilateral RAS.

Pyelonephritis

Etiology

Recurrent **urinary tract infection (UTI)** may lead to hypertension following scar formation in the kidney or reflux nephropathy that may develop as a result of accumulated pressure and infection. The decreased blood flow to the damaged kidney stimulates the renin-angiotensin-aldosterone axis, leading to hypertension.

The patient may have a **history of unexplained fevers** as an infant; as the child grows older, the signs and symptoms of UTI become more apparent.

Evaluation

Evaluation with **renal ultrasonography** may detect contractions in the renal mass due to scar formation. The most sensitive method for clinical detection of renal scarring is the **nuclear dimercaptosuccinic acid (DMSA) scan.**

Treatment

Most patients are treated with **antihypertensive medications.** Some patients may benefit from **partial nephrectomy.** Careful **monitoring** of urine **for infection** is required.

Pheochromocytoma

Clinical Features

This rare tumor may present with **hypertension, sweating, flushing, palpitations**, or **abdominal pain.** Tumors on the bladder may cause symptoms during urination.

Evaluation

Once pheochromocytoma is diagnosed, **palpation of abdominal tumors should be avoided** because doing so may release catecholamines, causing symptoms. **Urinary vanillylmandelic acid (VMA) level** measurement, **24-hour collection of catecholamines and metanephrines, metaiodobenzylguanidine**

(MIBG) scanning, and computerized tomography (CT) or magnetic resonance imaging (MRI) can help identify and localize the tumor.

Essential Hypertension

Etiology

In contrast to hypertension in the preteen patient, hypertension in **teenagers is rarely attributable to a specific cause.** Careful history taking might uncover a **large salt intake, high calorie intake, sedentary life-style** or the use of **medications** such as birth control pills, cocaine, corticosteroids, or sympathomimetics. **Obesity** contributes directly to the increasing incidence of hypertension in teenagers.

Clinical Features

Patients with essential hypertension are **asymptomatic** and an increased blood pressure reading is detected on routine physical examination. Teenagers with mild systolic hypertension most likely have essential hypertension. Because the odds of finding a renovascular or endocrine cause in teenagers are so low, **investigation should be delayed** until a **series of readings** are taken to confirm the hypertension.

Evaluation

Feeling for **femoral pulses** and measurement of **blood pressure in all four extremities** are part of the complete physical examination in hypertensive patients. In thin patients, the blood in the aorta may produce a normal sound that can be mistaken for a bruit if the stethoscope is applied too firmly.

    Falsely high readings stem from using a cuff that is too small, using incorrect technique, or taking a measurement while the patient is anxious or crying. **At least three measurements** should be obtained to ensure an accurate reading, and care should be taken to use a **blood pressure cuff that is the correct size.** The cuff should cover approximately two thirds of the upper arm as measured from the tip of the acromium to the antecubital fossa.

Treatment

Obese patients will profit from weight loss through **dieting, aerobic exercise,** and **control of salt intake,** which will relieve stress and strengthen the cardiovascular system.

▼ TREATMENT OF HYPERTENSION

Information about the entire patient's prescribed and over-the-counter medications must be obtained. The physician should consistently use a few **selected antihypertensive agents** (ACE inhibitors, angiotensin II receptor blockers, calcium channel blockers, beta blockers, diuretics, and vasodilators) and be familiar with their potentials, interactions, and side effects (Table 44.1) The patient and the parents must be **educated regarding side effects** of medications and idiosyncrasies of drugs (e.g., sudden cessation of a beta blocker can cause side effects). Drug doses should be maximized prior to adding a second agent. Use as few drugs per patient as possible and add or remove only one agent at a time.

TABLE 44.1. Commonly Used Antihypertensive Agents in Children

Category	Agent	Common Side Effects
Diuretics	Chlorothiazides	Hypokalemia, alkalosis, volume depletion, hyperuricemia, hyperlipidemia
	Furosemide	Volume depletion, hypokalemia, alkalosis, nephrocalcinosis
	Spironolactone	Hyperkalemia, mild acidosis, gynecomastia
Vasodilators	Hydralazine	Flushing, tachycardia, headaches
	Doxocin	Tachycardia, headaches
	Minoxidil	Hypotension, hirsutism
β blockers	Atenolol	Asthma, hypoglycemia
	Labetalol	Asthma, nightmares, tingling scalp
Calcium channel blockers	Nifedipine	Hypotension, peripheral edema, elevated liver enzymes
	Amlodipine	
	Diltiazem	Flushing
ACE inhibitors	Captopril, Enalapril	Hyperkalemia, dry cough, increase in serum creatinine, angioedema
ATIIR blockers	Losartan	Hyperkalemia, increase in serum creatinine

ACE = angiotensin-converting enzyme; ATIIR = angiotensin II receptor.

Suggested Readings

Deal JE, Shell MF, Buratt TM, et al: Renovascular disease in childhood. *J Pediatr* 121:378, 1992.

Ingelfinger JR: *Hypertension in Pediatric Kidney Disease,* 2nd ed. Boston, Little, Brown, 1992, p 1889.

Jung FF, Ingelfinger JR: Hypertension in childhood and adolescence. *Pediatr Rev* 14(5):169–179, 1993.

Lip GY, Beevers M, Beevers DG, Dillon MJ: The measurement of blood pressure and the detection of hypertension in children and adolescents. *J Hum Hypertens* 15(6):419–423, 2001.

Loggie JMH (ed): *Pediatric and Adolescent Hypertension.* Cambridge, MA, Blackwell, 1992.

Report of the Second Task Force on Blood Pressure Control in Children. *Pediatrics* 79:1, 1987.

Sorof JM. Systolic hypertension in children: benign or beware? *Pediatr Nephrol* 16(6):517–525, 2001.

Update on the 1987 Task Force Report on High Blood Pressure in Children and Adolescents: A Working Group Report from the National High Blood Pressure Education Program. *Pediatrics* 98:649–658, 1996.

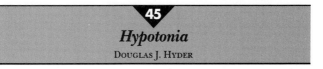

Hypotonia
DOUGLAS J. HYDER

▼ INTRODUCTION

Hypotonia is defined as **decreased resistance to passive movement.** The examiner determines tone by observing the **patient's posture** and feeling **resistance to movement** when flexing the patient's joints. It is important to **differentiate decreased tone from weakness and hyporeflexia.** A careful history and physical examination, including a thorough neurologic examination, frequently narrows the differential diagnosis enough to necessitate only confirmatory diagnostic tests.

▼ DIFFERENTIAL DIAGNOSIS LIST
Newborn

Infectious Causes

Abscess
Encephalitis
Meningitis
Sepsis

Genetic Causes

Angelman syndrome
Canavan disease
Cerebrohepatorenal (Zellweger) syndrome
Congenital myopathies
Galactosemia
Glycogen storage diseases
Niemann-Pick disease
Oculocerebrorenal (Lowe) syndrome
Prader-Willi syndrome
Tay-Sachs disease
Trisomy 21 (Down syndrome)

Anatomic Causes

Acute infarction
Aneurysm
Arteriovenous malformation (AVM)
Holoprosencephaly
Hydrocephalus
Increased intracranial pressure (ICP)
Lissencephaly
Myasthenia gravis
Schizencephaly
Spina bifida
Spinal muscular atrophy (Werdnig-Hoffmann disease)
Sturge-Weber syndrome
Tumor

Traumatic Causes

Brachial plexus injury (Erb palsy)
Carotid dissection
Carotid ligation
Epidural hematoma
Subarachnoid hemorrhage
Subdural hematoma

Miscellaneous Causes

Drug toxicity
Seizure
Hyperammonemia
Hyperbilirubinemia
Hyper- or hypocalcemia
Hypermagnesemia
Hypoglycemia
Hypoxia
Prematurity

Children

Infectious Causes

Abscess
Encephalitis
Meningitis
Myelitis
Myositis

Toxic Causes

Botulinum toxin
Drugs
Lead poisoning
Organophosphate poisoning

Neoplastic Causes

Brain tumor
Leukemia
Metastatic tumor

Traumatic Causes

Peripheral nerve trauma

Congenital or Vascular Causes

Acute cerebral or spinal cord infarction
Aneurysm
Carotid dissection
Spinal muscular atrophy

Metabolic or Genetic Causes

Adrenoleukodystrophy
Cerebrohepatorenal (Zellweger) syndrome
Congenital myopathies
Glycogen storage diseases

Hereditary motor and sensory neuropathy (Charcot-Marie-Tooth disease)
Leigh syndrome
Metachromatic leukodystrophy
Muscular dystrophy
Niemann-Pick disease
Organic acidemias
Tay-Sachs disease
Hyperammonemia
Hyperbilirubinemia
Hyper- or hypocalcemia
Hypermagnesemia
Hypoglycemia
Hypoxia

Inflammatory Causes

Guillain-Barré syndrome

Miscellaneous Causes

Dermatomyositis
Seizure
Migraine headache
Hydrocephalus
Increased ICP
Myasthenia gravis

▼ DIFFERENTIAL DIAGNOSIS DISCUSSION
Trisomy 21 (Down Syndrome)

Etiology

Trisomy 21 is the **most commonly observed** chromosomal abnormality, occurring in approximately 1 out of every 1000 births. The risk of trisomy 21 increases if the parents have previously had an affected child, when either parent has a translocation involving chromosome 21, and as the age of the mother increases.

Clinical Features

▼ **Shorter and heavier** than the norm for their age group
▼ The **head is small** and round with a flat occiput.
▼ The **palpebral fissures** slant upward and an inner epicanthal fold is present.
▼ The **eyes** may have **circumferential speckling** (Brushfield spots).
▼ The **nose and ears are small.**
▼ **Dermatoglyphic features** include a transverse palmar crease, distal triradius, and ulnar loops.
▼ The **hands are short** and **brachyclinodactyly** may be present.

⚄ HINT Growth charts designed for individuals with trisomy 21 should be used to monitor growth in these patients. Neurologic examination is significant for infantile hypotonia and mental retardation. Dementia usually affects individuals after the age of 30 years.

▼ Approximately 40% of individuals with trisomy 21 have **structural heart defects** [e.g., septal defects, patent ductus arteriosus (PDA), aortic arch defects].

▼ **Gastrointestinal problems** include structural abnormalities and Hirschsprung disease.

▼ **Seizures,** sometimes presenting as infantile spasms, occur in approximately 5% of affected individuals.

▼ **Sensorineural hearing loss** is seen more commonly than in the general pediatric population.

▼ **Increased risk of acute leukemia**

▼ **Atlantoaxial subluxation** occurs in approximately 15% of individuals, but most subluxations do not require treatment.

Evaluation

The condition can usually be diagnosed on the basis of a careful physical examination. **Genetic testing** is recommended to confirm the diagnosis of trisomy 21.

Treatment

Supportive care focuses on **cognitive development.** Optimal treatment of medical conditions is decided on a case-by-case basis. Currently, there is no accepted way of preventing the early dementia experienced by those with trisomy 21.

Prader-Willi Syndrome

Etiology

A **paternally inherited deletion in chromosome 15** results in the clinical features of Prader-Willi syndrome. When the deletion on chromosome 15 is **inherited from the mother,** the clinical features of **Angelman syndrome** are present.

Clinical Features

Newborn infants with Prader-Willi syndrome have **hypotonia, difficulty feeding,** and **hypogonadotrophic hypogonadism.** Other features include mental retardation, short stature, small hands and feet, hyperphagia, and obesity.

Evaluation

Prader-Willi syndrome may be suspected after careful physical examination, but **genetic testing** is recommended to confirm the diagnosis. Approximately 60% of individuals with Prader-Willi syndrome have a paternally inherited deletion in chromosome 15q11–q13. The remaining 40% do not have the deletion, but do have maternal uniparental disomy 15. (A phenotypically different condition called Angelman syndrome is also associated with a deletion in chromosome 15q11–q13, but this deletion is maternally inherited.)

Treatment

Treatment is **supportive** and focuses on **cognitive development.** Although difficult, **controlling obesity** is an important way to minimize the risk of obstructive apnea and the cardiopulmonary consequences of obesity.

Myasthenia Gravis

Etiology

Antibodies bind the acetylcholine receptor and impair neuromuscular transmission. In neonates, antibodies can be transferred from the mother. Older patients produce **autoantibodies,** leading to myasthenia gravis.

Clinical Features

The hallmark of myasthenia gravis is **weakness and fatigue of skeletal muscle** that **worsens with activity** and improves with rest. The muscular weakness may cause ptosis, diplopia, and difficulty in chewing and swallowing.

🖐 HINT Similar symptoms may develop secondary to congenital myasthenic syndromes because the patient has inherited transmembrane receptors, synaptic vesicles, or transjunctional enzymes that are dysfunctional.

Evaluation

On examination, **hypotonia and weakness** are present and **reflexes are decreased.** Muscle bulk, sensation, and pupillary constriction to light are normal. Hyperthyroidism, systemic lupus erythematosus (SLE), rheumatoid arthritis, insulin-dependent diabetes mellitus (IDDM), and thymoma are associated with myasthenia gravis, and signs of these disorders may be present on physical examination.

The **edrophonium (Tensilon) test** is a reliable way to diagnose myasthenia gravis. Because edrophonium impairs acetylcholine esterase, the concentration of acetylcholine increases in the neuromuscular junction so that the patient's weakness temporarily improves. If a congenital myasthenic syndrome is present, the edrophonium test usually does not improve the weakness.

Nerve conduction studies are normal, but **electromyography** demonstrates a decremental response with repetitive stimulation.

🖐 HINT Antibodies against the acetylcholine receptor are present in the sera of 75% of patients.

Treatment

During an acute exacerbation, it may be necessary to **support ventilation and nutritional needs.** Long-acting **acetylcholine esterase antagonists** (e.g., pyridostigmine, neostigmine) are used to improve the weakness. Usually, **glycopyrrolate,** an antimuscarinic agent, is administered simultaneously to counteract the diarrhea that is a side effect of acetylcholine esterase antagonists. Sometimes, **immunosuppression** with corticosteroids or azathioprine is necessary to improve the patient's weakness.

If a thymoma is present, or if the weakness is refractory to medications, a **thymectomy** is performed. It is important to avoid administering the **many medications** that can **exacerbate** myasthenia gravis (e.g., aminoglycoside antibiotics, β-adrenergic receptor antagonists, neuromuscular blocking agents).

Spinal Muscular Atrophy

Etiology

An **abnormality in chromosome 5p** is believed to be responsible for spinal muscular atrophy. Two genes, called survival motor neuron and neuronal apoptosis inhibitory protein, are abnormal and eventually cause the motor neurons in the brainstem and spinal cord to degenerate.

Clinical Features

Three recognized types of spinal muscular atrophy differ from one another on the basis of the age of onset, maximum muscular strength, and prognosis for survival.

▼ **Type I (Werdnig-Hoffmann disease).** Newborn infants may display hypotonia, weakness, and hyporeflexia. Pectus excavatum, secondary to intercostal muscle weakness, may be present. Weakness of the cranial nerves may make eye movement and swallowing difficult. Pupils are normally reactive to light. Tongue fasciculations may be present.

▼ **Type II (intermediate type).** Type II spinal muscular atrophy presents in children 1–2 years of age. These toddlers have hypotonia, difficulty attaining motor milestones, and weakness of the proximal limb muscles. The weakness is generally less severe than that seen in type I spinal muscular atrophy, but children generally require a wheelchair and attention to scoliosis.

▼ **Type III (Wohlfart-Kugelberg-Welander syndrome).** The mean age of onset is 9 years. Children are weak and have difficulty climbing stairs, jumping, and running. Gowers sign, muscle atrophy, hypotonia, and hyporeflexia are present. The abdomen frequently protrudes because the abdominal muscles are weak. Scoliosis may be present. This type of spinal muscular atrophy has a better long-term prognosis; some patients retain the ability to walk for many years after their diagnosis.

Evaluation

Electrodiagnostic studies show fibrillations and decreased nerve conduction velocity in motor nerves with normal conduction velocity in sensory nerves.

Treatment

There is **no cure** for any form of spinal muscular atrophy. **Support of respiratory, nutritional, and mobility needs** is important. Children with scoliosis may require **surgery.**

Brachial Plexus Injury (Erb Palsy)

Etiology

Traction on the head or arm during delivery injures the brachial plexus, resulting in a peripheral neuropathy of the fifth and sixth cervical nerves.

Clinical Features

The **affected arm is adducted** and **internally rotated,** with the **forearm extended** and **pronated,** and the **wrist flexed.** Tone, strength, and tendon reflexes are decreased in the deltoid, biceps, supinator, and wrist extensors.

Evaluation

Generally, no evaluation is necessary. An **electromyogram (EMG)** documents the extent of the neuropathy.

Treatment

Generally, **no treatment is necessary,** but recovery may take several months. The sleeve of the shirt on the affected side should be pinned to the front of the shirt to protect the arm from injury. Physical therapists use **passive range-of-motion exercises** to help keep the joints nimble during recovery. Rarely, surgical intervention is attempted to connect a severed nerve.

Treatment of a coincidental clavicle or humerus fracture may be necessary.

Botulinum Toxin

Etiology

In infants, ingestion of the spores of *Clostridium botulinum* produces a toxin in the intestine that prevents the release of acetylcholine at the neuromuscular junction. **Honey** is one of the sources of the spores, but infants who are nursed around **excavated land** are also prone to ingesting the spores. The acidity of the infant's stomach is not sufficient to kill the ingested spores. Older children and adults acquire botulism by ingesting preformed toxin, generally from contaminated food.

Clinical Features

Constipation is usually the first symptom, followed by **diplopia** and **progressive bulbar and extremity weakness. Swallowing and breathing** become progressively more difficult.

Evaluation

On physical examination, consciousness is normal. The **extraocular muscles are weak,** and the pupils usually do not constrict in response to light. **Generalized hypotonia, weakness,** and **hyporeflexia** are present. Sensation remains normal.

Lumbar puncture (LP) reveals normal cerebrospinal fluid (CSF). *C. botulinum* organisms or toxin can be detected in **stool samples.**

Electrophysiologic studies demonstrate normal nerve conduction velocity, decreased amplitude of evoked muscle potentials, and improved responses with repetitive stimulation of the nerve.

Treatment

Meticulous support of respiratory and nutritional needs is imperative. If the disease was caused via a wound or ingestion of contaminated food, use of an **antitoxin** should be considered. Because the antitoxin is derived from **equine sera,** care should be taken to test for **hypersensitivity** prior to administration.

Guillain-Barré Syndrome

Etiology

The **myelin sheaths around the peripheral nerves are destroyed** in response to an inflammatory infiltrate. Sometimes, nerve axons are also damaged. It is thought that an infection or immunization causes the **autoimmune response** that produces the inflammation, but the precise mechanism is unknown.

Peripheral nerves (which carry motor, sensory, and autonomic information) are all affected. The central nervous system (CNS) is not affected.

Clinical Features

Children usually present with an **ascending weakness** that **worsens** over the course of a few days and gradually involves all four limbs and the face. Usually, paraesthesia and discomfort occur simultaneously.

Evaluation

On physical examination, **hypotonia, hyporeflexia,** and **weakness** are present. The sensory examination shows decreased sensation to all modalities. **Autonomic dysfunction** may cause urinary retention, fluctuating blood pressures, and cardiac dysrhythmias.

The **CSF protein level is characteristically elevated,** with a minimum of leukocytes. **Nerve conduction velocity is decreased** in motor and sensory nerves.

Treatment

Supportive care is directed toward **maintaining ventilation** and **meeting nutritional needs.** A **catheter** needs to be placed in the bladder if urinary retention is present. It is important to **monitor** the patient's **vital capacity** and **cardiac electrical activity;** elective endotracheal intubation should be considered if the vital capacity falls below 10 ml/kg. Approximately 10% of patients require **endotracheal intubation and mechanical ventilation** because of difficulty breathing.

To modify the autoimmune response, **plasma exchange, intravenous immunoglobulin,** and **corticosteroids** have all been used with success, although no clinical trial has demonstrated superiority of one method over another.

▼ EVALUATION OF HYPOTONIA

Patient History

There are several important questions to seek answers to when assessing an infant or child with hypotonia to help narrow the differential diagnosis:

▼ **At what age did the symptoms first appear?**
▼ **Are the symptoms getting worse or staying the same?**
▼ **Was the onset of symptoms acute?** Infarction, seizure, and bleeding are associated with a rapid onset of symptoms. The onset of symptoms associated with infectious disorders and intoxication is generally subacute (i.e., evolving over several hours or days). Metabolic and immunologic conditions generally progress even more slowly.
▼ **How extensive are the symptoms?** Are all of the muscles involved, or is just one limb involved?
▼ **What is the birth history?** Things of note include a difficult pregnancy, decreased fetal movements, oligohydramnios on prenatal ultrasound, traumatic delivery, and premature delivery.

Physical Examination

Care should be taken to **examine the skin and the fundi carefully,** because abnormalities of these tissues occur with certain neurologic disorders.

A **complete neurologic assessment,** including assessment of mental status; cranial nerves; muscle bulk, tone, and strength; coordination; reflexes; and sensation, provides useful information. If possible the child should be examined when she is awake and relaxed, with head in the midline. Note the following:

▼ **The posture of the trunk and the extremities**
▼ **A "frog-leg" position** (i.e., hips abducted, flexed, and externally rotated)—seen in hypotonic infants
▼ **Muscle bulk and how the muscles feel when palpated**
▼ **Fasciculations of the tongue**—in an infant with suspected Werdnig-Hoffmann disease
▼ **Flexion and extension of the limbs at each of the joints**
▼ **Head lag**—if safe to do so, infants should be pulled from a supine to a sitting position to observe their head lag

---

▨ HINT Hypotonic infants seem to slip through the examiner's hands when held under the axillae, and drape over the examiner's hands when held in horizontal suspension. Subtle hypotonia in a child can be identified by asking the child to hold his hands above his head—the hypotonic arm will overpronate, and the forearm will drift toward the head.

Laboratory Studies

Care should be taken to gather as much information as possible with the history and physical examination before proceeding with laboratory assessment.

▼ **Blood work** generally includes a complete blood count (CBC); toxicology screen; electrolyte analysis; and serum glucose, calcium, magnesium, and bilirubin determinations. It is frequently useful to determine the arterial oxygen, pH, and ammonia content. When certain metabolic conditions are suspected, serum may be sent for amino acid determination.
▼ **Urinalysis** may be appropriate for organic acid analysis in some patients with suspected metabolic disorders.
▼ **CSF analysis.** If an LP can be performed safely, CSF analysis is indicated when infection or certain metabolic conditions are suspected.
▼ **Bone marrow analysis.** Abnormal cells in the bone marrow are seen with some metabolic conditions.
▼ **Chromosome analysis** is important with conditions such as trisomy 21 and Prader-Willi syndrome.
▼ **Enzyme analysis** can assist with the diagnosis of some conditions, such as Canavan disease.

Diagnostic Modalities

▼ **Electroencephalography.** An electroencephalogram (EEG) is helpful when considering the diagnosis of a seizure disorder.
▼ **Electromyography** or **muscle biopsy** is necessary when the differential diagnosis includes conditions that affect the peripheral nerves, neuromuscular junction, or muscles.
▼ **Computed tomography (CT).** If intracranial bleeding, hydrocephalus, or a skull fracture is suspected, a CT study of the head is indicated.
▼ **Magnetic resonance imaging (MRI)** of the brain or spine identifies most abnormalities that are caused by anatomic, metabolic, neoplastic, or vascular conditions.

▼ APPROACH TO THE PATIENT

Conditions that are amenable to rapid treatment (e.g., electrolyte imbalance, toxin exposure, seizure, infection, intracranial bleeding, hydrocephalus) must be excluded prior to entertaining the possibility of rarer conditions.

▼ **When symptoms are acute in onset,** intracranial bleeding, seizure, and infarction should be suspected: a CT study of the head and a neurology or neurosurgery consultation are wise.

▼ **When the symptoms are subacute or chronic,** the patient's respiratory and cardiovascular condition should be quickly assessed. Remember that many conditions associated with hypotonia also weaken the pharyngeal muscles, so the need for endotracheal intubation must be assessed. If the patient is swallowing secretions improperly, the examiner should maintain a high suspicion for aspiration pneumonia.

Because the differential diagnosis of hypotonia is broad, after the patient is stable, care should be taken to ascertain all of the **historical facts** and to perform a **complete examination.** A **neurology consult** is generally necessary to help narrow the differential diagnosis, assist with long-term care, or both.

Suggested Readings

Cassidy SB: Prader-Willi syndrome. *J Med Genet* 34(11):917, 1997.

Dubowitz V: Evaluation and differential diagnosis of the hypotonic infant. *Pediatr Rev* 6:237, 1985.

Hayes A, Batshaw ML: Down syndrome. *Pediatr Clin North Am* 40(3):523, 1993.

Jones HR: Childhood Guillain-Barré syndrome: clinical presentation, diagnosis and therapy. *J Child Neurol* 11:4, 1996.

Petersen MC, Palmer FB: Advances in prevention and treatment of cerebral palsy. *Ment Retard Dev Disabil Res Rev* 7:30, 2001.

Wiggington JM, Thill P: Infant botulism: A review of the literature. *Clin Pediatr* 32(11):669, 1993.

46

Infections, Newborn

Samir S. Shah

▼ NEONATAL SEPSIS

Overview

The most common classification of neonatal sepsis is by age at onset.

▼ **Early-onset infection.** Clinical manifestations of early-onset infection occur **within the first 7 days of life** (95% present within the first 72 hours). Frequently, **maternal complications of labor or delivery** lead to these infections. Organisms from the maternal genital tract during the intrapartum period colonize the infant's skin and gastrointestinal and respiratory tracts. The progression from colonization to infection, which is not well understood, includes bacteremia, pneumonia, and meningitis. The most common organisms are group B streptococci (GBS), *Escherichia coli*, and, occasionally, *Listeria monocytogenes*.

▼ **Late-onset infection.** Clinical manifestations of late-onset infection occur **between 7 and 30 days of life.** Infection may be the result of **colonization during birth or during hospitalization** in the intensive care unit. Although most infants do not become ill as a result of this colonization, necessary invasive procedures put them at increased risk for infection. Infections include bacteremia, pneumonia, and meningitis, as well as osteomyelitis, skin and soft tissue infection, endocarditis, and urinary tract infection. The most common organisms are coagulase-negative staphylococci, *Staphylococcus aureus*, *Enterococcus* spp., GBS, *E. coli*, *Klebsiella pneumoniae*, and *Candida* spp.

▼ **Late, late-onset infection.** The improved survival rate of **very low birth weight infants** (< 1500 g) has prompted the addition of this third category: late, late-onset infection. Although these infants are no longer neonates, their "corrected" gestational age (usually 28–34 weeks) and continued need for hospitalization because of complications of prematurity accord them "newborn" status. One-fourth of all very low birth weight infants who survive beyond 3 days of life will have at least one episode of late-onset or late, late-onset sepsis. These infants usually have **central venous catheters or endotracheal tubes** in place. Infection in this group is **nosocomially acquired** and often due to coagulase-negative staphylococci, *Pseudomonas aeruginosa*, *Enterobacter cloacae*, *Serratia marcescens*, and *Candida* spp.

Common Pathogens

Group B *Streptococcus* Infection

The maternal colonization rate for GBS is 15%–30%, and 50% of these women deliver infants who are **colonized at birth.** The risk of infection in a colonized baby is 1%. Risk factors for infection are shown in Table 46.1. The most common clinical manifestations for **early-onset infection are sepsis, pneumonia, and, less often, meningitis** (5%–10% of early-onset GBS cases). Early-onset GBS infection has a fulminant presentation; 50% of infected

---

TABLE 46.1. Select Risk Factors for Group B Streptococcal Infection

Maternal risk factors
  Prior infant with group B streptococcal sepsis
  Group B streptococcal bacteriuria
  Prolonged rupture of membranes (≥ 18 hours)
  Premature rupture of membranes (< 37 weeks gestation)
  Preterm labor (< 37 weeks gestation)
  Intrapartum fever > 37.9°C (100.4°F)

Fetal/neonatal risk factors
  Prematurity
  Meconium passed in utero
  Low 5-minute Apgar score (≤ 5)
  Male gender (sepsis four times more common in boys than in girls)

infants are symptomatic at birth. Initial manifestations include **respiratory distress, hypoxia, and shock.** The mortality rate of early-onset GBS infection is 5%–10%. **Late-onset infections** include **sepsis, meningitis** (30%–40% of late-onset GBS cases), and, occasionally, **skin or soft tissue infections, osteomyelitis, or septic arthritis.** The mortality rate of late-onset GBS infection is 2%–6%. **Permanent neurologic sequelae** occur in approximately 50% of patients with meningitis caused by GBS infection.

The use of **intrapartum antibiotics** to treat GBS colonized women has greatly decreased the incidence of early-onset GBS infection in neonates. Current American Academy of Pediatrics (AAP) and American College of Obstetrics and Gynecology (ACOG) recommendations include administering intrapartum **penicillin to women with any of the risk factors** listed in Table 46.1. Other pregnant women are **tested for anogenital GBS colonization at 35–37 weeks gestation** and offered intrapartum chemoprophylaxis if colonized. Other **factors that increase the risk** of neonatal sepsis include a **multiple gestation pregnancy and maternal chorioamnionitis.**

E. coli Infection

E. coli, like GBS, is passed from **mother to infant,** and the ratio of infected to colonized babies is similar. **Early-onset and late-onset infections** occur. Organisms that have the K1 surface antigen are more apt to cause infection, especially meningitis.

Coagulase-negative Staphylococcal Infection

Coagulase-negative staphylococci (primarily *S. epidermidis*) are most commonly associated with nosocomial infection. Risk factors include **prematurity** and the use of **indwelling catheters.** The organism produces a slime coating that allows it to adhere to the surfaces of synthetic polymers used to make central venous catheters and also enables it to evade the immune system. **Clinical manifestations** of staphylococcal sepsis are **often subtle** and a **high index of suspicion** is needed to diagnose the infection early.

Fungal Infection

Candida albicans has been the most common cause of neonatal fungal infection; however, *C. parapsilosis* and other non-*albicans Candida* species (*C. tropicalis, C. glabrata*) are becoming more prevalent. Risk factors for fungal infection have been identified (Table 46.2). Systemic infection occurs after hematogenous dissemination. The most commonly involved sites are the **heart** (15%), **retina** (6%), **kidneys** (5%), and **liver** (3%). *Malassezia furfur* **bloodstream infection** is associated with intralipid infusion.

TABLE 46.2. Risk Factors for Candidemia

Gestational age < 32 weeks
Indwelling vascular catheter
Endotracheal intubation > 7 days
Receipt of intralipids or parenteral nutrition
Broad-spectrum antibiotic use (> 5 days or > two antibiotics), especially third-generation cephalosporins

Evaluation of Sepsis

All infants with suspected sepsis should receive antibiotics while awaiting blood culture results. The remainder of the evaluation, including lumbar puncture (LP), can be completed once the infant has been stabilized. Table 46.3 summarizes the differential diagnosis for sepsis.

Patient History

▼ Are there maternal factors that place the infant at risk for sepsis (see Table 46.1)?
▼ Is there a family history of infection or other diseases in newborns?
▼ Does the infant have poor feeding, feeding intolerance (e.g., vomiting, abdominal distention), decreased activity, lethargy, or irritability?

Physical Examination

Signs of infection in the newborn infant are nonspecific and include the following disturbances:

▼ **Temperature**—fever (> 37.9°C) or hypothermia (< 36.0°C)
▼ **Neurologic**—bulging fontanelle, lethargy, irritability, weak suck or cry, hypotonia, hypertonia
▼ **Respiratory**—tachypnea (respiratory rate > 60/min), grunting, nasal flaring, retractions, hypoxemia, apnea
▼ **Cardiovascular**-tachycardia, bradycardia, hypotension (systolic blood pressure < 60 mm Hg in term infants), delayed capillary refill (> 2 seconds)
▼ **Cutaneous**—jaundice, mottled skin, cyanosis, or petechiae
▼ **Skeletal**—focal bone tenderness

Laboratory Studies

Table 46.4 lists the studies included in a standard sepsis work-up.

▼ **Complete blood count (CBC).** The range of normal values for the white blood cell (WBC) count and differential changes with the gestational and chronological age of the baby. The normal WBC count is 10,000–30,000/mm^3 at birth and decreases to 5,000–15,000/mm^3 by the second week of life. Although elevated total WBC and absolute neutrophil counts (ANC) are not helpful as single indicators of sepsis, neutropenia (ANC < 1500/mm^3) and an elevated immature-to-total WBC ratio > 0.2 are more often associated with infection. Positive and negative predictive values in large enough studies have not been established to use these values for treatment decisions. The initial WBC count may be normal in an infected newborn, with abnormalities developing 24–48 hours later.

⚡ HINT Remember that several noninfectious conditions can cause neutropenia in newborns, including pregnancy-induced hypertension, asphyxia, intraventricular hemorrhage, hemolytic disease, and alloimmune neutropenia.

▼ **Cerebrospinal fluid (CSF) analysis.** The CSF sample should be evaluated for the cell count and differential and protein and glucose levels. Newborns have higher CSF cell counts and protein levels than do older children and adults. The average CSF WBC count in an uninfected newborn is 6 WBCs/mm^3, and several studies have determined the normal range

TABLE 46.3. Differential Diagnosis of Sepsis

Category	Disorder	Associated Symptoms and Signs	Differentiating Features
Metabolic	Hypoglycemia	Respiratory distress, jitteriness, lethargy, seizures	Hypoglycemia can occur with sepsis; check blood glucose in sick infants; especially common in infants of diabetic mothers and small-for-gestational-age infants
	Hypocalcemia	Respiratory distress, jitteriness, seizures	Check calcium; especially common in infants of diabetic mothers and preterm infants
	Inborn error of metabolism	Lethargy, vomiting, seizures, tachypnea	Urea cycle defects and organic acidemias often present after the first few feedings
Pulmonary	Respiratory distress syndrome	Respiratory distress in preterm infant	CXR shows hazy, "ground glass" appearance; often indistinguishable from bacterial pneumonia
	Meconium aspiration	Respiratory distress in term infant	Classic CXR shows diffuse, patchy interstitial infiltrates with hyperinflation; may have severe cyanosis from pulmonary hypertension and right-to-left shunting
	Transient tachypnea of the newborn	Tachypnea without significant respiratory distress	CXR clear or with fluid in fissures; usually minimal supplemental oxygen requirement; usually seen after cesarean section delivery
Cardiac	Cyanotic congenital heart disease: tetralogy of Fallot, TGA, tricuspid atresia, truncus arteriosus, TAPVR	Tachypnea, cyanosis unresponsive to oxygen, cardiac murmur, extra heart sounds, or abnormal S_2	CXR without infiltrates but with abnormal pulmonary vasculature or cardiac silhouette; difference in pre- and postductal pulse oximetry; lack of response to hyperoxia test [$PaO_2 < 100$ mm Hg breathing 100% O_2]

	Congestive heart failure (VSD, patent ductus arteriosus, myocarditis, AVM—especially hepatic or cerebral)	Poor feeding, tachypnea, poor perfusion, hepatomegaly, S_3	Congestive heart failure from a left-to-right shunt is unusual in the immediate newborn period when the pulmonary vascular resistance is high; onset is gradual
	Ductal-dependent lesions (aortic coarctation, hypoplastic left heart, critical pulmonic stenosis)	Poor perfusion, tachypnea, metabolic acidosis, cyanosis	Often sudden in onset, from hours to weeks after birth; check arterial blood gas, four-extremity blood pressures, and pre- and postductal pulse oximetry
Neurologic	Hemorrhage	Pallor, hypotonia, tachycardia, hypotension	Especially common in preterm infants and following traumatic vaginal delivery
	Cerebral infarct	Seizures	May be associated with polycythemia or cocaine exposure; often idiopathic
GI	Necrotizing enterocolitis	Feeding intolerance, abdominal distention, bloody stools	Usually associated with prematurity; abdominal radiograph may show pneumatosis, portal venous air, or free air; associated laboratory findings may include metabolic acidosis and thrombocytopenia
	Malrotation, volvulus	Bilious emesis, abdominal distention, bloody stools, and shock	All newborns with bilious emesis should be evaluated for GI obstruction; **volvulus is a surgical emergency**
Hematologic	Profound anemia	Pallor, tachycardia, jaundice (if due to hemolysis)	Hemolysis, perinatal bleeding (vasa previa, placental abruption), or postnatal hemorrhage

AVM = arteriovenous malformation; CXR = chest radiograph; GI = gastrointestinal; PaO_2 = arterial oxygen tension; S_2 = second heart sound; S_3 = third heart sound; TAPVR = total anomalous pulmonary venous return; TGA = transposition of the great arteries; VSD = ventricular septal defect.

TABLE 46.4. Standard Sepsis Work-Up
Complete blood count with differential
Blood culture
Lumbar puncture (LP) and cerebrospinal fluid (CSF) analysis*
Urinalysis and urine culture†
Chest radiograph‡

* If the infant is clinically stable and has a platelet count of more than $50,000/mm^3$, an LP can be performed to obtain CSF for analysis of cell count, protein level, and glucose level, and for Gram stain and culture.

† If infant is > 72 hours of life.

‡ If respiratory symptoms are present.

to be up to 20 WBCs/mm^3. The average value for protein in the CSF is 90 mg/dl in full-term infants and 120 mg/dl in preterm infants. Normal babies may have CSF protein of 150–200 mg/dl. Traumatic ("bloody") LPs can give results that are difficult to interpret. The correction factor applied to a traumatic LP is based on the WBC:red blood cell (RBC) ratio in the CSF and in the peripheral blood. Unfortunately, it is often inaccurate in determining the true WBC and protein counts of the CSF.

▼ **Other studies.** Additional tests to consider include C-reactive protein, prothrombin time, partial thromboplastin time, hepatic function panel, serum electrolytes, glucose, serum enteroviral polymerase chain reaction, and viral cultures of nasopharyngeal secretions, rectal swabs, or CSF.

▼ **C-Reactive protein.** The level of C-reactive protein, an acute phase reactant, is often increased in response to infection. The negative predictive value of two C-reactive protein measurements < 1 mg/dl measured 24 hours apart and within 48 hours of birth was > 97% in one study. Routine use of C-reactive protein to guide initiation of antibiotic therapy in the asymptomatic newborn infant is not advocated because of insufficient data.

Treatment of Sepsis

Stabilization and Monitoring

One must always remember the ABCs: **airway, breathing, and circulation.** Close monitoring of the **respiratory status, perfusion, and urine output** is necessary in all newborns with sepsis.

Initial Empiric Antibiotic Therapy

Empiric antimicrobial therapy for suspected bacterial infections is guided by knowledge of pathogens suspected, associated focus of infection, and the antimicrobial susceptibility patterns in a particular intensive care unit. The standard therapy for suspected early-onset sepsis is **ampicillin** (which is effective against GBS, *L. monocytogenes,* most enterococci, and 50% of *E. coli* strains) plus **gentamicin** (provides good gram-negative coverage and is synergistic with ampicillin against many organisms). **Cefotaxime** may be used in place of gentamicin for treatment of meningitis or when resistance to aminoglycosides is suspected. **Vancomycin plus an aminoglycoside** (gentamicin, tobramycin, or amikacin) can be used as empiric therapy for nosocomial infections in the intensive care nursery. Obviously, the therapy should be altered appropriately when an organism is isolated and susceptibilities are available.

Specific Antibiotic Therapy

▼ **Group B *Streptococcus*.** Bacteremia or pneumonia can be treated with administration of ampicillin alone. If meningitis is present, aminoglycoside administration should be continued.

▼ ***L. monocytogenes*.** Ampicillin alone is generally adequate.

▼ ***E. coli* and *K. pneumoniae*.** Combination therapy with an aminoglycoside and a third-generation cephalosporin is generally recommended. A single agent may be used for an uncomplicated urinary tract infection.

▼ **Other gram-negative organisms.** Therapy is more complicated because of development of strains resistant to gentamicin and cephalosporins. Administration of a carbapenem and amikacin (or tobramycin) should be considered. This decision should be made in conjunction with a pediatric infectious diseases specialist. Cephalosporins should not be used as monotherapy to treat gram-negative rod bloodstream infections because of the risk of inducing resistant strains.

▼ **Coagulase-negative staphylococci.** Oxacillin can be used if sensitivity to this agent is demonstrated in vitro. Otherwise, vancomycin should be continued. Meningitis should be treated with a combination of vancomycin and an aminoglycoside.

▼ ***Candida albicans*.** Treat with amphotericin B. For meningitis, add oral flucytosine. For severe amphotericin B-associated toxicity (e.g., renal insufficiency), consider lipid amphotericin B or fluconazole. Removal of the infected catheter is an important part of treatment of candidemia. Failure to remove the catheter as soon as candidemia is detected results in prolonged duration of candidemia and increased mortality rates.

Duration of Antibiotic Therapy

Expected duration of therapy depends on many variables, including **virulence of pathogen, rapidity of clinical response, removal of infected catheter, and adequacy of drainage of purulent foci,** if present. Approximate duration of therapy for selected infections is presented in Table 46.5.

TABLE 46.5. Approximate Duration of Therapy for Selected Infections in the Newborn Infant

Site of Infection	Duration of Therapy (days)
Skin/soft tissue	7–10
Bacteremia	10
Bacteremia with CVC	10–14
Necrotizing enterocolitis	10–14
Pneumonia	10–14
Meningitis (gram-positive)	14
Meningitis (gram-negative)	21
Osteomyelitis/septic arthritis	28–42
Endocarditis	28–42
Fungemia (CVC removed)	14
Fungemia (disseminated)	>28

CVC = central venous catheter.

In cases of **bacterial meningitis**, a **repeat LP** should be performed several days into therapy to document sterilization of the CSF. Therapy should continue **2 weeks after obtaining a negative culture result for gram-positive meningitis** and **3 weeks after obtaining a negative culture result for gram-negative meningitis.**

Other Treatment Modalities

▼ **Blood products.** Some centers treat coagulation disorders with administration of fresh frozen plasma (15 ml/kg) to replenish clotting factors. Platelets should be given to maintain a count of more than $20,000/mm^3$ (or more than $50,000/mm^3$ if there is evidence of bleeding).

▼ **Alternative therapies.** Various strategies for prophylaxis or treatment of sepsis in the newborn have been studied, including exchange transfusion, neutrophil transfusion, administration of intravenous immunoglobulin, and cytokine therapy. Unfortunately, none has consistently proven effective for routine use. Hemopoietic colony-stimulating factors have been shown in recent trials to increase ANC and decrease mortality rates in critically ill neutropenic neonates.

Approach to the Asymptomatic Patient with Risk Factors for Sepsis

The decision on whether to evaluate an asymptomatic newborn for infection should be based on **maternal and fetal risk factors,** such as those listed in Table 46.1. In asymptomatic infants with gestational age > 35 weeks, the duration of intrapartum prophylaxis before delivery determines subsequent management. If **two or more doses of maternal prophylaxis** were given before delivery, **no laboratory evaluation or antimicrobial treatment** is required. These infants should be **observed in the hospital for at least 48 hours.** If **fewer than two doses** were given, the AAP and ACOG recommend a **limited evaluation** (CBC with differential and blood culture) and **at least 48 hours of observation** before discharge from the hospital.

Premature neonates have at least a **10-fold higher risk for early-onset GBS sepsis** compared with term neonates. Furthermore, as the degree of prematurity increases, clinical evaluation for signs and symptoms of sepsis are less reliable. Therefore, asymptomatic infants < 35 weeks gestation should receive **limited evaluation** (CBC with differential and blood culture) and **at least 48 hours of observation** prior to hospital discharge. Empiric antibiotic therapy is not required. If, during the period of observation, the clinical course **suggests systemic infection, complete diagnostic evaluation** and **administration of empiric antibiotic therapy** are indicated. This degree of surveillance and treatment is justified by the high morbidity and mortality rates associated with neonatal infection.

▼ CONGENITAL (TORCH) AND PERINATAL INFECTIONS
Overview

A congenital infection is acquired by the infant transplacentally during the first, second, or early third trimester. Table 46.6 lists the clinical features associated with these infections. The classic acronym for the agents that cause

TABLE 46.6. Clinical Features Suggesting Infection with TORCH Agents

Intrauterine growth retardation
Hydrops
Microcephaly, hydrocephalus, intracranial calcifications
Eye abnormalities (chorioretinitis, cataracts, glaucoma)
Cardiac malformations, myocarditis
Pneumonitis
Hepatosplenomegaly
Anemia, thrombocytopenia, petechiae
Jaundice (especially conjugated hyperbilirubinemia)
Bone abnormalities (osteochondritis, periostitis)

TORCH = toxoplasmosis, other (congenital syphilis and viruses), rubella, cytomegalovirus, and herpes simplex virus.

these congenital infections is TORCH. Infections that are acquired in the perinatal period are frequently included in this group:

Toxoplasmosis
Other (includes HIV, syphilis, enterovirus, parvovirus, hepatitis B virus, varicella-zoster virus)
Rubella
Cytomegalovirus (CMV)
Herpes simplex virus (HSV)

Common Infections

Cytomegalovirus (CMV) Infection

CMV is the **most common viral cause** of congenital infection. Approximately 50%–80% of women of childbearing age are seropositive for CMV, but the risk of reactivation during pregnancy causing fetal infection is small (less than 1%). Primary CMV infection occurs in 1%–4% of pregnancies and the fetus will be infected in 40% of these cases. Most affected infants are **asymptomatic at birth** and develop normally. Approximately **10%–15% of infected infants have symptoms at birth** and 90% of these infants develop sequelae (e.g., **mental retardation, hearing loss, seizures**).

Congenital CMV infection is diagnosed by **isolation of the virus from the urine** within 3 weeks of birth; after this time, a positive culture could indicate intrapartum or postnatal infection, which is usually not clinically significant unless the baby is premature.

Treatment of congenital CMV infection involves **supportive care** and close follow-up. Clinical trials studying the effectiveness of **ganciclovir** (for treatment) and **maternal vaccination** (for prevention) are in progress.

Syphilis

Congenital syphilis results from **transplacental passage** of the spirochete *Treponema pallidum;* rarely, infant contact with a maternal chancre results in perinatal transmission. Maternal syphilis in any stage can lead to fetal infection.

Fetal or perinatal death occurs in 40% of congenital syphilis infections. The **surviving infants** are **asymptomatic at birth** but, if not treated, **develop symptoms within the first few weeks of life.** The most common manifestations of early congenital syphilis are **hepatosplenomegaly, bone abnormalities, hemolytic anemia, and jaundice.** Less common findings include ocular involvement, bloody nasal discharge (snuffles), mucocutaneous rash, and pneumonia alba.

Maternal testing for syphilis involves **nontreponemal serology** using either the Venereal Disease Research Laboratory (VDRL) or the rapid plasma reagin (RPR) test. Treponemal test [i.e., the microhemagglutination-*Treponema pallidum* (MHA-TP) test or the fluorescent treponemal antibody absorbed (FTA-ABS) test] are positive for life; therefore, they indicate disease history, not activity at the time of the blood study. In many cities, the health department will have records of previous infection and treatments.

Indications for treatment of the infant vary; consult the latest Academy of Pediatrics Committee on Infectious Disease report, the *Red Book,* for recommendations. Maternal history of treatment and response to treatment by a fourfold drop in titers are major factors to consider in management plans. Testing of the newborn infant includes:

▼ **Serum RPR.** Umbilical cord testing can show false-positive results.
▼ **LP.** Send CSF for VDRL; CSF analysis reveals pleocytosis and elevated protein.
▼ **Radiographs of the long bones**

In the newborn period, the normally high CSF protein, WBCs up to 20 mg/dl and infrequency of abnormal bone finding make these criteria less absolute. Pregnancy can slightly elevate the RPR.

Infants should be treated for congenital syphilis if:

▼ They were born to a mother with untreated syphilis.
▼ There is evidence of maternal relapse or reinfection.
▼ There is physical, radiologic, or laboratory evidence of syphilis.
▼ Their CSF VDRL is reactive.
▼ Their serum quantitative nontreponemal titer is at least fourfold greater than the mother's titer.

Treatment of early asymptomatic infection prevents long-term clinical sequelae. **Penicillin G** (50,000 units/kg given intravenously every 12 hours for 10–14 days) is the treatment of choice. **Infants born to mothers treated in the last month of pregnancy** should be evaluated; if the work-up is normal, they may receive a single dose of **intramuscular benzathine penicillin G.** Detailed recommendations for the treatment of syphilis in pregnancy and infancy can be found in *2000 Red Book: Report of the Committee on Infectious Diseases,* published by the AAP.

⚚ HINT False-positive VDRL tests occur in patients with lupus. Patients with Lyme disease will have positive treponemal tests (MHA-TP or FTA-ABS) and negative VDRL.

Hepatitis B (HBV)

In utero infection with HBV rarely occurs; **perinatal transmission** is more common. Overall, there is a 60%–70% chance of perinatal transmission if the mother has acute symptomatic infection. If the mother is seropositive for hepatitis B e antigen (HBeAg), the perinatal transmission rate is 90%, as opposed to only 10% if the mother is HBeAg negative.

Infected infants are **asymptomatic at birth** but may develop **antigenemia** and an **increased level of transaminases by 2–6 months** of age.

Hepatitis B can be **prevented by either active or passive immunization.** Current recommendations include treating all infants born to mothers who are hepatitis B surface antigen positive with hepatitis B immune globulin and hepatitis B vaccine.

⚔ HINT Mothers with hepatitis B may breast-feed their infants.

Herpes Simplex (HSV)

Approximately 75% of neonatal HSV infections are caused by herpes simplex virus-type 2. Congenital infection with this organism is extremely rare; usually, the baby is infected via the maternal genital tract shortly **before or during delivery.** Primary maternal infection results in neonatal HSV infection in approximately 50% of cases, whereas recurrent infection poses a risk of approximately 5%. Transmission of HSV may be **prevented by cesarean delivery** when the mother has active genital lesions and the membranes have been ruptured for less than 4 hours.

Neonates with HSV infection manifest in three distinct clinical groups:

▼ Disease localized to the skin, eye, and/or mouth (SEM disease)
▼ Encephalitis with or without skin involvement (CNS disease)
▼ Disseminated disease that involves multiple organ systems, including the central nervous system (CNS), lung, liver, adrenals, skin, eye, and mouth

Disease onset occurs at < 24 hours of life in 9%, at days 1–5 in 30%, and at > 5 days in 60% of infants.

Skin lesions are seen in 60% of infants **with CNS or disseminated disease. Seizures** occur in 50% with CNS disease and in 20% with disseminated disease. **Pneumonia** occurs in 35%–40% of infants with disseminated disease. **Disseminated infection** appears **clinically similar to bacterial sepsis** (e.g., lethargy, poor feeding, temperature instability). As the disease progresses, **jaundice, disseminated intravascular coagulation, hepatosplenomegaly, and shock** develop. Common CSF findings include **pleocytosis** (with a lymphocyte predominance), an **increased RBC count,** and an **increased protein level.** Skin or conjunctival cultures are positive in more than 90% of neonates with any type of HSV infection.

Neonatal HSV infection is treated with **high-dose acyclovir** (60 mg/kg/day, divided, every 8 hours). Duration of treatment is **14 days for SEM disease** and **at least 21 days for CNS or disseminated disease.**

HIV

The risk of transmission of HIV from a seropositive mother to her fetus is approximately 20%–30%, although **treatment of the infected mother during pregnancy and delivery reduces the transmission** dramatically. The **risk increases** to approximately 50% **if the mother has AIDS or if she previously had a child who was infected.** It is not known whether cesarean section delivery reduces the probability of transmission. Because the virus can also be **transmitted through breast milk,** the current recommendation in the United States is to counsel HIV-positive mothers not to breast-feed.

For babies of mothers with **unknown HIV status,** antibody level is the initial screening. **If the mother is HIV positive, HIV DNA polymerase chain reaction**

(PCR) of the infants' blood should be performed at birth, 1 month, and 4 months of age and **blood for HIV culture** should be sent at **1 month** of age. HIV DNA PCR is positive in 30% of HIV-infected infants on the first day of life (the false-positive rate of HIV DNA PCR is 2%). The false-negative rate of HIV culture is approximately 0.5%. The combination of HIV culture and HIV DNA PCR will detect 98% of all positive infants by 1 month of age and > 99% by 4 months of age. **Infants with negative HIV DNA PCR** (at birth, 1 month, and 4 months of age) and HIV culture (at 1 month of age) should undergo **HIV antibody testing at 12, 15, and 18 months** of age to confirm that maternal HIV antibody is no longer present.

Opportunistic infections have been reported in young infants; therefore, **Bactrim prophylaxis** is usually **started at 6 weeks of age and discontinued at 4 months of age** if testing reveals that the infant does not have HIV. Clinical trials have shown that **treatment of HIV-positive women** with zidovudine during the **second and third trimesters** of pregnancy and **intrapartum**, followed by **treatment of the newborn** for the first 6 weeks of life, **decreases the rate of transmission** of infection from mother to infant to approximately 8%.

TABLE 46.7.   Clinical Findings in TORCH Infections

Toxoplasmosis
Hydrocephalus with generalized calcifications
Chorioretinitis, microphthalmia
Deafness

Rubella
Cataracts, glaucoma, pigmented retinopathy, microphthalmia
Deafness
Cardiac malformation (PDA, pulmonary artery stenosis)
"Blueberry muffin" appearance (extramedullary hematopoiesis)

CMV
Microcephaly with periventricular calcifications
Chorioretinitis
Inguinal hernias (boys)
Petechiae with thrombocytopenia

Herpes
Acute CNS findings
Keratoconjunctivitis
Skin, eye, mucous membrane vesicles

Syphilis
Interstitial keratitis, pigmentary retinopathy
Snuffles (persistent and often bloody nasal discharge)
Fissures (lips, nares) and mucous patches (mouth, genitalia)
Eczematoid skin rash
Osteochondritis and periostitis

Modified with permission from Stagno S, Pass RF, Alford CA: Perinatal infections and maldevelopment. In *The Fetus and the Newborn*, Volume 17, Series 1. Edited by Bloom AD, James LS. New York, Wiley-Liss, 1981.

CMV = cytomegalovirus; CNS = central nervous system; PDA = patent ductus arteriosus.

Evaluation of Congenital Infection

Patient History

Confirm the results of maternal serologic screening for rubella, hepatitis B, syphilis, and HIV.

Physical Examination

Examine the baby for organ system involvement, including funduscopic examination. Findings suggestive of particular infections are listed in Table 46.7.

Laboratory Studies

It is not necessary to perform a complete "TORCH evaluation" for every baby with suspected congenital infection. A **thorough history and physical examination** of the baby and **knowledge of maternal prenatal laboratory studies** (rubella, syphilis, hepatitis, and HIV serologies) can narrow the differential diagnosis. Studies to consider in the evaluation of an infant with a suspected TORCH infection are listed in Table 46.8.

TABLE 46.8. Evaluation of the Infant with a Suspected TORCH Infection

CSF studies
CSF cell count, protein, glucose (enterovirus, rubella, syphilis)
CSF DNA PCR (enterovirus, HSV)
CSF VDRL (syphilis)
CSF viral culture (enterovirus, HSV)

Serology
IgG (specify *Toxoplasma* or rubella—if positive, send IgM)
RPR (syphilis)
Hepatitis B surface antigen

Skin Lesions
Dark-field examination (syphilis)
Direct fluorescent antibody (HSV, varicella)
Tzanck smear (HSV)

Viral Culture
Conjunctiva (HSV)
Mouth or nasopharynx (HSV, enterovirus)
Rectum (enterovirus, HSV)
Skin (HSV)
Urine (CMV)

Other studies
Audiologic evaluation (rubella, toxoplasmosis)
Head CT (CMV, toxoplasmosis)
Ophthalmologic examination (toxoplasmosis, rubella, CMV, HSV, varicella, syphilis)
Radiograph of long bones (rubella, syphilis)

See text for evaluation of an infant for HIV.

CMV = cytomegalovirus; CSF = cerebrospinal fluid; CT = computed tomography; HSV = herpes simplex virus; PCR = polymerase chain reaction; RPR = rapid plasma reagin; VDRL = venereal disease research laboratory.

▼ **Serology.** Maternal IgG antibody crosses the placenta; therefore, the absence of rubella- or *Toxoplasma*-specific IgG in the infant excludes congenital infection. However, positive IgG titers in the infant for rubella or *Toxoplasma* are not diagnostic of congenital infection. If the serology is positive, check specific IgM titers. In suspected congenital syphilis, serum RPR and CSF VDRL should be tested.

▼ **Viral culture.** All infants with suspected HSV should have surface viral cultures performed. Urine viral culture to diagnose congenital CMV infection must be sent within 3 weeks of birth, otherwise postnatal acquisition cannot be excluded. Enteroviral culture of nasopharyngeal and rectal swabs and CSF may be indicated for a baby with myocarditis, hepatitis, or aseptic meningitis.

▼ **Other laboratory studies** include a CBC, bilirubin (conjugated and unconjugated), and transaminases. Darkfield examination of nasal discharge in patients with "snuffles" may reveal syphilis.

Suggested Readings

American Academy of Pediatrics: Revised guidelines for prevention of early-onset group B streptococcal (GBS) infection. *Pediatrics* 99:489–496, 1997.

Cole FS: Viral infections of the fetus and newborn. In: *Avery's Diseases of the Newborn*, 7th ed. Edited by Taeusch HW, Ballard RA. Philadelphia, WB Saunders, 1998, pp 467–489.

Kimberlin DW, Lin C-Y, Jacobs RF, et al: Natural history of neonatal herpes simplex virus infections in the acyclovir era. *Pediatrics* 108:223–229, 2001.

Nielsen K, Bryson YJ: Diagnosis of HIV infection in children. *Pediatr Clin North Am* 47:39–62, 2000.

Rowley AH, Stumos JK: Timely diagnosis of congenital infections. *Pediatr Clin North Am* 41:1017–1034, 1994.

Stoll BJ, Gordon T, Korones SB, et al: Late-onset sepsis in very low birth weight neonates: a report from the National Institute of Child Health and Human Development Neonatal Research Network. *J Pediatr* 129:63–71, 1996.

47

*Jaundice**

JAMES M. CALLAHAN

▼ INTRODUCTION

Jaundice (icterus) is a **yellow discoloration** of the skin, mucous membranes, and sclera caused by **increased levels of circulating bilirubin.** Jaundice signals either increased production or decreased elimination of bilirubin.

---

* The most common causes of jaundice in infants younger than 3 months of age are described in Chapter 48, "Jaundice, Newborn." Jaundice in children older than 3 months is always pathologic.

The major source of bilirubin is the breakdown of heme pigment released from degraded RBCs. Normally, the liver clears bilirubin from the circulation via conjugation, and then the bilirubin is excreted in bile and eliminated in the feces. **Hemolytic processes and diseases affecting the liver** are the major causes of jaundice.

▼ DIFFERENTIAL DIAGNOSIS LIST

Unconjugated Hyperbilirubinemia

Hemolytic Causes

Hemoglobinopathies
RBC defects
Autoimmune hemolytic anemia
Wilson disease

Hepatic Disorders

Gilbert disease
Crigler-Najjar syndrome

Conjugated Hyperbilirubinemia

Infectious Causes

Viral infections—hepatitis A–E, cytomegalovirus infection, Epstein-Barr virus (EBV) infection
Bacterial infections—sepsis, liver abscess, pneumonia, peritonitis

Toxic Causes

Amanita mushrooms
Carbon tetrachloride and other solvents
Drugs
Total parenteral nutrition

Metabolic or Genetic Causes

α_1-Antitrypsin (α_1-AT) deficiency
Wilson disease
Cystic fibrosis
Hemochromatosis (primary or secondary)

Inflammatory Causes

Autoimmune chronic active hepatitis
Primary sclerosing cholangitis

Vascular Causes

Budd-Chiari syndrome
Venoocclusive disease

Miscellaneous Causes

Biliary tract disorders—cholangitis, cholecystitis, choledochal cyst, cholelithiasis
Pancreatic disease
Kawasaki syndrome
Rare hepatic disorders

🏆 HINT If a toddler or an older child presents with yellowish discoloration of the skin, one must first determine whether jaundice actually exists. Children who eat a large amount of yellow, orange, or red vegetables or fruits can develop keratodermia (owing to ingestion of carotene-containing vegetables) or lycopenemia (owing to ingestion of certain red foods, such as tomatoes). In both conditions, the child is healthy, active, and without other significant findings. In these conditions, the sclerae remain white and the serum bilirubin levels are within normal limits.

▾ DIFFERENTIAL DIAGNOSIS DISCUSSION
Hemolytic Processes

A complete discussion of hemoglobinopathies, RBC defects, and autoimmune hemolytic anemia can be found in Chapter 40, "Hemolysis."

Gilbert Disease and Crigler-Najjar Syndrome

In the absence of hemolysis, **unconjugated hyperbilirubinemia in older children is usually attributable to a relative deficiency in glucuronyl transferase** and the resulting decrease in conjugation of bilirubin seen in Gilbert disease and Crigler-Najjar syndrome. Gilbert disease is diagnosed much more often in older children and adults than it is in infants. Gilbert disease and Crigler-Najjar syndrome are compared in Table 47.1.

Hepatitis
Etiology

The **most common cause of conjugated hyperbilirubinemia in older infants and children is an acute viral infection that causes hepatitis. Hepatitis A, B, C, D, and E viruses** are agents that specifically attack the liver. **Hepatitis A virus (HAV)** and **hepatitis E virus (HEV,** mainly found in developing countries) are usually passed by the fecal–oral route; day care center outbreaks of hepatitis A are not unusual.

Clinical Features

HAV is the most common cause of food-borne hepatitis in this country. It usually has a **2- to 6-week incubation period.** A **preicteric phase** characterized by

TABLE 47.1. Defects in Hepatic Bilirubin Conjugation

Disease	Defect	Genetics
Gilbert disease	Underactivity of the transferase, defective uptake of albumin-bound bilirubin from the plasma	Autosomal recessive
Crigler-Najjar syndrome		
Type I	Complete absence of the transferase enzyme	Autosomal recessive
Type II	Partial absence of the transferase enzyme (less severe than type I)	Autosomal dominant

fever, headache, malaise, and abdominal complaints (e.g., abdominal pain, nausea, vomiting, anorexia) may last up to 5 days. This phase is followed by the appearance of **dark urine and frank icterus,** usually as the fever begins to resolve (although children younger than 3 years may never develop jaundice). There is usually **hepatomegaly and right upper quadrant tenderness.** Other symptoms tend to lessen as the jaundice resolves (which may take as long as 1 month). **Complete resolution** without the development of chronic liver disease or a chronic carrier state **is characteristic.** However, **occasional patients** may **progress to liver failure and even death.**

Hepatitis B is usually **transmitted parenterally via contaminated blood products or by sexual contact with an infected person.** The incubation period is longer than for hepatitis A (**2–6 months**). There is a preicteric and an icteric phase in this illness, as with hepatitis A. The **preicteric phase** may be accompanied by **rash, arthritis, arthralgia, and even urticaria. Late sequelae** include **fulminant hepatitis, hepatic necrosis, cirrhosis, and hepatocellular carcinoma. Chronic carrier states** and **chronic active hepatitis** are **occasionally seen** after infection with hepatitis B virus (HBV). The **younger the patient** is at the time of infection, the **higher the likelihood of development of chronic infection**—infants infected at the time of delivery have a 60%–90% risk of developing a chronic infection.

Hepatitis C constitutes most of what was previously called non-A, non-B hepatitis. It is **transmitted parenterally or through sexual contact.** Cases of hepatitis C have been documented in teenage patients who have received **tattoos** and who use **intranasal crack cocaine** (because of sharing of glass paraphernalia). Intranasal crack cocaine use may also be associated with HBV infection. The **incubation period is 1–5 months,** and the disease usually has an insidious onset and produces a **mild clinical illness.** Jaundice occurs in only 25% of patients. Infection with hepatitis C virus (HCV) has been associated with **chronic liver disease and a chronic carrier state,** and it may lead to **cirrhosis or hepatocellular carcinoma.**

Hepatitis D occurs only as a **coinfection or superinfection** in patients with acute or chronic disease secondary to HBV infection. **Except for perinatal transmission,** hepatitis D virus is **acquired similarly to HBV. The incubation period is 3 weeks to 3 months. The onset is usually acute,** and the symptoms are usually more severe than with hepatitis B. A **chronic carrier state, chronic hepatitis, or cirrhosis** may develop, and the **mortality rate is higher than with hepatitis B** alone.

Hepatitis E is usually benign, although there has been a **high fatality rate in pregnant women** infected with HEV. HEV is mainly seen in **developing countries with poor sanitation.**

Evaluation

When viral hepatitis is suspected, **evaluation to determine the causative agent** is appropriate. A **history of exposures** [e.g., shellfish (hepatitis A) or blood transfusions (hepatitis B)] may guide testing.

Testing for **IgM antibody to hepatitis A, hepatitis B surface antigen (HBsAg), and IgM antibody to hepatitis B core antigen (IgM-HBcAg),** as well as for **EBV** and possible **noninfectious causes** is indicated. **Hepatic transaminases** (alanine aminotransferase, aspartate aminotransferase), **γ-glutamyl transferase,** and the **prothrombin time** should be obtained and monitored.

▼ During infection with HAV, hepatic transaminase levels peak at about the time that jaundice appears. Hepatitis A antibody is present at the onset of disease. IgM antibody predominates initially, but within several months, it is completely replaced by IgG.

▼ With HBV infection, hepatic transaminase and bilirubin levels increase rapidly after the onset of symptoms. HBsAg is detectable one to several weeks before the onset of symptoms and the rapid increase in hepatic transaminase and bilirubin levels. HBcAb appears about 1 week after the onset of increased transaminase levels and is initially predominantly of the IgM class. HBsAg usually disappears about 2 months after the onset of symptoms. Some time after this, antibody to HBsAg becomes detectable. The intervening period has been known as the "window phase." Positive results on IgM-HBcAb testing during this phase confirm the diagnosis of hepatitis B.

▼ Diagnosis of HCV infection is accomplished by detection of anti-HCV antibodies. A positive polymerase chain reaction for HCV RNA is a confirmatory test.

Treatment

Treatment for hepatitis A, B, and C is **mainly supportive. Intravenous fluids** may be required to ensure adequate hydration. Patients with **progressive cases of hepatitis B and hepatitis C may benefit from α-interferon administration,** although success rates have been low in the few studies performed.

Epstein-Barr Virus (EBV) Infection

Clinical Features

EBV, the agent that **causes infectious mononucleosis,** can be associated with hepatic involvement and jaundice. Children with this disease often have a **high fever,** and the illness is usually associated with **splenomegaly** as well as **hepatomegaly, pharyngitis, and lymphadenopathy.** The course of this disease is usually **benign;** often, jaundice does not develop at all.

Treatment

Treatment is **supportive. Steroids** may be administered if **tonsilloadenoidal hypertrophy or lymphadenopathy threatens airway patency.**

Hepatotoxicity

Etiology

Many drugs (Table 47.2) **and environmental toxins** can produce hepatic injury, elevated transaminases, and cholestasis. **Acetaminophen overdose,** either accidental or intentional, is probably the **most common drug-induced cause** of hepatic toxicity in children and adolescents.

Clinical Features

The clinical picture in a patient with drug- or toxin-induced hepatotoxicity **is similar to** that seen in patients with **infectious hepatitis;** however, there is **no prodrome** before the onset of hepatitis. **Liver failure usually occurs late** in the clinical course unless there is an overwhelming drug or toxin exposure or a continued exposure that is unrecognized. **Occasionally,** a toxic exposure can lead to **fulminant hepatic failure,** including coagulopathy and encephalopathy. **Acetaminophen overdose rarely causes acute symptoms;** liver

TABLE 47.2. Commonly Used Pediatric Medications That May Cause Cholestasis and Hepatotoxicity

Anticonvulsants
  Phenobarbital
  Diphenylhydantoin
  Carbamazepine
  Valproic acid

Antimicrobials
  Tetracycline
  Erythromycin (estolate preparations)
  Sulfonamides
  Ketoconazole
  Isoniazid
  Rifampin
  Griseofulvin

Immunosuppressants
  Cyclosporine
  Azathioprine
  Methotrexate

Steroids
  Corticosteroids
  Androgens
  Oral contraceptives

Miscellaneous drugs
  Acetaminophen
  Salicylates
  Chlorpromazine
  Cimetidine
  Iron preparations (with overdosage)

A large number of less commonly encountered agents, including antineoplastic agents, antidepressants, antipsychotics, and tranquilizers can also cause cholestasis and hepatotoxicity.

injury becomes evident 2–4 days after ingestion. In **iron toxicity, gastrointestinal symptoms** (e.g., vomiting, diarrhea, hematochezia) **predominate early,** and hepatotoxicity and cholestasis occur during the late stages.

Evaluation

The patient's **medication, social, and psychiatric histories** should be obtained. The **absence of prodromal symptoms and the acute onset of symptoms** can be clues to a possible toxic exposure.

Transaminase levels, the bilirubin level, and coagulation studies should be followed. An **acetaminophen level** (or a qualitative toxicology screen for acetaminophen) should be obtained **for any adolescent who has attempted suicide by ingestion with any substance** because acetaminophen is often an unrecognized co-ingestant.

Treatment

Acetaminophen and iron are the only agents in Table 47.2 for which **specific antidotes are available.** N-Acetylcysteine is a specific **antidote for acetaminophen poisoning,** which, if used early, can **prevent hepatic failure and death.** Similarly, prompt recognition of the symptoms of **iron ingestion** and appropriate **treatment with deferoxamine** prevents most late complications, including hepatotoxicity and cholestasis. When there is **no available antidote** for the toxin, **withholding the toxic agent and supportive care** are the only available treatments. **Liver transplantation** has been successfully used for patients who have developed frank liver failure.

Alpha₁-Antitrypsin (α_1-AT) Deficiency

Etiology

α_1-AT deficiency is a **genetic disorder** characterized by decreased serum concentrations of α_1-AT, an **important protease inhibitor.** There are **many**

phenotypic variants denoted by "Pi-typing." Individuals with a homozygous Pi ZZ phenotype are at risk for developing hepatic dysfunction. Patients with heterozygous phenotypes have intermediate serum levels of α_1-AT.

Clinical Features

Patients may develop **premature pulmonary emphysema, chronic liver disease, and nephritis in infancy;** however, if the disease is not detected at that time, some or all of these **manifestations may appear in later life. Progressive liver disease,** characterized by jaundice, hepatomegaly, and acholic stools, occurs in 10%–20% of patients. **Cirrhosis and hepatic failure** may develop by late childhood.

Evaluation

Diagnosis is established by finding **decreased serum levels of α_1-AT.** Phenotype determination and characteristic findings on **liver biopsy** confirm the diagnosis.

Treatment

There is **no specific treatment** for individuals who have this disorder and progressive liver disease. **Infusions of the deficient serum protein have slowed the progression of lung disease in adult patients,** but have not been shown to be helpful in pediatric patients with hepatic dysfunction. There is hope that gene therapy will be available in the future. Presently, **hepatic transplantation** is the only hope for children who develop hepatic failure as a result of α_1-AT deficiency.

Wilson Disease

Wilson disease is discussed in detail in Chapter 42, "Hepatomegaly." Wilson disease may present as isolated hemolysis and unconjugated hyperbilirubinemia. More often, it presents with signs of **hepatic involvement** (including conjugated hyperbilirubinemia) **and neurologic involvement.**

Autoimmune Chronic Active Hepatitis

Autoimmune chronic active hepatitis is discussed in Chapter 42, "Hepatomegaly."

Hepatobiliary Tract Disorders

Etiology

Hepatobiliary tract disease is **rare in most pediatric patients;** however, **patients with variants of hemolytic anemia** (especially sickle cell disease) **often develop cholelithiasis (gallstones).** Although rare, **choledochal cysts** may present in late childhood.

Clinical Features

The **acute onset of right upper quadrant pain or recurring episodes** of right upper quadrant pain in a patient with a **history of ongoing hemolysis** should prompt consideration of the possibility of cholelithiasis. If **fever** is present, **acute cholecystitis** may be complicating the picture. A **palpable right upper quadrant mass** may be felt.

Usually, patients with **choledochal cysts** complain of **right upper quadrant pain or diffuse abdominal pain and vomiting.**

Evaluation

Abdominal ultrasonography demonstrates the presence of gallstones or anatomic abnormalities.

⚄ HINT Cholestasis can also be associated with hydrops of the gallbladder in patients with Kawasaki syndrome. Other manifestations of this multisystem disease should be evident. Hydrops can be demonstrated on an abdominal ultrasound.

⚄ HINT Patients with pancreatic disease and abdominal tumors can have hepatobiliary obstruction and cholestasis. Patients with vascular disease (e.g., Budd-Chiari syndrome in patients with hypercoagulable states or vasoocclusive disease in patients following bone marrow transplantation) may have hepatic vein obstruction and resultant jaundice, ascites, and hepatomegaly. An ultrasound or computed tomography scan of the abdomen demonstrates these obstructions.

▼ EVALUATION OF JAUNDICE
Patient History

Important questions to ask when evaluating a patient with jaundice include:

- ▼ Has the child eaten a large amount of yellow, red, or orange vegetables (suggestive of keratodermia or lycopenemia)?
- ▼ Is there a past history or a family history of a blood disorder (suggestive of hemolysis)?
- ▼ Is the jaundice acute in onset and associated with right upper quadrant pain (suggestive of cholelithiasis or cholecystitis, especially in patients with a history of a hemolytic disorder)?
- ▼ Were there prodromal symptoms before the onset of jaundice (suggestive of an infectious cause)?
- ▼ Was the onset acute in the absence of prodromal symptoms (suggestive of toxic injury)?
- ▼ What is the patient's medication history?
- ▼ Is there a history of psychiatric illness or social stress (suggestive of intentional ingestion)?
- ▼ Is there a history of behavioral changes, diminished school performance, or other subtle neurologic changes (suggestive of Wilson disease)?
- ▼ Is there a family history of unexplained psychiatric, neurologic, or hepatic disease (suggestive of Wilson disease or another genetic cause)?
- ▼ Has the patient had symptoms of chronic illness, such as weight loss or pruritus (suggestive of an inflammatory or metabolic process)?
- ▼ Has the patient complained of unusual bleeding or a marked change in mental status (suggestive of hepatic failure)?

Physical Examination

- ▼ **Hepatomegaly and splenomegaly** are common associated findings in patients with viral hepatitides or inflammatory liver disease.

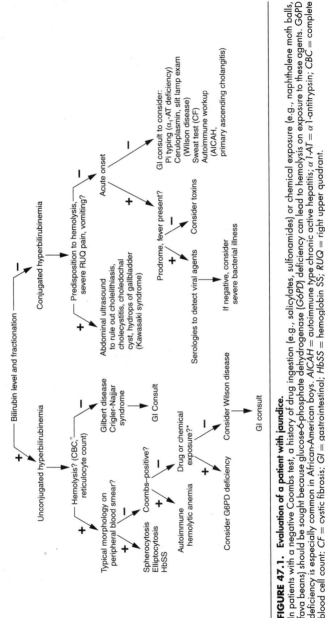

FIGURE 47.1. Evaluation of a patient with jaundice.

In patients with a negative Coombs test, a history of drug ingestion (e.g., salicylates, sulfonamides) or chemical exposure (e.g., naphthalene moth balls, fava beans) should be sought because glucose-6-phosphate dehydrogenase (G6PD) deficiency can lead to hemolysis on exposure to these agents. G6PD deficiency is especially common in African-American boys. $AICAH$ = autoimmune type chronic active hepatitis; $\alpha1\text{-}AT$ = α 1-antitrypsin; CBC = complete blood cell count; CF = cystic fibrosis; GI = gastrointestinal; $HbSS$ = hemoglobin SS; RUQ = right upper quadrant.

▼ **Tenderness over the liver,** but not marked hepatomegaly, is often seen in patients with hepatotoxicity.

▼ **Right upper quadrant tenderness or a mass** can be seen with biliary tract disease. A mass may not be distinguishable from a finding of hepatomegaly.

▼ **Signs of systemic or chronic disease** may be present if hepatic involvement is a component of a more protean disorder. Rash, fever, adenopathy, oral lesions, and changes in the hands and feet are seen with Kawasaki disease. Cachexia, edema, palmar erythema, pruritus, and spider angiomata may be detected in patients with autoimmune chronic active hepatitis. Digital clubbing and pulmonary symptoms may be found in patients with cystic fibrosis and hepatic involvement.

▼ **Abnormal bleeding and a decreased level of consciousness** are worrisome findings in jaundiced patients because these findings may herald the onset of hepatic failure.

▼ TREATMENT OF JAUNDICE

Until the cause of the jaundice is determined, treatment is supportive and may entail:

▼ Administration of intravenous fluids

▼ Administration of vitamin K, clotting factors, or both

▼ Intubation (for patients with a decreased level of consciousness)

▼ Administration of lactulose and neomycin for treatment of hepatic encephalopathy in patients with hepatic failure

▼ APPROACH TO THE PATIENT (FIGURE 47.1)

Suggested Readings

D'Agata ID, Balistreri WF: Evaluation of liver disease in the pediatric patient. *Pediatr Rev* 20:376–390, 1999.

Donnelly LF, Bisset GS III: Pediatric hepatic imaging. *Radiol Clin North Am* 36:413–427, 1998.

Krugman S: Viral hepatitis: A, B, C, D, and E—Infection. *Pediatr Rev* 13:203–212, 1992.

Krugman S: Viral hepatitis: A, B, C, D, and E—Prevention. *Pediatr Rev* 13:245–246, 1992.

Mews C, Sinatra FR: Chronic liver disease in children. *Pediatr Rev* 14:436–443, 1993.

Park RW, Grand RJ: Gastrointestinal manifestations of cystic fibrosis. *Gastroenterology* 81:1143–1161, 1981.

Pashankar D, Schreiber RA: Jaundice in older children and adolescents. *Pediatr Rev* 22:219–226, 2001.

Shah U, Habib Z, Kleinman RE: Liver failure attributable to hepatitis A virus infection in a developing country. *Pediatrics* 105:436–438, 2000.

Udall JN, Jr, Dixon M, Newman AP, et al: Liver disease in α-1-antitrypsin deficiency: a retrospective analysis of the influence of early breast vs. bottle feeding. *JAMA* 253:2679–2682, 1985.

Walker WA, Mathis RK: Hepatomegaly: an approach to differential diagnosis. *Pediatr Clin North Am* 22:929–942, 1975.

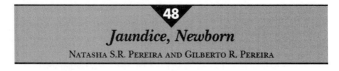

Jaundice, Newborn
NATASHA S.R. PEREIRA AND GILBERTO R. PEREIRA

▼ INTRODUCTION

Jaundice is the **most prevalent problem** in the newborn period, with up to 65% of full-term neonates having visible jaundice resulting from excessive accumulation of bilirubin in blood and tissues. Accumulation of bilirubin in the tissues may be caused by **overproduction** of bilirubin, **immaturity of the liver conjugation system,** or an **abnormality of biliary excretion** of conjugated bilirubin. All of these factors can be involved to a variable degree in neonatal jaundice.

▼ DIFFERENTIAL DIAGNOSIS LIST
Increased Bilirubin Production or Absorption
Hemolytic Causes

Isoimmune hemolysis—Rh, ABO, other blood antigens
Inherited red blood cell (RBC) membrane defects—elliptocytosis, pykno-
cytosis, stomatocytosis
RBC enzyme deficiency—pyruvate kinase, glucose-6-phosphate dehydro-
genase (G6PD), hexokinase, 2–3 diphosphoglycerate (DPG) mutase de-
ficiency
Hemoglobinopathy—α-thalassemia
Acquired RBC defects—infection, drugs, microangiopathy

Gastrointestinal Causes

Intestinal obstruction
Pyloric stenosis
Hirschsprung disease
Meconium ileus

Miscellaneous Causes

Sequestered blood
Swallowed blood
Polycythemia
Breast milk jaundice
Diabetic mother
Jaundice of prematurity

Decreased Bilirubin Uptake or Excretion
Infectious Causes

Sepsis
Neonatal hepatitis
Cytomegalovirus (CMV) infection
Herpes
Rubella

Toxoplasmosis
Hepatitis B

Metabolic or Genetic Causes

Decreased Y protein
Galactosemia
Hypothyroidism
Tyrosinosis
Galactosemia
Hypermethionemia

Obstructive Causes

Alagille syndrome
Biliary atresia
Choledochal cyst
Bile duct obstruction

Toxic Causes

Total parenteral nutrition—induced cholestasis

Decreased Bilirubin Conjugation

Metabolic or Genetic Causes

Gilbert disease
Crigler-Najjar syndrome
Hypothyroidism
Galactosemia
Acquired transferase deficiency

Miscellaneous Causes

Physiologic jaundice

▼ DIFFERENTIAL DIAGNOSIS DISCUSSION
Isoimmune Hemolytic Disease

Blood group incompatibility between fetal and maternal blood can lead to hemolysis in the fetus and newborn baby if maternal IgG antibodies are transmitted to the fetal blood stream via the placenta.

Rh Incompatibility

Rh incompatibility is the **most serious of the isoimmune hemolytic disorders.** Fifteen percent of Caucasians, five percent of African-Americans, and one percent of Asians are negative for the D antigen, which is the most potent of the Rh antigens. **Previous pregnancy or** another type of **contact with Rh-positive blood sensitizes the Rh-negative mother** to the Rh antigen. In subsequent pregnancies, **transplacentally derived antibodies coat the fetal RBCs,** which are then lysed by the reticuloendothelial tissues, leading to excessive **hemolysis** and **bilirubin production.**

Affected infants appear **pale,** and the **liver and spleen may be enlarged** as a result of excessive extramedullary hematopoiesis. Infants afflicted with **hydrops fetalis,** a potentially severe complication resulting from severe anemia and congestive heart failure, may have **cardiopulmonary signs** (i.e., tachycardia, tachypnea).

Infants have a **positive Coombs test,** an **elevated reticulocyte count,** and **rapidly increasing serum bilirubin levels** (peaking on the third or fourth day of life).

Management involves **correcting the anemia** and **preventing an excessive increase in bilirubin levels,** which can lead to **kernicterus.** [Kernicterus (bilirubin encephalopathy), a complication of unconjugated hyperbilirubinemia, is discussed in detail later in the chapter in the section titled "Complications of Neonatal Jaundice."] **Phototherapy** converts unconjugated bilirubin to harmless products, and **exchange transfusion** removes potential sources of bilirubin. Guidelines for the use of phototherapy and exchange blood transfusion are provided in Table 48.1.

With the introduction of **anti-D immunoglobulin G (RhoGAM) inoculation,** the antepartum sensitization rate of Rh-negative mothers has been lowered from 2% to 0.17%. **Rh factor sensitization should be diagnosed prenatally** by identifying the anti-D antibody in the mother's plasma.

ABO Incompatibility

ABO incompatibility occurs in 12% of all pregnancies, and 1% of newborns experience severe hemolysis. The transplacental passage of anti-A or anti-B IgG antibodies generally **causes less severe disease than does Rh incompatibility.** Because A and B antigens are common in nature, group O mothers are previously sensitized to these antigens and **hemolysis may occur in a first pregnancy.**

The presentation is similar to that seen with Rh incompatibility, although it is usually much less severe, because the A and B antigens are ubiquitously distributed in fetal tissues and these antigens are weaker than the Rh antigens.

▼ **Physical examination findings can be unremarkable** unless the degree of hemolysis is severe.
▼ **Jaundice presents early** in affected newborns.
▼ **The serum bilirubin level increases rapidly in the first 24 hours of life.**

TABLE 48.1. Guidelines for the Use of Phototherapy and Exchange Blood Transfusions

| | Age or Birth Weight | Serum Bilirubin Level | |
		Phototherapy	Exchange Blood Transfusion
Healthy full-term infant	25–48 hours	> 15 mg/dl	> 25 mg/dl*
	49–72 hours	> 18 mg/dl	> 25 mg/dl
	> 72 hours	> 20 mg/dl	> 25 mg/dl
Ill full-term infant†	< 24 hours	10–14 mg/dl	20 mg/dl
	> 24 hours	15 mg/dl	20 mg/dl
Preterm infant	< 1250 g	5–7 mg/dl	10–13 mg/dl
	1250–1499 g	7–10 mg/dl	13–16 mg/dl
	1500–1999 g	10–12 mg/dl	16–18 mg/dl
	2000–2499 g	12–14 mg/dl	18–20 mg/dl

* Exchange blood transfusion should be implemented when the serum bilirubin level is 20 mg/dl if phototherapy has been tried but unsuccessful.

† An infant with hemolysis, hypoglycemia, acidosis, sepsis, or hypoxemia.

▼ **Anemia may be absent, mild, or late** (occurring weeks after birth).

▼ **The Coombs test may be negative or only weakly positive** in these infants, because newborns have fewer A and B antigenic sites on their erythrocytes than do adults.

▼ **Spherocytes may be present** on a peripheral smear because of removal of a portion of the RBC membrane in the spleen.

Most affected babies can be managed with **phototherapy** (see Table 48.1). Patients with ABO incompatibility and severe jaundice require the same **aggressive management** as do patients with Rh disease because these patients are at an **increased risk for** the development of **bilirubin encephalopathy.**

Other Forms of Isoimmune Hemolysis

Other blood groups that could present problems in the neonatal period are the **Kell, Duffy, and Kidd groups.** These conditions are **diagnosed prenatally** when the mother is found to have antibodies to these antigens. In affected infants, the clinical presentation is **between that of Rh and ABO incompatibility,** depending on the severity of the condition. As with Rh and ABO incompatibility, these conditions may be associated with an **increased risk of kernicterus.**

Inherited Nonimmune Hemolytic Disease

Hereditary Spherocytosis (HS)

HS is an autosomal dominant disease, with 25% of cases arising sporadically as new mutations. The incidence is 1 in 5000. There is usually a **family history** significant for **splenectomy, gallbladder surgery,** and **anemia.**

The clinical presentation depends on the degree of hemolysis. There may be **hepatosplenomegaly** as a result of extramedullary hematopoiesis. Both **anemia and jaundice are moderate.**

The peripheral blood smear shows **microcytic RBCs with an increased mean corpuscular hemoglobin concentration.** The diagnosis is confirmed with **abnormal results** on an **osmotic erythrocyte fragility test.**

Treatment is **supportive** and entails a **packed RBC transfusion** to address the anemia, **and phototherapy** to address the jaundice.

G6PD Deficiency

G6PD deficiency, the most common RBC enzyme deficiency, is an **X-linked recessive disease** seen in **African-Americans,** people of **Mediterranean descent, Sephardic Jews,** and **Asians.** It is proposed to have a high incidence in certain ethnic groups because it confers resistance to malaria. It afflicts 13% of African-American men and 2% of African-American women in the United States. Affected RBCs are **deficient in the enzyme G6PD** and **lyse readily** under oxidant stresses.

A family history that includes similarly affected siblings may lead to the diagnosis. A **maternal history of ingestion of oxidants** (e.g., antipyretics, sulfonamides, antimalarials) is important, but hemolysis may arise without an obvious precipitant. Physical examination findings vary according to the degree of hemolysis. The **complete blood count (CBC)** and **reticulocyte index** may indicate hemolysis. The diagnosis is confirmed by means of an **RBC enzyme assay.**

Treatment is **supportive** and includes **avoidance of oxidant stresses.** Jaundice may persist until the third week of life. **Severe hemolysis** is associated with an increased **risk of kernicterus.**

Physiologic Jaundice

Etiology

Many physiologic factors contribute to hyperbilirubinemia in neonates:

▼ A larger RBC mass
▼ A decreased RBC lifespan (70–90 days in neonates versus 120 days in adults)
▼ Increased intrahepatic circulation of RBCs
▼ Reduced uridine diphosphate glucuronyl transferase activity (< 1% that of adults in the first 10 days of life)
▼ Decreased bilirubin uptake from plasma as a result of reduced binding protein (ligandin) levels
▼ Absent or low levels of the bacteria necessary to convert bilirubin to urobilinogen prior to excretion in the urine and feces
▼ Delayed meconium passage leading to enterohepatic recirculation, and consequent reabsorption, of bilirubin
▼ An immature hepatic bilirubin conjugation system, which does not become efficient until day 3 or 4 in term babies and days 5, 6, or 7 in preterm babies

In utero, unconjugated bilirubin easily crosses the placenta and is conjugated and excreted by the mother. After birth, **97% of newborns become chemically hyperbilirubinemic in the first 3 days of life,** although the hyperbilirubinemia only becomes clinically apparent when the **bilirubin level is higher than 5 mg/dl.** Hyperbilirubinemia **peaks on day 3** (at 12 mg/dl) **in term babies** and **on days 5, 6, or 7** (at 15 mg/dl) **in preterm babies.**[*] The adult level of conjugation is not achieved until the baby reaches 6–14 weeks of age.

Evaluation

Physiologic jaundice is a **diagnosis of exclusion.** No laboratory testing is indicated beyond serum bilirubin determination. Conditions under which jaundice should be considered nonphysiologic include:

▼ Jaundice in the first day of life, which is always pathological and suggests excessive hemolysis, internal hemorrhage, or infection
▼ A bilirubin level that increases faster than 5 mg/day or 0.5 mg/dl/hr
▼ A conjugated bilirubin level greater than 1.5 mg/dl or 10% of the total bilirubin
▼ A bilirubin level of greater than 13 mg/dl in a term baby or 15 mg/dl in a preterm baby
▼ Jaundice that persists beyond the first week of life in term babies or beyond 2 weeks in preterm babies
▼ Jaundice accompanied by hepatosplenomegaly and anemia
▼ Jaundice in the presence of a family history of hemolytic disease
▼ Associated findings of lethargy, vomiting, a high-pitched cry, dark urine, or light feces

---

[*] East Asian and Native American infants have mean maximum serum bilirubin concentrations twice that of Caucasian infants, and African-American infants have concentrations that are less than those of Caucasian infants. Thus, ethnicity should be taken into account when determining the threshold for further work-up of a jaundiced newborn.

Treatment

In cases of **physiologic jaundice,** hyperbilirubinemia **resolves within 8 days** without sequelae.

Breast Milk Jaundice

Etiology

Approximately 13% of breast-fed babies (as compared with 4% of formula-fed babies) attain a bilirubin level of more than 12 mg/dl within 1 week of birth. The bilirubin level commonly peaks at 10–30 mg/dl and persists 4–10 days at that level before declining slowly to adult values by 3–12 weeks of age. This condition has been arbitrarily divided into **early-onset (breast-feeding) jaundice,** which occurs **2–4 days after birth,** and **late-onset (breast milk) jaundice,** which develops later, on **days 4–7.** There is much **overlap** between the two conditions. The hyperbilirubinemia results from alterations in the conjugation and excretion of bilirubin:

▼ **Early-onset (breast-feeding) jaundice** may be related to suboptimal total fluid and calorie intake before full establishment of lactation. In addition, breast-fed neonates pass fewer meconium stools and their stools contain less bilirubin than those of formula-fed infants.

▼ **Late-onset (breast milk) jaundice** has been postulated, but not proved, to be caused by inhibition of hepatic excretion of bilirubin by lipase and by the nonesterified long-chain fatty acid of breast milk. Also, β-glucuronidase, present in breast milk, is believed to hydrolyze conjugated bilirubin to the unconjugated lipid-soluble form. The latter is easily reabsorbed, thereby increasing enterohepatic circulation of bilirubin.

Treatment

Once pathological causes of jaundice have been ruled out, patients can be **managed conservatively. Interrupting breast-feeding** by eliminating oral feeding **for up to 24 hours** will markedly bring down the bilirubin level. Upon resumption of nursing, the bilirubin level increases, but it does not attain the previous high level. It is also possible to control late-onset (breast milk) jaundice with **phototherapy** without interrupting nursing.

Total Parenteral Nutrition–Associated Jaundice

Etiology

Cholestatic jaundice associated with total parenteral nutrition is the most commonly encountered cause of conjugated hyperbilirubinemia in infants in intensive care nurseries. It usually arises after **2–3 weeks of hyperalimentation** and is associated with **prematurity.** The exact pathophysiology is unknown, but the protein load in total parenteral nutrition may be a contributing factor. Prolonged fasting also seems to play a role, because babies maintained on minimal enteral feeds are less prone to the development of cholestasis.

Clinical Features and Evaluation

The diagnosis is usually apparent from the clinical situation. **Biliary sludge or stones** may be visible on **ultrasound.** Histopathological features seen on liver biopsy include **bile stasis, portal inflammation,** and **bile duct proliferation.** Serum bile acid and γ-glutamyltransferase levels are both increased.

Treatment

The **jaundice usually clears within 1–3 months** of instituting enteral nutrition.

Biliary Atresia

Etiology

Extrahepatic biliary atresia occurs in approximately 1 in 10,000 live births in North America and is the **most common treatable cause of neonatal cholestasis.** The cause is unknown, although certain infectious agents (reovirus 3, rotavirus, CMV, and rubella virus) have been postulated as causative agents.

Clinical Features

Affected infants usually present for evaluation **between the second and sixth weeks of life** with **jaundice, acholic stools, and dark urine.** There may be **hepatomegaly** and the **liver may feel hard** on examination.

Evaluation

In the **newborn period,** it may be **difficult to distinguish biliary atresia from idiopathic neonatal hepatitis,** even using liver function studies, abdominal ultrasonography, and radionuclide studies. In infants with a serum bilirubin level greater than 10 mg/dl, a **biliary scan following 5 days of phenobarbital administration** demonstrates **normal hepatocyte uptake** of isotype, but **failure to excrete it into the intestine.**

Treatment

Surgical correction with the Kasai procedure (hepatoportoenterostomy) is successful in 80% of patients when the diagnosis is made within 90 days of birth.

Idiopathic Neonatal Hepatitis

Clinical Features and Evaluation

Idiopathic neonatal hepatitis, a **diagnosis of exclusion,** accounts for 30%–40% of all instances of neonatal cholestasis in infants. The presentation is **similar to that seen in biliary atresia,** but the development of **acholic stools is variable.** Affected neonates have **prolonged jaundice** with no evidence of congenital infection or metabolic disease. Histopathological examination of **liver biopsy** specimens reveals areas of **necrosis and inflammation** and **hepatocytes** that have undergone **multinucleated giant cell transformation.**

Treatment

Sixty to ninety-four percent of affected infants recover without persistent liver disease. Treatment is **supportive, with replacement of fat-soluble vitamins.**

Congenital Infection

Clinical Features

Congenital infections often cause **mild jaundice** (as a result of conjugated and unconjugated hyperbilirubinemia) during the neonatal period. Jaundice is rarely the sole manifestation of these conditions, however; the most common infections (toxoplasmosis, rubella, syphilis, coxsackievirus B, CMV infection, and herpes simplex) usually leave other stigmata in the form of **growth retardation, microcephaly, hepatosplenomegaly, thrombocytopenia, cerebral calcifications, chorioretinitis, and retinal hemorrhages.**

Evaluation

Maternal and infant titers for **TORCH infections** should be obtained.

Treatment

Treatment depends on the causative agent.

▼ COMPLICATIONS OF NEONATAL JAUNDICE

The **most severe complication** of jaundice in the newborn **is kernicterus** (bilirubin encephalopathy). Fortunately, this complication is quite rare. Kernicterus occurs in the setting of **very high unconjugated hyperbilirubinemia, an injured blood–brain barrier, and the presence of molecules that compete with bilirubin for albumin binding.** The lower the birth weight, the lower the threshold for kernicterus. The unconjugated bilirubin **disrupts neuronal metabolism and function,** particularly in the basal ganglia.

Kernicterus is **unusual with a bilirubin level of less than 25 mg/dl except in the presence of coexisting conditions** (e.g., hypoxemia, hypercarbia, hypothermia, hypoglycemia, hypoalbuminemia, hyperosmolality) that "open up" the blood–brain barrier. At one time, data associating kernicterus with bilirubin levels as low as 9 mg/dl led to overzealous treatment of infants. However, recent studies performed on premature infants have shown an uncertain association of maximum serum bilirubin levels and developmental outcomes.

Kernicterus usually manifests **within 2–5 days of birth** in term babies. **Clinical features** may be **indistinguishable from** those seen in **sepsis, asphyxia, intraventricular hemorrhage, or hypoglycemia** (Table 48.2). If the infant survives, the clinical features seem to **resolve by age 2 months, except for residual muscle rigidity, opisthotonos, and convulsions.** The child may be ultimately left with **choreoathetosis, mental retardation, enamel dysplasia, sensorineural deafness, strabismus, defective upward gaze, and dysarthric speech.**

Early signs may be reversed by instituting exchange transfusion.

TABLE 48.2. Signs of Kernicterus	
Age	**Signs**
1–4 days of age	Lethargy
	Poor feeding
	Hypotonia
	Blunted Moro reflex
4–7 days of age	Fever
	Hypertonia
	High-pitched cry
	Emesis
	Depressed tendon reflexes
	Depressed respiration
Older than 1 week	Opisthotonic posturing
	Bulging anterior fontanelle
	Pulmonary hemorrhage
	Fever
	Generalized tonic–clonic seizures

▼ EVALUATION OF JAUNDICE IN THE NEWBORN

⚕ HINT In general, jaundice presenting at or within 24 hours of birth is pathological (Table 48.3).

Patient History

▼ **Family history.** Obtain information about hematologic disorders, splenectomy, gallbladder problems, previously affected children, and maternal blood type and antibody status.
▼ **Pregnancy, labor, and delivery history.** A traumatic delivery may indicate the possibility of hemolysis because of sequestered blood.
▼ **Medication history**

Physical Examination

In addition to scleral, mucous membrane, and skin icterus, physical examination may reveal pallor, hepatosplenomegaly, and other evidence of hemolysis.

▼ **Ascites, pleural effusion,** and **severe hepatomegaly** may be seen in patients with severe cases of isoimmunization or anemia.
▼ **Signs of shock** (e.g., hypotension, tachycardia, prolonged capillary refill) may be associated with severe anemia.
▼ **Dark urine** and **acholic feces** may be seen in infants with cholestatic jaundice.
▼ **Splenomegaly** may be present, especially in patients with congenital infection or biliary atresia.

⚕ HINT Jaundice has a cephalopedal progression. If the jaundice is restricted to the face and trunk above the umbilicus, the serum bilirubin level should be less than 12 mg/dl.

TABLE 48.3. Common Causes of Jaundice According to Age

Time of Presentation	Most Common Causes
Within 24 hours of birth	Erythroblastosis fetalis
	Concealed hemorrhage
	Congenital infection
	Intrauterine transfusion
	ABO incompatibility
Days 2–3	Physiologic jaundice
Days 4–7	Congenital infection
	Polycythemia
	Extensive ecchymosis
	Hematoma
1 week or longer after birth	Breast milk jaundice
	Biliary atresia
	Viral hepatitis
	Galactosemia
	Congenital spherocytosis
	G6PD deficiency or other RBC enzyme deficiencies

G6PD = glucose-6-phosphate dehydrogenase; RBC = red blood cell.

Laboratory Studies

Laboratory work-up is reserved for babies **with a bilirubin level that exceeds 15 mg/dl, a rapidly increasing bilirubin level, or history or physical findings suggestive of hemolysis.** The first step is fractionation of the bilirubin level into conjugated, unconjugated, and delta bilirubin (conjugated bilirubin bound to albumin).

Unconjugated Hyperbilirubinemia

Figure 48.1 suggests the laboratory tests that should be ordered to distinguish pathological hyperbilirubinemia from exaggerated physiologic jaundice.

▼ **A direct Coombs test** is routinely performed on the cord blood of babies delivered to Rh-negative mothers. The baby's blood group should be determined, because babies with evidence of hemolysis who are delivered to ABO-incompatible mothers are at increased risk for the development of bilirubin encephalopathy.

▼ **A CBC and peripheral blood smear.** Chronic hemolysis is indicated by a mean corpuscular volume of less than $100 : \mu m^3$, anemia, and an increased reticulocyte count (more than 10%).

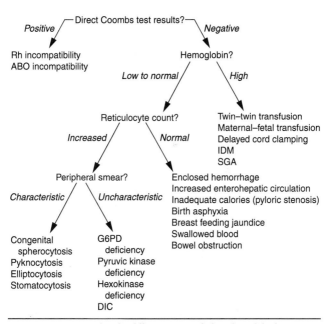

FIGURE 48.1. Procedure for differentiating pathologic hyperbilirubinemia from physiologic jaundice in a patient with unconjugated hyperbilirubinemia. *DIC* = disseminated intravascular coagulation; *G6PD* = glucose-6-phosphate dehydrogenase; *IDM* = infant of diabetic mother; *SGA* = small for gestational age.

▼ **An enzyme assay for G6PD** may be indicated in selected babies to detect nonimmune hemolysis.

Conjugated Hyperbilirubinemia

Elevation of conjugated bilirubin is never physiologic. Any infant with conjugated hyperbilirubinemia (defined as a conjugated bilirubin fraction greater than or equal to 2 mg/dl or greater than 20% of the total bilirubin value) must be evaluated immediately. Laboratory tests and diagnostic modalities that may be necessary include:

▼ **Blood and urine cultures**
▼ **Viral titers**
▼ **Thyroid hormone levels**
▼ **Sweat chloride determination**
▼ α_1**-Antitrypsin (α_1-AT) phenotyping**
▼ **Liver function tests**
▼ **CBC**
▼ **Urinalysis** (to aid in diagnosing galactosemia)
▼ **Radionuclide scans** (to rule out biliary atresia)
▼ **Abdominal ultrasonography** (to evaluate the extrahepatic biliary tract and the homogeneity of hepatic tissue)
▼ **Percutaneous liver biopsy** (to confirm the diagnosis of biliary atresia or idiopathic neonatal hepatitis)
▼ **Duodenal fluid analysis** (to detect bile pigment in a 24-hour collection sample)

▼ TREATMENT OF JAUNDICE IN THE NEWBORN

Management of hyperbilirubinemia **depends on its cause and severity** and on the **degree of accompanying anemia.** A high unconjugated bilirubin level can be neurotoxic in the newborn period. On the other hand, jaundice that is physiologic usually does not reach toxic levels and thus does not require treatment. **Careful monitoring of eating, activity, and bilirubin levels** is mandatory if no active treatment is instituted. Table 48.4 delineates follow-up guidelines for early discharge of infants.

Phototherapy

Following absorption of light at wavelengths of 425–475 nm, **unconjugated bilirubin is converted to polar photoisomers** that are less lipophilic than bilirubin and are **readily excretable** through the bile and the urine, thereby

TABLE 48.4. Discharge Guidelines		
	Bilirubin Level (mg/dl)	**Guidelines**
24-hour	< 5	Follow up in 24 hours
	5–8*	Repeat bilirubin test in 12–24 hours
	> 8	Mandatory evaluation in 12 hours
48-hour	< 8	Follow up in 48 hours
	8–12*	Repeat bilirubin test in 12–24 hours
	> 12	Mandatory evaluation in 12 hours

* Or ABO-incompatible.

bypassing the liver conjugating system. Blue lights and tungsten halide lights produce the most optimal results and the **exposed skin surface area** should be **as large as possible.** The efficacy of treatment is related to the dose of light given. Phototherapy is **more effective than exchange transfusion** for achieving a prolonged reduction of bilirubin level. **Temperature and hydration status should be routinely monitored.** The bilirubin level usually rebounds by 1–3 mg/dl following discontinuation of phototherapy, although in a recent study of healthy newborns weighing more than 1800 g, rebound hyperbilirubinemia after discontinuation of phototherapy was found to be rare. Whether this finding can be extrapolated to smaller preterm infant or infarction with hemolysis is not clear.

Side effects of phototherapy include:

▼ Insensible water loss and dehydration
▼ Diarrhea
▼ Photosensitization
▼ Overheating
▼ Hyperpigmentation
▼ Retinal injury (if the eyes are not covered with a patch)
▼ Maculopapular skin rash
▼ Riboflavin deficiency
▼ Hypocalcemia
▼ Decreased tryptophan level
▼ Genotoxicity
▼ Delay of newborn–mother bonding (as a result of physical separation)

Exchange Blood Transfusion

Exchange blood transfusion is used when phototherapy does not control the bilirubin level (see Table 48.1). **Small amounts** (5–20 ml) **of whole blood, cross-matched with mother and infant,** are **infused** following the withdrawal and disposal of equal amounts of the infant's blood. The procedure removes 85% of the infant's RBCs, maternal antibodies, and unconjugated bilirubin. Although posttransfusion bilirubin levels are approximately 45% of pretransfusion levels, there is usually a **rebound effect** to 60% of the pretransfusion level **within 30 minutes. Complications** include **transfusion reaction, infection, vessel perforation, hemorrhage, hypotension, and necrotizing enterocolitis.**

Pharmacological Therapy

Pharmacological agents may be used as adjuncts to phototherapy or exchange blood transfusion therapy.

▼ **Agar and charcoal,** agents that bind to bilirubin and interrupt the enterohepatic circulation, have been modestly beneficial in clinical trials.
▼ **Several inhibitors of heme oxygenase** (e.g., tin mesoporphyrin, tin protoporphyrin, zinc porphyrin, cobalt protoporphyrin) have been used with some success in reducing bilirubin production. The only untoward effects of their use are transient erythema during phototherapy and the fact that none of these products are available for oral administration.
▼ **Flumecinol,** a nonsedating inducer of the bilirubin conjugating enzymes, has been used.
▼ **Phenobarbital** may be used to induce the uptake, conjugation, and excretion of bilirubin.

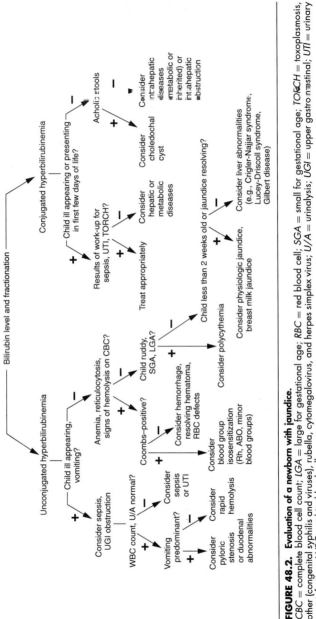

FIGURE 48.2. Evaluation of a newborn with jaundice.
CBC = complete blood cell count; LGA = large for gestational age; RBC = red blood cell; SGA = small for gestational age; $TORCH$ = toxoplasmosis, other (congenital syphilis and viruses), rubella, cytomegalovirus, and herpes simplex virus; U/A = urinalysis; UGI = upper gastrointestinal; UTI = urinary tract infection; WBC = white blood cell.

▼ APPROACH TO THE PATIENT (FIGURE 48.2)

Suggested Readings

Bhutani VK, Johnson L, Silvieri EM: Predictive ability of a predischarge hour-specific serum bilirubin for subsequent significant hyperbilirubinemia in healthy term and near term newborns. *Pediatrics* 103;493–495, 1999.

Connolly AM, Volpe JJ: Clinical features of bilirubin encephalopathy. *Clin Perinatol* 17(2):371–380, 1990.

Gourley GR: Pathophysiology of breast milk jaundice. In *Fetal and Neonatal Physiology*. Edited by Polin RA, Fox WW. Philadelphia, WB Saunders, 1992, pp 1173–1179.

Maisels MJ: Jaundice. In *Neonatology: Pathophysiology and Management of the Newborn*. Edited by Avery GB, Fletcher MA, MacDonald MG. Philadelphia, Lippincott-Raven, 1994, pp 630–725.

Martinez JC, Maisels MJ, Otheguy L, et al: Hyperbilirubinemia in breast-fed newborns: a controlled trial of four interventions. *Pediatrics* 91:470–473, 1993.

Newman TB, Maisels MJ: Evaluation and treatment of jaundice in the term newborn: a kinder, gentler approach. *Pediatrics* 89:809–818, 1992.

Oski FA: Disorders of bilirubin metabolism. In *Diseases of the Newborn*. Edited by Taeusch HW, Ballard RA, Avery ME. Philadelphia, WB Saunders, 1991, pp 747–752.

Rosenthal P: Bilirubin metabolism in the fetus and neonate. In *Fetal and Neonatal Physiology*. Edited by Polin RA, Fox WW. Philadelphia, WB Saunders, 1992, pp 1154–1164.

Watchko JF, Oski FA: Kernicterus in preterm newborns: past, present, future. *Pediatrics* 90:707–715, 1992.

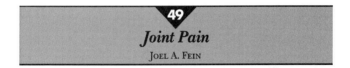

49
Joint Pain
JOEL A. FEIN

▼ INTRODUCTION

Arthritis is defined as limitation of motion of a joint with associated **swelling, pain with motion, tenderness, or warmth. Arthralgia** is joint pain in which there is **no limitation of range of motion** and in which **none of the other associated findings** is present. Arthritis or arthralgia may present as **polyarticular** (multiple joint), **pauciarticular** (few joints), or **monoarticular** (one joint).

▼ DIFFERENTIAL DIAGNOSIS LIST

Traumatic Causes

Recent trauma—sprain, fracture
Foreign body synovitis
Overuse syndromes—stress fracture, apophysitis (tendinitis), Osgood-Schlatter disease

Degenerative—slipped capital femoral epiphysis (SCFE), Legg-Calvé-Perthes disease, patellofemoral pain syndrome, chondromalacia patella, osteochondritis dissecans

Infectious Causes

Osteomyelitis
Septic arthritis
Viral arthritis
Postinfectious arthritis—acute rheumatic fever (ARF), Lyme disease, post-streptococcal arthritis, postdysenteric arthritis (Reiter syndrome)

Inflammatory Causes

Toxic synovitis
Systemic lupus erythematosus
Dermatomyositis
Polyarteritis nodosa
Henoch-Schönlein purpura
Behçet syndrome
Psoriatic arthropathy

Immunologic Causes

Serum sickness
Stevens-Johnson syndrome
Erythema multiforme
Inflammatory bowel disease
Juvenile rheumatoid arthritis (JRA)

Congenital Causes

Hemophilia
Sickle cell disease (SCD)
Hypermobility syndromes
Multiple epiphyseal dysplasia

Neoplastic Causes

Bone tumors
Leukemia
Neuroblastoma

Miscellaneous Causes

Functional (growing pains)

▼ DIFFERENTIAL DIAGNOSIS DISCUSSION

Fractures and Sprains

Etiology

Fractures located **near the growth plate** are a common cause of posttraumatic joint pain.

Clinical Features and Evaluation

The growth plate is often the **weakest portion of the joint** in children. For this reason, it is difficult to diagnose anything but the most minor joint injuries as "sprains" in patients whose growth plates have not yet fused. Fractures near the growth plate can be classified by their radiographic appearance and severity.

Treatment

Injuries that reveal **localized or "point" tenderness** at a child's joint require **immobilization and orthopedic follow-up, even if radiographs fail to reveal an obvious fracture site** (Salter I fracture classification).

Foreign Body Synovitis

Etiology

Splinters, glass, or other **foreign material located near a joint space** can induce an **inflammatory response,** causing **synovitis or tendinitis.** This process can occur over a period of months, or it can develop earlier if it is complicated by infection.

Clinical Features and Evaluation

Diagnosis is based on a **high index of suspicion** and a **review of the history. Plain radiographs** are helpful **only with radiopaque foreign materials,** such as glass.

Treatment

Treatment consists of **surgical exploration and removal** of the foreign material.

Overuse Injury

Overuse injuries occur when a **small amount of stress** is placed on the joint **for a long period of time.** Although these injuries are **most common in the knee joint,** overuse injuries of other joints can occur secondary to exercise of inappropriate rate, intensity, or both (e.g., "Little Leaguer's elbow").

Stress Fractures

Stress fractures occur most commonly in the **lower extremity** and may be difficult to diagnose without a **bone scan.**

Apophysitis

Apophysitis is **inflammation of a tendon or ligament at its insertion site near the bone.** It occurs more commonly in children than does pure tendinitis. In apophysitis, the tenderness is usually **localized to the area just above or below the bone,** and radiographs are generally normal.

Osgood-Schlatter Disease

Osgood-Schlatter disease is thought to be either **apophysitis or an avulsion of the tibial tubercle secondary to recurrent traction of the patellar tendon.** The patient, usually an **active preadolescent or adolescent,** complains of **tenderness below the patella** and has **pain on extension of the knee against force. Radiographs** may be normal but can reveal **irregularity** and, possibly, **fragmentation** of the tibial tubercle. Treatment consists of **limiting activity until the natural fusion of the tubercle** occurs during midadolescence.

Degenerative Disease

Legg-Calvè-Perthes Disease

Legg-Calvè-Perthes disease is an avascular necrosis of the femoral head that can produce **hip or thigh pain.** The diagnosis should be considered in **5- to 10-year-old boys** with an **indolent presentation of limp** and with **painful abduction and internal rotation of the affected hip.** Plain **radiographs** might reveal changes in the femoral head on the affected side; a **bone scan** allows earlier detection of the disease. Other causes of avascular necrosis include sickle cell disease (SCD) and **chronic steroid use.**

Slipped Capital Femoral Epiphysis (SCFE)

SCFE, **displacement of the femoral head from the femoral neck,** is commonly seen in **obese school-aged children.** These children complain of **hip or thigh pain** and walk with the **affected leg externally rotated. Hip radiographs** are diagnostic. **Orthopedic referral is mandatory.**

Patellofemoral Pain Syndrome

Patellofemoral pain syndrome results from **recurrent transmission of force onto a malaligned patella.** The common scenario is an adolescent girl who complains of pain on flexion of a previously rested knee joint, pain when traveling down an incline, or **weakness,** causing the **knee to "give out** from under her." **Damage to the articular cartilage** (i.e., idiopathic adolescent anterior knee pain syndrome) can occur. Radiographs are frequently normal. **Exercise that strengthens the medial quadriceps muscles** may help realign the patella. **Surgical realignment** may be necessary.

Osteochondritis Dissecans

Osteochondritis dissecans is a **degenerative** process in which **cartilage replaces bone at an articular surface,** usually the **lateral epicondyle of the distal femur, the radial capitellum, or the talus.** It can develop as a result of **acute trauma** or as a result of the **repeated application of smaller forces,** which cause a **small subchondral fracture.** Osteochondritis dissecans is most common in children undergoing a **growth spurt.** Radiographs may be normal early in the course of the disease. **Immobilization in a non–weight-bearing cast** frequently alleviates the problem. However, **surgical removal of the avulsed fragment** occasionally is necessary.

Osteomyelitis

Etiology

Osteomyelitis in children can present with symptoms **similar** to those of **septic arthritis: fever, limp, or refusal to use an extremity in younger children,** or, **discrete localized pain in older children.** Although the pathophysiology of osteomyelitis differs from that of septic arthritis, the **predominant causative bacteria** remain the same. Occasionally, **viral, fungal, and mycobacterial causes** have been reported.

Clinical Features

Because osteomyelitis tends to affect the metaphyseal portion of the bone, symptoms can often be confused with joint pain. However, in contrast to septic arthritis, **isolated movement of the affected joint** in an older child with osteomyelitis **does not cause as much pain as does palpation of the** affected portion of the bone. The **C-reactive protein and the erythrocyte sedimentation rate (ESR) are usually increased** and are helpful in monitoring the response to therapy.

Evaluation

The triple-phase bone scan is a sensitive and specific test of osteomyelitis, except in neonates.

▼ **Plain radiographs** may reveal periosteal elevation or bone destruction 10–21 days after the onset of illness.
▼ **Magnetic resonance imaging** can be used to detail the extent and degree of bone and soft tissue injury, and to define the presence of a bone abscess ("Brodie abscess").
▼ **Blood culture results** identify the causative organism in up to 60% of patients.
▼ **Needle aspiration of metaphyseal bone** identifies the organism in 80% of patients.

Treatment

High-dose antibiotic therapy is required to ensure adequate penetration of the bone and complete eradication of the bacterial nidus. A **combination of intravenous and oral antibiotics** may be required for a longer total course than in patients with septic arthritis. However, recent evidence suggests that **shorter courses of intravenous and oral antibiotics** can be administered to successfully treat osteomyelitis caused by *Staphylococcus aureus*.

Septic Arthritis

Etiology

The cause is predominantly **bacterial,** occurring by **hematogenous delivery, direct extension from osteomyelitis, or from a penetrating injury** to the joint. *S. aureus* and *Haemophilus influenzae* are the most commonly involved organisms; however, the latter organism is becoming less prevalent as a result of recent immunization practices. Other bacterial causes include group B streptococcus and gram-negative organisms in neonates, *Neisseria gonorrhoeae* in adolescents, and *Salmonella* in patients with SCD. **Pyogenic infection** in the joint space causes increased pressure within the joint capsule, resulting in **derangements of the vascular and lymphatic supply. Bacterial and leukocyte proliferation** may also occur, causing the release of proteolytic enzymes. These changes can rapidly **damage cartilage and bone tissue.**

Clinical Features

Seventy-five percent of patients with septic arthritis develop **fever** within the first few days of infection. If the **hip or shoulder joints** are involved, the patient will hold the extremity **slightly flexed, abducted, and externally rotated** to relieve the pressure within the joint. The **knee and elbow,** if affected, will be **slightly flexed,** and the **ankle** will be **plantar flexed.** The **application of pressure** to the joint **or movement of the joint** through **any range of motion** will **produce pain.** This finding contrasts with that found in purely traumatic injuries, which may be asymptomatic through a small range of motion. Normal ranges of motion for each major joint are delineated in Table 49.1. **Erythema, heat, and swelling** may be present, but are difficult to detect in

TABLE 49.1. Range of Motion of Major Joints

	Flexion	Extension	Abduction	Adduction	Internal Rotation	External Rotation
Hip	120°	30°	50°	30°	35°	45°
Knee	135°	5°	0°	0°	10°	10°
Ankle	50°	20°	10°	20°	5° (eversion)	5° (inversion)
Shoulder	90°	45°	180°	45°	55°	45°
Elbow	135°	5°	0°	0°	90° (supination)	90° (pronation)
Wrist	80°	70°	20° (radial)	30° (ulnar)	0°	0°

the hip and shoulder joints because these joints are relatively deep beneath the skin surface.

Neisseria infections can produce either **monoarticular or polyarticular** disease. Gonococcal arthritis may begin as polyarthralgia, with a progression to monoarticular arthritis within a few days. These **symptoms** begin within 2–4 weeks of the initial urethritis and commonly **increase in severity 1 week following the menstrual period** in girls. Acute cases may be associated with **fever, malaise, or dermatitis. Tenosynovitis** (painful tendon sheaths) may also be present.

Evaluation

Plain radiographs may not be helpful early in the course of illness, but they may reveal distortion of the normal fat pads and dislocation of the bone from the joint.

Although the peripheral leukocyte count is not often helpful, the **ESR** will be greater than 30 mm/hr in more than 95% of patients. The joint fluid may appear turbid and will reveal a large number of leukocytes and a low fluid:serum glucose ratio, as described in Table 49.2.

Joint fluid cultures identify the causative organism in more than 70% of patients. In contrast, blood culture results are positive in only 30% of all patients. Joint fluid culture results are more likely to reveal the organism **within the first week of infection. Chronic meningococcemia** presents a **similar clinical picture** to gonococcal joint disease; however, **joint fluid cultures** are usually **sterile.**

Treatment

Septic arthritis is a **medical emergency.** Management of septic arthritis involves **evacuation of the purulent material** from the joint space **as soon as possible. Open surgical drainage** is preferred for the hip joint and remains an option for other joints that contain thick purulent material as well. **Parenteral antibiotic therapy** directed at the causative organism should be initiated soon after the diagnosis is made. A combination of **intravenous therapy and oral therapy** is given for at least **4 weeks** after diagnosis.

Viral Arthritis

Young children **under the age of 5 years** can often present with pain caused by **infection of the joint by viruses. Parvovirus and adenovirus** are two of the

TABLE 49.2. Characteristics of Synovial Fluid

	Appearance	WBC/mm³	% Neutrophils	Glucose Synovial Fluid	Blood
Normal	Clear	< 2000	< 40	> 50	> 0.5
Infectious	Turbid	> 75,000	> 75	< 50	< 0.5
Inflammatory (JRA, SLE)	Clear or turbid	5000–75,000	50	≥ 50	> 0.5
Traumatic	Bloody or clear	< 5000	< 50	> 50	> 0.5

JRA = juvenile rheumatoid arthritis; SLE = systemic lupus erythematosus; WBC = white blood cell.

more common culprits, and the **fever, rash and polyarthritis** is frequently **preceded by an upper respiratory infection.**

Postinfectious Arthritis

Acute Rheumatic Fever (ARF)

The **arthritis** of ARF is **migratory** and involves **several large joints in quick succession.** Commonly, each joint is **affected for less than 1 week,** and the entire polyarthritis rarely lasts more than 1 month. The **arthralgia** is also migratory but is differentiated from the arthritis by the **absence of swelling, redness, and decreased range of motion** in an otherwise **painful joint.** One **cannot use both the arthritis and arthralgia as criteria** for diagnosis.

Because the joint manifestations of ARF occur **within 5 weeks** of the initial streptococcal infection, **antistreptococcal antibody levels** are almost always **increased** during this period. Children with **poststreptococcal reactive arthritis do not fulfill the Jones criteria for ARF** (Table 49.3) but may still complain of **prolonged polyarthritis** after group A hemolytic streptococcal infection. These children may still develop **recurrent arthritis** and are thought to carry a **greater risk** of development of a subsequent **"second attack" of rheumatic fever.** Some physicians therefore treat these patients similarly to those with acute rheumatic fever. Treatment consists of **antistreptococcal and anti-inflammatory medications.** The arthritis associated with ARF responds dramatically to treatment with **aspirin.**

Lyme Disease

Approximately 60% of patients with documented Lyme disease complain of **painful joints** at some point during their illness. The knee is the most frequently affected joint. Initially, many patients suffer from **polyarthralgias** within the first few weeks of illness. **Frank arthritis** of one or more large

---

TABLE 49.3. Revised Jones Criteria for Diagnosis of Acute Rheumatic Fever

Major Criteria	Minor Criteria
Carditis	Fever
Arthritis	Arthralgia
Rash (erythema marginatum)	Elevated ESR, CRP
Chorea (Sydenham)	Prolonged PR interval on ECG
Subcutaneous nodules	History of prior attack of rheumatic fever or rheumatic heart disease

Diagnosis is likely with the presence of two major and one minor criteria, or one major and two minor criteria. Supporting evidence of a preceding streptococcal infection includes a history of recent scarlet fever, a positive throat culture for group A *Streptococcus*, and an increased antistreptolysin O (ASO) titer (or titers for other streptococcal antibodies).

Adapted from The Report of the ad hoc Committee of the American Heart Association Council on Rheumatic Fever and Congenital Heart Disease. *Circulation* 69:204A–208A, 1984.

CRP = C-reactive protein; ECG = electrocardiogram; ESR = erythrocyte sedimentation rate.

joints can occur **2 weeks to 2 years after the onset** of disease, and episodes of **arthritis and arthralgia** can recur over **subsequent years in untreated patients.** Each episode usually lasts a few weeks but can last as long as 1 year.

Many patients will **not report a history of deer tick bite** and **will not exhibit the pathognomonic rash** of erythema chronicum migrans. The diagnosis, albeit difficult to confirm, is supported by the finding of **concurrent clinical manifestations and serologic evidence** of recent infection. Examination of **synovial fluid** for polymerase chain reaction to the *Borrelia* antigens can be diagnostic.

Intravenous therapy is warranted only for cases of arthritis that do not respond to treatment with **amoxicillin (or tetracycline in children older than** the age of **8 years)** for 1 month.

Postdysenteric Arthritis

Occasionally, patients who have recently suffered **acute gastroenteritis** will experience **subsequent aseptic arthritis** affecting the large joints. This may occur days to weeks after the infection. It is most common after *Yersinia, Campylobacter,* and *Shigella* infections. In some patients, the **arthritis lasts for years** and may produce **destructive changes** in the joint. **Reiter syndrome,** which consists of **arthritis, urethritis, and uveitis,** may present similarly after gastrointestinal or chlamydial infections in HLA-B27–positive patients.

Toxic (Transient) Synovitis

Etiology

The cause of transient synovitis is **unknown,** but it has been associated with **upper respiratory infections.**

Clinical Features

The child with transient synovitis is most commonly a boy **3–9 years** of age who has a **preceding or concurrent upper respiratory infection.** The **hip** is the most commonly affected joint, causing a **limp** as well as **hip, thigh, or knee pain.**

Evaluation

Differentiation from septic arthritis and osteomyelitis is based on the child's **nontoxic appearance** and his **ability to move the hip through some range of motion without pain.**

Treatment

Treatment of transient synovitis includes **rest** of the affected extremity, **administration of oral analgesic medications,** and **follow-up** to assure resolution within 1 week.

Immunologic Causes

Serum Sickness

Serum sickness is an antigen–antibody mediated disease of **immune complex** deposition. It commonly occurs 1–2 weeks after **exposure to viral antigens or to certain medications,** such as cephalosporin or sulfa drugs. However, many **other infectious or medicinal agents** have been implicated. Symptoms consist of an **urticarial rash, arthralgias in the large joints, and constitutional symptoms, such as fever.** The **rash may turn purple** within a few days. **Steroid treatment** is reserved for the most severe cases.

Erythema Multiforme and Stevens-Johnson Syndrome

Erythema multiforme is an illness with causes similar to those of serum sickness, **in which erythematous target lesions found over the entire** body are accompanied by **pauciarticular arthritis. Stevens-Johnson syndrome is a more severe, potentially fatal form** of this entity and includes **mucosal lesions** on the **conjunctiva, lips, oral cavity,** and, potentially, the **intestine. Herpes simplex virus** is a common inducing agent.

Inflammatory Bowel Disease

Inflammatory bowel disease can present **initially as a form of arthritis.** There are multiple forms of arthritic manifestations of inflammatory bowel disease, the most common being the **pauciarticular enteropathic arthritis of large joints** that is **associated with erythema nodosum.** The attacks can last up to 6 weeks and coincide with the acute exacerbations of inflammatory bowel disease.

Ankylosing Spondylitis

Ankylosing spondylitis is a less common form of arthritis **associated with inflammatory bowel disease in HLA-B27–positive children.**

Juvenile Rheumatoid Arthritis (JRA)

JRA is a **systemic illness** with arthritis as one of its manifestations. It carries an incidence of approximately 3 in 100,000 children, with a female predominance of 2:1.

The clinical presentation of JRA may be divided into three types: **pauciarticular, polyarticular, and systemic.** Within these types, the age of onset and the presentation of illness may vary, as delineated in Table 49.4.

The key to the diagnosis of JRA is the **presence of symptoms for at least 6 weeks,** with a **fluctuating** clinical course. The diagnosis is made primarily from **historical** and **physical examination** findings. Laboratory analysis should be guided toward the evaluation of other illnesses that may be causing the joint pain, but **antinuclear antibody (ANA) testing** can be included.

TABLE 49.4. Main Subsets of JRA and Their Characteristics

Subset Frequency	Number of Joints	Gender	Age	+ANA	+RF	Uveitis	Outcome
Pauciarticular	1–4	F	2 yrs	++	–	Yes	Good
Polyarticular	≥5	F	3 & 9	+	–	Yes	Poor
Polyarticular RF+	≥5	F	Teens	+	+	No	Very poor
Systemic	Any	Either	0–16	–	–	No	Very poor*

* Intriguingly, it is excellent in some patients.

(Reprinted with permission from Polin A. and Ditmar M.: Pediatric Secrets, 3rd ed. Philadelphia: Hanley & Belfus, Inc., 2001, p. 681.)

Rheumatoid factor testing is usually not helpful and it is positive only in older girls with polyarticular manifestations. The ESR is often normal in all patients but those with systemic JRA. A thorough **search for other illnesses with similar manifestations** should ensue before diagnosing this condition. **Anti-inflammatory drugs** are the mainstay of treatment for the arthritis of JRA. **Intraarticular corticosteroid injections, low-dose methotrexate, and biological agents that act as tumor necrosis factor receptors** have been successful in alleviating symptoms in children with JRA.

Primary Bone Tumors

Etiology

Primary bone tumors are uncommon in children; however, they can cause joint pain if they are localized to the proximal or distal portions of the bone.

▼ **Osteogenic sarcoma (osteosarcoma)** is the most common primary bone tumor in children and can spread to the joint space by direct extension or as a "skip" lesion.

▼ **Ewing sarcoma,** another malignant bone tumor in children, involves the joint space less often than does osteogenic sarcoma.

▼ **Eosinophilic granuloma,** a benign bone lesion that can cause joint pain, often mimics the more malignant tumors.

▼ **Osteoid osteoma,** another benign bone lesion that can cause joint pain, has a predilection for the femur or tibia and may present as nighttime bone pain that awakens the child from sleep and responds dramatically to anti-inflammatory drugs.

Clinical Features

Frequently, the symptoms are **subtle,** with **progressive development of bone or joint pain,** a **soft tissue mass,** and possibly **recurrent fevers.** The patient or parents may relate the symptoms to a **single episode of trauma,** and **pathological fractures** may occur when minor trauma causes a break in a bone that is weakened by the presence of tumor.

Evaluation

The diagnosis is usually made after review of the **plain radiographs,** which reveal the tumor and corresponding bony changes.

Leukemia and Lymphoma

Leukemia and lymphoma can cause either **bone or joint pain** in children. Most often, the patient presents with **arthralgias** in conjunction with **other systemic problems.** The concomitant findings include **hepatomegaly or splenomegaly, petechiae, lymphadenopathy, anemia, and fever.** The joint pain is usually **chronic and remitting. Peripheral blood smear** and **bone marrow aspiration or lymph node biopsy** are diagnostic.

Limb Pain of Childhood

"Growing pains" result from **muscle overuse.** The pain lasts **less than a few hours,** frequently **awakens the child at night,** and is usually **localized to the muscles of the lower extremities.** The pain is **rarely (if ever) localized to the joint.**

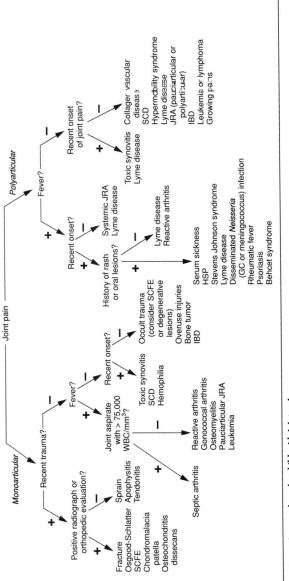

FIGURE 49.1. Approach to the child with joint pain.
GC = gonococcus; HSP = Henoch-Schönlein purpura; IBD = inflammatory bowel disease; JRA = juvenile rheumatoid arthritis; SCD = sickle cell disease; SCFE = slipped capital femoral epiphysis; WBC = white blood cell.

▼ EVALUATION OF JOINT PAIN

Patient History

The medical history should include questions regarding the presence of **rash, fever, or recent illness.** In addition, the **time course** of the joint pain should be elicited. A **history of trauma** can account for any acute event, or be the disclosing event in a more chronic problem, such as slipped capital femoral epiphysis (SCFE), chondromalacia patella, stress fractures, bone tumors, and hemophilia.

Physical Examination

Physical examination should concentrate on the **range of motion** of each joint in comparison with the corresponding contralateral joint. A thorough **neurologic examination** should be performed, with attention to **muscle strength and tone** as well as careful observation of the **child's gait.** The remainder of the physical examination may reveal specific rashes, mucosal lesions, lymphadenopathy, or fever.

Laboratory Studies

- ▼ ESR
- ▼ C-reactive protein
- ▼ Joint fluid analysis
- ▼ Plain radiographs
- ▼ Bone scans
- ▼ EKG
- ▼ WBC

▼ APPROACH TO THE PATIENT (FIGURE 49.1)

Although many of the illnesses that cause joint pain can be diagnosed and treated by the pediatrician or family physician, **referral to an orthopedist, a rheumatologist, or an oncologist** may be necessary.

Suggested Readings

Adebajo AO: Rheumatic manifestations of infectious diseases in children. *Curr Opin Rheumatol* 9:68–74, 1997.

Ansell BM: Rheumatic disease mimics in childhood. *Curr Opin Rheumatol* 12:445–447, 2000.

Carek PJ, Dickerson LM, Sack JL: Diagnosis and management of osteomyelitis. *Am Fam Physician* 63:2413–2420, 2001.

Del Beccaro MA, Champoux AN, Bockers T, et al: Septic arthritis versus transient synovitis of the hip: the value of screening laboratory tests. *Ann Emerg Med* 21:1418–1422, 1992.

Oudjhane K, Azouz EM: Imaging of osteomyelitis in children. *Radiol Clin North Am* 39:251–266, 2001.

Peltola H, Unkila-Kallio L, Kallio MJT, and the Finnish Study Group: Simplified treatment of acute staphylococcal osteomyelitis of childhood. *Pediatrics* 99:846–850, 1997.

Sherry DD: What's new in the diagnosis and treatment of juvenile rheumatoid arthritis. *J Pediatr Orthop* 20:419–420, 2000.

Sorokin R, Ward SB: Joint pain. *Med Clin North Am* 79:247–260, 1995.

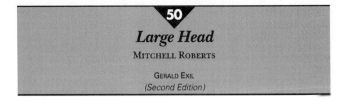

50
Large Head
MITCHELL ROBERTS

GERALD EXIL
(Second Edition)

▼ INTRODUCTION

Macrocephaly is defined as a head circumference that is **two standard deviations above the mean** for age. Serial measurements are often necessary for a complete evaluation. Normal head growth velocities (according to age) are given in Table 50.1. Gender must also be considered.

Enlargement of any of the four major constituents of the head can lead to macrocephaly: **enlarged ventricles** (hydrocephalus), **enlarged brain mass** (megalencephaly), **increased skull thickness** (osteodysplasia), or **subdural, subgaleal, or subperiosteal fluid collections.**

Hydrocephalus may be congenital or acquired. **Congenital hydrocephalus** generally arises secondary to central nervous system (CNS) malformations or aqueductal stenosis, whereas **acquired hydrocephalus** is produced by conditions that lead to excessive cerebrospinal fluid (CSF) production or that obstruct a CSF pathway. **Intraventricular pathway obstruction** produces **noncommunicating hydrocephalus. Extraventricular pathway blockage** (impaired absorption at the arachnoid villi) results in communicating hydrocephalus. Causes of communicating hydrocephalus include intraventricular hemorrhage; infection or inflammation (e.g., bacterial, tuberculous, or cryptococcal meningitis; viral encephalitis); meningeal infiltration by tumor; and associated metabolic conditions, including mucopolysaccharidosis deposition at the leptomeninges (e.g., Hurler syndrome).

▼ DIFFERENTIAL DIAGNOSIS LIST
Congenital Hydrocephalus

Infectious Causes

Cytomegalovirus infection
Toxoplasmosis
Mumps
Rubella

Anatomic Causes

Chiari malformation
Hydranencephaly
Aqueduct stenosis

Neoplastic Causes

Medulloblastoma
Choroid plexus papilloma
Meningioma

TABLE 50.1. Head Growth Velocity

Full-Term		Preterm	
Rate of Growth	Age	Rate of Growth	Age
2 cm/month	0–3 months	1 cm/wk	0–2 months
1 cm/month	3–6 months	0.5 cm/wk	2–4 months
0.5 cm/month	7–12 months	1 cm/month	> 4 months

Acquired Hydrocephalus

Neoplastic Causes

Posterior fossa tumor—medulloblastoma, ependymoma, cerebellar astrocytoma
Intraventricular tumor—ependymoma, choroid plexus papilloma, giant
cell astrocytoma, meningioma
Intraparenchymal mass—cyst, abscess, tumor

Traumatic Causes

Cephalohematoma
Subdural collections
Subgaleal collections

Congenital or Vascular Causes

Aneurysm of the vein of Galen
Intraparenchymal bleed
Intraventricular hemorrhage

▼ DIFFERENTIAL DIAGNOSIS DISCUSSION
Congenital Hydrocephalus

Patients with congenital hydrocephalus usually present during the newborn
period or early infancy. In some cases, the diagnosis can be made during
intrauterine life by means of prenatal ultrasound examination.

Some patients with hydrocephalus and other CNS abnormalities are asymptomatic at birth, but infants with congenital hydrocephalus usually present
with **lethargy or irritability, vomiting, poor feeding, poor weight gain, and
instability of arterial blood gases.** Signs of **increased intracranial pressure**
(ICP) include apnea, bradycardia, a tense and bulging fontanelle, split sutures, the setting sun sign (i.e., downward deviation of the eyes), vomiting,
sixth nerve palsies, and increased blood pressure with bradycardia. The scalp
veins may be prominent and tortuous.

✄ HINT Papilledema is uncommon in infancy because fontanelles are open
and relieve pressure.

Evaluation is with serial head measurements and imaging. In patients with
progressive hydrocephalus, treatment entails ventriculoperitoneal shunting.

Chiari Malformations

There are **four types of Chiari malformations,** classified according to severity. In **type II (Arnold-Chiari malformation),** the **cervical canals of both the brain stem and the cerebellum** are **displaced downward,** the **fourth ventricle is elongated,** and **hydrocephalus** results from obstruction of the flow of CSF through the foramina of Magendie and Luschka.

At birth, some patients already have advanced hydrocephalus, while others show rapid head enlargement during the first weeks of life. In addition to the signs and symptoms of hydrocephalus with increased ICP, patients with complicated Chiari malformations usually exhibit signs and symptoms related to **brain stem dysfunction: lower cranial nerve findings, breathing difficulty** (stridor), **apnea, poor feeding, swallowing problems** (drooling), **poor gag reflex,** and **tongue fasciculations.** Seizures are not uncommon.

▼ **Magnetic resonance imaging (MRI)** of the head confirms the diagnosis.
▼ **Testing of brain stem auditory evoked responses** complements the MRI assessment.
▼ **Electroencephalography** is indicated for selected patients.
▼ **Serial head circumference measurements** also need to be performed.

✂ HINT　Macrocephaly in a patient with a very prominent occiput raises suspicion of a Dandy-Walker malformation with hydrocephalus.

Congenital Infection

Congenital infection is discussed in detail in Chapter 46, "Infections, Newborn." Calcification seen on a computed tomography (CT) scan of the head increases the suspicion for congenital infection.

Genetic Syndromes

Fifty percent of patients with trisomy 13 syndrome have **meningomyelocele with hydrocephalus.** In Warburg syndrome, an autosomal recessive disorder, findings include hydrocephalus, retinal lesions, Dandy-Walker cyst, occipital encephalocele, agyria, and pachygyria.

Hydranencephaly

In hydranencephaly, the **cortex is replaced by a hugely enlarged ventricle,** presumably secondary to massive intrauterine infarctions. **Initially, the infant may appear normal,** with a normal head circumference and intact primitive reflexes. Later, **developmental arrest** and **long tract signs** become evident. **Positive transillumination and percussion of the skull** (transmitted sound) confirm the diagnosis. Many patients **die in early infancy.**

Acquired Hydrocephalus

Neoplasia

The most common tumors in patients younger than 2 years are **choroid plexus papilloma, ependymoma,** and **medulloblastoma.** Children with a **posterior fossa mass** (e.g., medulloblastoma, ependymoma, cerebellar astrocytoma) present for evaluation with signs of **increased ICP, ataxia, papilledema, and stiff neck. Persistent torticollis** in a child should increase the physician's suspicion of the presence of a tumor.

Intraventricular tumors (e.g., choroid plexus papilloma) can lead to the development of **hydrocephalus,** either by increasing CSF production or blocking the CSF pathways. A **CT or MRI scan** of the head is diagnostic. Treatment is by **surgical resection** of the tumor.

Intraventricular Hemorrhage

Intraventricular hemorrhage is **common in low-birth-weight infants** because of the degree of anatomic development and the immature vascularity of the germinal matrix. Perinatal and neonatal stresses (e.g., respiratory distress syndrome, hypoxemia, shock) are triggering factors.

Low-grade intraventricular hemorrhage is **usually asymptomatic. Grade III or IV hemorrhages** may result in **acute or progressive hydrocephalus** with a rapidly increasing head circumference. In some cases, there is only mild to moderate ventricular enlargement without signs of increased ICP (arrested hydrocephalus).

Infection and Inflammation

Inflammation and seeding (from tumor cells) of the meninges results in **communicating hydrocephalus.** The clinical picture is dominated by the underlying disease. **Patchy cranial nerve abnormalities** may result from entrapment of the nerves at their exit foramina at the base of the skull. In some cases (e.g., bacterial meningitis), **massive subdural effusion or empyema** may contribute to the head enlargement. **MRI** with gadolinium reveals hydrocephalus with enhanced basal cisterns.

Trauma

Cephalohematoma and subdural collections may result from **traumatic delivery,** which can be spontaneous or secondary to forceps or vacuum delivery.

Patients with a large subdural collection may experience **rapid head enlargement.** The presenting signs and symptoms and the prognosis are variable, depending on the severity of the trauma. In **severe cases,** the patient presents with an acute encephalopathy characterized by **lethargy, poor feeding, vomiting, signs of increased ICP, and seizures.**

CT of the head should be performed immediately in all symptomatic infants with a history of traumatic birth injury, because diagnostic failure can be fatal in some cases. A large collection may result in an increase in the occipitofrontal circumference measurement. In this setting, CT of the head is recommended to rule out associated skull fracture and intraparenchymal insult.

Large, symptomatic, subdural collections may require **neurosurgical intervention.**

Megalencephaly

Familial Megalencephaly

These patients have a **family history of a large head,** a normal intelligence quotient, and a normal neurologic examination. The head circumference is more than two standard growth deviations for age and remains parallel to the expected percentile over time. No work-up is necessary, although if neuroimaging is performed, one finds that the ventricles and the subarachnoid spaces tend to be top normal in size or mildly enlarged.

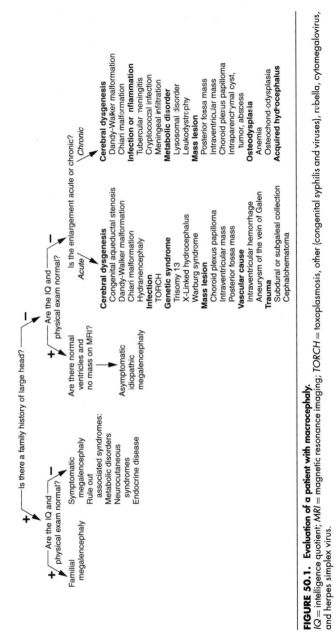

FIGURE 50.1. Evaluation of a patient with macrocephaly.
IQ = intelligence quotient; *MRI* = magnetic resonance imaging; *TORCH* = toxoplasmosis, other (congenital syphilis and viruses), rubella, cytomegalovirus, and herpes simplex virus.

⚔ HINT   A review of family photographs can be a major help in diagnosing this condition.

Sotos Syndrome

Characteristics of this syndrome are **cerebral gigantism with excessive somatic growth, advanced bone age, megalencephaly, and mild mental retardation.**

Idiopathic Megalencephaly

In these patients, there is no identifiable cause or associated syndrome, and there is no family history of macrocephaly. The **diagnosis is by exclusion. MRI** shows normal or mildly dilated ventricles.

Symptomatic Megalencephaly

In these patients, **megalencephaly is associated with a syndrome or has another identifiable cause.** For example, degenerative diseases (e.g., Tay-Sachs disease, Canavan disease, Alexander disease) as well as certain neurocutaneous syndromes (e.g., neurofibromatosis, tuberous sclerosis) are often associated with macrocephaly.

Osteodysplasia

Increased skull thickness can be **caused by anemia, osteochondrodysplasia** (characterized by short limbs, flat vertebrae, a large cranium, and a low nasal bridge), or **rickets.**

▼ APPROACH TO THE PATIENT (FIGURE 50.1)

Suggested Readings

Alper G, Ekinci G, Yilmaz Y, et al: Magnetic resonance imaging characteristics of benign macrocephaly in children. *J Child Neurol* 14(10):678–682, 1999.

Archibald SL, Fennema-Notestine C, Gamst A, et al: Brain dysmorphology in individuals with severe prenatal alcohol exposure. *Dev Med Child Neurol* 43(3):148–154, 2001.

Babson S: Growth of low birth weight infants. *J Pediatr* 77:11, 1970.

Charney E: Management of Chiari II complications. *J Pediatr* 3(3):364–371, 1989.

Mercuri E, Ricci D, Cowan FM, et al: Head growth in infants with hypoxic-ischemic encephalopathy: correlation with neonatal magnetic resonance imaging. *Pediatrics* 106(2 Pt 1):235–243, 2000.

Mochida GH, Walsh CA: Molecular genetics of human microcephaly. *Curr Opin Neurol* 14(2):151–156, 2001.

Sher PK, Brown SB: A longitudinal study of head growth in preterm infants. I: Normal rates of head growth. *Dev Med Child Neurol* 17:705–710, 1975.

Sher PK, Brown SB: A longitudinal study of head growth in preterm infants. II: Differentiation between "catch up" head growth and early infantile hydrocephalus. *Dev Med Child Neurol* 17:711–718, 1975.

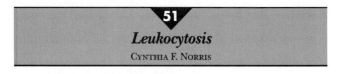

51
Leukocytosis
CYNTHIA F. NORRIS

▼ INTRODUCTION

Leukocytosis is defined as an **increased white blood cell (WBC) count, usually more than 12,000/mm³.** (The age of the patient needs to be considered, since the normal range varies with age.) Leukocytosis may result from an increase in any of the types of WBCs found in the bone marrow. **Neutrophilia is most common,** but lymphocytosis, monocytosis, basophilia, eosinophilia, and atypical lymphocytosis can also occur. **Lymphoblasts or myeloblasts** can be seen in abundance in the peripheral blood in **leukemia,** causing leukocytosis. **Leukemoid reactions,** which consist of benign but excessive leukocytosis (WBC counts of more than 50,000/mm³) associated with an **increase in the number of immature myeloid cells** (blasts, promyelocytes, myelocytes, and metamyelocytes) in the peripheral blood, can also occur. Most other forms of leukocytosis are characterized by WBC counts of less than 50,000/mm³.

▼ DIFFERENTIAL DIAGNOSIS LIST
Neutrophilia (Absolute Neutrophil Count > 8000/mm³)

Infectious Types

Abscesses
Tonsillitis
Otitis media
Pneumonia, pleuritis
Meningitis
Pericarditis
Arthritis, osteomyelitis
Peritonitis, appendicitis

Infectious Causes

Bacterial Infection

Staphylococcus
Streptococcus
Gonococcus
Meningococcus
Escherichia coli
Pseudomonas
Corynebacterium diphtheriae
Pasteurella

Viral Infection

Herpes zoster
Varicella
Rabies

Poliomyelitis
Epstein-Barr virus (infectious mononucleosis)

Fungal Infection

Actinomyces
Coccidioides

Mycobacterial Infection

Tuberculosis

Rickettsial Infection

Spirochetal Infection

Leptospira
Lyme disease
Syphilis

Other Infection

Kawasaki disease

Toxic/Drug/Hormonal Causes

Corticosteroids, adrenocorticotrophic hormone
Mercury, lead, kerosene, camphor
Insect venom—black widow spider
Epinephrine, norepinephrine, serotonin, histamine, acetylcholine

Neoplastic Causes

Tumors—lymphoma
Leukemia

Metabolic Abnormalities

Acidosis—diabetic ketoacidosis and others
Eclampsia
Uremia
Anorexia

Inflammatory Causes

Collagen vascular diseases—e.g., rheumatoid arthritis
Acute rheumatic fever
Generalized—vasculitis, dermatitis, myositis
Localized—nephritis, colitis, pancreatitis, thyroiditis, periodontitis

Hematologic Causes

Hemolysis—associated with both acute hemolysis, as in autoimmune
hemolytic anemia, and chronic hemolysis, as in sickle cell anemia
Acute blood loss
Myeloproliferative disorders
Surgical or functional asplenia
Leukemoid reaction

Miscellaneous Causes

Physical Stimuli

Burns
Pain
Electric shock
Trauma/surgery

Physiologic

Pregnancy/labor
Ovulation/menstruation
Vigorous exercise
Emotional stress

Eosinophilia (> 4% of Total WBC Count)

Infectious Causes

Ascaris infestation
Hookworm infestation
Strongyloides infestation
Trichinosis
Visceral larva migrans
Filariasis
Malaria
Toxoplasmosis
Pneumocystis carinii
Schistosomiasis
Scabies
Scarlet fever
Aspergillosis
Coccidioidomycosis

Toxic Causes

Drug hypersensitivity reaction
Postirradiation

Neoplastic Causes

Leukemia
Hodgkin and non-Hodgkin lymphoma
Brain tumors
Myeloproliferative disorders

Inflammatory/Allergic/Immune Conditions

Polyarteritis nodosa
Sarcoidosis
Goodpasture syndrome
Milk precipitin disease
Enteritis/ulcerative colitis
Environmental allergies
Asthma
Hay fever
Urticaria

Miscellaneous Causes

Skin disorders—eczema, atopic dermatitis, dermatitis herpetiformis, psoriasis, pemphigus, pemphigoid

Hereditary eosinophilia

Idiopathic hypereosinophilic syndromes—Loeffler syndrome, eosinophilic leukemia, pulmonary infiltration with eosinophilia (PIE syndrome)

Tropical eosinophilia (syndrome of pulmonary infiltrates, asthma-like symptoms, lymphadenopathy, and eosinophilia thought to be secondary to an unidentified filarial parasite)

Peritoneal dialysis

Chronic renal or liver disease

Immune deficiency syndromes

Monocytosis (> 8%–10% of Total WBC Count in Childhood; > 2% of Total WBC Count in Newborn Period)

Infectious Causes

Tuberculosis
Syphilis
Brucellosis
Malaria
Bacterial endocarditis
Rocky Mountain spotted fever
Kala azar
Typhoid fever

Neoplastic Causes

Preleukemia
Acute myelogenous leukemia—myelomonocytic and monocytic forms
Chronic myelogenous leukemia
Hodgkin and non-Hodgkin lymphoma

Inflammatory Causes

Systemic lupus erythematosus
Rheumatoid arthritis
Ulcerative colitis/Crohn disease
Sarcoidosis

Miscellaneous Causes

Chronic neutropenia syndromes (e.g., Kostmann syndrome)
Postsplenectomy
Recovery phase after myelosuppressive chemotherapy

Basophilia (> 1% of Total WBC Count)

Infectious Causes

Varicella
Tuberculosis
Influenza

Neoplastic Causes

Chronic myelogenous leukemia
Hodgkin disease

Inflammatory Causes

Ulcerative colitis
Rheumatoid arthritis

Miscellaneous Causes

Asthma
Drug hypersensitivity reaction
Chronic hemolytic anemia
Postsplenectomy or postradiation

Lymphocytosis

Infectious Causes (Associated with an Increased Number of Atypical Lymphocytes)

Bacterial Infection

Pertussis[*]
Tuberculosis
Brucellosis
Typhoid fever

Viral Infection

Infectious mononucleosis (Epstein-Barr virus)[†]
Cytomegalovirus[†]
Acute viral lymphocytosis (with common viral infections)[*]
Infectious hepatitis (A, B, or C)[†]
Rubeola
Rubella
Mumps
Varicella

Other Infection

Syphilis
Toxoplasmosis

Miscellaneous Causes

Physiologic lymphocytosis (percentage of lymphocytes is greater than percentage of polymorphonuclear leukocytes from age 2–5 years)
Relative lymphocytosis (secondary to neutropenia)
Endocrine—thyrotoxicosis, Addison disease
Drug hypersensitivity reaction
Crohn disease/ulcerative colitis
Leukemia

---

[*] Frequently associated with very *high* lymphocyte counts.
[†] Frequently associated with high *atypical* lymphocyte counts.

> **▨ HINT** Normal lymphocyte counts vary according to age. The following guidelines may be useful in assessing lymphocyte count abnormalities: more than 4000/mm³ in adults; more than 7,200/mm³ in adolescents; and more than 9000/mm³ in young children and infants.

▼ DIFFERENTIAL DIAGNOSIS DISCUSSION
Neutrophilia

Neutrophilia is the **most common type of leukocytosis.** The cause of neutrophilia is **most frequently an infection,** although drugs, inflammation, and other conditions listed in the differential diagnosis can be responsible. Neutrophilia is a result of one or more of the following mechanisms:

▼ Increased neutrophil production by the bone marrow
▼ Increased release of neutrophils from bone marrow storage
▼ A shift of neutrophils from the marginating to the circulating pool
▼ Prolonged neutrophil survival owing to decreased neutrophil entry into tissue or decreased removal by the spleen

Some forms of neutrophilia develop within minutes of exposure to the stimulus. For example, the neutrophilia that follows exposure to epinephrine is a result of neutrophils shifting from the marginating to the circulating pool. Other forms of neutrophilia take longer to develop because they occur by a combination of these mechanisms. The **duration of neutrophilia is usually days to weeks,** although in some instances it may persist for months.

> **▨ HINT** Healthy newborn infants normally experience a period of neutrophilia associated with a "left-shifted" differential (an increase in the percentage of early myeloid forms in the peripheral blood). The peak WBC count occurs during the first few days of life and decreases to adult levels within the first few weeks.

Eosinophilia

Normal eosinophil counts vary with age, reaching the adult value by 6–8 years of age. **Boys have slightly higher counts than girls,** and most individuals experience a **diurnal variation** in eosinophil count, with the **peak being at night.** Most eosinophils reside in the tissues (especially in areas exposed to the external environment, such as the gastrointestinal and respiratory tracts), and their **release into the bloodstream is the primary cause** of eosinophilia. Histamine release in allergic conditions or chronic inflammation tends to make blood vessel walls permeable, resulting in a release of eosinophils into the peripheral blood. By far the **most common cause** of eosinophilia is **an allergic reaction,** although skin diseases, parasitic infections, and conditions associated with chronic inflammation can also be factors. The **hypereosinophilic syndromes** are a poorly understood grouping of disorders characterized by persistent profound neutropenia (often less than 1500/mm³) of unclear cause.

Acute Lymphoblastic Leukemia
Incidence

Acute lymphoblastic leukemia (ALL) is the **most common malignancy** seen in the pediatric population. The peak age for development of acute lymphoblastic leukemia is approximately 4 years, although all ages can be affected. Certain individuals, such as those with **Down syndrome** or **ataxia–telangiectasia,** are at **increased risk** of development of this disorder.

Etiology

The **cause is unknown,** although genetic, environmental, infectious, and immune-mediated factors have all been implicated.

Clinical Features

Symptoms at presentation may include **pallor, fatigue, fever, bleeding, or bruising.** Bone pain is common, and young children may present for evaluation with a **limp or refusal to walk.** Physical findings include **bruises, petechiae, lymphadenopathy, and hepatosplenomegaly.**

Evaluation

Laboratory evaluation may reveal **leukocytosis, anemia, and thrombocytopenia.** In approximately 50% of patients, the WBC count is more than $10,000/mm^3$ at the time of diagnosis, and in 20% of patients, it is more than $50,000/mm^3$. **Neutropenia** (absolute neutrophil count of less than $500/mm^3$) is also frequently seen. **Lymphoblasts** can be found **in the peripheral blood,** but the inexperienced observer may report them as atypical lymphocytes. Definitive diagnosis of leukemia is made by a **bone marrow aspiration** that demonstrates **greater than 25% lymphoblasts. Immunologic, cytogenetic, and biochemical characterization of the cells** should also be performed. The **spinal fluid** also needs to be examined because the central nervous system is a sanctuary site of extramedullary disease.

Treatment

Prognostic factors such as the initial WBC count and the patient's age dictate the treatment indicated. High-risk patients require more intensive therapy. Most treatment plans last **2–3 years** and begin with a **remission induction phase intended to decrease the detectable leukemic burden to less than 5%.** The following phases of therapy aim to decrease and eventually eliminate all leukemic cells from the body.

▼ **Central nervous system preventive therapy** is incorporated into all protocols.
▼ **Multiagent chemotherapy** is the mainstay of treatment, although irradiation to the central nervous system is used for some high-risk patients.
▼ **Bone marrow transplantation** is another treatment approach used for the child who has experienced a relapse in the bone marrow.

Other sites of relapse include the central nervous system and the testes. The prognosis for long-term disease-free survival with current therapy is approximately 75% for all risk groups.

▓ **HINT** Tumor lysis syndrome (a metabolic triad of hyperuricemia, hyperkalemia, and hyperphosphatemia) is a complication of therapy that occurs when leukemic cells lyse in response to cytotoxic chemotherapy and release their intracellular contents into the bloodstream. This occurs commonly in cells with a high-growth fraction (T-cell leukemia/lymphoma and Burkitt lymphoma). Aggressive hydration, alkalinization, and allopurinol administration before initiating chemotherapy may alleviate serious renal dysfunction. The first two maneuvers promote uric acid and phosphate excretion, and allopurinol reduces uric acid formation. Potassium should not be added to hydration fluids. By monitoring the electrolyte concentrations and renal function closely, one can often avoid the development of renal failure.

Acute Nonlymphocytic Leukemia

Incidence

Acute nonlymphocytic leukemia (ANLL) represents approximately 15%–20% of all cases of leukemia seen in the pediatric population. It is slightly more common in older children but affects all ages. ANLL also represents the **majority of congenital leukemias** (mainly because acute lymphoblastic leukemia is rare at this age). It affects both sexes equally. The **incidence is increased in** individuals with **Down syndrome, Fanconi anemia, and Bloom syndrome.** It is also a **common "secondary malignancy"** resulting from **prior exposure to chemotherapy** (especially regimens that included alkylating agents).

Etiology

The **cause is unknown.** Predisposing factors include the earlier mentioned syndromes, exposure to large doses of **ionizing radiation,** and exposure to certain **chemicals.**

Clinical Features

Symptoms at presentation are similar to those of acute lymphoblastic leukemia and include **pallor, fatigue, fever, infection, bruising, and bleeding.** The physical examination may reveal **hepatosplenomegaly, lymphadenopathy, bruises, or petechiae. Leukemic infiltration of the skin** (leukemia cutis) may occur; it appears as colorless or slightly purple lesions. **Localized tumors or chloromas** can also be seen.

Evaluation

Laboratory evaluation typically reveals **neutropenia, anemia, and thrombocytopenia.** The WBC count is variable, although approximately 25% of children will have a WBC count of more than $100,000/mm^3$ at the time of diagnosis. Blasts can be seen in the peripheral blood. The definitive diagnosis is made by examination of the **bone marrow aspirate,** which demonstrates **greater than 25% blasts.** As in acute lymphoblastic leukemia, the **spinal fluid** must also be examined for evidence of leukemia. Up to 15% of patients will have evidence of blasts in the spinal fluid at the time of diagnosis.

Based on morphologic characterization and the result of histochemical staining, ANLL is divided into **seven subgroups.** The FAB (French-American-British system) subclasses are:

▼ **M1, acute myeloblastic leukemia without differentiation**
▼ **M2, acute myeloblastic leukemia with differentiation**
▼ **M3, acute promyelocytic leukemia**
▼ **M4, acute myelomonocytic leukemia**
▼ **M5, acute monocytic leukemia**
▼ **M6, erythroleukemia**
▼ **M7, acute megakaryoblastic leukemia**

The subclasses differ from each other in their method of presentation, associated chromosome abnormalities, and prognosis. **Poor prognostic variables** include having a **high WBC count at the time of diagnosis** and the M5 subtype.

Treatment

Standard treatment consists of **multiagent chemotherapy** that includes central nervous system preventive therapy. **Allogeneic bone marrow** transplanted **from a matched sibling donor during first remission** is the **treatment of choice.** Despite advances in ANLL therapy, the **prognosis remains poor,** with long-term disease-free survival rates of approximately 40%. In addition, ANLL therapy is generally more toxic than is therapy for acute lymphoblastic leukemia. **Serious infection rates** are higher during therapy, and the **late effects of treatment** can be problematic.

Complications

Three complications of ANLL deserve mention:

▼ Disseminated intravascular coagulation (DIC)
▼ Leukostasis
▼ Tumor lysis syndrome (mentioned previously)

💥 HINT Disseminated intravascular coagulation can occur with any subtype of ANLL but is especially common in the M3 and M5 subtypes. Aggressive treatment with platelet and fresh frozen plasma transfusions is often indicated. The initiation of chemotherapy frequently causes the coagulopathy to worsen before it improves.

💥 HINT Leukostasis (intravascular WBC clumping) rarely occurs unless the WBC count is more than 200,000/mm^3. Since myeloblasts are larger and more "sticky" than lymphoblasts, leukostasis occurs more frequently in ANLL than in acute lymphoblastic leukemia. The most commonly involved organs are the brain and the lungs. Central nervous system hemorrhage or stroke can occur. The pulmonary involvement is manifested by tachypnea and development of a need for supplemental O_2. Treatment consists of leukophoresis and prompt initiation of cytotoxic therapy. Red blood cell transfusion should be used with caution, since it can increase whole blood viscosity. (Hemoglobin level should not exceed 10 g/dl.)

▓ **HINT** Children with Down syndrome deserve special mention. Neonates with Down syndrome may develop a transient myeloproliferative syndrome that mimics congenital leukemia in every way except that it regresses spontaneously without therapy. For older children with Down syndrome and ANLL, there is also a better prognosis than for the average child with ANLL. The reasons are unclear.

Chronic Myelocytic Leukemia (CML)

Incidence and Etiology

Chronic myelocytic leukemia (CML) accounts for approximately 3% of all pediatric cases of leukemia. Individuals of any age can be affected, but most cases occur in late childhood. The disease is relatively **indolent** as compared with the acute leukemias. The **cause is unknown.**

Clinical Features

The patient is often **asymptomatic** and presents with a **high WBC count or splenomegaly** that was discovered at a routine well-child visit. However, symptoms such as **fever, night sweats, abdominal pain, or bone pain** can occur. Physical examination reveals impressive splenomegaly. **Hepatomegaly** can also be present.

Evaluation

Laboratory evaluation typically reveals impressive **leukocytosis, thrombocytosis, and mild anemia.** The bone marrow is hypercellular but with normal myeloid maturation. An abundance of blasts is not seen. In approximately 90% of cases, the characteristic cytogenetic hallmark of chronic myelocytic leukemia is seen: the **Philadelphia chromosome.** This is associated with the classic t(9;22).

Treatment

There are **three phases** of chronic myelocytic leukemia: **chronic phase, accelerated phase, and blast crisis.** The **chronic phase** may last for years and represents **hyperproliferation of mature myeloid elements.** Treatment during this phase is aimed at **cytoreduction** to decrease the risk of development of leukocytosis and massive splenomegaly. Administration of **hydroxyurea** is the mainstay of cytoreductive treatment. With time, **all patients will enter the accelerated and blast phases,** developing frank leukemia. In most instances, **myeloblasts** are seen morphologically, but **lymphoblast transformation** can also occur. **Once the blast phase has begun, the prognosis is poor. Bone marrow transplantation** is the only curative therapy and should be undertaken while the patient is still **in the chronic phase.**

General Therapy Guidelines For Leukemia

▼ **Prevent bleeding.** Aim to keep the platelet count higher than $20,000/mm^3$ by means of platelet transfusions. Watch for signs of DIC, which is especially common in the M3 and M5 subtypes of ANLL.

▼ **Treat anemia.** Most oncologists aim to keep the hemoglobin level higher than 8 g/dl (but not more than 10 g/dl if hyperleukocytosis is present). Some oncologists treat anemia only if the patient is symptomatic.

▼ **Identify and treat infection.** Because all neutropenic patients are at increased risk for development of an infection, fever should be treated aggressively. Blood should be drawn for culturing, and use of broad-spectrum antibiotics (to cover both gram-positive and gram-negative organisms) should be instituted. Prolonged fever in the neutropenic host raises the question of the existence of fungal disease.

▼ **Watch for tumor lysis.** This was described in the discussion of ALL.
▼ **Watch for complications of hyperleukocytosis.** This was described in the discussion of ANLL.
▼ **Begin definitive chemotherapy promptly,** once the diagnosis has been established.

Leukemoid Reactions

Etiology

Leukocytosis that develops in **response to an infection** or other stimuli can occasionally become **exaggerated,** often with WBC counts of more than 50,000/mm³. If the **white cells are not malignant blasts,** this syndrome is termed a leukemoid reaction (Table 51-1). Frequently, there is an associated **increase in the number of immature myeloid or lymphoid precursors** in the peripheral blood. Examination of the bone marrow typically reveals **myeloid hyperplasia** with normal maturation. Myeloid leukemoid reactions (comprising two-thirds of all cases) most often occur in association with **bacterial infection.** The etiologic agents most frequently involved are *Staphylococcus, Haemophilus, Neisseria meningitidis, Meningococcus,* and *Salmonella.* Lymphoid leukemoid reactions (which comprise one-third of all cases) occur most commonly in individuals infected with *Bordetella pertussis* or in common acute viral infections. **Other causes** of a leukemoid reaction include **granulomatous disease, severe hemolysis, vasculitis, drugs, and the presence of a tumor that metastasizes to the bone marrow.**

TABLE 51.1. Features of Leukemoid Reactions, ALL, and CML (Chronic Phase)

	Leukemoid Reaction	ALL	CML
Common physical examination findings	Evidence of infection	Hepatospleno-megaly or lym-phadenopathy	Splenomegaly
Predominant WBC morphological characteristics	Myelocytes or lymphocytes	Lymphoblasts	Myelocytes
WBC count	> 50,000/mm³	Wide range	> 100,000/mm³
Other cell lines	Normal hemo-globin and platelet counts	Anemia and thrombocyto-penia	Mild anemia and thrombocytosis

ALL = acute lymphoblastic leukemia; CML = chronic myelocytic leukemia; WBC = white blood cell.

Evaluation

Distinguishing a leukemoid reaction from chronic myelogenous leukemia in the chronic phase may be difficult. The acute leukemias may also exhibit excessive leukocytosis, usually composed of predominantly blast forms.

Suggested Readings

Ebb DH, Weinstein HJ: Diagnosis and treatment of childhood acute myelogenous leukemia. *Pediatr Clin North Am* 44:847, 1997.

Kelly KM, Lange B: Oncologic emergencies. *Pediatr Clin North Am* 44:809, 1997.

Pui CH: Acute lymphoblastic leukemia. *Pediatr Clin North Am* 44:831, 1997.

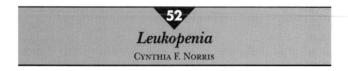

52

Leukopenia

CYNTHIA F. NORRIS

▼ INTRODUCTION

Leukopenia is defined as a **decrease in the total white blood cell (WBC) count, usually to below 4000/mm^3**. Neutropenia is defined as a **decrease in the number of circulating neutrophils** (both segmented and band forms). An absolute neutrophil count (ANC) of **less than 1500/mm^3** is considered neutropenia. The absolute neutrophil count is calculated by multiplying the total white blood cell count by the sum of the percent of segmented neutrophils plus the percent of band forms in the differential count. For example, if the WBC count is 4000, with 12% segmented neutrophils/polymorphonuclear leukocytes, 10% bands, 60% lymphocytes, and 18% monocytes, the ANC will be 880 [4000 × (0.12 + 0.10)]. The differential diagnoses of isolated leukopenia and neutropenia are similar; the two conditions will therefore be considered as one entity for the purpose of this chapter. Their pathogenesis is summarized in Table 52-1.

▼ DIFFERENTIAL DIAGNOSIS LIST

Infectious Causes

Bacterial Infection

Sepsis syndrome, bacteremia (especially group B streptococcal disease in neonates)

Tuberculosis

Brucellosis

TABLE 52.1. Pathogenesis of Isolated Neutropenia

Decreased bone marrow production of cells
Increased utilization of cells
Sequestration of cells in the spleen
Immune destruction of cells

Tularemia
Typhoid
Paratyphoid

Viral Infection

Hepatitis A or B
Parvovirus B19
Respiratory syncytial virus
Influenza A or B
Rubeola
Varicella
Rubella
Infectious mononucleosis (Epstein-Barr virus)
HIV
Cytomegalovirus

Protozoal Infection

Malaria
Kala azar (visceral leishmaniasis)

Rickettsial Infection

Scrub typhus
Sandfly fever

Toxic Causes

Drugs (Table 52.2)
Ionizing radiation

TABLE 52.2. Drugs That Can Induce Leukopenia

Chemotherapy agents
    Alkylating agents (e.g., cyclophosphamide)
    Antimetabolites (e.g., methotrexate)
    Anthracyclines (e.g., doxorubicin)
Antibiotics
    Sulfonamides (e.g., co-trimoxazole)
    Penicillin
    Chloramphenicol
Antipyretic agents
    Aspirin
    Acetaminophen
Antirheumatic agents
    Gold
    Penicillamine
    Phenylbutazone
Sedatives
    Barbiturates (e.g., phenobarbital)
    Benzodiazepines (e.g., diazepam, lorazepam)
Phenothiazines
    Chlorpromazine (Thorazine)
    Promethazine (Phenergan)

Congenital Causes

Kostmann syndrome
Cyclic neutropenia
Chronic benign neutropenia of childhood
Reticular dysgenesis
Schwachman-Diamond syndrome (neutropenia and exocrine pancreatic insufficiency)
Neutropenia associated with X-linked agammaglobulinemia
Neutropenia associated with dysgammaglobulinemia type I (neutropenia, absent IgA and IgG, and increase in IgM)
Neutropenia associated with metabolic disease—hyperglycemia, isovaleric acidemia, propionic acidemia, methylmalonic acidemia
Neutropenia as part of bone marrow failure syndrome—Fanconi anemia, dyskeratosis congenita

Immune-Mediated Causes

Autoimmune neutropenia (due to IgG-mediated destruction of neutrophils)
Felty syndrome (triad of neutropenia, splenomegaly, and rheumatoid arthritis)
Secondary to collagen vascular disease—juvenile rheumatoid arthritis or systemic lupus erythematosus
Isoimmune neonatal neutropenia (antibody derived from mother)

Miscellaneous Causes

Idiopathic aplastic anemia
Hypersplenism
Malnutrition
Copper deficiency
In association with megaloblastic anemia—B_{12} or folate deficiency
Preleukemia, leukemia
Bone marrow infiltration—with tumor, osteopetrosis, Gaucher disease

▼ DIFFERENTIAL DIAGNOSIS DISCUSSION

Neutropenia Associated with Infection

Infection, usually viral, is the most common cause of neutropenia in childhood. Typically, neutropenia develops during the first few days of infection and persists for 3–6 days. **Neonates** are at especially **high risk** for developing neutropenia because they have only a small neutrophil reserve in their bone marrow, and they release neutrophils too quickly into the circulation when stressed. The mechanism by which an infection causes neutropenia is not well understood; it seems to vary with the type of infection. Management consists of **treating the underlying infection.**

Drug-Induced Neutropenia

Etiology

Drug-induced neutropenia may be due to a cytotoxic effect or may be an idiosyncratic reaction. Neutropenia can be a result of:

▼ **Increased sensitivity** of myeloid precursors to appropriate drug concentrations

▼ **Altered drug metabolism** resulting in toxic levels of the drug in the bone marrow

▼ An **immunologic response** that occurs after exposure to the drug, resulting in neutrophil destruction.

Clinical Features

Fever, chills, and fatigue occur commonly in **immune-mediated drug-induced neutropenia.** These symptoms typically develop **7–14 days after exposure** to the drug. The duration of the neutropenia is usually brief (6–8 days).

Drug-induced neutropenia that is **not immune mediated is less predictable.** It may present several days to more than a month after exposure to the drug. The duration may be brief, or it may last months or years.

A list of drugs that may cause neutropenia can be found in Table 52-2.

Treatment

Treatment consists of **prompt discontinuation** of the offending drug.

Kostmann Syndrome

Etiology

Kostmann syndrome, a **severe congenital neutropenic disorder** of **unknown cause,** is inherited as an autosomal recessive trait, although a familial autosomal dominant form has been reported.

Clinical Features

Children with this disorder frequently present for medical care in the **first few months of life. Fever, cellulitis, stomatitis, and perirectal abscesses** are the most common findings. These children are **at risk for** developing severe bacterial infections, which may be **life threatening.**

Evaluation

Laboratory test results reveal **profound neutropenia** (absolute neutrophil count of **less than 200/mm^3**) with or without leukopenia. The differential count may reveal **monocytosis and eosinophilia.**

Bone marrow biopsy findings are variable. Usually, there is normal myeloid maturation up to the promyelocyte or myelocyte stage but **no evidence of mature neutrophils** (maturational arrest). Erythroid precursors and megakaryocytes are present in normal numbers, with a normal maturational sequence noted.

Treatment

The natural course of this disease is **death at an early age secondary to overwhelming infection.** Prophylactic antibiotics are not beneficial. Therapeutic use of the **cytokine granulocyte colony-stimulating factor (G-CSF)** has resulted in an improvement in the neutrophil count, decreased risk of development of serious infections, and improved survival in many patients with Kostmann syndrome.

Autoimmune Neutropenia

Etiology

Autoimmune neutropenia is **analogous to autoimmune hemolytic anemia or idiopathic thrombocytopenic purpura.** For reasons that are not well understood, children with this disorder develop **IgG, IgA, or IgM antibodies against** their own neutrophils. This disorder affects individuals of all ages, but young children seem most susceptible.

Clinical Features

Clinical manifestations are usually **mild. Skin infections, oral ulcerations, and pharyngitis** are the most common complaints. Some children will have mild to moderate **splenomegaly** on physical examination.

Evaluation

Laboratory testing results reveal n**eutropenia** (absolute neutrophil count of 0–1000/mm^3) **and monocytosis.** Bone marrow examination typically reveals normal cellularity with **myeloid hyperplasia** and a **paucity of mature neutrophils.** Diagnosis is made by demonstrating **antineutrophil antibodies** in the serum or on the surface of the neutrophil.

Treatment

In most children with this disorder, the neutrophil count will increase in response to infection. Although the prognosis is good, **aggressive treatment of infections** is recommended. Most children will experience an improvement in their symptoms as they grow older. In many children, the WBC count will completely normalize within 1–3 years.

Cyclic Neutropenia

Etiology

Cyclic neutropenia, a **rare** problem in children, is characterized by regular **oscillation in the number of circulating neutrophils** in the peripheral blood. The periodicity is usually every 21 days, but cycles as short as 14 days and as long as 28–36 days have been described. The **cause is unknown.** Studies suggest, however, that there may be a **regulatory defect in stem cell precursors.**

Clinical Features

Symptoms usually appear before the age of 10 years. Diagnosis is made from analysis of **serial complete blood counts** and **differential counts** (two to three times a week for 3–4 weeks). Clinical findings include **stomatitis, oral ulcers, pharyngitis with lymph node enlargement, and skin infection.** Laboratory test results reveal **severe neutropenia. Monocytosis and eosinophilia** occur in some patients. The **platelet and reticulocyte counts may also fluctuate,** although not consistently in the same direction. The **morphological characteristics of the bone marrow change** according to the time in the cycle, varying from normal to hypocellular, with maturational arrest of the myeloid line. The **ANC is low for 3–10 days and then begins to increase.**

Symptoms disappear as the ANC returns to normal. The **severity of infection varies** with each child and with the ANC. Some children do not have infections despite profound neutropenia, although there are reports of death in up to 10% of patients.

Treatment

Therapeutic use of G-CSF has been demonstrated to decrease the risk of infection.

Schwachman-Diamond Syndrome

Etiology

Schwachman-Diamond syndrome is a **rare congenital form of neutropenia** inherited as an autosomal recessive trait. The syndrome consists of neutropenia with **exocrine pancreatic insufficiency.** Some children also have metaphyseal **chondrodysplasia and dwarfism.**

Clinical Features

The symptoms of **weight loss, diarrhea, steatorrhea, and failure to thrive** usually develop in infancy, resembling the **clinical presentation of cystic fibrosis.** Patients experience **recurrent infections;** the mortality rate from infection or bone marrow failure is 15%–25%.

Evaluation

The sweat electrolyte values are normal in this syndrome, however. The neutrophil count is usually 200–400/ml.

Chronic Benign Neutropenia of Childhood

Chronic benign neutropenia of childhood is a **poorly understood** disorder. Symptoms of **skin infections** usually appear in early childhood and vary with the degree of neutropenia. Laboratory test results reveal **severe neutropenia and associated monocytosis.** The diagnosis is essentially one of **exclusion** and should be considered in any child with **persistent chronic neutropenia, a benign clinical course, and no evidence of another neutropenic disorder.** The prognosis is good.

▼ EVALUATION OF LEUKOPENIA

Patient History

▼ Does the child have a fever? (This raises the question of infection, especially in a neutropenic patient. It may also give a clue to the cause, since some infections can cause neutropenia.)

▼ Does the child have any skin infections? (Abscesses and cellulitis require prompt treatment in the setting of neutropenia.)

▼ Has the child previously had a normal complete blood cell count (CBC)? (If so, this will exclude congenital causes of neutropenia, such as Kostmann syndrome.)

▼ Has the child recently taken any medication (e.g., sulfonamides, penicillin, phenothiazines)?

▼ Does the child have any symptoms of a systemic infection, such as fever, rash, and upper respiratory symptoms? (This could indicate infectious mononucleosis, rubeola, rubella, or varicella.)

▼ Does the child have any symptoms of the following infections: tuberculosis, brucellosis, tularemia, or malaria?

▼ Is there a history of jaundice (seen in hepatitis A and B)?

▼ Is the child a sick neonate? (This could indicate group B streptococcal infection or isoimmune neonatal neutropenia.)

▼ Does the child have a history of recurrent skin infections or oral ulcerations? (This suggests a more chronic, perhaps congenital neutropenia such as cyclic neutropenia or Kostmann syndrome.)

▼ Does the child have an unusual diet or look malnourished? (This could indicate malnutrition or an isolated B_{12}, folate, or copper deficiency.)

▼ Is there a family history of neutropenia, recurrent infection, or death at an early age from infection? (This would be seen in any of the congenital neutropenia syndromes—Kostmann syndrome, chronic benign neutropenia, or familial aplastic anemia.)

▼ Is there any bruising or bleeding? Is the child pale or fatigued? (If the answer is yes, this suggests that other cell lines are involved, such as in aplastic anemia, leukemia, or megaloblastic anemia.)

Physical Examination

▼ Is the child ill appearing? (Infection, either as the cause or the result of neutropenia, is likely and should be treated promptly.)

▼ Is there evidence of cellulitis, perirectal abscesses, labial abscesses, or pharyngitis? (All are seen in neutropenic patients and require prompt treatment.)

▼ Are there oral ulcerations or swollen red gums (common in many neutropenic disorders)?

▼ Are there bruises, petechiae, or pallor (suggesting leukemia or aplastic anemia)?

▼ Is there splenomegaly (found in hypersplenism, Felty syndrome, and leukemia)?

▼ Is there hepatomegaly (occurring in hepatitis, leukemia, and infectious mononucleosis)?

▼ Are there phenotypic abnormalities, such as thumb anomalies (Fanconi anemia), dwarfism (Schwachman-Diamond syndrome or cartilage-hair hypoplasia), or skin hyperpigmentation (Fanconi anemia, dyskeratosis congenita)?

▼ Are there joint findings suggesting arthritis (seen in juvenile rheumatoid arthritis, systemic lupus erythematosus, or Felty syndrome)?

▼ Is there fever or rash? (See corresponding list in "Patient History")

Laboratory Studies

▼ CBC, differential count (sometimes serially)
▼ Bone marrow aspirate $+/-$ biopsy
▼ Antineutrophil antibodies

Factitious Causes of Leukopenia (False–Positive Test Result)

▼ Delay in testing blood sample drawn from the patient
▼ Excessive leukocyte clumping (in the presence of cold agglutinins, increased immunoglobulin levels, or certain paraproteins)
▼ Leukocyte fragility (due to certain drugs or leukemia)

**Results of a WBC count determined manually should identify the last two conditions.

HINT In African-Americans, the total WBC count normally may be as low as 3600/mm³, and the ANC may be as low as 1000/mm³.

✄ HINT In infants, the total WBC count is higher than in later childhood. Lymphocytes are the predominant WBC form in children 2–5 years of age. Neutrophils are the predominant WBC form in infants and again in children greater than 5 years of age.

▼ TREATMENT OF LEUKOPENIA

Antibiotics

Prompt treatment of infection with antibiotics is indicated.

Cytokines

G-CSF

G-CSF is a **hematopoietic growth factor** produced by recombinant DNA technology that stimulates the growth of committed neutrophil progenitors. G-CSF has been approved for use in treating the neutropenia that results from **cancer chemotherapy.***

Granulocyte-Macrophage Colony-Stimulating Factor (GM-CSF)

GM-CSF is another **hematopoietic growth factor** produced by recombinant DNA technology. GM-CSF is a **multilineage growth factor** that stimulates the growth of neutrophils, eosinophils, monocytes, macrophages, and megakaryocytes. GM-CSF has been approved for use **following autologous bone marrow transplant for lymphoid and other malignancies** to enhance bone marrow recovery.*

Granulocyte Transfusions

Granulocyte concentrates are usually prepared by **leukapheresis of a single donor.** Each unit contains some lymphocytes, platelets, red blood cells, and plasma in addition to granulocytes. The indications for a granulocyte transfusion are few and include:

▼ Gram-negative sepsis not responding to antibiotics in a neutropenic host
▼ Prolonged neutropenia and sepsis in the neonate since they may quickly deplete their marrow reserve of neutrophils
▼ Life-threatening infections in a neutropenic patient who shows no sign of bone marrow recovery

Complications are many and include the **risks of infection, allergic or febrile transfusion reactions and graft-versus-host disease.** A hematologist or blood bank physician should be involved in this decision.

✄ HINT WBC concentrates should not be run through a leukoreduction filter.

▼ APPROACH TO THE PATIENT

▼ If the child is ill appearing, the work-up should be delayed while administration of appropriate antibiotics is started. If the cause of the fever is not evident, broad-spectrum antibiotics should be chosen.

---

* Other indications for G-CSF or GM-CSF that are still under investigation include aplastic anemia, Kostmann syndrome, cyclic neutropenia, and chronic benign neutropenia. Complications include the potential to stimulate the growth of leukemia, lymphoma, or nonhematopoietic tumor cells.

▼ If a recent infection or drug exposure is noted in the history and the child is clinically well with isolated neutropenia, close follow-up with performance of several repeat CBCs and differentials may be all that is indicated.

▼ If the neutropenia is chronic or if there is a history of recurrent infection, a more extensive work-up should be initiated which includes (a) bone marrow aspirate and biopsy; (b) serial complete blood counts and differential counts two to three times a week for 3–4 weeks; and (c) analysis of antineutrophil antibodies. More specific testing is dictated by the history and physical examination findings.

Suggested Readings

Anonymous: Standardization of definitions and criteria of causality assessment of adverse drug reactions. Drug-induced cytopenia. *Int J Clin Pharmacol Ther Toxicol* 29:75, 1991.

Bernini JC: Diagnosis and management of chronic neutropenia during childhood. *Pediatr Clin North Am* 43:773, 1996.

Calhoun DA, Christensen RD: Recent advances in the pathogenesis and treatment of nonimmune neutropenias in the neonate. *Curr Opin Hematol* 5:37, 1998.

Kostmann R: Infantile genetic agranulocytosis: a review with presentation of ten new cases. *Acta Paediatr Scand* 64:362, 1975.

Shastri KA, Logue GL: Autoimmune neutropenia. *Blood* 81:1984, 1993.

Welte K, Gabrilove J, Bronchud MH, et al: Filgrastim (r-metHuG-CSF): the first 10 years. *Blood* 88:1907, 1996.

Zeidler C, Boxer L, Dale DC: Management of Kostmann syndrome in the G-CSF Era. *Br J Haematology* 109:490, 2000.

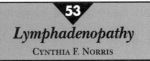

53

Lymphadenopathy

CYNTHIA F. NORRIS

▼ INTRODUCTION

Healthy children frequently have **palpable lymph nodes,** most commonly in the cervical, axillary, and inguinal areas. Although not found in infants, palpable lymph nodes normally become more prominent as the child approaches puberty and then tend to regress as the child approaches adulthood. **Benign lymph nodes should be small, soft, and freely mobile.** Nodes that are **greater than 1 cm** in diameter or that are **firm, hard, erythematous, tender, warm, fluctuant, or fixed** in position **require further attention.** In addition, **adenopathy in the supraclavicular, posterior auricular, epitrochlear, or popliteal areas is always abnormal.** A thorough physical examination will determine whether the enlarged node is isolated to one region or is part of a generalized adenopathy. This will help to narrow the differential diagnosis.

▼ DIFFERENTIAL DIAGNOSIS LIST
Generalized Lymphadenopathy

Infectious Causes

Bacterial Infection

Bacteremia, sepsis
Scarlet fever
Syphilis
Tuberculosis (TB)
Subacute bacterial endocarditis
Brucellosis
Leptospirosis
Typhoid fever
Plague
Lyme disease
Tularemia

Viral Infection

Epstein-Barr virus (EBV)
HIV
Varicella
Cytomegalovirus (CMV)
Rubeola
Rubella
Infectious hepatitis
Influenza

Fungal Infection

Histoplasmosis
Coccidioidomycosis

Parasitic Infection

Toxoplasmosis
Malaria

Toxic Causes—phenytoin, isoniazid
Neoplastic Causes

Primary Lymphoid Neoplasm

Hodgkin disease
Non-Hodgkin lymphoma

Metastatic Neoplasm

Acute lymphocytic leukemia
Acute myelogenous leukemia
Neuroblastoma

Metabolic Causes

Gaucher disease
Niemann-Pick disease

Immunologic Causes

Systemic lupus erythematosus
Juvenile rheumatoid arthritis
Vasculitis syndromes
Serum sickness
Autoimmune hemolytic anemia

Endocrine Causes

Hyperthyroidism

Miscellaneous Causes

Skin disorders
Atopic dermatitis
Histiocytosis X
Chronic granulomatous disease
Chediak-Higashi syndrome
Sarcoidosis
Nonspecific reactive hyperplasia

Regional Lymphadenopathy

Cervical

Infectious Causes

Viral Infection

Upper respiratory tract infections
Systemic viral infections (rubeola, rubella, varicella, CMV, EBV)

Bacterial Infection

Pharyngitis (streptococcal, diphtheria)
Primary adenitis (staphylococcal, streptococcal)
Infections of head/neck
Systemic bacterial infections (tularemia, brucellosis, leptospirosis)
TB
Atypical mycobacterium
Cat-scratch disease (*Bartonella henselae*)

Fungal Infection

Histoplasmosis

Parasitic Infection

Toxoplasmosis

Other Infection

Kawasaki syndrome

Neoplastic Causes

Hodgkin disease
Non-Hodgkin lymphoma
Carcinoma of thyroid
Rhabdomyosarcoma
Neuroblastoma

Other Causes

Sinus histiocytosis (benign)
Sarcoidosis

Occipital

Tinea capitis
Seborrheic dermatitis

Preauricular

Conjunctivitis (viral, bacterial, chlamydial)
External ear infections
Cat-scratch disease (*Bartonella henselae*)
Tularemia

Submaxillary/Submental

Herpetic gingivostomatitis
Dental infections

Epitrochlear

Local infection of hand/forearm
Rheumatologic disease of fingers/wrist
Tularemia
Cat-scratch disease (*Bartonella henselae*)

Axillary

Infectious Causes

Local infection of upper extremity, chest wall, or breast
Cat-scratch disease (*Bartonella henselae*)

Neoplastic Causes

Rhabdomyosarcoma of extremity

Other Causes

Postvaccination (when administered in arm)
Chronic inflammation of skin (rash) or joints (juvenile rheumatoid arthritis) of upper extremity

Mediastinal

Infectious Causes

TB
Histoplasmosis
Coccidioidomycosis
Blastomycosis

Inflammatory Causes

Sarcoidosis

Neoplastic Causes

Hodgkin disease
Non-Hodgkin lymphoma

Supraclavicular

Hodgkin disease
Lung, mediastinal, or abdominal malignancy

Inguinal

Venereal Disease Causes

Genital herpes
Syphilis
Chancroid
Chlamydia
Lymphogranuloma venereum

Local Infection of Lower Extremity

Chronic Inflammation of Lower Extremity

Skin—diaper dermatitis, insect bites
Joints—juvenile rheumatoid arthritis

Neoplastic Causes

Rhabdomyosarcoma of extremity
Neuroblastoma

Popliteal

Local infection of lower leg/foot

⚡ HINT   Are your physical examination or radiographic findings truly consistent with lymphadenopathy? For a list of possible entities confused with adenopathy, see Table 53.1.

▼ DIFFERENTIAL DIAGNOSIS DISCUSSION
Non-Hodgkin Lymphoma

Incidence

Non-Hodgkin lymphoma, the third most common pediatric cancer, is a **heterogeneous group of lymphomas** whose incidence increases with age. The incidence of non-Hodgkin lymphoma varies with geographic area. **Africa and the Middle East** have the highest rates of non-Hodgkin lymphoma, with Burkitt lymphoma being especially prevalent in Africa.

Etiology

EBV has been recovered from many of these tumors, raising the question of its role in the etiology of the tumor. Risk factors for development of non-Hodgkin lymphoma include **genetically determined immunodeficiency syndromes** (ataxia–telangiectasia, Wiskott-Aldrich syndrome, severe combined immunodeficiency disease, and X-linked lymphoproliferative disease) **and acquired immunodeficiency syndromes** (AIDS and postrenal/cardiac/bone marrow transplant).

TABLE 53.1. Possible Entities Confused with Adenopathy

Cervical area
Thyroglossal cyst
Branchial cleft cyst
Epidermal cyst
Cystic hygroma
Ectopic thyroid tissue
Anterior mediastinum
Thymic neoplasm/thymoma
Teratoma/dermoid cyst
Cystic hygroma
Rhabdomyosarcoma
Lymphangioma/hemangioma
Bronchogenic cyst
Foreign body
Middle mediastinum
Neuroblastoma
Bronchogenic cyst
Teratoma
Pericardial cyst
Foreign body
Posterior mediastinum
Neurogenic tumor
Bronchogenic cyst
Ewing sarcoma
Rhabdomyosarcoma
Thoracic meningocele

Clinical Features

Childhood non-Hodgkin lymphoma is divided into **three main histologic patterns: lymphoblastic** (40%), **small noncleaved cell** (including Burkitt and non-Burkitt lymphoma) (40%), **and large cell** (20%).

▼ **Lymphoblastic.** Most lymphoblastic lymphomas are of T-cell origin. The patient may present with **cervical adenopathy and respiratory distress.** A chest radiograph frequently reveals a **mediastinal mass** and **pleural effusions. Superior vena cava syndrome is a life-threatening emergency** that may arise in this setting. The mediastinal mass compresses the superior vena cava and/or trachea, impeding blood return and air flow. Symptoms include **cough, dyspnea, and difficulty lying down secondary to respiratory distress.** Physical findings include **edema and cyanosis of the face, neck, and upper extremities and wheeze or stridor. Immediate therapy with radiation or chemotherapy** may obscure the diagnosis but may be life saving.

▼ **Small noncleaved cell.** Most patients with small noncleaved cell lymphomas present with abdominal findings. **Abdominal pain and swelling** are common complaints. Physical findings include a **rapidly enlarging abdominal mass and inguinal adenopathy.** Signs of **intestinal obstruction** may be present.

▼ **Large cell lymphomas.** Large cell lymphomas have various clinical presentations.

Evaluation

Work-up should include a **complete blood cell count (CBC) with white blood cell (WBC) differential, serum lactate dehydrogenase, serum uric acid, and examination of the bone marrow and spinal fluid.** Chest radiography or computed tomography (CT) of the chest should be performed to evaluate supradiaphragmatic disease; **abdominal ultrasonography or CT** should be performed to evaluate subdiaphragmatic disease. Ascites, pleural, or pericardial fluid can also be used to establish the diagnosis.

Treatment

Because this tumor grows rapidly, prompt diagnosis is vital so that treatment can be initiated. **Combination chemotherapy** is the mainstay of treatment. These patients are at increased **risk for tumor lysis syndrome** [see discussion of leukemia in Chapter 51, "Leukocytosis"], as a result of the tumor's high growth rate and sensitivity to chemotherapy. **Prognosis is good,** except in patients with advanced disease (bone marrow or central nervous system [CNS] involvement).

Hodgkin Disease

Etiology

Hodgkin disease is a form of lymphoma most frequently seen in **late adolescence.** Although it can occur at other ages, it is especially rare in those younger than the age of 5 years. The etiology is unknown.

Clinical Features

The patient usually presents with **painless cervical or supraclavicular adenopathy,** although other nodes may be involved. Systemic symptoms include **fever, weight loss, night sweats, anorexia, and fatigue.**

Evaluation

Physical examination reveals **firm, nontender lymph nodes** in the areas mentioned earlier. **Hepatosplenomegaly** is a common finding and may indicate advanced disease.

If Hodgkin disease is suspected, a **chest radiograph should be obtained promptly** because two-thirds of patients have some degree of **mediastinal involvement.** The **airway should be assessed** for evidence of tracheal compression before any procedures are performed. **Lymph node biopsy** will establish the definitive diagnosis, revealing the **characteristic Reed-Sternberg cell and one of four histologic patterns** (nodular sclerosing, lymphocytic predominance, lymphocytic depletion, and mixed cellularity). Further work-up is necessary for staging purposes and to establish a baseline for following response to treatment. Studies should include a **CBC with differential, erythrocyte sedimentation rate, chest and abdominal CT scans, bone scan, and bone marrow aspirate/biopsy. Gallium scans and staging laparotomies** are helpful in some instances.

Treatment

Treatment consists of **combination chemotherapy and/or radiation therapy,** based on the patient's age, pubertal status, and stage of disease. Long-term survival continues to improve but still varies greatly with stage of disease.

Infectious Mononucleosis

Etiology

Epstein-Barr virus (EBV), a member of the herpesvirus group, is the causative agent in infectious mononucleosis. EBV is also **associated with nasopharyngeal carcinoma** and some cases of **Burkitt lymphoma.** The virus, **transmitted by saliva,** gains entry through the pharynx and spreads throughout the lymphatic system.

Clinical Features

Primary infection may occur at an early age in developing countries and in lower socioeconomic groups. The **primary infection** is frequently **asymptomatic.** Individuals who experience primary infection in adolescence or young adulthood are more likely to develop the clinical syndrome of infectious mononucleosis. After an **incubation period of 4–8 weeks,** the patient begins to experience **fatigue, anorexia, headache, and malaise. Fever and sore throat** usually develop within 1 week, bringing the patient to medical attention.

Physical findings at presentation include **pharyngitis, lymphadenopathy, and hepatosplenomegaly.** Not uncommonly, the patient is **misdiagnosed with streptococcal pharyngitis** and treated with ampicillin. For reasons that are unclear, **80%–100% of patients** with infectious mononucleosis **treated with ampicillin will develop a pruritic maculopapular rash,** which can prove very helpful in making the diagnosis. Symptoms usually persist for **several weeks,** although **fatigue and malaise may persist for months. CNS complications** include aseptic meningitis, encephalitis, Bell palsy, and Guillain-Barré syndrome. Other complications include splenic rupture, autoimmune hemolytic anemia, thrombocytopenia, granulocytopenia, myocarditis, interstitial pneumonitis, and airway obstruction.

Evaluation

Diagnosis is suggested by the **clinical triad of fever, lymphadenopathy, and pharyngitis combined** with the laboratory finding of **atypical lymphocytosis.** If the clinical presentation is unclear, **serologic testing** is available. **Heterophile antibodies** (an abnormal antibody directed against antigens from certain animal tissues found in individuals with infectious mononucleosis) can be measured in several ways. **EBV titers** are a quantitative measure and **rapid slide agglutination tests** (which yield a positive or negative result) are qualitative. Most children with infectious mononucleosis will have a positive rapid slide agglutination test, although the test is less reliable in those younger than the age of 5 years.

Treatment

Treatment is **supportive** because the disease is **self-limiting.** Patients should be advised to **avoid contact sports for 6–8 weeks** to decrease the risk of splenic rupture.

Tuberculosis

Incidence

The incidence of TB has risen in recent years. **Early detection and prompt treatment** are becoming increasingly important to prevent spread of the disease. The highest rates of infection are currently seen in minority populations, in urban settings, and in association with crowded living conditions. **Patients with HIV infection** are especially likely to present with active disease. Transmission of the etiologic agent *Mycobacterium tuberculosis* is by inhalation of infected droplets. The **incubation period** from time of infection to the development of a positive skin test is 2–10 weeks. Clinical disease develops in a minority of infected patients. When disease does develop, it is usually within the first 2 years after infection.

Clinical Features

Patients most commonly present with either an **asymptomatic infection or pulmonary disease.** Those with a positive skin test and no evidence of clinical disease should have a **screening chest radiograph.** Individuals with pulmonary disease may have symptoms that include **fever, weight loss, and cough** and physical examination may reveal **lymphadenopathy. A chest radiograph** will reveal an **infiltrate or hilar adenopathy. Extrapulmonary disease** (miliary, meningeal, lymph node, bone/joint disease, and so on) can also occur in a minority of patients.

Evaluation

An infection is diagnosed by a **positive skin test or by culture** (which will take months to grow) from infected **body fluids** (sputum, gastric washings). The tuberculin preparation recommended for skin testing is the purified protein derivative (PPD). The standard dose is 5 tuberculin units in 0.1 ml of solution, which should be injected intradermally on the forearm. A positive reaction is defined as greater than 10 mm of induration after 48–72 hours. Tine tests should not be used for definitive diagnosis and are of questionable value for screening.

Treatment

Treatment of patients with asymptomatic infection consists of **isoniazid for 9 months.** Patients with clinical disease should be treated with **multiple-drug regimens.**

Cat-Scratch Disease

Etiology

Cat-scratch disease is a benign **self-limited regional adenitis** that occurs following the scratch or bite of a cat. Cervical, axillary, or epitrochlear nodes are most commonly involved. The etiologic agent is a gram-negative bacillus (*Bartonella henselae*).

Clinical Features and Evaluation

The presenting symptom is usually a **large swollen, erythematous, painful solitary lymph node.** History usually reveals an **erythematous papule** that appeared approximately **2 weeks earlier** in the area drained by the lymph node. Most patients recall a cat scratch or bite approximately 10 days before papule formation. **Suppuration of the involved node** occurs in 30% of cases. In most instances, the nodes **regress within 8 weeks without intervention.** Occasionally drainage is required. Atypical presentations of the disease include encephalitis, Parinaud oculoglandular syndrome (granulomatous conjunctivitis and unilateral preauricular node enlargement), erythema nodosum, osteolytic lesions, and thrombocytopenic and nonthrombocytopenic purpura.

Cervical Lymphadenitis

Etiology

Cervical lymphadenitis is a problem frequently encountered in the pediatric population. It represents a **primary infection of the lymph node and should not be confused with lymphadenopathy,** which is lymph node enlargement in response to infiltration (e.g., malignancy or storage disease) or drainage of distal structures that have become infected or inflamed. The causative organism frequently gains entry to the body via the **pharynx, nares, dentition, or a break in the skin.** The cause is most often **bacterial,** with *Staphylococcus aureus* being the organism most frequently isolated. Other pathogens that may be found include group A streptococci, *Mycobacterium tuberculosis,* atypical mycobacteria, gram-negative bacilli (thought to be etiologic agents in cat-scratch disease), *Haemophilus influenzae,* anaerobic bacteria, *Francisella tularensis,* and *Yersinia pestis.*

Clinical Features

Physical examination usually reveals a **tender, warm, erythematous firm lymph node. Fluctuance** is present in about 25% of cases. Fever and elevated WBC count occur occasionally, most often in the younger child.

Evaluation and Treatment

Aspiration often reveals the cause and may provide symptomatic relief if the lymph node is large or in an awkward position. In uncomplicated cases, treatment with an **antibiotic** such as oxacillin or cephalexin is frequently all that is needed. Children who appear clinically ill or have an underlying immunodeficiency and infants should be admitted to the hospital for **IV antibiotics.** Placement of a **PPD skin test** at the time of presentation would be prudent in all cases.

Reactive Lymph Node Hyperplasia

Etiology

Reactive hyperplasia of lymph nodes represents the body's **response to antigenic stimuli** (foreign material, cellular debris, or infectious organisms and their toxic products).

Clinical Features

The resulting lymphadenopathy can be **acute or chronic.** The cervical, axillary, and inguinal nodes are most commonly involved and can sometimes grow to be quite large. The nodes clinically enlarge secondary to infiltration with histiocytes or plasma cells. Acute cellular infiltration and edema causes distention of the capsule, producing **tenderness when the lymph node is palpated.**

Evaluation

▼ **In the acute setting,** lymph node biopsy frequently reveals prominent lymphoid follicles and large germinal centers. No infectious organism is isolated, and malignant cells are not observed.

▼ **In chronic situations,** three pathological patterns are seen: follicular hyperplasia, paracortical lymphoid hyperplasia, and sinus histiocytosis. Lymph node hyperplasia can pose a diagnostic dilemma, especially in chronic situations. Lymph node biopsy may be helpful. Reactive hyperplasia is the most common histologic diagnosis seen in children undergoing lymph node biopsy.

Treatment

Because reactive hyperplasia represents the body's normal response to stimuli, treatment is not indicated. The nodes usually **regress** with time.

▼ EVALUATION OF LYMPHADENOPATHY

Patient History

▼ When were the swollen glands first noted? (the longer the duration, the more worrisome)
▼ Are they getting larger? (in general, the larger the node, the more worrisome)
▼ Is the node red, tender or painful? (lymphadenitis)
▼ Has there been fever, weight loss, night sweats? (lymphoma, TB)
▼ Is there any bruising or bleeding? Is the child fatigued or pale? (leukemia)
▼ Is there fever, rash, systemic symptoms? (scarlet fever, rubeola, rubella, infectious mononucleosis, Kawasaki disease)
▼ Are there joint complaints? (juvenile rheumatoid arthritis, systemic lupus erythematosus)
▼ Is there a history of a cat scratch (cat-scratch disease), tick bite (Lyme disease), or other animal exposure (tularemia)?
▼ Has there been exposure to an individual with TB?
▼ Is there a history of high-risk sexual behavior, substance abuse, or transfusion? Does a parent have any of these risk factors? (HIV)
▼ Is the child taking any medications? (dilantin, isoniazid)
▼ Is there a history of travel? (malaria)

Physical Examination

▼ Are the nodes generalized or regional? (see "Differential Diagnosis" section at beginning of this chapter)
▼ What size are the nodes? (baseline measurement is important to ensure proper follow-up)
▼ Are the nodes erythematous, tender, warm, fluctuant? (lymphadenitis)
▼ Are the nodes firm/hard and fixed in position? (malignancy)
▼ Is there fever, rash? (scarlet fever, rubeola, rubella, infectious mononucleosis, Kawasaki disease)
▼ Is there pharyngitis? (streptococcal disease)
▼ Is there hepatosplenomegaly? (infectious mononucleosis, leukemia)
▼ Are there bruises, petechiae, pallor? (leukemia)
▼ Are there joint findings? (juvenile rheumatoid arthritis, systemic lupus erythematosus)
▼ Is there a palpable abdominal mass? (neuroblastoma)
▼ Is there any skin infection, inflammation? (tinea, atopic dermatitis)

Laboratory Studies

▼ CBC, differential count
▼ PPD skin test
▼ Chest radiograph
▼ Lymph node biopsy

▼ APPROACH TO THE PATIENT

▼ Do you have a probable diagnosis (e.g., fever, sore throat, cervical lymphadenopathy, exudative pharyngitis, probable streptococcal pharyngitis) after completing the history and physical examination? If so, perform appropriate diagnostic tests (throat culture) and begin treatment (penicillin) if indicated.

▼ Are you unsure of the diagnosis in a patient who looks ill or is febrile without a clear cause? Consider admission to the hospital and a more extensive laboratory screen for infectious or malignant causes.

▼ Are you unsure of the diagnosis in a patient who looks well and does not have any high-risk symptoms or physical findings? See following; consider close follow-up with serial examinations.

▼ Does the patient exhibit any particularly worrisome symptoms or physical findings, such as the following?
   ▼ Supraclavicular adenopathy
   ▼ Hard, matted adenopathy
   ▼ Fever, constitutional symptoms of greater than 1 week duration without infectious cause identified
   ▼ Cervical nodes that continue to increase in size despite adequate antibiotic therapy
   ▼ A node that continues to increase in size after 1–2 weeks
   ▼ An enlarging node that does not regress in size after 4 weeks

▼ If the answer to one or more of these questions is yes, these children should all have a CBC with differential, PPD skin test, and a chest radiograph. Lymph node biopsy should be considered.

Suggested Readings

Bass JW, Vincent JM, Person DA: The expanding spectrum of *Bartonella* infections: II. Cat-scratch disease. *Pediatr Infect Dis J* 16:163, 1997.

Bodenstein L, Altman RP: Cervical lymphadenitis in infants and children. *Semin Pediatr Surg* 3:134, 1994.

Hudson MM, Donaldson SS: Hodgkin's disease. *Pediatr Clin North Am* 44:891, 1997.

Jenson HB: Acute complications of Epstein Barr virus infectious mononucleosis. *Curr Opin Pediatr* 12:263, 2000.

Kelly CS, Kelly RE Jr: Lymphadenopathy in children. *Pediatr Clin North Am* 45:875, 1998.

Kelly KM, Lange B: Oncologic emergencies. *Pediatr Clin North Am* 44:809, 1997.

Peter J, Ray CG: Infectious mononucleosis. *Pediatr Rev* 19:276, 1998.

Schutze GE: Diagnosis and treatment of *Bartonella henselae* infections. *Pediatr Infect Dis J* 19:1185, 2000.

Shad A, Magrath I: Non-Hodgkin's Lymphoma. *Pediatr Clin North Am* 44:863, 1997.

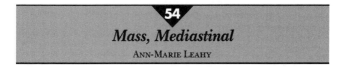

54
Mass, Mediastinal
ANN-MARIE LEAHY

▼ INTRODUCTION

> **HINT** Approximately 52% of mediastinal masses are caused by malignant tumors, and this percentage is higher if the patient is symptomatic.

The mediastinum (i.e., the space between the two pleural cavities) is divided into anterior, middle, and posterior regions. The location of the mass often suggests the cause.

▼ **Anterior mediastinum.** The anterior mediastinum is bounded by the first rib superiorly, the posterior surface of the sternum anteriorly, the anterior border of the upper dorsal vertebra posteriorly, and by an imaginary curved line that follows the cardiac border and extends backward until it reaches the border of the dorsal vertebra. This area contains the thymus, lymph nodes, and, rarely, extensions of the thyroid gland. The superior vena cava is a thin-walled vessel with a low intraluminal pressure that is surrounded by the lymph nodes and thymus.

▼ **Posterior mediastinum.** The posterior mediastinum is bounded posteriorly by the anterior surface of the curve of the ribs, anteriorly by the posterior border of the pericardium, and inferiorly by the diaphragm. This area contains the sympathetic ganglia and esophagus, among other structures.

▼ **Middle mediastinum.** The middle mediastinum is the area between the anterior and posterior regions; the diaphragm forms its base. This region contains the trachea, bronchi, heart, and great vessels, as well as lymph nodes.

> **HINT** Often, large anterior mediastinal masses extend into the middle mediastinum.

▼ DIFFERENTIAL DIAGNOSIS LIST
Anterior Mediastinum

Lymphoma—non-Hodgkin lymphoma (NHL), Hodgkin lymphoma
Germ cell tumor
Thymus hyperplasia or cyst
Lymphangioma (cystic hygroma)
Hemangioma
Histiocytosis
Lipoma
Thymoma
Substernal thyroid

Middle Mediastinum

Lymph node granuloma
Histoplasmosis
Tuberculosis (TB)
Sarcoidosis
Bronchogenic cyst
Pericardial cyst
Fibromatosis

Posterior Mediastinum

Tumors of neurogenic origin—neuroblastoma, ganglioneuroblastoma,
    ganglioneuroma
Thoracic meningocele
Esophageal duplication cyst

General

Ewing sarcoma
Rhabdomyosarcoma

▼ DIFFERENTIAL DIAGNOSIS DISCUSSION
Superior Vena Cava Syndrome/Superior Mediastinal Syndrome

Etiology

Superior vena cava and superior mediastinal syndromes are **life-threatening complications of anterior mediastinal masses. Superior vena cava syndrome** implies **venous obstruction** from compression or thrombosis. When **coupled with tracheal compression,** the syndrome is called **superior mediastinal syndrome.** Tracheal compression without signs of venous obstruction is more common than the full-blown syndrome, but is equally worrisome. The mediastinal mass compresses the superior vena cava, the trachea, or both, impeding blood return and air flow and producing the signs and symptoms summarized in Table 54.1.

These are rare syndromes; only 10%–15% of pediatric patients with malignant anterior mediastinal tumors have superior vena cava syndrome or

TABLE 54.1. Signs and Symptoms of Superior Vena Cava Syndrome or Superior Mediastinal Syndrome

History	Physical Examination
Cough, especially when supine	Retractions
Dyspnea or orthopnea	Wheezing or stridor
Headache	Papilledema
Dizziness or syncope, especially when symptoms are exacerbated with Valsalva maneuver	Prominence of neck or chest veins Suffusion or edema of conjunctiva
Facial swelling	Cyanosis or plethora
Visual changes	Anxiety or confusion
Sense of fullness in ears	

superior mediastinal syndrome. However, it is **critical to recognize these patients** because their condition can **deteriorate dramatically** with disastrous consequences. **Immediate consultation with an oncologist** is always appropriate.

⚔ HINT Most, but not all, symptomatic anterior mediastinal masses in children are malignant.

Lymphoma

⚔ HINT Lymphoma is the most common cause of superior vena cava syndrome and superior mediastinal syndrome in children.

Non-Hodgkin Lymphoma (NHL)

Mediastinal masses in patients with NHL are almost exclusively caused by lymphoblastic lymphoma (see Chapter 53, "Lymphadenopathy"). Approximately 60% of patients with lymphoblastic lymphoma present with a mediastinal mass, and often have pleural effusions as well.

Hodgkin Lymphoma

Although NHL has a slightly higher incidence than does Hodgkin lymphoma, the mediastinum is more often the primary site of involvement in Hodgkin disease. **Cervical adenopathy** is the most common clinical presentation, but approximately 52%–65% of patients with Hodgkin lymphoma also present with a mass consisting of **anterior mediastinal, paratracheal, and tracheobronchial lymph nodes. Tracheobronchial compression** has been observed on chest radiographs in 50% of newly diagnosed children with Hodgkin lymphoma. Half of these patients also have systemic symptoms of Hodgkin disease, including **fever, night sweats, and weight loss** of greater than 10% in the previous 6 months. (Hodgkin lymphoma is discussed in detail in Chapter 53, "Lymphadenopathy.")

Germ Cell Tumors

The **anterior mediastinum** is the second most common site of extragonadal germ cell tumors [i.e., teratomas, germinomas, embryonal carcinomas, endodermal sinus (yolk sac) tumors, and choriocarcinomas].

⚔ HINT Klinefelter syndrome has been reported in 20% of boys with mediastinal germ cell tumors.

Teratomas

Teratomas are classified on a histologic basis as follows:

▼ **Mature teratoma.** The tumor is composed of well-differentiated tissues derived from the three germinal layers of the embryo (i.e., endoderm, mesoderm, and ectoderm).
▼ **Immature teratoma.** In addition to mature elements, the mass contains embryonic-appearing elements. In infants, immature teratomas behave as mass lesions, but in adolescents, they behave as highly malignant tumors.

▼ **Teratoma with malignant germ cell tumor components.** These teratomas contain one or more of the components of germinomas, embryonal carcinomas, endodermal sinus tumors, or choriocarcinoma, in addition to characteristics of either a mature or immature teratoma.

Germinoma

Germinomas histologically **resemble primordial germ cells.** Previously, germinomas were designated "seminomas" when they occurred in the testes and "dysgerminomas" when they occurred in the ovaries.

Embryonal Carcinoma

Embryonal carcinomas histologically **resemble a poorly differentiated or anaplastic carcinoma with extensive necrosis.** These tumors are most commonly found in the **testes of young adults.**

Endodermal Sinus (Yolk Sac) Tumor

Endodermal sinus tumors are **the most common malignant germ cell tumors in children.** They are most commonly found in the **sacrococcygeal area.** Patients test **positive for α-fetoprotein** (the principal serum protein of the fetus, with a structure and function similar to that of albumin). The half-life of α-fetoprotein is 5–7 days.

Choriocarcinoma

Choriocarcinoma is rare in children, but two forms have been described: **gestational** (arising from the placenta) and **nongestational.** β-Human chorionic gonadotropin is invariably produced and has a half-life of only 45 minutes.

Thymus Hyperplasia

An enlarged thymus is the most common cause of a widened anterior mediastinum in neonates. These patients are **asymptomatic** unless the hyperplastic thymus is located in an abnormal position. Thymic enlargement is sometimes the result of a **thymic cyst,** which can be delineated by computed tomography (CT).

Lymphangioma (Cystic Hygroma)

Lymphangiomas are **rarely localized to the mediastinum** but can extend into the mediastinum from a neck lesion and cause symptoms. Lymphangiomas are almost always noted by the time the patient reaches 3 years of age. **Surgical resection** is necessary.

Hemangioma

Like lymphangiomas, hemangiomas have been reported in all portions of the mediastinum, but approximately **75% occur in the anterior mediastinum.** Many are **asymptomatic,** but they may cause **airway compression** or, rarely, **bleeding into the pleural cavity.** Mediastinal hemangiomas have been associated with hemangiomas at other sites in the body. Generally, hemangiomas **grow during the first and second year of life and then slowly regress. Steroids** are considered first-line therapy for symptomatic patients once a diagnosis has been established, because surgery is often difficult or impossible.

Histiocytosis

Histiocytosis is an increase in the number of mononuclear phagocytic cells (histiocytes) **of bone marrow origin.** Rarely, patients with Langerhans cell histiocytosis (which is caused by immunologic stimulation of the normal antigen-processing Langerhans cell in an uncontrolled manner) present with a mediastinal mass.

Thymoma

A neoplasm of the thymus is not considered a thymoma unless it contains **neoplastic epithelial components.** Such tumors are rare in adults and even rarer in children. Thymomas are slow-growing tumors that extend locally and rarely metastasize. Rarely, **autoimmune disorders** (e.g., myasthenia gravis, systemic lupus erythematosus, rheumatoid arthritis, cytopenias, thyroiditis) have been reported in **association with thymomas.**

Histoplasmosis

✔ HINT Mediastinal lymph node granulomas, usually from histoplasmosis, are the second most common cause of mediastinal masses.

This disease is caused by the fungus *Histoplasma capsulatum.* It is endemic in the Mississippi, Ohio, and Missouri River valleys, where up to 80% of the population have a positive histoplasmin skin test by the age of 20 years. The diagnosis is best made by either noting a fourfold increase in the complement fixation titer between acute and convalescent sera (using *Histoplasma* yeast and mycelial antigens) or by performing a tissue diagnosis.

Tuberculosis (TB)

This mycobacterial disease commonly affects **mediastinal lymph nodes** in children. Infection of nodes without significant pulmonary involvement is more common in primary pulmonary TB than in reactivation of the disease. Of note, as many as 20% of patients with culture-proven TB have negative Mantoux skin test reactions during the early phase of their illness (even when the skin testing is performed with 250 tuberculin units). A definitive diagnosis requires **histologic and bacteriologic confirmation.**

Sarcoidosis

This **chronic, multisystemic disease** of obscure origin is uncommon in patients younger than 10 years and is more common in **African-American children.** The pathological lesion is a noncaseating granuloma; the **lung** is the most frequently affected organ. **Hilar and paratracheal adenopathy** is often found in association with parenchymal infiltrates and may be far more dramatic than the parenchymal lesions. **Biopsy** of the affected tissue is the most valuable diagnostic tool.

Bronchogenic Cysts

These cysts, which are lined with ciliated epithelium, can be found in any portion of the mediastinum, but most often are found **near the carina in the middle mediastinum.** Cysts can become **symptomatic** either **by becoming infected or by enlarging in size,** thereby compromising the function of an adjacent airway. **Surgical excision is curative.**

Fibromatosis

This **nonmalignant** (but often **locally aggressive**) **lesion** has been reported as a rare cause of a **middle mediastinal mass.**

Tumors of Neurogenic Origin

⚏ HINT Most posterior mediastinal masses in children are neurogenic in origin.

Neuroblastoma, a malignant tumor, may arise **anywhere along the sympathetic nervous system chain.** Approximately 15% of neuroblastomas arise in the paraspinal ganglion of the thorax. **Thoracic neuroblastomas** are almost always attached to the **intervertebral foramina** and thus can cause **spinal cord compression.** Interestingly, **less than gross total resection of such lesions can provide a cure.**

Differentiation of neuroblasts into benign ganglion cells occurs both **spontaneously and after therapy.** The term **ganglioneuroma** refers to such differentiated lesions. **Ganglioneuroblastoma** refers to **lesions containing malignant cells and benign ganglion cells.**

Esophageal Duplication Cysts

Approximately 10% of alimentary tract duplications are esophageal, and two-thirds are **right sided.** Alimentary tract duplications have been discovered in patients as old as 13 years. The **duplication does not communicate with the esophagus** unless there is ulceration of the gastric mucosa within the cyst.

Neurenteric cysts are esophageal duplication cysts that **contain glial elements;** vertebral anomalies usually accompany these cysts.

Ewing Sarcoma

This **small, round, blue-cell tumor** rarely occurs in children younger than 5 years and has a very low incidence in African-American children. Ewing sarcoma most frequently involves the **axial skeleton,** and some "mediastinal" masses actually originate from the chest wall (or a rib). True mediastinal involvement occurs rarely at diagnosis but is not infrequent in advanced cases.

Ewing sarcoma must be **differentiated from** other small, round, blue-cell tumors, including **neuroblastoma, lymphoma, and rhabdomyosarcoma.** Previously a diagnosis of exclusion, Ewing sarcoma can now be **diagnosed by demonstrating the characteristic t(11;22) by polymerase chain reaction.**

Rhabdomyosarcoma

This sarcoma, which arises from **primitive mesenchymal cells,** is the **most common soft tissue sarcoma in children.** However, in large series, only 1% of these tumors arise in the mediastinum, and these series do not stratify masses into the anterior, posterior, or middle mediastinum. Most patients with mediastinal rhabdomyosarcomas are **boys (65%)** with a mean age of 10 years. Metastatic disease has been seen in the **lungs (including pleura), bone, and bone marrow** of these patients.

▼ EVALUATION OF MEDIASTINAL MASS

⚔ HINT As many as one-third of masses in the mediastinum are found accidentally when radiographs are performed to evaluate fever or other complaints.

History and Physical Examination

Important features of the history and physical examination that should be specifically addressed to **rule out an emergency** are listed in Table 54.1. The **presence or absence of hepatosplenomegaly, adenopathy, systemic signs of a malignant tumor** (e.g., fever, weight loss), **or neurologic signs** (e.g., Horner syndrome, signs of cord compression) are equally important.

Laboratory Studies

Laboratory tests are tailored to the individual, but the following may be appropriate:

▼ **Complete blood count with differential.** The presence of lymphoblasts on smear or cytopenias from marrow infiltration may allow the physician to establish the diagnosis without biopsying tissue from the mediastinal mass.

▼ **Chemistry panel, including uric acid.** A high uric acid level, lactate dehydrogenase (LDH) level, or both are often seen in patients with lymphoblastic lymphomas.

▼ α-**Fetoprotein** and β-**hCG levels** are helpful in suggesting the diagnosis of germ cell tumor and useful in following the response to therapy.

▼ **Quantitative vanillylmandelic (VMA) and homovanillic acid (HVA) analysis.** Elevations of these substances in the urine are suggestive of neuroblastoma, but some thoracic tumors do not show elevated VMA or HVA.

▼ **Histoplasma complement fixation titers** should be obtained in endemic areas.

Other Diagnostic Modalities

▼ **CT and magnetic resonance imaging (MRI).** A CT scan can delineate the cystic nature of a lesion and reveals calcifications in 95% of patients with neuroblastomas and 35% of patients with germ cell tumors. Visualization of a tooth is pathognomonic of a teratoma. CT is more sensitive for bony erosion than MRI, but MRI is more helpful for detecting intraspinous extension and should be considered for patients with posterior mediastinal masses.

⚔ HINT Before performing CT or MRI, a careful history should be taken for orthopnea because injudicious positioning of a patient with superior mediastinal syndrome can cause disaster.

▼ **Bone marrow aspirate.** Performed while the patient is sitting, bone marrow aspirate is indicated for ill patients in whom the diagnosis of lymphoma or another disease involving the marrow is suspected.

▼ **Pleurocentesis or pericardiocentesis.** It is usually possible to make a definitive diagnosis of lymphoblastic lymphoma by assessing cells collected during these procedures.

▼ **Biopsy** may be necessary to make a definitive tissue diagnosis and requires general anesthesia.

⚅ HINT Before considering a biopsy to definitively make a tissue diagnosis, an echocardiogram (preferably upright and supine) and a (pulmonary) flow–volume loop should be obtained. Patients who do not tolerate these procedures are not candidates for general anesthesia. Cardiopulmonary changes associated with general anesthesia can aggravate superior vena cava syndrome and superior mediastinal syndrome, leading to total airway obstruction, cardiac arrest, or both. Particularly worrisome is the fact that these complications can develop in patients with mild or no preoperative symptoms.

▼ TREATMENT OF MEDIASTINAL MASS

Thirty years ago it was stated "early, vigorous treatment, designed to cause rapid shrinkage of the tumor, should not be delayed by an overly diligent pursuit of the diagnosis." This is equally true today. **If a patient is critically ill and cannot tolerate a definitive diagnostic procedure, empiric chemotherapy, emergency radiation therapy, or both are indicated.** One must be aware, however, that **steroids or even low-dose radiotherapy** (200 cGy) **may render definitive diagnosis impossible**—even if a biopsy is done only 24 hours later. Biopsy of a node that is out of the field or intentionally shielded is, of course, still possible after the patient has been stabilized.

Some authors recommend **concurrent treatment with steroids** during radiotherapy because patients can transiently worsen, presumably as a result of edema. A significant percentage of patients improve within 12 hours of the first dose of radiation. **Chemotherapy with steroids, cyclophosphamide, or both in combination with vincristine or an anthracycline** is a reasonable **alternative empiric approach,** although this too can render the subsequent histologic picture uninterpretable. Even when the histologic diagnosis is lost, **continued treatment of the diagnosis that best fits the clinical picture** usually results in long-term disease-free survival.

Suggested Readings

Bhatia S, Robison LL, Oberlin O, et al: Breast cancer and other second neoplasms after childhood Hodgkin's disease. *N Engl J Med* 334:745–751, 1996.

Durand C, Baudain P, Nugues F, et al: Mediastinal and thoracic MRI in children. *Pediatr Pulmonol Suppl* 18:60, 1999.

Filler RM, Simpson JS, Ein SH: Mediastinal masses in infants and children. *Pediatr Clin North Am* 14:677, 1979.

Glick RD, La Quaglia MP: Lymphomas of the anterior mediastinum. *Semin Pediatr Surg* 8(2):69–77, 1999.

Issa PY, Brihi ER, Janin Y, et al: Superior vena cava syndrome in childhood: report of ten cases and review of the literature. *Pediatrics* 71:337, 1983.

Murphy SB, Fairclough DL, Hutchinson RE, et al: Non-Hodgkin's lymphomas of childhood: an analysis of the histology staging and response to treatment of 338 cases at a single institution. *J Clin Oncol* 7:186–193, 1989.

Ricketts RR: Clinical management of anterior mediastinal tumors in children. *Semin Pediatr Surg* 10(3):161–168, 2001.

Saenz NC: Posterior mediastinal neurogenic tumors in infants and children. *Semin Pediatr Surg* 8(2):78–84, 1999.

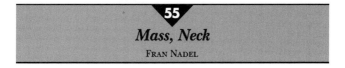

Mass, Neck
FRAN NADEL

▼ INTRODUCTION

Neck masses are a common clinical problem in children. Although the list of potential causes is extensive, most are due to **benign processes** that can be readily diagnosed after a complete history and physical examination. **Close follow-up** is important to ensure that less common causes in children such as malignancy are not overlooked.

▼ DIFFERENTIAL DIAGNOSIS LIST

Infectious Causes

Cervical Adenitis

Bacterial infection-*Streptococcus pyogenes, Staphylococcus aureus,* Group B *Streptococcus,* oral anaerobes, *Pasteurella multocida*
Cat scratch disease
Tularemia
Nocardia

Mycobacterium tuberculosis

Atypical mycobacterium

Reactive Adenopathy

Viral infection—upper respiratory viruses, mumps, measles, Epstein-Barr virus (EBV), cytomegalovirus (CMV), HIV
Bacterial infection—syphilis, brucellosis
Fungal infection—histoplasmosis, coccidioidomycosis, tinea
Parasitic infection—toxoplasmosis
Other infections—head and neck infections (tonsillitis, otitis media, tinea capitis)

Toxic Causes

Drug-related adenopathy—e.g., phenytoin

Neoplastic Causes

Malignant neoplasms—Hodgkin lymphoma, non-Hodgkin lymphoma, rhabdomyosarcoma, fibrosarcoma, thyroid carcinoma, neuroblastoma, metastatic deposits
Benign neoplasms—lipoma, fibroma, neurofibroma, teratoma, osteochondroma, hemangioma

Traumatic Causes

Hematoma
Congenital muscular torticollis
Subcutaneous emphysema
Cervical spine fracture

Congenital or Vascular Causes

Thyroglossal duct cyst
Branchial cleft cyst
Cystic hygroma
Laryngocele
Dermoid
Cervical thymic cyst
Arteriovenous fistula

Metabolic or Genetic Causes

Goiter
Thyroid nodule

Inflammatory Causes (Cervical Adenopathy)

Kawasaki syndrome
Systemic lupus erythematosus
Sinus histiocytosis
Sarcoidosis

▼ DIFFERENTIAL DIAGNOSIS DISCUSSION

Reactive Adenopathy

Familiarity with regional anatomy helps to narrow the differential diagnosis in a child who presents with a neck mass. Because **most neck masses in infants and children are enlarged lymph nodes,** it is important to be familiar with areas of lymphatic drainage. In addition, certain masses present in typical locations that help to identify the cause. The neck is divided into the anterior and posterior triangles, with the sternocleidomastoid muscle (SCM) forming the posterior border of the anterior triangle (Figure 55.1).

It is **important to distinguish adenopathy from adenitis.** Adenopathy is defined by nodal enlargement. In adenitis, the swelling is usually accompanied by signs of inflammation such as warmth, tenderness, and erythema. The vast majority of children with adenopathy have a **benign viral or easily treatable bacterial cause.** However, **follow-up is important** to assess resolution of symptoms and progressive reduction in size so as not to miss unusual infectious, inflammatory, or oncological processes. A more detailed review of this topic is covered in Chapter 53, "Lymphadenopathy."

✄ HINT Epitrochlear, popliteal, supraclavicular, or occipital nodes in children under 2 years are rarely due to benign lymph node hyperplasia. These nodes, as well as any palpable nodes in the newborn infant, deserve further investigation.

Congenital Malformations

Thyroglossal Duct Cyst (TGDC)

Etiology

TGDC results from the cellular proliferation of **embryonic remnants of the thyroglossal duct.**

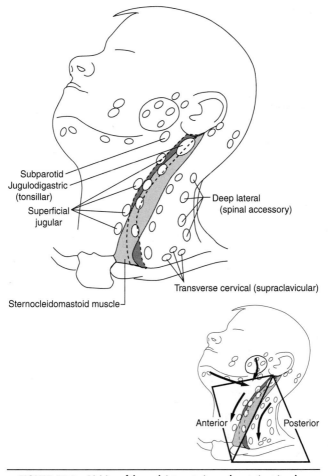

FIGURE 55.1. Division of the neck into anterior and posterior triangles.

Clinical Features and Evaluation

TGDC is the **most common congenital neck mass** and usually presents in the **first decade of life.** TGDC may become apparent during an upper respiratory infection that causes cyst inflammation. Physical examination is best done with the **neck fully extended** and will reveal a **midline or paramedian swelling of the anterior neck.** The location can be anywhere along the embryonic pathway from the base of the tongue to the thyroid cartilage. The **mass is round and changes position when the child swallows or sticks out his tongue.** Children with TGDC should be **referred to an otorhinolaryngologist** for further evaluation. The surgeon may consider further testing to confirm normal thyroid function and location.

Treatment

Almost all TGDC require **surgical excision** for definitive diagnosis and to prevent recurrent infections of the cyst.

Branchial Cleft Cyst/Fistula/Sinus (BCC)

Etiology

The embryological branchial clefts give rise to the structures of the face and neck. Cysts result from the **proliferation of the remnants of these clefts, usually involving the second cleft.**

Clinical Evaluation

Branchial cleft remnants are the **second most common congenital neck mass.** A fistula or sinus will be obvious in the newborn; however, a cyst often does not become clinically apparent until early school age. Second BCCs are found **anterior to the lower third of the sternocleidomastoid muscle as a small, round, soft mass.** An upper respiratory infection or infection of the cyst itself may lead to an **inflammatory appearance.** Diagnosis should be suspected if a **mass lateral to the SCM persists or recurs despite antibiotic treatment** for an adenitis.

Treatment

If there is evidence of cyst infection, an **antibiotic** that covers skin flora should be initiated. Definitive treatment requires **surgical excision,** which can be done electively.

Cystic Hygroma

Etiology

Cystic hygromas arise from the **nonmalignant proliferation of lymphatic tissue that does not connect with normal lymphatic drainage.** These sacs become **filled with lymphatic fluid** secreted by the endothelial lining. They can compress or stretch surrounding tissues.

Clinical Evaluation

Cystic hygromas are the **third most common congenital neck mass.** The vast majority of hygromas are found in the **posterior cervical triangle** and most are diagnosed within the first year of life. The mass is **soft, easily compressible, and, if not secondarily infected, will transilluminate.** Upper respiratory infections or trauma may cause a rapid increase in size. **Encroachment on the airway may lead to respiratory symptoms such as stridor.** Diagnosis is usually clinical, but **ultrasound or computed tomography (CT) imaging** may be necessary to delineate the extent of the lesion.

Treatment

Spontaneous regression is rare. Currently, **staged surgical excision** is the mainstay of therapy. **Sclerosing agents** and other therapies may have an adjunctive role. Timing of surgery will depend on the location of the lesion, age of the child, and involvement of vital structures. **Tracheostomy and gastric tube feedings** are sometimes required.

Dermoid

Dermoids consist of ectoderm and mesoderm and are considered **true developmental neoplasms.** This rare midline mass is often **doughy, nontender, mobile,** and is found **above the level of the hyoid bone.** It may initially be confused with a TGDC; however, it **will not change position with tongue protrusion.** Signs of **inflammation** may occur with cyst infection. **Ultrasound and CT imaging** will help delineate the nature and extent of the lesion. **Surgical excision** is required.

Laryngocele

Laryngocele is an **extremely rare** congenital anomaly. It is an **air-filled mass that arises from the larynx.** External extension through the thyrohyoid membrane will result in a **compressible mass,** lateral to midline, that will **increase in size with a Valsalva maneuver.** Lateral radiographs may demonstrate the air-filled sac. **Surgical excision** is required.

Oncological Masses

See Chapter 53, "Lymphadenopathy," Chapter 43, "Hilar Adenopathy," and Chapter 36, "Goiter" for more details on this topic.

⚡ HINT Fortunately, neck masses in children are rarely due to an oncological process. A mass that is rapidly growing, found in a neonate, adherent to underlying tissues, ulcerated, greater than 3 cm in size, or located in the posterior triangle is more of a concern for malignancy.

Lymphoma

Hodgkin lymphoma is the **most frequent malignant neck mass** in children. Hodgkin lymphoma often presents with a **unilateral slowly enlarging mass of the neck,** whereas **non-Hodgkin lymphoma is more often bilateral.** Systemic symptoms of **fatigue, fever, weight loss, night sweats, and respiratory distress** may be present. Findings related to **bone marrow dysfunction, mediastinal involvement, and spinal cord impingement** may also be found. **Node biopsy** is necessary for diagnosis. **Immediate referral to a pediatric oncologist** is indicated to plan the diagnostic and therapeutic evaluation.

Neuroblastoma

Neuroblastoma of the cervical region may present in a child **5 years old or younger with a neck mass and Horner syndrome** (miosis, ptosis, and anhidrosis). Neuroblastoma may also **metastasize** from other regions to the neck, but neurologic symptoms will be absent until the mass causes nerve compression.

Thyroid Masses

See Chapter 36, "Goiter."

Traumatic Causes

Congenital Muscular Torticollis (Fibromatosis of Infancy)

Etiology

The exact mechanism of this condition is not clear. **Birth trauma that causes injury and bleeding into the SCM** and subsequent fibrosis and contracture probably plays an important role. An **intrauterine position that obstructs SCM venous outflow** may also cause muscle injury and contracture.

Clinical Evaluation

Parents usually notice a neck mass or torticollis in the baby's **first month of life.** Physical examination reveals a **nontender, mobile mass within the SCM.** The **head will be in lateral flexion** and the **chin will be pointed away from the mass.** Diagnosis can usually be made clinically. **Cervical spine radiographs** and **ultrasound** may assist in ruling out other less common causes.

Treatment

Delayed diagnosis and treatment may lead to irreversible asymmetric development of facial features. The vast majority of children improve with **passive stretching exercises.** If the torticollis persists past 6–12 months, a **surgical release of the muscle** may be necessary.

Inflammatory Causes

These disease processes may have **associated cervical adenopathy.** It is rare that cervical adenopathy is the first or only presenting finding.

Kawasaki Disease (Mucocutaneous Lymph Node Syndrome)

Sinus Histiocytosis (Rosai-Dorfman Syndrome)

This is an **extremely rare disorder** of unknown etiology. The typical patient is a young **African-American child** who presents with **prolonged fever** and **massive bilateral cervical adenopathy.** Diagnosis depends on characteristic findings on **lymph node biopsy.** Treatment may include **chemotherapeutic agents,** and these patients should be **referred to an oncologist.**

▼ APPROACH TO THE PATIENT

Most neck masses in children are benign. A thorough history and physical examination coupled with a follow-up visit will be sufficient to diagnose most masses. **Systemic symptoms, persistence or recurrence of a mass, or a history of exposure to an infectious agent** such as tuberculosis should prompt **further evaluation.** Further evaluation may include a **CBC, purified protein derivative tuberculin test, other pathogen-specific assays, or imaging with ultrasound or computed tomography.** **Biopsy** should be considered in a patient whose mass has increased in size at 2 weeks, unchanged in size in 4–6 weeks, or not returned to normal at 8–12 weeks. **Inpatient evaluation and treatment** will often be necessary for neonates or for patients who are ill appearing, have signs of impending airway compromise, are immunocompromised, or have failed outpatient oral antibiotic treatment.

Suggested Readings

Chesney PJ: Cervical adenopathy. *Pediatr Rev* 15:276–283, 1994.

May M: Neck masses in children: diagnosis and treatment. *Pediatr Ann* 5:518–535, 1976.

Nagy M, Backstrom J: Comparison of the sensitivity of lateral neck radiographs and computed tomography scanning in pediatric deep-neck infections. *Laryngoscope* 109(5):775–779, 1999.

Pounds LA: Neck masses of congenital origin. *Pediatr Clin North Amer* 28: 841–844, 1981.

Wetmore RF, Mahboubi S, Soyupak SK: Computed tomography in the evaluation of pediatric neck infections. *Otolaryngol Head Neck Surg* 119(6): 624–627, 1998.

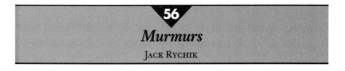

56
Murmurs
JACK RYCHIK

▼ INTRODUCTION

A murmur is an **auditory vibration produced by turbulent flow within the cardiac structures.** A murmur may be **physiologic** (i.e., a normal finding) or **pathologic.**

Heart Sounds

Variations in the normal heart sounds, as well as **adventitious** heart sounds, may be associated with murmurs and are essential clues to diagnostic interpretation of the murmur.

First Heart Sound (S₁)

The S_1 is produced by **closure of the mitral and tricuspid valves, in that order.** The mitral component and tricuspid component are **best heard at the apex and the lower sternal border region,** respectively.

▼ The intensity of the S_1 is accentuated in conditions characterized by increased cardiac output and a short PR interval, because in these circumstances maximal excursion of the leaflets occurs during closure.

▼ Wide splitting of the S_1 with a delayed tricuspid component may normally be noted during inspiration in infants and young children; in patients with tricuspid stenosis, Ebstein anomaly, and right bundle branch block; and when pacing the left ventricle.

Second Heart Sound (S₂)

The S_2 is produced by **closure of the aortic valve (A_2) immediately followed by closure of the pulmonic valve (P_2)** and is **best heard at the base** of the heart. The P_2 **is normally softer than the A_2** and is **less widely transmitted. Splitting of the S_2** is normally appreciated **during quiet respiration.** Inspiration results in two physiologic phenomena: an **increased capacitance of the lung vasculature,** with a greater systolic "hang-out" time for the right ventricle relative to the left ventricle, and **increased venous return to the right-sided structures.** Both of these phenomena result in **delayed closure of the pulmonic valve.**

▼ In mild forms of aortic or pulmonic stenosis, the A_2 or the P_2, respectively, is soft.

▼ The S_2 is single and loud in the following circumstances: when there is fusion of the two components, such as in severe pulmonary hypertension; when there is only one semilunar valve, such as in atresia of either the aortic or pulmonic valves or truncus arteriosus; and when the P_2 is inaudible because of an anteriorly positioned aorta, such as in tetralogy of Fallot or transposition of the great arteries.

▼ Abnormally wide splitting of the S_2 is noted in the conditions listed in Table 56.1.

TABLE 56.1. Common Causes of Abnormally Wide Splitting of the Second Heart Sound (S_2)

> Atrial septal defect
> Mild pulmonic stenosis
> Complete right bundle branch block
> Left ventricular paced beats
> Massive pulmonary embolus

Third Heart Sound (S_3) and Fourth Heart Sound (S_4)

Heart sounds are occasionally heard during ventricular diastole. **Early rapid filling of the ventricle,** which follows the opening of the atrioventricular valve, **may produce the third heart sound (S_3); ventricular filling related to the forceful expulsion of blood from the atrium into the ventricle** with atrial contraction **may produce the fourth heart sound (S_4).** These sounds are **best heard at the apex with the bell of the stethoscope. An audible S_3 may be normal in infants and young children,** whereas an **audible S_4 is distinctly abnormal.**

▼ Conditions that cause ventricular volume overload produce an abnormally prominent S_3 and are summarized in Table 56.2.
▼ Conditions that result in ventricular hypertrophy produce an S_4 and are summarized in Table 56.3.

Characteristics of a Murmur

▼ **Phase.** The murmur is described as occurring either during systole (following S_1, corresponding with ventricular contraction), diastole (following S_2, corresponding with ventricular relaxation), or continuously (throughout the cardiac cycle).
▼ **Length and timing.** The murmur is described as being of short, medium, or long duration and occurring in the early, mid-, or late part of the cardiac cycle. The terms "holosystolic" and "pansystolic" refer to a murmur that begins with S_1 and ends with S_2.
▼ **Peak intensity (grade)** is summarized in Table 56.4.
▼ **Variation in intensity.** The term "crescendo" implies that the murmur starts low and builds to a peak, while "decrescendo" implies that the murmur starts at its greatest intensity and subsequently diminishes. The term "crescendo–decrescendo" is used to describe a murmur that starts low, builds to a peak, and then diminishes over the course of the murmur (i.e., a "diamond-shaped" murmur).

TABLE 56.2. Conditions Causing a Prominent Third Heart Sound (S_3)

Physiologic (infants and children)
Congestive heart failure
Ventricular septal defect, with large pulmonary to systemic flow ($\dot{Q}p:\dot{Q}s$) ratio
Mitral insufficiency
Tricuspid insufficiency
Hyperdynamic ventricle with high output (e.g., anemia, thyrotoxicosis, arteriovenous fistula)

TABLE 56.3. Conditions Causing a Prominent Fourth Heart Sound (S₄)

Left ventricular outflow tract obstruction (e.g., aortic stenosis)
Right ventricular outflow tract obstruction (e.g., pulmonic stenosis)
Hypertrophic cardiomyopathy
Heart block (atrium contracting against a closed valve)

▼ **Location and radiation.** The location of the murmur is described in relation to a chest wall landmark such as the sternum or intercostal spaces (e.g., the left upper sternal border second intercostal space). The direction of projection (i.e., the radiation) is also noted (e.g., originating at the apex of the heart and radiating toward the left axilla).

Physical Maneuvers

The following maneuvers can alter the characteristics of a murmur:

▼ **Supine position.** Having the patient lie supine increases venous return to the heart and augments murmurs that are volume dependent (e.g., those associated with aortic stenosis or pulmonic stenosis; functional murmurs). Pericardial rubs are diminished when the patient is supine because the visceral and parietal membranes move away from each other when the heart shifts posteriorly in the chest.
▼ **Valsalva maneuver.** Forced exhalation against a closed glottis or straining with the mouth and nose closed increases the intrathoracic pressure and reduces venous return to the heart. During the Valsalva maneuver, the two components of S₂ become single, and volume-dependent murmurs are attenuated.

▼ DIFFERENTIAL DIAGNOSIS LIST

Heart murmurs can be categorized into three groups: **functional or innocent** murmurs, which are **normal; physiologic** murmurs, which are caused by an **abnormality of flow not of primary cardiac origin;** and **pathological** murmurs, which are caused by an **abnormality of primary cardiac origin.**

Functional or Innocent Murmurs

Still murmur
Cervical venous hum

TABLE 56.4. Grading of Murmurs

Grade	Description
I	Very soft, no thrill
II	Easily audible, of moderate intensity, no thrill
III	Prominent intensity, but no thrill
IV	Loud murmur accompanied by a thrill
V	Very loud murmur accompanied by a thrill; heard with the stethoscope partially off the chest wall
VI	Very loud murmur accompanied by a thrill; heard with the stethoscope completely off the chest wall

Physiologic Murmurs

High cardiac output states
Arteriovenous fistula
Peripheral pulmonic stenosis

Pathological Murmurs

Ventricular septal defect (VSD)—nonrestrictive and restrictive
Atrial septal defect (ASD)
Patent ductus arteriosus (PDA)
Pulmonic stenosis
Aortic stenosis
Coarctation of the aorta

▼ DIFFERENTIAL DIAGNOSIS DISCUSSION

Still Murmur (Innocent "Flow" Murmur)

Etiology

This sound, described in the early twentieth century by Dr. George Frederick Still of Great Ormond Street Children's Hospital, London, is **one of the most common findings in the physical examination of a normal child.** It is heard in children **between the ages of 2 years and early adolescence** and may even persist into adulthood. Although its **cause is uncertain,** some evidence points to turbulent flow across the left ventricular outflow tract as the source.

Clinical Features and Evaluation

The Still murmur is a **systolic murmur, grade II–III** (never associated with a thrill), and **heard best at the left lower sternal border.** It is described as **vibratory, scratchy, or musical,** and is **accentuated when the patient is supine** (i.e., with increased venous return to the heart). The **intensity and splitting of the S_2 are always normal.** Additional testing is usually not indicated if the murmur fits this description.

Cervical Venous Hum

Turbulent flow may occur **at the junction of the subclavian vein and head vessels as they join to form the superior vena cava,** resulting in a **continuous murmur** called a venous hum. It is **low pitched** and **heard best just beneath the right clavicle** while the child is **sitting up. Turning the patient's head to either the extreme right or left,** placing the patient in **supine position,** or **applying gentle pressure in the supraclavicular fossa** may dramatically **eliminate the murmur,** and is **pathognomonic.** This murmur **may be confused with a patent ductus arteriosus (PDA),** although the latter does not change with position and is best heard in the left clavicular region. Venous hums **usually disappear during adolescence,** but may persist in thin adults.

Murmurs Associated with a High Cardiac Output State

Etiology

Murmurs secondary to a high cardiac output state (e.g., **fever, anemia, thyrotoxicosis**) are usually caused by a **relative stenosis of normal-sized structures** in relation to increased blood flow.

Clinical Features

These murmurs are usually located at the **left mid- to upper sternal border,** are **grade II–III,** are of **medium pitch,** and are **ejection type,** in that the timing and intensity follow the upstroke and downstroke of the systolic pressure curve. An S_3 **may be audible,** creating a gallop sound.

Evaluation

A **chest radiograph** may show **cardiac enlargement secondary to an increased end-diastolic volume,** but the **EKG should be normal.** In patients with **chronic anemia** (e.g., those with sickle cell disease), high-output physiology may lead to **compensatory left ventricular hypertrophy,** which will be evident on EKG.

Treatment

Because the murmur is caused by an increased volume of flow, **treatment of the primary problem** (e.g., with **antipyretics** or **blood transfusion**) diminishes the intensity of the murmur.

Arteriovenous Fistula

Etiology

Congenital anomalous connections between arteries and veins may occur in the **lung, head, or liver.** Because of the constant pressure differential between the artery and vein, the **potential exists for a torrential amount of shunting** to occur, leading to **increased venous return to the right chambers** of the heart.

Clinical Features

A **continuous murmur** is heard over the site of the anomalous arteriovenous connection. In addition, increased flow across the pulmonic and aortic outflow tracts results in a **systolic murmur,** usually of **grade II–III,** along the **left mid- or upper sternal border.**

Evaluation

Auscultation over the liver and the head should be a routine part of the **evaluation of all newborn infants with a heart murmur.** Chest radiographs may reveal a **giant heart with increased pulmonary arterial markings.**

Peripheral Pulmonic Stenosis

Etiology

This murmur is **heard only in newborn infants,** primarily **premature** ones, and involves a **relative stenosis of the branch pulmonary arteries** in relation to the amount of pulmonary blood flowing across them.

Clinical Features

The murmur of peripheral pulmonic stenosis is a **low-pitched systolic** murmur with **occasional decrescendo run-off into diastole,** and is heard **loudest in the back over both the right and left lung** fields. At times the murmur is heard **equally in both the right and left axillae. No thrill** is present and the S_2 is normal.

Evaluation

Most infants **outgrow this murmur by the age of 12–18 months,** but if it persists, an **echocardiogram** may be indicated **to rule out a fixed anatomic stenosis of the branch pulmonary arteries.**

Nonrestrictive (Large) Ventricular Septal Defect (VSD)

Etiology

In **nonrestrictive VSD,** a **large communication between the lower pumping chambers** allows blood to flow from the left to the right ventricle, resulting in **increased blood flow to the lungs** and **increased pulmonary venous return to the left ventricle.** Hence, in a large VSD, the **volume demand is exerted on the left ventricle.**

✄ HINT A murmur related to a large VSD is heard as soon as a significant difference is reached in the level of resistance between the pulmonary and systemic vascular circuits. Because the natural decrement in pulmonary vascular resistance may not reach a point that would allow for a substantial amount of blood to flow across the defect until after the first few weeks of life, a murmur related to a large VSD may become evident only at the 2- or 4-month postnatal visit.

Clinical Features

The murmur of a large VSD is **holosystolic,** reflecting the persistent pressure differential between the right and left ventricles throughout systole. It is **heard best at the left lower sternal border,** frequently **radiating to the right lower sternal border.** A **thrill is not palpable** because the defect is large and nonrestrictive, producing little turbulence. **As the pulmonary vascular resistance continues to drop during the first 6 months of life, a greater amount of blood flow ("shunt") across the defect occurs,** so that **two to three times the amount of blood exiting the aorta** may end up **circulating through the lungs.**

A **low-pitched diastolic rumble murmur** may be **heard at the apex.** This rumble murmur is caused by a **relative mitral stenosis secondary to the increased blood volume returning to the left atrium** via the normal-sized mitral valve.

Evaluation

In patients with a large VSD, the **EKG reveals left ventricular hypertrophy initially** and **biventricular hypertrophy over time.** A **chest radiograph** reveals a **large heart with increased pulmonary vascular markings.** If a large VSD is suspected, an **echocardiogram** to assess the location and anatomy of the defect is indicated. **Cardiac catheterization** may be necessary if complete anatomic detail is not satisfactorily delineated on the echocardiogram, or if hemodynamic information is needed to aid in the decision making.

Treatment

A large VSD does not undergo spontaneous closure; therefore, **surgery is required.** A VSD with a **pulmonary to systemic flow ($\dot{Q}p:\dot{Q}s$) ratio of greater than 2:1** (as calculated by cardiac catheterization) is considered physiologically large and **requires closure.**

Restrictive (Small) Ventricular Septal Defect (VSD)

By definition, small defects are **not hemodynamically significant,** but **may produce a very prominent murmur.**

Clinical Features

Small defects in the muscular portion of the ventricular septum produce a **short, high-pitched, systolic** murmur **heard best along the left lower sternal**

border or apex of the heart. The murmur may be **truncated**—not extending to the end of systole—and may even **abruptly stop at midsystole.** This occurs when the defect is closed off by its muscular borders at the peak of ventricular contraction. Because of the potential for tremendous turbulence across a restrictive narrow orifice in small muscular defects, a **thrill** may be appreciated, and the murmur **may be as loud as grade VI.** The natural tendency is for **muscular defects to become smaller with time,** and hence it is not uncommon for the **murmur to get louder with subsequent examinations.**

A small defect may also be noted in the **inlet portion of the ventricular septum adjacent to the septal leaflet of the tricuspid valve;** this is called a **perimembranous or conoventricular VSD.** A small perimembranous VSD produces a **high-pitched holosystolic** murmur, **heard best at the left lower sternal border and radiating to the right lower sternal border.** The septal leaflet of the tricuspid valve may fill in the defect, and **aneurysmal tissue may develop,** surrounding the VSD. This may produce an **early systolic click** that precedes the onset of the murmur. Additional **growth of aneurysmal tissue** adjacent to a perimembranous VSD **may result in its spontaneous closure.**

Evaluation

In a small VSD, the **S_2 is normal, as are the EKG and chest radiographs.** Over 50% of small VSDs undergo **spontaneous closure** by the time the patient reaches **2 years of age.**

Atrial Septal Defect (ASD)

Etiology

ASD allows for **passive low-pressure flow of blood from the left to the right atrium,** resulting in a volume load on the right ventricle and causing a **relative pulmonic stenosis** (i.e., normal-size pulmonic structures, but increased flow) and a **murmur similar to that heard in** patients with **pulmonic stenosis.** The murmur in an ASD is therefore not caused by flow at the defect site; rather, it is a **physiologic consequence of increased flow at the pulmonic valve** level.

Clinical Features

The murmur is **systolic, ejection type, usually grade II–III,** and **low to medium pitched.** It is **heard best at the left upper sternal border and second intercostal space,** with **occasional radiation to the lung fields in the back.**

A **pathognomonic** finding is a **widely split S_2 caused by the large right ventricular ejection volume.** The S_2 **does not vary with respiration** because the usual effect of inspiration on right-sided volume is equilibrated in the presence of a large communication.

In the presence of a **large shunt,** a **diastolic rumble murmur** may be heard at the **right lower sternal border** relating to **increased flow across the tricuspid valve** (normal flow returning via the superior and inferior vena cavae plus flow across the ASD).

Evaluation

Typically, the **EKG shows a mild right ventricular conduction delay** [i.e., an rSR' pattern in the anterior precordial leads (V_{3R}, V_{4R}, V_1]. A **chest radiograph** reveals a **normal to slightly enlarged heart** with a **prominent pulmonary artery bulge along the left heart border.** Pulmonary vascular markings are **normal or slightly increased.** An **echocardiogram** is sufficient to confirm the diagnosis; cardiac catheterization is rarely indicated.

Patent Ductus Arteriosus (PDA)

Etiology

Persistence in patency of the ductus arteriosus is a common cause of murmurs within the **first year of life.** In utero, the ductus arteriosus functions as the **conduit through which blood from the right ventricle is shunted away from the lungs to the descending aorta.** This structure is **highly sensitive to oxygen, and usually undergoes spontaneous closure within 24 hours of birth.** In some infants, a stimulus (e.g., **prematurity, sepsis, volume overload**) may be identified as the **cause of the PDA.**

Clinical Features

Classically, the murmur heard in a PDA is a **continuous rumbling murmur,** at times even **harsh and machine-like.** It is **best heard in the left upper sternal border area and under the left clavicle.** The continuity of the murmur is caused by the **persistent pressure differential** that exists **between the aorta and pulmonary artery,** both in systole and diastole, leading to **continuous left-to-right shunting** throughout the cardiac cycle. The S_2 **is normal** and may be **masked by the murmur.**

When **patients present** at the nadir of the pulmonary vascular resistance decrement (**between the ages of 3 and 6 months,** earlier in premature infants), the **amount of shunting from aorta to pulmonary artery may lead to left ventricular volume overload and congestive heart failure (CHF).** In these patients, a **diastolic rumble** may be apparent at the **apex** as a result of increased flow across the mitral valve, and the **EKG** may show left **ventricular hypertrophy.** The diagnosis is confirmed on **echocardiogram.**

Treatment

Treatment consists of **close observation during the first 6 months,** because **spontaneous closure** in this period is **still possible.** In patients who are **older than 6 months,** or in whom **CHF is present** and is **poorly controlled** with anticongestive medication (e.g., digoxin, diuretics), **surgical ligation** is recommended. In **premature infants, indomethacin treatment** has been reported as being extremely successful, although it is less effective after the age of 2 weeks.

Pulmonic Stenosis

Etiology

Dysplasia of the pulmonary valve leaflets or a bicuspid pulmonary valve may cause pulmonic stenosis.

Clinical Features

When **stenosis is severe,** the infant may present with **cyanosis** from **impedance of flow** out of the right ventricle **and right-to-left shunting** at the level of the foramen ovale. **Emergent intervention** in this circumstance is necessary.

In patients with **mild to moderate** pulmonary stenosis, the typical presentation is a murmur noted on physical examination in a child without symptoms. The murmur is **systolic, low pitched, crescendo–decrescendo,** and **best heard at the second intercostal space at the left upper sternal border.** An early, dull-sounding systolic ejection click may be appreciated at the **left upper sternal border.** Frequently, the murmur **radiates along the course of the branch pulmonary arteries** and may be **heard over the lungs in the right and left back.** The S_2 **may split widely,** with normal respiratory variation, but the P_2 **component is soft.**

Evaluation

The **EKG and chest radiograph** may be **normal** in patients with **mild to moderate** pulmonic stenosis.

Treatment

In cases of **mild stenosis, treatment is not necessary;** however, in **moderate or severe stenosis, cardiac catheterization with balloon valvuloplasty** is the procedure of choice. Although pulmonic insufficiency is always created at the time of balloon valvuloplasty, the insufficiency is well tolerated as long as the tricuspid valve remains competent.

Aortic Stenosis

Etiology

Dysplasia, or more commonly, fusion, of the aortic leaflets may cause aortic stenosis. A **bicuspid aortic valve,** in fact, is the **most common form of congenital heart "disease" in the older child** and adult and often results in **very mild or no obstruction.**

Clinical Features

> ✂ **HINT**   Severe aortic stenosis seen in infancy may not cause a murmur if obstruction to aortic outflow is of such a degree that a PDA is present to supply the systemic circulation.

In an **older child** aortic stenosis **always produces a murmur.** The murmur is typically **systolic crescendo–decrescendo,** at times **harsh,** and **heard best at the right upper sternal border at the second intercostal space radiating along the course of the aortic arch up into the carotid vessels.**

A **thrill** may be palpable in the **suprasternal notch.** The S_2 **is softer than normal** and may be **single.** In patients with **mild to moderate cases** of aortic stenosis, a **high-pitched ejection click** may be heard in **early systole,** just preceding the onset of the murmur. Of note is the fact that the click is best appreciated at the **apex of the heart,** not at the base, and its cause may relate more to inertial forces in the left ventricular outflow tract than to the opening of the aortic valve.

> ✂ **HINT**   Aortic stenosis may be a progressive disease. Increased harshness of the murmur as well as disappearance of the click may indicate an increased gradient across the aortic valve.

Evaluation

EKG findings of left ventricular hypertrophy and cardiac enlargement on the chest radiograph are present when the aortic stenosis is hemodynamically significant.

Coarctation of the Aorta

Etiology

A **narrowing or shelf-like protuberance in the aortic arch distal to the left subclavian artery** is called a coarctation of the aorta. In **infancy,** the coarctation is usually a **diffuse narrowing** of the area just **proximal to the insertion of the ductus arteriosus** (isthmus of the aortic arch). In **older children, a discrete** shelf is more commonly found and is thought to relate to remnants of ductal tissue within the aorta.

Clinical Features

The murmur in a coarctation is **long systolic** and **heard best along the left upper sternal border.** It is **loudest in the interscapular region in the back.** Frequently, an **early systolic ejection click** can be heard at the **base** of the heart; it is caused by a **bicuspid aortic valve,** which is found in 80% of patients.

In **older patients** with longstanding coarctation, **continuous murmurs** may be appreciated along the **lateral chest wall.** These are caused by intercostal collateral flow to the portion of the aorta distal to the narrowing.

Evaluation

On physical examination, **relative hypertension of the upper extremities** in comparison with the lower extremities is present, as well as **diminished femoral pulses.** An EKG may show **left ventricular hypertrophy.** A **chest radiograph** is either **normal or reveals mild cardiomegaly.** Occasionally, **poststenotic dilatation of the descending aorta distal to the coarctation** can be seen.

Suggested Readings

Asprey DP: Evaluation of children with heart murmurs. *Lippincotts Prim Care Pract* 2(5):505–513, 1998.

Birkebaek NH, Hansen LK, Elle B, et al: Chest roentgenogram in the evaluation of heart defects in asymptomatic infants and children with a cardiac murmur: reproducibility and accuracy. *Pediatrics* 103(2):E15, 1999.

Braunwald E: The physical examination. In *Heart Disease: A Textbook of Cardiovascular Medicine.* Edited by Braunwald E. Philadelphia, WB Saunders, 1992, pp 13–42.

Duff DF, McNamara DG: History and physical examination of the cardiovascular system. In *The Science and Practice of Pediatric Cardiology,* 2nd ed. Edited by Garson A Jr, Bricker JT, Fisher DJ, et al. Baltimore, Williams & Wilkins, 1998, pp 693–713.

Haney I, Ipp M, Feldman W, et al: Accuracy of clinical assessment of heart murmurs by office based (general practice) paediatricians. *Arch Dis Child* 81(5):409–412, 1999.

McCrindle BW, Shaffer KM, Kan JS, et al: Cardinal clinical signs in the differentiation of heart murmurs in children. *Arch Pediatr Adolesc Med* 150(2):169–174, 1996.

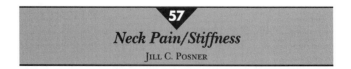

57

Neck Pain/Stiffness

JILL C. POSNER

▼ INTRODUCTION

In children, the chief complaint of neck pain often may represent neck stiffness or torticollis. **Torticollis** describes a **characteristic malpositioning of the head and chin** in which the head is tilted to one direction and the chin points oppositely. It is a sign of an underlying disease process, and does not imply a specific diagnosis. The head and neck regions are highly complex anatomically, and there are many structures within these areas that can give rise to symptoms. **Pain or stiffness can arise from structures within the neck** such as the cervical musculature, the vertebral bones or lymph nodes. Alternatively, **pain from the scalp, ear, oropharynx or mandible** can refer and be perceived in the neck region. **Pressure** originating from the head either external to the dura or from within the brain or spinal cord can cause neck pain or stiffness. Finally, processes involving the upper thorax (e.g., clavicular fracture or upper lobe pneumonia) can also cause pain that might radiate to the neck region.

▼ DIFFERENTIAL DIAGNOSIS LIST

Trauma

Fracture of cervical spine
Subluxation of cervical spine
Spinal cord injury without radiographic abnormality (SCIWORA) syndrome
Atlantoaxial rotary subluxation
Muscular contusions/spasm
Subarachnoid hemorrhage
Epidural hematoma of cervical spine
Clavicular fracture

Infectious

Meningitis
Retropharyngeal abscess
Peritonsillar abscess
Epiglottitis
Osteomyelitis
Discitis
Epidural abscess
Cervical adenitis
Pharyngitis
Upper respiratory tract infection
Upper lobe pneumonia
Viral myositis
Otitis media/mastoiditis

Inflammatory

Atlantoaxial rotary subluxation
Grisel syndrome
Collagen vascular diseases
Juvenile intervertebral disc calcification

Congenital

Congenital muscular torticollis
Skeletal malformations
Klippel-Feil syndrome
Atlantoaxial instability

Toxic Metabolic

Dystonic reaction
Tetanus
Lead poisoning

Neurologic

Space-occupying lesions
    Brain tumor
    Spinal cord tumor
    Arnold-Chiari malformation
    Syringomyelia
    Arteriovenous malformation (AVM)
Strabismus
Cranial nerve palsies
Myasthenia gravis
Migraine headaches

Miscellaneous

Benign paroxysmal torticollis
Gastroesophageal reflux (Sandifer syndrome)
Psychogenic

▼ DIFFERENTIAL DIAGNOSIS DISCUSSION
Major Trauma

Etiology

Cervical spine fracture, subluxation of the vertebral bodies, or **spinal cord injury without radiographic abnormality (SCIWORA)** syndrome may result from high-risk mechanisms of injury (e.g., motor-vehicle collision, pedestrian struck by motor vehicle, falls from heights, high-impact sports activities). The larger head size, weaker neck muscles, and increased ligamentous laxity render children more likely to sustain injury in the **upper cervical area** as compared with adults, who are more likely to sustain lower cervical injuries.

Clinical Features

Cervical spine injury should be **suspected in the patient with a high-risk mechanism of injury or suggestive signs or symptoms:** pain on neck palpation, neck muscle spasm, limited range of motion, torticollis, transient or persistent sensory changes, hyporeflexia, muscle weakness or flaccidity, priapism, bladder or bowel dysfunction, or hypotension with bradycardia (spinal shock). In addition, in the **nonverbal or uncooperative child** or the child who has an **altered mental status** or an **associated severe head injury,** the physical examination may be difficult or unreliable. In these children, the possibility of cervical spine injury should be considered at the outset of the evaluation and **spinal immobilization and precautions maintained until proved otherwise.**

Evaluation

Suspected cervical spine injury generally requires **emergent evaluation.** The child should be immobilized with a rigid cervical collar and pediatric spine board.

▼ **The evaluation should begin by assessing the patient's respiratory and hemodynamic status.** In some alert, verbal, and cooperative children, an attempt to "clinically clear" the cervical spine may be made through a careful physical examination.

▼ **A complete sensory and motor neurologic exam** should be performed and must be without deficits.

▼ **A careful examination of the cervical spine with the collar removed,** but with manual immobilization maintained, should yield no tenderness or deformity.

At this point, the patient may be allowed to attempt **active** (not passive) **neck flexion, extension,** and **lateral rotation.** Any limitation or complaint of pain with range of motion should prompt the immediate reinstitution of cervical spine immobilization and cervical radiography.

▼ The **radiographic evaluation** should include a minimum of three views: the lateral, anterior-posterior, and open-mouth (odontoid) radiographs. Flexion and extension views are used to assess for ligamentous injury in a child with persistent neck pain after normal three-view series.

▼ **Computed tomography (CT) scan** provides excellent bone detail, whereas **MRI scan** is used to evaluate the soft tissues and spinal cord.

Treatment

In addition to **supportive care,** a treatment adjunct for spinal cord injury with associated neurologic abnormality is the administration of **methyl-prednisolone,** 30 mg/kg over 15 minutes followed by 5.4 mg/kg/hour for 23 hours. Based on studies in adults, this treatment is most effective if given within 8 hours of the injury.

Atlantoaxial Rotary Subluxation

Etiology

The odontoid process of the second cervical vertebrae is normally positioned squarely within the ring of C1, and the two vertebrae are secured by the transverse and alar ligaments. The increased laxity and longer lengths of the ligaments renders **children more susceptible** to traumatic cervical spine injury than their adult counterparts.

As the name implies, in patients with rotary subluxation, **C1 and C2** are **rotationally malpositioned.** This commonly results from a **minor traumatic mechanism,** as might occur during light wrestling or gymnastics. Some conditions such as **tonsillectomy** (Grisel syndrome), **upper respiratory infections,** or **juvenile rheumatoid arthritis** may cause inflammation and laxity of the transverse ligament, resulting in C1–C2 instability with rotary subluxation. Additionally, certain conditions such as **Down syndrome** or **congenital odontoid dysplasias** may predispose to rotary subluxation.

Clinical Features

Patients commonly present with **neck pain** or **stiffness.** Physical examination reveals **torticollis, tender paracervical muscles,** and **decreased range of motion** of the neck. The torticollis results as the ipsilateral sternocleidomastoid muscle attempts to reestablish normal positioning. Rotary subluxation is a **stable cervical spine injury,** rarely causing spinal cord impingement, and neurologic signs are infrequently encountered.

The lateral radiograph may be normal or show distorted anatomy. Particular attention should be paid to check the **peridental space** that may be widened. The diagnostic modality of choice, however, is the **static and dynamic neck CT scan.** A static CT scan usually shows the asymmetric location of the dens within the anterior arch of C1. In the dynamic CT, the rotation of C2 on C1 is fixed, persisting despite lateral rotation of the head to both directions.

Treatment

Most patients have resolution of symptoms with **supportive care with a soft collar** and the administration of nonsteroidal **anti-inflammatory drugs.** Orthopedic referral is suggested for the patients with persistent symptoms who may require reduction and stabilization with traction.

Meningitis

Meningitis is discussed in Chapter 21, "Coma."

Retropharyngeal Abscess, Peritonsillar Abscess, Epiglottitis, Cervical Adenitis, Pharyngitis

Retropharyngeal abscess, peritonsillar abscess, epiglottitis, cervical adenitis, and pharyngitis are discussed in Chapter 75, "Sore Throat."

Discitis

Etiology

Infectious discitis is a **rare illness** with an unclear etiology. In approximately 50% of patients with discitis, an aspirated culture of the affected area will yield a bacterial pathogen (*Staphylococcus aureus* in most, also coagulase-negative *Staphylococcus, Kingella, Salmonella*), which has led some to believe that the process is **infectious** in etiology. Yet, the outcome in patients is the same with or without antimicrobial treatment. Others suggest a **traumatic or inflammatory** etiology, theorizing that a preceding traumatic event induces the release of tissue enzymes from the disc, resulting in inflammation. Discitis more commonly affects the **lumbar area** but can occur in the cervical region.

Clinical Features

The clinical presentation is **gradual in onset** with few constitutional symptoms. The patient may present with mild irritability or more obvious pain. The physical exam is often near normal except that the child may refuse to move his neck.

The peripheral white blood count and differential are usually normal. **Nonspecific indicators of inflammation [erythrocyte sedimentation rate (ESR), C-reactive protein (CRP)] are almost always elevated.** Blood cultures are rarely positive. Radiographs are usually normal early in the course of the illness, but may demonstrate erosion of the adjacent vertebral plates by 4 to 8 weeks after the onset. **Repair and residual sclerosis** is the typical progression. **Bone scan** may detect disease earlier, showing increased uptake in the disc and vertebral bodies.

Treatment

The management of discitis is **controversial.** Supportive treatment with immobilization and analgesia generally renders patients free of discomfort in about 48 hours. The role of parenteral antibiotics remains unclear.

Epidural Abscess

Epidural Abscess is discussed in Chapter 59, "Paraplegia."

Congenital Muscular Torticollis (CMT)

Etiology

CMT is a relatively common entity, occurring with a prevalence of 3–19 per 1000 newborns. The **etiology is unknown,** although several theories exist. The **intrauterine theory** suggests that abnormal fetal positioning results in a shortened sternocleidomastoid muscle. Another theory contends that **birth trauma** during difficult deliveries leads to bleeding into the sternocleidomastoid muscle with subsequent compartment syndrome, fibrosis, and contracture. There is no genetic predisposition.

Clinical Features

CMT is **often undetected** in the **immediate newborn period.** The head tilt becomes more obvious, however, as the infant develops head control. The **head tilts** toward the shorted muscle and the chin points away. A **mass** can be palpated in the inferior portion of the sternocleidomastoid muscle in about one-third of cases. Rarely, other musculoskeletal anomalies are associated, including hip dysplasia, metatarsus adductus, and talipes equinovarus.

Evaluation

A thorough **physical examination** to eliminate other causes of torticollis should be performed. **Radiographic evaluation** of the cervical spine can identify rare congenital vertebral anomalies such as Klippel-Feil syndrome (congenital fusion of any number of cervical vertebrae).

Treatment

Treatment is usually **nonsurgical** with **strengthening and stretching exercises.** Early **physical therapy** referral correlates with improved outcome. **Recurrence** of torticollis may occur in 11% of patients and can happen years later.

Paroxysmal Torticollis

Etiology

The etiology is unclear but felt to be either a **migraine** variant or related to **vestibular dysfunction.**

Clinical Features

The syndrome, generally presenting in the **first few months of life,** is characterized by **recurrent episodes of head tilt,** often alternating in sides. Torticollis is rarely the only finding. Other **associated symptoms** may include **vomiting, pallor, irritability,** and **ataxia.** While frightening for the parents to witness, paroxysmal torticollis is a **benign, self-limited process.** The frequency of attacks progressively decreases and ultimately it resolves in 1 to 5 years.

Evaluation and Treatment

Evaluation of the initial episode consists of a careful history and physical examination to **rule out other causes of vomiting** and **ataxia** such as central nervous system processes or intoxication. Subsequent attacks are managed by **supportive therapy** including intravenous fluid hydration if necessary. Pharmacologic treatment has not been well studied.

Dystonic Reactions

Etiology

Antiemetics, neuroleptics, and **other medications** with dopamine receptor antagonism can cause dystonia when taken either in overdose or in therapeutic doses.

Clinical Features

Patients with dystonic reactions experience a **severe, uncomfortable contraction of the sternocleidomastoid muscle.** Often the **facial muscles,** and sometimes the muscles of the **extremities and trunk,** are also involved.

Evaluation and Treatment

The administration of **diphenhydramine** (1.25 mg/kg) can be both diagnostic and therapeutic. The response is **rapid and dramatic.** The offending agent should be discontinued, and diphenhydramine continued every 6 to 8 hours for several days to avoid recurrence.

Neurologic Causes

Central nervous system (CNS) processes can induce torticollis via a variety of mechanisms. **Space-occupying lesions** exerting pressure on the dura can cause irritation that can cause neck stiffness. Alternatively, **tonsillar herniation** may cause stretching or irritation of the accessory nerve, which then induces sternocleidomastoid spasm. In addition, a child with diplopia secondary to **cranial nerve dysfunction or strabismus** may attempt compensation through tilting his head to realign the visual axis. This head tilt may be perceived by the examiner as torticollis. The evaluation of the child with neck stiffness or torticollis must include a **careful neurologic examination** to assess for the presence of a neurologic cause.

Atlantoaxial Rotary Subluxation

Inflammatory conditions involving the transverse ligament of C1 and C2 can result in torticollis as described earlier.

Juvenile Rheumatoid Arthritis (JRA)

The **cervical spine** is involved in 50% of patients with JRA. It is rarely an early complication of the disease and is usually found in patients with greater than 6 months of illness.

Juvenile Intervertebral Disc Calcification (JIDC)

Etiology

This uncommon disease entity has an **unknown etiology** but has been postulated to arise from developmental changes in the water content, blood supply, and cellular matrix of the nucleus of the disc. There are several distinguishing features of JIDC, and therefore it is felt to be a **different** entity **than adult IDC.**

▼ **The location of involvement in children is distinct from that in adults.** In JIDC, the cervical region is most commonly involved and the calcification occurs within the nucleus. In adults, the annulus of the discs in the thoracic or lumbar regions is affected.

▼ **Childhood disease may be either asymptomatic or transiently symptomatic.** Adults generally have asymptomatic, permanent calcification.

Clinical Features

Patients with JIDC may be divided into **symptomatic** and **asymptomatic** groups, depending on clinical features. It is unknown what triggers the development of symptoms. Many asymptomatic patients never develop symptoms, but resolution does not occur without a symptomatic period. In most symptomatic patients, symptoms develop over 24–48 hours and most commonly consist of **neck pain, torticollis,** and **fever.** Neurologic symptoms and signs are rare.

Evaluation and Treatment

In the symptomatic patient, **nonspecific laboratory evidence of inflammation** is apparent in one-third to one-half of patients (leukocytosis, elevated ESR). Blood cultures are negative. Radiographs of the spine demonstrate **intervertebral disc calcification** of the nucleus pulposus. During the acute episode, the involved **interspace may widen** and then normalize as the symptoms resolve. **Extruded calcified disc material** may be seen posteriorly within the spinal canal or within the prevertebral soft tissues. There is no destruction of the adjacent vertebral bodies and the retropharyngeal space is not enlarged. MRI can be used to evaluate for canal compromise that is secondary to disc herniation.

Given that the disease is usually benign and self-limited, treatment is generally **supportive** with bedrest, analgesics, heat, and muscle relaxants. Operative removal of the disc is usually not indicated. Symptoms resolve in 3 weeks (67%) to 6 months (95%). **Complete radiographic resolution** is the rule.

▼ EVALUATION OF NECK PAIN

A child who presents with neck pain may have a **potentially life-threatening illness.** The immediate priority is to ensure the adequacy of the **airway, breathing,** and **circulation.** The possibility of **cervical spine injury** is **considered early** and spinal immobilization and precautions are instituted if warranted. Most diagnoses are made based on the history and physical examination findings alone. Further evaluation with laboratory and radiographic tests will be based on these findings.

History

In the history, it is important to characterize the nature of the chief complaint, **distinguishing neck pain from stiffness or torticollis.** Is the pain acute or chronic in nature? Is it constant or intermittent? Has there been any response to any home therapies? It is particularly important to elucidate any evidence of acute or chronic **central nervous system pathology** such as weakness, paresthesias, loss of bowel or bladder continence, or loss of developmental milestones. There should be a careful probing for any **symptoms of increased intracranial pressure** such as headaches, vomiting, or changes in school performance. Preceding **major trauma** is usually evident, but the possibility of **minor trauma** should be explored. Has the patient had fever, sore throat, cough, upper respiratory symptoms, or ear or mouth pain? Is the patient, or are any household contacts, taking any medications, either prescription or over the counter?

Physical Examination

A **general review of all systems** should occur. The diagnosis of meningitis usually can be excluded by physical examination. When in doubt, a **lumbar puncture** should be performed. The examination of the neck begins with **observation of positioning.** If **palpation** of the cervical spinous processes yields **localized tenderness or deformity,** a **cervical collar** should be placed and no further manipulation done until a **radiographic evaluation** shows the absence of fracture, subluxation, or ligamentous injury. Barring this, the rest of the neck should be carefully palpated for masses and muscle spasm. At this point, the child should be allowed to attempt **active (not passive) neck flexion, extension, and lateral rotation.**

Diagnostic Evaluation

The diagnostic evaluation is selective and based on history and physical examination clues to the diagnosis. **Laboratory studies** such as a complete blood count, ESR, CRP, and blood culture may provide nonspecific evidence for an infectious or inflammatory etiology. **Radiographic studies** such as plain films, CT, MRI, and nuclear medicine scans can be useful in selected circumstances.

▼ TREATMENT OF NECK PAIN

Until the cause of the neck pain is established, treatment is **supportive** and may entail:

▼ Administration of analgesics, usually in the form of nonsteroidal anti-inflammatory drugs
▼ Application of warm compresses
▼ Administration of antipyretic agents

Suggested Readings

Ballock RT, Song KM: The prevalence of nonmuscular causes of torticollis in children. *J Pediatr Orthop* 16(4):500–504, 1996.

Bredenkamp JK, Maceri DR: Inflammatory torticollis in children. *Arch Otolaryngol Head Neck Surg* 116:310–313, 1990.

Dias MS, Pang D: Juvenile intervertebral disc calcification: recognition, management, and pathogenesis. *Neurosurgery* 28(1):130–135, 1991.

Fernandez M, Carrol CL, Baker CJ: Discitis and vertebral osteomyelitis in children: an 18 year review. *Pediatrics* 105(6):1299–1304, 2000.

Gupta AK, Roy DR, Conlan ES, et al: Torticollis secondary to posterior fossa tumors. *J Pediatr Orthop* 16(4):505–507, 1996.

Hall DE, Boydston W: Pediatric neck injuries. *Pediatr Rev* 20(1):13–19, 1999.

Parker C: Complicated migraine syndromes and migraine variants. *Pediatr Ann* 26:417–421, 1997.

Robin NH: In brief: congenital muscular torticollis. *Pediatr Rev* 17(10):374–375, 1996.

Singer JI: Evaluation of the patient with neck complaints following tonsillectomy or adenoidectomy. *Pediatr Emerg Care* 8(5):276–279, 1992.

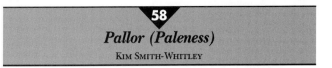

58
Pallor (Paleness)
KIM SMITH-WHITLEY

▼ INTRODUCTION

Pallor (paleness) results from a **decreased amount of circulating hemoglobin or vasoconstriction of dermal blood vessels.** Causes can be classified as hematologic or nonhematologic.

▼ DIFFERENTIAL DIAGNOSIS LIST
Hematologic Causes
Increased Red Blood Cell (RBC) Destruction

RBC membrane defects—see Chapter 40, "Hemolysis"
RBC enzyme defects—see Chapter 40, "Hemolysis"
Qualitative hemoglobin disorders
Quantitative hemoglobin disorders
Isoimmune or alloimmune hemolytic anemia
Autoimmune hemolytic anemia
Microangiopathic hemolytic anemia
Drugs
Toxins
Infections

Bone Marrow Failure

Pure red cell aplasia
Diamond-Blackfan anemia
Congenital dyserythropoietic anemia
Transient erythroblastopenia of childhood
Aplastic crisis with underlying congenital hemolytic anemia
Anemia associated with systemic illness
Drug-related anemia
Infection
Pregnancy
Fanconi anemia
Dyskeratosis congenita
Aplastic anemia—idiopathic or secondary to drugs, chemicals, viruses, radiation, pregnancy
Transient bone marrow suppression—caused by viral or bacterial infection, drugs, pregnancy, radiation

Bone Marrow Infiltration

Leukemia or neoplasm metastatic to bone marrow
Infection
Osteopetrosis
Histiocytosis

Myelofibrosis
Storage diseases

Nutritional Deficiencies

Iron deficiency
Folate deficiency
Vitamin B_{12} deficiency

Blood Loss

Hemorrhage
Bleeding disorder

Nonhematologic Causes

Infectious Causes

Bacterial process leading to shock, anemia, or both

Toxic Causes

Lead poisoning

Neoplastic Causes

Pheochromocytoma

Traumatic Causes

Head trauma resulting in a closed head injury or cerebral hemorrhage

Congenital Causes

Constitutional skin color

Metabolic or Genetic Causes

Hypoglycemia

Inflammatory Causes

Atopic dermatitis
Other chronic systemic diseases

Miscellaneous Causes

Shock
Skin edema (myxedema, as in thyroid disease)
Uremia
Cystic fibrosis
Seizures
Syncope
Lack of sun exposure

▼ DIFFERENTIAL DIAGNOSIS DISCUSSION
Blood Loss

Etiology

Blood loss, acute and chronic, is one of the most common causes of anemia in the pediatric patient. Chronic blood loss may be caused by **gastrointestinal bleeding, excessive menstrual bleeding, or a bleeding disorder** characterized by frequent bleeding episodes.

Clinical Features

Patients with chronic blood loss may present with **pallor,** usually noted by an observer who has not seen the child recently. **Chronic blood loss** may be **difficult to recognize** because the hemoglobin level diminishes slowly.

Evaluation

Initial laboratory studies should include a **complete blood count (CBC), blood type and cross-match, prothrombin time (PT), and partial thromboplastin time (PTT).** In a patient with anemia secondary to **chronic blood loss,** a peripheral smear will show **hypochromic, microcytic RBCs** from iron deficiency. In a patient with **acute blood loss,** it will show **normocytic, normochromic RBCs.**

Treatment

If bleeding is **massive or life threatening, intravenous access should be established, active bleeding controlled, and albumin administered intravenously** until blood for transfusion is available. If the **child is in shock,** the physician should not wait for cross-matching to be completed; **type O-negative, uncross-matched packed cells should be transfused.** Rarely, in the previously transfused, alloimmunized child, minor blood group antigen incompatibility results in **severe delayed hemolytic transfusion reactions** following the administration of O-negative uncross-matched packed cells.

Iron-Deficiency Anemia

> ✄ **HINT** Nutritional deficiencies may be caused by decreased oral intake, increased requirements, decreased absorption, or ineffective transport or metabolism of the element. The specific deficiency should be determined as well as the underlying cause to provide optimal treatment.

Etiology

Iron deficiency, which is the most common cause of anemia in childhood, can occur at any age, although children between the ages of 6 and 36 months and 11 and 17 years are at increased risk. Iron deficiency in childhood is caused by **rapid growth in the presence of inadequate dietary intake, chronic or massive blood loss, or poor gut absorption.** Infants with iron deficiency usually have a history of **consuming large amounts of cow's milk** and other food substances low in iron.

> ✄ **HINT** Iron deficiency is less common in breast-fed infants. Although the iron content of breast milk is lower than that of cow's milk-based formula, iron absorption is improved.

> ✄ **HINT** Pica may be a symptom of iron deficiency, or a risk factor for iron deficiency. Children who eat dirt should be evaluated for lead poisoning.

Clinical Features

Children with severe iron deficiency are commonly **pale, irritable, and have little appetite.** In addition to signs of anemia, **spooning of the nails, angular stomatitis, and splenomegaly** may be present.

Laboratory Evaluation

The degree of iron deficiency can be estimated by the abnormalities found on laboratory studies. The following laboratory abnormalities occur progressively: **decreased serum ferritin, decreased serum iron, increased microcytosis, and decreased hemoglobin with a normal or decreased reticulocyte count.** The **platelet count** may be markedly **increased.** The peripheral blood smear shows **hypochromic, microcytic RBCs with increased variation in RBC size** (anisocytosis) **and shape** (poikilocytosis). **Increased** numbers of **elliptocytes and ovalocytes** may be noted.

Treatment

Treatment of iron deficiency includes **iron supplementation,** as well as **treatment of the underlying cause** with **nutritional counseling** when appropriate. Oral iron replacement is achieved with **ferrous sulfate** (6 mg/kg/day of elemental iron in two or three divided doses). Although absorption is better on an empty stomach, gastric irritation is lessened if the iron is given **with meals.**

In patients with severe anemia, the hematologic response to ferrous sulfate administration can be documented by obtaining a **reticulocyte count within 7–10 days.** The reticulocyte count increases earlier than the hemoglobin level, which may not reach a normal level until 2 months after starting iron therapy, depending on the degree of anemia.

Many physicians believe that because iron deficiency is so common, the healthy child or adolescent with a **microcytic, hypochromic anemia** is appropriately managed using a **trial of iron supplementation without additional laboratory evaluation.** If a patient is managed this way, **close follow-up** should be provided. If the microcytic anemia persists, a comprehensive evaluation for other causes (e.g., thalassemia, anemia of chronic disease, chronic blood loss, sideroblastic anemia) should be performed.

Megaloblastic Anemias

Etiology

Megaloblastic anemias are often caused by **folate and vitamin B_{12} deficiencies,** which result in **abnormal DNA synthesis.** Folate deficiency in the United States is **primarily caused by malabsorption of folate, increased RBC turnover, and drugs.** Vitamin B_{12} deficiency may be **caused by malabsorption or pernicious anemia,** a rare disease caused by an inability to secrete the intrinsic factor required for normal vitamin B_{12} absorption.

Evaluation

Megaloblastic anemias are characterized by **macrocytic RBCs and a mean corpuscular volume (MCV) value greater than 95 μm^3.** The **reticulocyte count is low** and in advanced cases, **pancytopenia** may exist. Analysis of a **bone marrow aspirate and biopsy sample** shows **dyssynchrony** between **nuclear and cytoplasmic maturation** with increased cellularity.

Serum folate may be decreased but measurement of **RBC folate levels** provides a more accurate picture of chronic folate deficiency. In pernicious anemia, **serum vitamin B_{12} levels are reduced** and the **Schilling test** for evaluation of the **presence of intrinsic factor is abnormal.**

Therapy

Therapy includes **supplemental folate or vitamin B_{12}** administration, as well as **treatment of the underlying cause** of the deficiency.

Transient Erythroblastopenia of Childhood

Clinical Features

Transient erythroblastopenia of childhood is characterized by the **acute onset of anemia** in a previously healthy child **between the ages of 6 months and 4 years.** There may be a history of a **viral prodrome.** The physical examination is normal except for signs of anemia.

Evaluation

The hemoglobin and reticulocyte values vary according to the stage of disease. **Early in the illness, the hemoglobin and reticulocyte count are low,** whereas **in the recovery stage** the hemoglobin may be low but the **reticulocyte count is increasing.** Therefore, **serial reticulocyte counts** should be used **in conjunction with serial hemoglobin values** to clarify the stage of disease.

Other laboratory findings include **neutropenia** (25% of patients) and a **normal platelet count.** The bone marrow aspirate shows a marked **decrease in erythroid precursors** early in the disease.

Treatment

Because of the potential severity of the anemia and the need for serial testing, these patients are initially managed more appropriately in a **hospital inpatient setting.** Transient erythroblastopenia of childhood usually **resolves in 1–2 months.** No medications have been shown to accelerate bone marrow recovery. **RBC transfusion** is sometimes necessary.

Diamond-Blackfan Anemia (Congenital Hypoplastic Anemia)

Etiology

Diamond-Blackfan anemia is a **congenital disorder** characterized by **pure RBC aplasia.**

Clinical Features

Most patients become anemic within the first 6 months of life. **Congenital anomalies** occur in 25% of patients, including **radial anomalies** (triphalangeal thumbs); **short stature;** and **eye, palate, heart, and kidney anomalies.**

Evaluation

The disease is characterized by a **macrocytic anemia,** although a normocytic anemia with a decreased reticulocyte count is seen early in life. Bone marrow aspirate shows **normal cellularity** with isolated **decreased RBC precursors. Hemoglobin F is increased** in a heterogeneous fashion.

Treatment

Approximately 60%–70% of patients with Diamond-Blackfan anemia respond to corticosteroids and do not require chronic transfusions. Steroid-unresponsive patients receive **RBC transfusions** each month and have a poorer prognosis because of the long-term complications associated with chronic blood transfusion (e.g., iron overload). **Splenectomy** has also been attempted in steroid-unresponsive patients with mixed success. Some patients are cured by **bone marrow transplantation.**

Congenital Hemolytic Anemia with Aplastic Crisis

Etiology

Children with congenital hemolytic anemias can experience a **transient aplastic crisis as a result of parvovirus infection.**

Evaluation

Transient erythroblastopenia of childhood, Diamond-Blackfan anemia (congenital pure RBC aplasia), **and an aplastic crisis** in the presence of a previously undiagnosed hemolytic anemia can be **difficult to distinguish** from one another. Children with congenital hemolytic anemia may have the following:

▼ **A history of intermittent scleral icterus** with intercurrent illnesses
▼ **Family members with anemia** or family members **who have required splenectomy or cholecystectomy** before adulthood. Children with transient erythroblastopenia of childhood or Diamond-Blackfan anemia do not have this history as frequently.
▼ **Splenomegaly** on physical examination, which is absent in patients with transient erythroblastopenia of childhood, but may be present in those with Diamond-Blackfan anemia
▼ **Peripheral RBC morphology that suggests the diagnosis of hereditary spherocytosis, hereditary elliptocytosis, or sickle cell disease (SCD).**

If the RBC morphology is normal but the history is suspicious for a congenital hemolytic anemia, hemoglobin electrophoresis, measurement of RBC enzyme levels, and evaluation of membrane abnormalities should be performed (prior to transfusing the patient).

Children with congenital hemolytic anemia and aplastic crisis usually have a **febrile viral prodrome** and may have **profound anemia and reticulocytopenia.** Serum should be obtained for parvovirus IgM and IgG evaluation (see Chapter 40, "Hemolysis").

Aplastic Anemia

Etiology

Aplastic anemia (i.e., bone marrow failure characterized by decreased bone marrow cellularity and pancytopenia) is **usually acquired.** Acquired aplastic anemia may be idiopathic or secondary to a number of processes (Table 58.1). Acquired aplastic anemia of childhood is usually idiopathic; 30%–50% of the patients have no antecedent cause. Most reported pediatric cases of aplastic anemia with definable causes result from **exposure to drugs, chemicals, or other toxic substances.**

Clinical Features

Patients with aplastic anemia usually present with signs of **thrombocytopenia** (e.g., petechiae, ecchymoses, abnormal bleeding); however, signs of **anemia** are not uncommon. Hepatosplenomegaly and lymphadenopathy are usually absent on physical examination.

Evaluation

Laboratory findings demonstrate **moderate to severe anemia, thrombocytopenia, and neutropenia. Reticulocytopenia** occurs with corrected reticulocyte counts of less than 2%.

TABLE 58.1. Causes of Acquired Aplastic Anemia

Drugs
    Chloramphenicol
    Sulfa drugs
    Anticonvulsants
    Cancer chemotherapeutic agents
Chemicals
    Benzenes
    Gold
    Insecticides (DDT)
    Lindane (active ingredient in shampoos used to treat pediculosis)
Pregnancy
Viral infection
    Hepatitis A, hepatitis B, hepatitis C
    Epstein-Barr virus
Radiation
Paroxysmal nocturnal hemoglobinuria
Inherited disorders
    Fanconi anemia
    Dyskeratosis congenita
    Reticular dysgenesis
    Schwachman-Diamond syndrome
Immunologic disorders
    Severe combined immunodeficiency disorder with graft-versus-host disease
    Systemic lupus erythematosus
    Eosinophilic fasciitis
    Thymoma
    Hypogammaglobulinemia

Analysis of a **bone marrow aspirate and biopsy sample** is necessary to establish a diagnosis. Bone marrow aspirate shows a **paucity of RBC, white blood cell (WBC), and platelet precursors** as well as an **absence of bone marrow infiltration** with malignant cells. Bone marrow biopsy shows a **decrease in overall bone marrow cellularity and replacement with fatty tissue.** A bone marrow biopsy that demonstrates normal cellularity does not eliminate the possibility of aplastic anemia because these patients may have patchy foci of normal bone marrow activity. In these patients, **magnetic resonance imaging** may be useful to demonstrate bone marrow replacement with fat, especially in the spine.

Treatment

Once the diagnosis of aplastic anemia has been established and a full evaluation has been performed to identify possible causes, potential treatment options should be evaluated. Initial management of the pediatric patient with pancytopenia should be directed toward **treating life-threatening bleeding, infection, and anemia-related congestive heart failure.** Supportive measures include **irradiated RBC and platelet transfusions** (when necessary) and **antimicrobial administration** to treat or prevent severe infections.

The majority of cases of aplastic anemia can be **cured by bone marrow transplantation or pharmacological regimens.** Any patient with severe aplastic anemia and an **HLA-identical sibling** should first be evaluated for bone marrow transplantation. If there is no HLA-identical sibling, pharmacological treatment includes the administration of immunosuppressive agents such as **antithymocyte globulin, cyclosporine, and corticosteroids.** Recently, success with high-dose **cyclophosphamide** has been reported. Other options include **androgens and growth factors.** Despite therapeutic interventions, a small number of patients with aplastic anemia do not respond, or develop leukemia.

Fanconi Anemia

Etiology

Fanconi anemia is a rare autosomal recessive disorder characterized by **pancytopenia, bone marrow hypoplasia, and chromosomal instability.**

Clinical Features

Fanconi anemia may occur **with or without congenital anomalies** such as thumb and radial abnormalities, short stature, and hyperpigmentation. The age of presentation is **between 6 and 10 years,** and boys are affected slightly more often than girls.

Evaluation

Hematologic abnormalities are not always present at the time of diagnosis. **Thrombocytopenia usually develops first, then neutropenia, followed by anemia.** The RBC morphology is **macrocytic.** The diagnosis is confirmed by identifying **increased chromosomal breakage patterns in peripheral lymphocytes.**

Treatment

Patients with Fanconi anemia are at **increased risk for developing leukemia and other malignancies.** Treatment entails **supportive care** as well as specific therapy. **RBC and platelet transfusions** should be leukoreduced because alloimmunization may complicate bone marrow transplantation if it is needed. **Corticosteroids, androgens, bone marrow transplantation, and growth factors** have been used with variable success to treat patients with Fanconi anemia.

Bone Marrow Infiltration

Etiology

Malignant diseases that can infiltrate or replace bone marrow include **leukemia, rhabdomyosarcoma, neuroblastoma, retinoblastoma, Ewing sarcoma, lymphoma, and histiocytosis syndromes. Nonmalignant diseases** that infiltrate and replace bone marrow include **storage diseases, osteopetrosis, infections** such as tuberculosis, **and fibrous tissue replacement.**

Evaluation

Bone marrow infiltration with malignant or abnormal cells can cause **pancytopenia.** Peripheral blood smears may show predominant **teardrop-shaped RBCs** and **increased RBC and WBC precursors.**

Treatment

Treatment is directed toward **management of the causative disorder.** Supportive measures include **antibiotic therapy** and **RBC and platelet transfusions.**

▼ EVALUATION OF PALLOR (TABLE 58.2)
Patient History

The following information should be sought:

▼ Patient's age. The differential is slightly different for neonates (Table 58.3).
▼ A complete prenatal history, birth history, and family history, including information regarding the need for transfusion, a childhood history of splenectomy or cholecystectomy, or abnormal bleeding (if excessive blood loss is the cause of anemia)
▼ Symptoms of anemia (e.g., pallor with or without scleral icterus)
▼ Symptoms of cardiovascular compromise [e.g., easy fatigability, shortness of breath (at rest or with exercise), orthopnea, headache, mental status changes]
▼ Presence of other systemic symptoms (e.g., fever)
▼ History of chronic disease
▼ History of seizures, syncope, or head trauma
▼ Dietary history

Physical Examination (see Table 58.2)

In addition to a general physical examination, care should be taken to **examine the skin and mucosa.** In a dark-skinned child, pale conjunctivae, palmar creases, nail beds, and oral mucosa help confirm the presence of pallor.

Cardiovascular findings often include **tachycardia** and a **systolic ejection (flow) murmur.** Signs of **congestive heart failure** caused by severe anemia include **extreme tachycardia, a third heart sound (S_3) cardiac gallop, rales, hepatomegaly** (possibly accompanied by splenomegaly), **pedal edema (rare), and shock.**

Laboratory Studies (see Table 58.2)

Appropriate laboratory studies may include:

▼ CBC
▼ Peripheral blood smear
▼ Bone aspirate and/or biopsy
▼ Serum electrolyte panel
▼ Blood urea nitrogen and creatinine levels
▼ Glucose level
▼ Blood culture
▼ Blood type and cross-match

🏅 HINT Pallor caused by anemia (i.e., a decrease in RBC mass) can only be confirmed by a CBC, which includes estimates of the RBC mass: the volume of packed RBCs, the hematocrit, and the hemoglobin level. Because expansion of the intravascular volume can decrease the hematocrit, hemoglobin or hematocrit values should be interpreted with the patient's intravascular volume status in mind.

▼ APPROACH TO THE PATIENT

A child who presents with pallor and appears ill could have a **potentially life-threatening illness.** Most patients with **shock** are **pale and lethargic and often have cool extremities.** After the patient is stabilized, **routine blood work**

TABLE 58.2. Clinical Evaluation of Pediatric Patients with Pallor

Question	If the Answer is "Yes," Consider. . .
History	
Has the child been lethargic with a sudden onset of pallor?	An acute process such as head trauma, bacterial infection, hypoglycemia, an acute anemia
Has the child had a slow onset of pallor with other major systemic symptoms?	A chronic illness such as cystic fibrosis, nephrotic syndrome, malignancy
Does the child have a known chronic disease?	Anemia of chronic disease
Is the child an infant whose diet primarily consists of cow's milk?	Iron-deficiency anemia
Is the child African-American?	G6PD deficiency, SCD, thalassemia syndromes
Is the child of Mediterranean or Asian descent?	G6PD deficiency, thalassemia syndromes
Are the child's parents pale without a history of anemia?	Constitutional pallor
Is the child a neonate?	Acute or chronic blood loss, hemolytic disease of the newborn
Physical examination	
Are there tongue abnormalities?	Nutritional deficiencies
Are there congenital anomalies?	Fanconi anemia, Diamond-Blackfan anemia, congenital infections
Is the child ill-appearing with lymphadenopathy and hepatosplenomegaly?	Chronic systemic illness, congenital infection, malignancy
Does the child have jaundice and hepatosplenomegaly?	A hemolytic process
Does the child have petechiae, ecchymoses, or excessive bleeding?	A platelet or coagulation disorder
Does the child have hepatomegaly or a gallop on cardiovascular examination?	Congestive heart failure
Laboratory studies	
Is the MCV low for age?	Iron-deficiency anemia, thalassemia, sideroblastic anemia, anemia of chronic disease
Is the MCHC low with microcytic, hypochromic RBC morphology?	Iron-deficiency anemia, thalassemia, sideroblastic anemia, anemia of chronic disease
Is the MCV elevated?	Megaloblastic anemia, reticulocytosis, hypothyroidism, trisomy 21, liver disease
Is there a normocytic, normochromic anemia?	Acute or chronic blood loss, hemoglobinopathies, early iron-deficiency anemia, infection, RBC membrane or enzyme abnormalities, hypersplenism
Is there an elevated RDW?	SCD, iron-deficiency anemia, megaloblastic anemias, thalassemia
Are the BUN and creatinine levels elevated?	Uremia, hemolytic-uremic syndrome

Continued

TABLE 58.2. Clinical Evaluation of Pediatric Patients with Pallor (continued)

Question	If the Answer is "Yes," Consider. . .
Are there prominent target cells?	Liver disease, thalassemia, hemoglobinopathies
Are there prominent burr cells?	Liver disease, renal disease, dehydration, pyruvate kinase deficiency, artifact
Are there prominent schistocytes?	Severe hemolytic anemia, microangiopathic hemolytic process, Kasabach-Merritt syndrome, hemolytic-uremic syndrome, thrombotic thrombocytopenic purpura
Are there prominent elliptocytes?	Hereditary elliptocytosis, iron-deficiency anemia, normal variant
Is there prominent basophilic stippling?	Consider iron-deficiency anemia, lead poisoning, thalassemias, unstable hemoglobins
Are there prominent blister cells?	G6PD deficiency
Are there prominent Howell-Jolly bodies?	Postsplenectomy patient, megaloblastic anemia

BUN = blood urea nitrogen; G6PD = glucose-6-phosphate-dehydrogenase; MCHC = mean corpuscular hemoglobin concentration; MCV = mean corpuscular volume; RBC = red blood cell; RDW = red blood cell distribution width index; SCD = sickle cell disease.

TABLE 58.3. Causes of Anemia in Neonates

Blood loss
  Fetomaternal hemorrhage
  Placental abnormalities
    Abruptio placentae
    Placenta previa
  Twin-to-twin transfusion
  Excessive blood loss due to a coagulation disorder
  Cord abnormalities
  Hemorrhage
    Cephalohematomas
    Hepatic hematomas
    Intracerebral hemorrhage
    Delivery trauma involving the placenta, the umbilical cord, or both

Hemolytic anemia
  Blood group incompatibility
  Red blood cell membrane or enzyme abnormalities
  Hemoglobinopathies
  Microangiopathic processes

Hypoplastic anemia
  Infections
    Cytomegalovirus infection
    Syphilis
    Toxoplasmosis
    Rubella
    Severe bacterial infections
  Diamond-Blackfan anemia

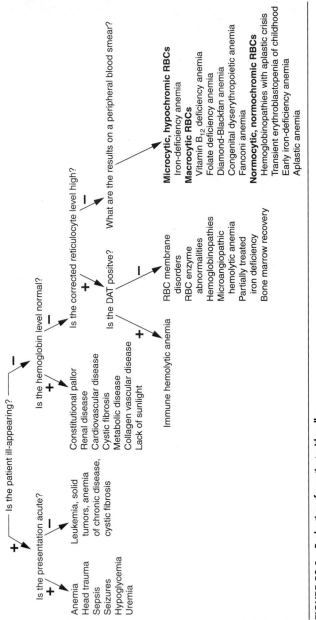

FIGURE 58.1. Evaluation of a patient with pallor.
DAT = direct antibody test; *RBC* = red blood cell.

should be obtained, including a CBC; serum electrolyte panel; serum BUN, creatinine and glucose levels; blood culture; and blood type and cross-match. The brief history should **focus on head trauma** and the presence of **seizures, syncope, prior illness, or fever.**

A child who is pale and well appearing should also have a **CBC, reticulocyte count, and a serum chemistry panel, including bilirubin estimates.** If the hemoglobin is low, the reticulocyte count is high, and the indirect bilirubin fraction is high, then a hemolytic anemia is very likely. A **Coombs or direct antibody test** should be obtained to determine whether the hemolysis is immune mediated.

A **peripheral blood smear** should be examined in all children with anemia. Variations in the RBC shape (poikilocytosis) and size (anisocytosis) should be documented. Laboratory values such as the **MCV and mean corpuscular hemoglobin** should be included in the assessment. The **RBC distribution width** confirms the degree of anisocytosis and is increased in patients with iron-deficiency anemia, SCD, and megaloblastic anemias.

Once the differential diagnosis is narrowed (Figure 58.1), specific tests should be obtained as necessary. For example, iron studies should be obtained for a well-appearing, milk-drinking toddler with a microcytic, hypochromic anemia. Children with a **chronic anemia,** a **severe anemia** with no cause, or an **anemia that is unresponsive** to definitive therapy should be referred to a **pediatric hematologist.**

Suggested Readings

Cohen AR: Pallor. In *Pediatric Emergency Medicine*, 3rd ed. Edited by Fleisher GR, Ludwig S. Baltimore, Williams & Wilkins, 1993, pp 388–396.

Graham EA: The changing face of anemia in infancy. *Pediatr Rev* 15:175, 1994.

Molteim RA: Perinatal blood loss. *Pediatr Rev* 12:47, 1990.

Oski FA: Transient erythroblastopenia. *Pediatr Rev* 4:25, 1982.

Reeves JD, Vichinsky E, Addlego J, et al: Iron deficiency in health and disease. *Adv Pediatr* 30:281, 1984.

Segel GB: Anemia. *Pediatr Rev* 10:77, 1988.

59
Paraplegia
AMY R. BROOKS-KAYAL

▼ INTRODUCTION

Paraplegia is any **weakness of the lower extremities** caused by dysfunction of the nervous system at the level of the peripheral nerves, spinal cord, or brain. Some paraplegias have **congenital causes** (tethered cord, syringomyelia, familial spastic paraparesis, spastic diplegia). Those that are **acquired** are grouped by timing of onset:

▼ **Acute** (evolving over minutes to hours)—trauma, spinal cord infarction
▼ **Subacute** (evolving over hours to days)—transverse myelitis, viral myelitis, epidural abscess, Guillain-Barré syndrome
▼ **Chronic** (evolving over weeks to months)—tumors

▼ DIFFERENTIAL DIAGNOSIS LIST
Infectious Causes

Epidural abscess
Viral myelitis
Discitis
Polyradiculoneuropathy
Tubercular osteomyelitis

Neoplastic Causes

Astrocytoma
Ependymoma
Neuroblastoma
Other—e.g., glioma, ganglioglioma, meningioma, neurofibroma

Traumatic Causes

Contusion
Transection
Epidural hematoma

Congenital or Vascular Causes

Spastic diplegia
Cord infarction
Arteriovenous malformation (AVM)
Congenital malformations—myelomeningocele, tethered cord, syringomyelia

Genetic/Metabolic Causes

Familial spastic paraparesis
Adrenal myeloneuropathy (rarely presents in childhood)

Inflammatory Causes

Transverse myelitis
Guillain-Barré syndrome (acute inflammatory demyelinating polyneuropathy)
Chronic inflammatory demyelinating polyneuropathy (CIDP)

Psychosocial Causes

Conversion disorder

▼ DIFFERENTIAL DIAGNOSIS DISCUSSION
Trauma
Etiology

Spinal cord injury is usually associated with major force, such as occurs with **significant trauma.** The most common causes of traumatic paraplegia are **motor vehicle accidents** and **sports-related injuries,** although **gunshot injuries** are increasingly more common. Trauma can result in contusion, acute edema, compression secondary to epidural hematoma, or actual transection.

Clinical Features

Initial examination shows **weak, flaccid muscles; absent reflexes;** and **sensory loss** below the level of the lesion (spinal shock). **Bowel and bladder dysfunction** is typical. **Autonomic disturbance** (e.g., sweating, piloerection) is usually found below the level of the lesion. Over a period of weeks to months, **flaccidity evolves into spasticity, hyperreflexia,** and **extensor plantar responses.**

Evaluation

The **neck must be stabilized** in a cervical collar until the stability of the cervical spine is established. **Magnetic resonance imaging (MRI)** should be done to differentiate contusion or transection from epidural hematoma. Plain radiographs or **computed tomography (CT)** of the spine may also be helpful to evaluate for vertebral fractures and dislocations.

Treatment

▼ **Spinal-dose steroids** (i.e., intravenous methylprednisolone, 30 mg/kg over 1 hour) should be initiated immediately (within 8 hours of injury). The initial dose is followed with 5.4 mg/kg/hr for 24 hours (if treatment is initiated less than 3 hours after injury) or 48 hours (if treatment is initiated 3–8 hours after injury).

▼ **Neurosurgical intervention** may be required for decompression of epidural hematomas or reduction and stabilization of vertebral fracture.

▼ **Meticulous supportive care,** including good bowel and bladder management and deep venous thrombosis (DVT) prophylaxis with sequential compression stockings is essential. Subcutaneous heparin 5000 units twice a day or low-molecular-weight heparin may be added in patients at particularly high risk for DVT.

Spinal Cord Infarction

Etiology

Spinal cord infarction is usually the result of **occlusion** of the **anterior spinal artery,** which supplies blood to the ventral two-thirds of the cord. The most common causes in children are dissection secondary to **trauma, infection, emboli** in patients with cardiac disease, or **thrombosis** in patients with hypercoagulable states.

Clinical Features

Patients with spinal cord infarction present with **flaccid motor paralysis, areflexia,** and **dissociated sensory loss** (loss of pain and temperature sensation with sparing of vibration and position sense) below the level of arterial occlusion. **Bowel and bladder dysfunction** are usual. **Back pain** is sometimes present. Over weeks to months, **flaccidity evolves** into **spasticity,** with hyperreflexia, clonus, and extensor plantar responses.

Evaluation

An **MRI** of the spine should be performed to look for evidence of cord infarction. A **spinal arteriogram** should also be considered. Evaluations for cardiac disease and hypercoagulable states should be performed if there is no obvious cause for the occlusion.

Treatment

Intravenous corticosteroids should be administered early to minimize cord edema, which may result in additional ischemia. **Anticoagulation** should be considered in **selected patients,** including those with hypercoagulable states, cardiogenic emboli, or vascular dissection.

Transverse Myelitis

Etiology

Transverse myelitis is an **acute inflammatory, demyelinating disorder** of the cord. It can occur as a complication of systemic **viral infections** (infectious mononucleosis [EBV], varicella, mumps, rabies, rubella, rubeola, influenza, HIV) or **bacterial infections** (cat scratch disease, *Mycoplasma pneumoniae*), **autoimmune disorders** (lupus), **immunizations** (rare), and **multiple sclerosis** (MS).

Clinical Features

The mean age of onset is 9 years. The patient presents with **thoracic back pain, lower extremity numbness, leg weakness** (symmetric or asymmetric), and **progressive urinary retention or incontinence.** Initial findings include weak, flaccid muscles (symmetric or asymmetric); absent reflexes; and sensory loss below the level of the lesion. Optic disc swelling and decreased vision or vision loss are often present in patients with Devic disease (i.e., transverse myelitis accompanied by optic neuritis), although the ocular symptoms may occur after the onset of spinal symptoms. Spasticity, hyperreflexia, clonus, and extensor plantar responses are seen later in the course of the disease.

Evaluation

A **lumbar puncture (LP)** should be performed to check for cerebrospinal fluid (CSF) opening pressure (normal to slightly elevated), protein level (usually increased) and electrophoresis (looking for oligoclonal bands), and cell count (usually a mixed pleocytosis of less than 200 cells/mm^3). **Spinal MRI** often shows swelling and abnormal signal at the level of the lesion. **Head MRI** should also be performed to look for other areas of demyelination suggestive of MS. **Viral serologies** (including HIV) may be helpful in identifying a triggering viral infection. **Antinuclear antibody panel and complement levels** should be considered as a screen for an autoimmune disorder.

Treatment

Usual therapy is a 3- to 5-day course of **high-dose intravenous methylprednisolone** (15 mg/kg/day, maximum 1 gm/day) followed by a **4-week prednisone taper.** Use of intravenous immunoglobulin has also been reported. **Supportive care** and intensive **physical therapy** are critical.

Viral Myelitis

Etiology

Viral myelitis is the **acute segmental infection of anterior horn cells.** Viruses most commonly responsible include poliovirus, group B coxsackievirus, and echoviruses.

Clinical Features

The patient usually has a history of **malaise, myalgias, low-grade fever,** and **upper respiratory tract symptoms progressing to severe headache** and **nuchal rigidity.** **Areflexia** and **flaccidity** and weakness of the muscles (usually asymmetric) are often heralded by pain in the spine and affected limbs. **Bulbar weakness** may also be present. There are usually no sensory symptoms.

Evaluation

The **most important diagnostic test is the LP,** which demonstrates pleocytosis (50–200 cells/mm^3). The predominance of polymorphonuclear cells is replaced by lymphocytes after the first week. CSF protein may be normal or slightly elevated, and CSF glucose is usually normal. **Viral isolation from CSF, stool, and nasopharyngeal swabs,** as well as **acute and convalescent viral titers,** can help confirm the diagnosis.

Treatment

Treatment of viral myelitis is **supportive.**

Epidural Abscess

Etiology

Epidural abscess is most commonly caused by the hematogenous spread of **bacteria,** usually *Staphylococcus aureus* in older children. The most common location is the **dorsal surface** of the **midthoracic** or **lower lumbar spine.**

Clinical Evaluation

Characteristically, the history includes **severe, localized back pain** (worse with cough or flexion) and **fever,** often associated with **headache, vomiting,** and a **stiff neck. Radiating pain** begins 3–6 days after the onset of back pain, followed by progressive **paraplegia** and **bladder dysfunction.** Examination shows localized spinal tenderness, lower extremity hyperreflexia, and spasticity (in patients with thoracic lesions) or hyporeflexia and decreased tone (in patients with lower lumbar lesions).

Evaluation

If epidural abscess is suspected, LP should not be performed because it can result in iatrogenic meningitis. **MRI,** on the other hand, is safe and demonstrates the lesion well.

Treatment

Initial treatment is with a **broad-spectrum intravenous antibiotic** with antistaphylococcal activity. Once a specific organism has been identified and sensitivities established, antibiotic therapy can be tailored to the patient. **Surgical drainage** may be required if there is evidence of cord compression.

Guillain-Barré Syndrome

Etiology

Guillain-Barré syndrome is an immune-mediated, acute, **inflammatory demyelinating polyneuropathy.** Approximately 50% of patients with Guillain-Barré syndrome have a history of antecedent viral infection.

Clinical Features

The syndrome can present at any age, but is **uncommon in children younger than 3 years.** Often the first symptoms are **transient dysesthesias** and **muscle aches.** A typical feature is rapidly progressive, symmetric motor weakness beginning distally and ascending proximally. **Areflexia** is the rule, and may precede significant weakness (e.g., biceps and triceps jerks may be lost while the arms are only minimally weak). **Facial weakness** and other cranial nerve involvement may be present in up to half of patients. Weakness can progress to include **respiratory muscles** with resultant hypoventilation. Although mild, symmetric, length-dependent sensory changes are common, extensive sensory loss or a sensory level should not be present. **Autonomic instability** (e.g., unstable blood pressure, cardiac arrhythmia) may occur.

Evaluation

On **LP,** patients with Guillain-Barré syndrome demonstrate **elevated CSF protein** with a paucity of cells (seen after the first week of illness). **Nerve conduction studies** show **reduced nerve conduction velocities** and **motor conduction block.** **Vital capacity** and **negative inspiratory potentials** should be monitored closely as indicators of impending respiratory failure.

Treatment

Meticulous **supportive care** (particularly of **respiratory function**) is critical. **Plasmapheresis** or **intravenous immune globulin** (2 g/kg divided over 2–5 days) is indicated if the patient loses the ability to ambulate independently.

▓ **HINT** Initially, it can be very difficult to distinguish transverse myelitis, viral myelitis, epidural abscess, and Guillain-Barré syndrome from one another. It may not be possible to get a good sensory examination in an uncooperative child, and all four disorders can initially present with flaccid weakness and areflexia in the lower extremities. Furthermore, many of the diagnostic tests are not helpful until approximately 1 week into the course of the disease; for example, nerve conduction studies and CSF protein levels can both be normal for up to 1 week in Guillain-Barré syndrome. Although the following clues may help, ultimately, the "tincture of time" and repeating studies after 1 week may be required to make a definitive diagnosis.

▼ **A high fever, severe back pain or tenderness,** and an **increased peripheral white blood cell (WBC) count** are suggestive of epidural abscess.
▼ **Reflexes.** If the reflexes are down in the arms as well as the legs, think Guillain-Barré syndrome. Mild symmetric facial weakness (facial diplegia) and diminished gag reflex may also be present in Guillain-Barré syndrome, but should not be seen in a spinal cord process.
▼ **Distribution of weakness.** The weakness in viral myelitis is often asymmetric, whereas Guillain-Barré syndrome and transverse myelitis usually cause symmetric weakness. In transverse myelitis, there is often a complete, uniform paralysis below the level of the lesion; in Guillain-Barré syndrome, the distal muscles tend to be weaker than the proximal muscles.
▼ **Bowel and bladder dysfunction** are suggestive of epidural abscess or transverse myelitis first, but remember that patients with Guillain-Barré syndrome occasionally also have bowel and bladder involvement.

Tumors

Etiology

Astrocytomas and **ependymomas** are the most common intrinsic spinal cord tumors, and **neuroblastoma** is the tumor that most commonly results in extrinsic cord compression (from extension of a paraspinal tumor through the neural foramen).

Clinical Features

Paraplegia caused by tumors presents with **slowly progressive leg weakness, gait difficulty,** and **sensory loss.** Often there is associated **back pain** and **bowel and bladder dysfunction.** Findings on physical examination depend on the location of the tumor: thoracic lesions produce spastic paraplegia with hyperreflexia; tumors involving the conus medullaris and cauda equina produce weak, flaccid muscles with decreased or absent reflexes. **Sensory loss** is present below the level of the tumor. **Scoliosis** is frequently seen in association with intrinsic cord tumors.

Evaluation

Spinal MRI is the diagnostic test of choice for detection of tumors.

Treatment

Initial therapy consists of **dexamethasone** (0.25 mg/kg every 6 hours) to decrease surrounding edema. Definitive treatment depends on the type, extent, and location of the tumor, but usually consists of some combination of **surgery, radiation,** and **chemotherapy.**

Tethered Cord

Etiology

In pediatric patients with tethered cord, the **conus medullaris** is **anchored** to the **base of the vertebral column** by a thickened filum terminale, lipoma, dermal sinus, or other site of traction. As the child grows, the spinal cord is stretched and lumbosacral segments become increasingly ischemic.

Clinical Features

Symptoms can occur at any time between infancy and young adulthood. Typical symptoms are **progressive clumsiness of gait, constipation,** and **urinary incontinence.**

Evaluation

Findings on general examination may include **scoliosis, stunted leg growth,** or **foot deformity** (pes cavus), **pigmentation, tufts of hair,** or a **deep dermal sinus** over the **lower spine.** On neurologic examination, **spastic leg weakness, hyperreflexia,** and **extensor plantar responses** are present.

Treatment

Surgery is required to release the cord.

Syringomyelia

Etiology

Syringomyelia is a **cavity within the spinal cord,** usually resulting from a congenital neural tube malformation. This condition most commonly occurs in the cervical and lumbar spinal cord segments.

Clinical Features

Syringomyelia often presents in adolescence or later with **progressive weakness** and **sensory loss.** Motor examination results depend on the **location of the lesion. Cervical lesions** show flaccid paralysis and hyperreflexia of the arms with spasticity and hyperreflexia in the legs; **lumbar lesions** present with flaccid paralysis of the legs with hyporeflexia, fasciculations, and muscle atrophy. Interruption of the **crossing spinothalamic fibers** in the central cord produces a "cape distribution" of pain and temperature sensation loss with relative sparing of light touch and proprioception.

Evaluation

The diagnostic test of choice is an **MRI.**

Treatment

Symptomatic congenital cord malformations are treated **surgically.**

Familial Spastic Paraparesis

Etiology

Familial spastic paraparesis is an **inherited progressive spastic paraparesis.** The genetics are complex, with autosomal dominant transmission seen in 70% of patients, but autosomal recessive and X-linked recessive transmission also reported. The mean age of onset in childhood type I familial spastic paraparesis is 11–16 years.

Clinical Features

Toe walking and **slowly progressive gait disturbance** are typical. One-third of patients present with **urinary symptoms.** On examination, **spasticity** is out of proportion to weakness. **Hyperreflexia** involves all four extremities, and **ankle clonus** may be present. One-third of patients have **pes cavus deformity.** The autosomal recessive form can also be associated with ataxia, sensory neuropathy, and pseudobulbar palsy.

Evaluation

Genetic testing for familial spastic paraparesis is of limited clinical utility at present. **Exclusion** of other, treatable disorders is critical. **MRI** of the spine can be useful to rule out structural disorders (e.g., vascular malformation, tumor, syringomyelia) or demyelination. **Vitamin B_{12}, vitamin E,** and **very-long-chain fatty acid levels** should be obtained. Eliciting a **family history** of similarly affected individuals is critical.

Treatment

No specific treatment is available.

Spastic Diplegia

Etiology

In this form of cerebral palsy (CP), **all four extremities** are involved to some degree; however, the lower extremities are affected much more significantly than the upper extremities.

Clinical Features

In early infancy (younger than 4 months), muscle tone is usually normal or hypotonic. Between the ages of 4 months and 1 year, there is an **insidious** onset of lower extremity spasticity, often associated with delay in sitting, crawling, and walking. **Toe walking** is common. On examination, there is **spasticity** and **hyperreflexia,** involving the legs more than the arms. **Scissoring** of the legs, ankle clonus, and extensor plantar responses are common.

Evaluation

Historical information suggesting premature birth or possible perinatal injury could be significant. **Brain MRI** may demonstrate evidence of periventricular leukomalacia or other evidence of perinatal injury.

Treatment

Supportive therapy often includes **physical and occupational therapy, bracing,** and, if needed, **botulinum toxin injections** or **surgical release** for treatment of contractures.

▼ EVALUATION OF PARAPLEGIA
Patient History

The history should include the following information:

▼ Timing of onset of symptoms (acute, subacute, or chronic)
▼ Trauma
▼ Fever
▼ Back pain
▼ Changes in sensation—if so, in what distribution?
▼ Bowel and bladder dysfunction
▼ Visual problems—past or present
▼ Previous weakness, numbness, or other neurologic symptoms
▼ Family history of leg weakness

Physical Examination

The following should be sought on physical examination:

▼ **General examination**—evidence of head, neck, or back trauma; scoliosis; stunted leg growth; foot deformity (pes cavus); or pigmentation, tufts of hair, or a deep dermal sinus over the lower spine
▼ **Cranial nerve examination**—look for papillitis (associated with transverse myelitis in Devic disease); eye movement abnormalities (associated with transverse myelitis secondary to MS); Horner syndrome (associated with cervical cord trauma); facial diplegia and decreased gag reflex (associated with Guillain-Barré syndrome).
▼ **Motor strength, tone, and reflexes in arms and legs**—weak, flaccid leg muscles and absent reflexes (associated with acute cord processes and Guillain-Barré syndrome); spasticity, hyperreflexia, and extensor plantar responses (associated with chronic spinal cord processes)
▼ **Sensation to all sensory modalities**—a sensory level (associated with spinal cord problems); mild distal sensory changes (associated with Guillain-Barré syndrome)
▼ **Autonomic disturbances**—associated with cord processes (usually found below the level of the lesion) or Guillain-Barré syndrome.

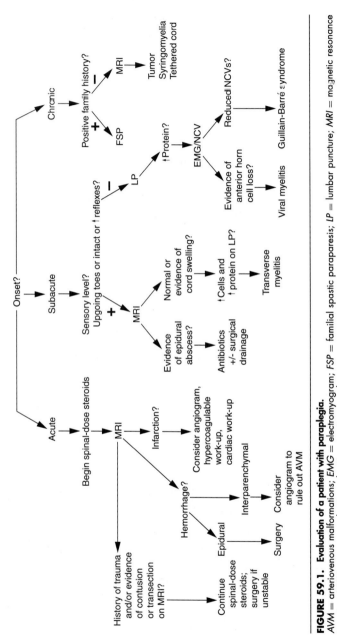

FIGURE 59.1. Evaluation of a patient with paraplegia.

AVM = arteriovenous malformations; EMG = electromyogram; FSP = familial spastic paraparesis; LP = lumbar puncture; MRI = magnetic resonance imaging; NCV = nerve conduction velocities; ↑ = increased.

Laboratory Studies and Diagnostic Modalities

The usual work-up for a patient with paraplegic symptoms includes a **MRI,** an **electromyogram (EMG), nerve conduction velocity studies,** and an **LP.** Several timing factors may cause false-negative results (e.g., CSF protein levels and nerve conduction studies may be normal for up to 1 week in patients with Guillain-Barré syndrome; MRI may not demonstrate cord swelling or signal changes in the first 24 hours in patients with transverse myelitis or cord infarction).

▼ TREATMENT OF ACUTE PARAPLEGIA

If there is any suspicion of cord trauma, the **neck should be stabilized** and spinal-dose **steroids** should be administered. **DVT prophylaxis with sequential compression stockings** is essential. **Subcutaneous heparin** 5000 units twice a day or low-molecular-weight heparin may be added in patients at particularly high risk of DVT, but only after hemorrhage has been ruled out. Urinary retention is common, so an **indwelling bladder** (Foley) **catheter** should be placed or intermittent bladder catheterizations should be performed. **Histamine blockers** should be administered to prevent gastritis. Autonomic instability may be a problem, so careful monitoring of heart rate and **blood pressure** are essential.

▼ APPROACH TO THE PATIENT (FIGURE 59.1)

Suggested Readings

Bracken MB, Shepard MJ, Holford TR, et al: Administration of methylprednisolone for 24 or 48 hours or tirilazad mesylate for 48 hrs in the treatment of acute spinal cord injury. *JAMA* 277:1597–1604, 1997.

Goldstein EM: Spasticity management: an overview. *J Child Neurol* 16(1):16–23, 2001.

Jones HR Jr: Guillain-Barré syndrome: perspectives with infants and children. *Semin Pediatr Neurol* 7(2):91–102, 2000.

Rust RS: Multiple sclerosis, acute disseminated encephalomyelitis, and related conditions. *Semin Pediatr Neurol* 7(2):66–90, 2000.

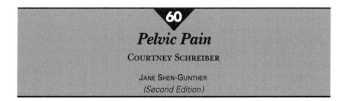

60
Pelvic Pain
COURTNEY SCHREIBER

JANE SHEN-GUNTHER
(Second Edition)

▼ INTRODUCTION

Knowledge regarding the location of organs in the female pelvic region and how they may be involved to cause discomfort is key to the evaluation of pelvic pain in female patients. The main areas of concern are **uterine and ovarian infection and inflammation.**

▼ DIFFERENTIAL DIAGNOSIS LIST
Reproductive Tract Causes

Infectious causes—pelvic inflammatory disease (PID), postabortion endometritis

Traumatic causes—falls, accidents, sexual molestation

Neoplastic causes—ovarian tumors (neoplastic, nonneoplastic), ovarian cysts (with or without rupture, hemorrhage, torsion), uterine fibroids

Congenital causes—obstructive müllerian tract anomalies

Gynecologic causes—endometriosis, dysmenorrhea, mittelschmerz, adhesions, adenomyosis

Pregnancy-related causes—abortion in progress, ectopic pregnancy, labor, postpartum endometritis

Intestinal Tract Causes

Infectious causes—acute appendicitis, Meckel diverticulitis, giardiasis

Inflammatory causes—mesenteric adenitis, regional enteritis, ulcerative colitis, pancreatitis

Congenital causes—midgut malrotation

Metabolic causes—lactose malabsorption

Miscellaneous causes—volvulus, intestinal obstruction, chronic constipation

Neoplasia

Urinary Tract Causes

Infectious causes—cystitis, pyelonephritis

Congenital causes—ureteropelvic junction obstruction

Miscellaneous causes—ureteral calculus, interstitial cystitis, detrusor instability

Other Causes

Pelvic bone and joint infections

Slipped femoral epiphysis

Abdominal wall trigger points

Acute intermittent porphyria

Henoch-Schönlein purpura

Abdominal epilepsy

Psychologic or emotional causes

Herpes zoster

▼ DIFFERENTIAL DIAGNOSIS DISCUSSION
Ovarian Cysts
Etiology

During puberty, gonadotropin-releasing hormone (GnRH) secretion from the hypothalamus resumes and **levels of the gonadotropins** (follicle-stimulating hormone and luteinizing hormone) **rise.** The surge in gonadotropins usually is **not cyclical** in adolescents, as it is in adults. The **constant stimulus of gonadotropins on the ovaries results in multiple follicular cysts** that may range from a few millimeters to 8 cm in diameter. Pain is caused by follicular distention, rupture, hemorrhage, or ovarian torsion, and peritoneal irritation.

Clinical Features

Most follicular cysts are **asymptomatic. Large follicular cysts** may cause a **vague, constant, dull sensation or a heaviness in the pelvis. Extreme distention with rupture or torsion of the cyst and ovary** may result in **acute, severe pelvic pain.**

Evaluation

Tender, slightly enlarged ovaries may be appreciated. Rarely, a large cystic ovary is identified.

A **CBC** is obtained to **rule out rupture and internal hemorrhage. A pregnancy test** is ordered to rule out pregnancy. **Pelvic ultrasound** may reveal ovarian cysts or fluid in the cul-de-sac.

Treatment

For **mildly symptomatic** patients, **reassurance** may be all that is necessary. The cyst should be observed using **serial ultrasound.** When observation is unsatisfactory, **nonsteroidal anti-inflammatory drugs (NSAIDs), oral contraceptives, or both** may be prescribed to relieve pain and suppress the cysts. **Laparoscopy** is indicated in the presence of a hemorrhagic cyst, ovarian torsion, or a persistent cyst.

Pelvic Inflammatory Disease (PID)

PID is discussed in Chapter 73, "Sexually Transmitted Diseases."

Adnexal Torsion

Etiology

Adnexal torsion is the **twisting of a fallopian tube or both the fallopian tube and the ovary on its pedicle.** This results in **vascular occlusion, ischemia, and tissue death.** A normal tube or ovary cannot "twist" without **predisposing factors** (e.g., ovarian cysts or tumors, tubal neoplasm, parovarian cysts). **Enlargement of the ovary** puts it at **risk for torsing,** especially if it is larger than 5 cm.

Clinical Features

Abdominal pain may develop **suddenly or gradually.** It is usually **paroxysmal and intermittent.** It tends to be **unilateral** and **localized** to the involved adnexa. As the ischemia becomes more extensive, the **pain worsens and becomes persistent.** Associated symptoms include **nausea, vomiting, and a sense of fullness in the lower abdomen.**

Evaluation

The patient usually appears in **acute distress. Mild tachycardia** (i.e., a heart rate greater than 100 beats/min) and a **slight elevation of temperature** ($< 38°C$) may be present. The abdominal examination may reveal **tenderness in the iliac fossa.** With increasing ischemia and peritoneal irritation, **guarding, rebound tenderness, and decreased bowel sounds** may be noted. On pelvic examination, a **tender adnexal mass** may be noted. On **rectal examination of the prepubertal child,** a **tender mass** may be felt in the **lower abdomen.**

The WBC count is normal or slightly elevated. Urinalysis is normal. **Pelvic ultrasonography** reveals an **adnexal mass** in most patients, and a **lack of blood flow to the torsed adnexa.**

Treatment

Evidence of an acute surgical abdomen warrants **laparoscopy** and possibly **exploratory laparotomy.** If the **ovary and tube are strangulated and infarcted, removal without untwisting** the pedicle is indicated. If the **torsion is incomplete** and the adnexa appears to be viable, the **adnexa may be preserved.**

Endometriosis

Etiology

Endometriosis is the presence of **endometrial tissue outside of the uterus.** Theories of pathogenesis include retrograde menstruation, direct implantation, coelomic metaplasia, and lymphatic and hematogenous spread. A polygenic multifactorial mode of inheritance has also been demonstrated. The major distinction between endometriosis in adolescents and adults is its **association with congenital anomalies of the reproductive tract in the pubertal patient.** Premenarchal patients are not affected by this disease because the **onset of menses must precede the development of endometriosis.**

Clinical Features

Characteristically, the pelvic pain is described as **cramping in the pelvic or sacral region** that is **aggravated during menstruation.** The pain may also be **intermittent, chronic, and not related to the menstrual cycle.** Other symptoms in the adolescent may include **abnormal bleeding, amenorrhea, dyspareunia, and gastrointestinal or urinary complaints.**

Evaluation

Examination under anesthesia may be necessary for an adequate pelvic examination **in the virginal adolescent.** A search for **anomalies of the hymen, vagina, cervix, uterus, and adnexa** is mandatory. In **older patients,** the finding of **pain on palpation of the adnexa** (i.e., the ovary and fallopian tube), **in the cul-de-sac, or along the uterosacral ligaments** suggests the possibility of endometriosis. Occasionally, **enlargement of the ovary** (endometrioma) or **fixation of the pelvic organs as a result of adhesions** may be noted.

Endocervical cultures for gonorrhea and chlamydia are obtained to rule out the possibility of pelvic infection. The **cancer antigen 125 test titer** may be elevated but is not sensitive or specific for endometriosis. A **pregnancy test** is obtained to rule out pregnancy.

Pelvic ultrasonography is useful when examination is difficult and is indicated when a palpable pelvic mass is noted. **Magnetic resonance imaging (MRI)** is helpful in delineating the pelvic anatomy and establishing the diagnosis of congenital müllerian anomalies. **Laparoscopy with visualization or biopsy** of endometriosis lesions is essential to confirm or eliminate the diagnosis of endometriosis.

Treatment

NSAIDs remain the first line of medical therapy for pain control. **Calcium-channel blockers** are also effective for adolescent dysmenorrhea. When pain persists or NSAIDs are contraindicated, **low-dose** (35 μg) **estrogen oral contraceptives** may be prescribed to suppress ovulation. GnRH agonists can cause osteoporosis, so their use is limited in younger patients. When medical therapy fails, **laparoscopy** is indicated to evaluate for pelvic pathology. Surgical treatment of endometriosis entails **laparoscopic fulguration or laser**

vaporization of endometriosis and **lysis of adhesions.** Patients with outflow obstruction require **corrective or reconstructive surgery** to create a patent genital tract.

Ectopic Pregnancy

Etiology

An ectopic pregnancy is one in which a **fertilized ovum implants itself outside the uterine cavity (most often in the fallopian tube)** as a result of **delayed passage** of the fertilized ovum into the uterine cavity. **Abdominal, cervical, and ovarian ectopic pregnancies** can also occur. Delayed passage of the fertilized ovum into the uterine cavity usually results from a **condition that interferes with tubal structure or function** (e.g., chronic salpingitis, pelvic adhesive disease, tubal surgery, congenital abnormalities of the fallopian tube, intrauterine devices).

Clinical Features

The **classic triad of symptoms** consists of **abdominal pain, amenorrhea, and intermittent, scanty vaginal bleeding.** The abdominal pain may develop **suddenly or gradually.** In **unruptured ectopic pregnancies,** the pain tends to be **unilateral, colicky, and localized** to the involved adnexa. If **rupture** has occurred, the pain becomes **diffuse, intense, and prostrating.** Referred shoulder pain occurs in the presence of hemoperitoneum. **Dizziness and syncope** are the result of anemia and hypotension.

Evaluation

▼ **Abdominal examination.** Localized tenderness may be revealed in the lower quadrant. With rupture and intra-abdominal bleeding, rebound tenderness and guarding are elicited. On pelvic examination, the cervix and uterus may be soft and tender from the effects of pregnancy hormones. Adnexal fullness or a discrete, tender mass may be noted in some patients.

▼ **CBC.** The hemoglobin and hematocrit values may be low in patients with acute or gradual intraperitoneal hemorrhage; in the absence of bleeding, they are usually normal.

▼ **Type and screen.** Rh status is assessed in case blood replacement is necessary.

▼ **A pregnancy test** [β-human chorionic gonadotropin (β-HCG)] is positive and the quantitative beta HCG should be drawn.

▼ **Vaginal ultrasonography** can detect an intrauterine gestational sac as early as 5 weeks' gestation and may show an adnexal mass or complex free fluid in the pelvis. An adnexal mass seen on ultrasound further substantiates the diagnosis of an ectopic pregnancy. Free fluid in the cul-de-sac seen on ultrasound suggests hemoperitoneum and the necessity of early surgical intervention.

HINT A positive pregnancy test and an empty uterus beyond 5–6 weeks' gestation, calculated by the last menstrual period, is presumptive evidence of an ectopic pregnancy.

Treatment

Surgical diagnosis and treatment via **laparoscopy or laparotomy** is almost always indicated to manage an ectopic pregnancy, although medical treatment with **methotrexate** may be indicated for an **unruptured** ectopic pregnancy. **Early gynecologic consultation** is recommended.

Congenital Obstructive Müllerian Malformations

Etiology

The differentiation and development of the urogenital system in the embryo and fetus is complex. Developmental errors may occur along this sequential process, resulting in distinctive structural abnormalities. Obstructive müllerian malformations include **imperforate hymen, transverse vaginal septum, and various types of uterine anomalies.**

Clinical Features

Often obstructive müllerian abnormalities are **asymptomatic** and not diagnosed **until an adolescent girl presents with primary amenorrhea and recurrent pelvic pain.** The obstruction, leading to **increasing collection of menstrual fluid,** causes **distention of the uterus and vagina** and results in **monthly cyclic pain.**

Evaluation

A **genital or rectal examination** is essential whenever a child complains of pelvic or abdominal symptoms. A **pediatric vaginoscope, otoscope, or nasal speculum** may be used to visualize the vagina and cervix. The child can be examined in either the **lithotomy or knee-chest position.** An **imperforate hymen** is diagnosed by **simple inspection.** In **infants and children, the hymen** may be **bulging and distended by mucus.** In **adolescents, menstrual blood fills the vagina.** The **transverse vaginal septum** may be **complete or incomplete** and is recognized on vaginoscopy. Uterine anomalies are more difficult to detect unless an abnormally shaped uterus or pelvic mass is noted on examination.

⚡ HINT   Prior to puberty, rectal examination is often the best method for evaluation of the upper genital tract.

Laboratory studies are nondiagnostic. **Pelvic ultrasonography and MRI** are helpful in the detection of uterine anomalies. Because the embryonic differentiation and development of the urologic system occurs around the same time as that of the genital system, **errors in development of the urologic system** must be sought using **intravenous pyelography.**

Treatment

An imperforate hymen is **opened surgically. In infants,** the hymenal membrane is tented and excised centrally with scissors. **In postmenarchal patients,** a portion of the membrane should be excised. In complete transverse vaginal septum, a simple incision is made to allow the egress of secretions in premenarchal patients. The **definitive surgical treatment,** which involves excision of the vaginal septal membrane with a surrounding ring of dense connective tissue, should be **delayed until after puberty,** because technical difficulties may be encountered if the surgery is performed on immature structures.

Anomalies of the uterus (e.g., a blind rudimentary uterine horn) **should not be resected until the patient is postmenarchal.**

Dysmenorrhea

Etiology

Primary dysmenorrhea is **painful menstruation with no demonstrable cause.**

▼ **Patients with primary dysmenorrhea** have a greater endometrial production of prostaglandins, which causes uterine contractions, uterine ischemia, and pelvic pain.

▼ **Secondary dysmenorrhea** results from various pathological conditions (e.g., endometriosis, salpingitis, or congenital müllerian anomalies).

Clinical Features

Symptoms of **primary dysmenorrhea** usually begin **6–12 months after menarche** when ovulation is established. The pain is described as **crampy, lower abdominal pain,** starting within **several hours of the onset of menses.** The pain usually lasts for **1–2 days.** Associated symptoms include **headache, nausea, vomiting, diarrhea, and backache.** The symptoms of **secondary dysmenorrhea** are **similar** to those described for primary dysmenorrhea, although they are **not associated with menarche.**

Evaluation

In patients with **primary dysmenorrhea** the **physical examination is normal.** Findings in **secondary dysmenorrhea** are related to the **underlying cause.**

A **CBC, erythrocyte sedimentation rate (ESR),** and **endocervical cultures for gonorrhea and chlamydia** are obtained to evaluate for possible infection. A **pregnancy test** is obtained to rule out pregnancy.

MRI is helpful in the diagnosis of müllerian abnormalities. **Pelvic ultrasonography** is useful for delineating the internal pelvic anatomy when examination is difficult.

Treatment

If the pelvic examination is normal, treatment is aimed at **symptomatic relief. Mild analgesics** (e.g., aspirin, acetaminophen, ibuprofen) may be used. Initially, if pain relief is unsatisfactory, the next step is to prescribe one of the **NSAIDs** (e.g., ibuprofen, naproxen sodium, mefenamic acid, meclofenamate). These medications should be initiated at or before the onset of menses and continued for the first 1–2 days of the menses. If dysmenorrhea persists, a course of **low-dose oral contraceptives** may be initiated to suppress ovulation. When the pain is refractory to all medical therapy, **laparoscopy** is indicated to evaluate for pelvic pathology, such as endometriosis, adhesions, or ovarian cysts.

▼ EVALUATION OF PELVIC PAIN

Patient History

The causes of acute and chronic pelvic pain are numerous (Table 60.1 and Table 60.2). The most important tool for making the correct diagnosis is a detailed history. The following information should be sought:

▼ Menstrual history, sexual history, and gynecologic history, including method of contraception (in postmenarchal patients)

TABLE 60.1. Age-related Prevalence of Principal Laparoscopic Findings in 121 Adolescent Females 11 to 17 Years Old with Acute Pelvic Pain (The Children's Hospital, Boston, 1980–1986)

	Number of Patients		
Diagnosis	Age 11–13	Age 14–15	Age 16–17
Ovarian cyst	12 (50%)	16 (35%)	19 (37%)
Acute pelvic inflammatory disease	4 (17%)	7 (16%)	10 (19%)
Adnexal torsion	0 (0%)	7 (16%)	2 (4%)
Endometriosis	0 (0%)	2 (4%)	4 (7%)
Ectopic pregnancy	0 (0%)	3 (7%)	1 (2%)
Appendicitis	3 (13%)	4 (9%)	6 (12%)
No pathology	5 (20%)	6 (13%)	10 (19%)
Total	24 (20%)	45 (37%)	52 (43%)

Reprinted from Goldstein DP: Acute and chronic pelvic pain. *Pediatr Clin North Am* 36(3):576, 1989.

▼ Psychosocial history (to assess the possibility of stress, substance abuse, or sexual or physical abuse)
▼ A detailed description of the pain (onset, location, character, frequency, duration, intensity, progression, exacerbating and relieving factors)

Physical Examination

The following should be sought on physical examination:

▼ Structural abnormalities
▼ The reproduction of pain on palpation of specific abdominopelvic structures
▼ Signs of peritonitis (guarding, rigidity, rebound tenderness)

TABLE 60.2. Age-Related Incidence of Laparoscopic Findings in 129 Adolescent Females 11 to 21 Years Old with Chronic Pelvic Pain (The Children's Hospital, Boston, 1980–1983)

	Number of Patients				
Diagnosis	Age 11–13	Age 14–15	Age 16–17	Age 18–19	Age 20–21
Endometriosis	2 (12%)	9 (28%)	21 (40%)	17 (45%)	7 (54%)
Postoperative adhesions	1 (6%)	4 (13%)	7 (13%)	5 (13%)	2 (15%)
Serositis	5 (29%)	4 (13%)	0 (0%)	2 (5%)	0 (0%)
Ovarian cyst	2 (12%)	2 (6%)	3 (5%)	2 (5%)	0 (8%)
Uterine malformation	1 (6%)	0 (0%)	1 (2%)	0 (0%)	1 (0%)
Others	0 (0%)	1 (3%)	2 (4%)	1 (3%)	0 (0%)
No pathology	6 (35%)	12 (37%)	19 (36%)	11 (29%)	3 (23%)

Reprinted from Goldstein DP: Acute and chronic pelvic pain. *Pediatr Clin North Am* 36(3):580, 1989.

Laboratory Studies

In the patient with a suspected acute abdomen, the following laboratory studies should be ordered:

▼ CBC
▼ Blood chemistries
▼ Blood type and screen
▼ Pregnancy test (β-HCG)
▼ Urinalysis
▼ Urine culture
▼ Cervical cultures (as indicated)

Suggested Readings

Arbel-DeRowe Y, Tepper R, Rosen DJ, et al: The contribution of pelvic ultrasonography to the diagnostic process in pediatric and adolescent gynecology. *J Pediatr Adolesc Gynecol* 10(1):3–12, 1997.

Carrico CW, Fenton LZ, Taylor GA, et al: Impact of sonography on the diagnosis and treatment of acute lower abdominal pain in children and young adults. Am J Roentgenol 172(2):513–516, 1999.

Goldstein DP: Acute and chronic pelvic pain. *Pediatr Clin North Am* 365:573–580, 1989.

Khoiny FE: Pelvic inflammatory disease in the adolescent. *J Pediatr Health Care* 3(5):230–236, 1989.

Ozaksit G, Caglar T, Zorlu CG, et al: Chronic pelvic pain in adolescent women. Diagnostic laparoscopy and ultrasonography. *J Reprod Med* 40(7):500–502, 1995.

Reese KA, Reddy S, Rock JA: Endometriosis in an adolescent population: the Emory experience. *J Pediatr Adolesc Gynecol* 9(3):125–128, 1996.

Sanfilippo JS: Dysmenorrhea in adolescents. *Female Patient* 18:29–33, 1993.

United States Department of Health and Human Services: 1998 Guidelines for Treatment of Sexually Transmitted Diseases. *MMWR* 47 (RR-1):1–118, 1997.

Vercellini P, Fedele L, Arcaini L, et al: Laparoscopy in the diagnosis of chronic pelvic pain in adolescent women. *J Reprod Med* 34(10):827–830, 1989.

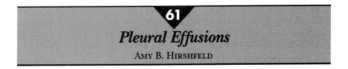

61
Pleural Effusions
AMY B. HIRSHFELD

▼ INTRODUCTION

A pleural effusion is an **accumulation of fluid between the parietal and visceral pleura.** Normally, fluid is produced by the capillaries of the parietal pleura and absorbed by the capillaries of the visceral pleura; only a trivial amount of fluid is left within the pleural space. The Starling relationship governs the net flow of fluid at each capillary bed:

$$F = k[(Pcap - Ppl) - \sigma(\Pi cap - \Pi pl)]$$

Where:

F = the rate of fluid movement
P = the hydrostatic pressure
Π = the oncotic pressure
k = the filtration coefficient
σ = the osmotic reflection coefficient for protein

Lymphatic drainage normally removes excess fluid from the pleural space. Accumulation of a pleural effusion may result from **increased capillary hydrostatic pressure, decreased hydrostatic pressure in the pleural space, decreased capillary oncotic pressure, capillary leak, lymphatic obstruction, movement of fluid from the peritoneal space, or a combination** of these factors.

Pleural effusions are classified according to their etiology as transudative or exudative. Pleural fluid analysis can often distinguish a transudate from an exudate (see "Laboratory Studies" section) and serves as the first step in the differential diagnosis.

▼ **Transudative effusions** are usually secondary to increased hydrostatic pressure or decreased oncotic pressure. The differential diagnosis is relatively straightforward.

▼ **Exudative effusions** are typically seen in diseases that injure the capillary membrane or impair lymphatic drainage. A broad differential diagnosis is implied by an exudative effusion and may require more extensive work-up.

▼ DIFFERENTIAL DIAGNOSIS LIST

Transudative Effusion

Congestive heart failure
Hepatic cirrhosis
Venous hypertension
Nephrotic syndrome
Peritoneal dialysis
Urinothorax
Atelectasis

Exudative Effusions

Infectious Causes

Bacterial infection—parapneumonic effusion/empyema, upper abdominal abscess
Viral infection—e.g., adenovirus
Mycoplasma infection
Mycobacterial infection—*Mycobacterium tuberculosis,* atypical *Mycobacterium*
Legionella infection
AIDS-related infection
Fungal infection—e.g., *Aspergillus, Coccidioides, Histoplasma, Cryptococcus* (latter seen most often in immunocompromised patients)

Parasitic infection—e.g., *Paragonimus westermani*, *Entamoeba histolytica*, *Echinococcus granulosus*, *Pneumocystic carinii*

Neoplastic Causes

Acute lymphoblastic leukemia
Lymphoma
Endodermal sinus tumor
Cervical teratoma
Pleural mesothelioma
Pheochromocytoma
Wilms tumor
Ewing's sarcoma, rhabdomyosarcoma, clear-cell sarcoma
Malignant histiocytosis
Squamous cell carcinoma

Inflammatory Causes

Acute pancreatitis
Pancreatic pseudocyst
Esophageal rupture
Trapped lung
Pulmonary embolism and infarct—e.g., sickle cell disease

Immunologic Causes

Rheumatoid arthritis, lupus pleuritis, sarcoidosis, Wegener granulomatosis
Postcardiac injury syndrome
Kawasaki disease

Lymphatic Causes

Chylothorax—postsurgical, traumatic
Obstruction of lymphatic drainage due to malignancy
Yellow nail syndrome
Congenital lymphangiectasis
Noonan syndrome

Iatrogenic Causes

Radiation therapy
Extravasation from subclavian or jugular central venous lines
Pharmacologic therapy
Surgery—e.g., post lung transplant
Esophageal sclerotherapy
Narrow-bore feeding tube placement

▼ DIFFERENTIAL DIAGNOSIS DISCUSSION

If the etiology of the effusion is unclear, the distinction should be made between a transudate and an exudate by thoracentesis and pleural fluid analysis (see "Laboratory Studies" section).

Transudative Effusions

Transudative effusions usually **resolve with treatment of the underlying disease process.**

Exudative Effusions: Infectious Causes

Parapneumonic Effusions

A parapneumonic effusion is any effusion that occurs in the **presence of pneumonia, lung abscess, or bronchiectasis.** Between 50% and 70% of pleural effusions in hospitalized children are parapneumonic.

Bacterial Infections

The most common bacterial causes of parapneumonic pleural effusions and empyema are *Streptococcus pneumoniae, Staphylococcus aureus,* and *Streptococcus pyogenes. Haemophilus influenza* type B was a major cause in the preimmunization era. Oral anaerobes can be causal in neurologically impaired children. Gram-negative rods are seen in neonates and chronically ventilated children.

A minority of bacterial parapneumonic effusions **progress to empyema** (gross pus in the pleural space), leading to **deposition of fibrin** in the pleural space; loculation of the effusion making clearing the infection difficult; and ultimately **development of a fibroblast "peel"** on the visceral and parietal pleural surfaces. Parapneumonic effusions are thus classified as uncomplicated, that is, those that will resolve with systemic antibiotic therapy alone, and complicated, that is those that require drainage for resolution. Pleural fluid analysis can be helpful in predicting which parapneumonic effusions are likely to be complicated.

Viral Infections

Pleural effusions occur in 10%–15% of patients with viral infections. **Adenoviral infection** is the most common cause of virus-related effusions. Effusions rarely occur with influenza, cytomegalovirus, herpes simplex virus, Epstein-Barr virus, or hepatitis virus infections. The effusion usually **resolves spontaneously** within a few weeks.

Other Causes

The frequency of various causes of pleural effusion in two hospital-based series is given in Table 61.1.

▼ EVALUATION OF PLEURAL EFFUSION

Physical Examination

The clinical findings in a patient with a pleural effusion vary, depending on the size and cause of the effusion. With **small effusions,** patients may be **asymptomatic** or have a **cough, chest pain, fever, or a combination** of the three. **As fluid accumulates** and the lung becomes compressed, the patient may **develop shallow, rapid respirations.** With **extreme effusions,** cyanosis may be seen as intrapulmonary shunting occurs.

Examination of the chest reveals **decreased breath sounds** and **dullness to percussion** on the affected side. If the lung is compressed by the effusion, **egophony** ("E to A" changes) may also be noted.

TABLE 61.1. Causes of Pleural Effusions in Hospitalized Children

Cause	Alkrinawi and Chernick* n = 127 Number (%)	Hardie et al.† n = 210 Number (%)
Parapneumonic	64 (50%)	143 (68%)
Congenital heart disease	22 (17%)	
Malignancy	13 (10%)	10 (5%)
Renal	11 (9%)	
Liver failure		7 (3%)
Trauma	9 (7%)	
Sickle cell disease		7 (3%)
Ruptured appendix		6 (3%)
Miscellaneous	8 (6%)	14 (7%)

* Alkrinawi S, Chernick V: Pleural fluid in hospitalized pediatric patients. *Clin Pediatr* 35:5–9, 1993.

† Hardie W, BoKulic R, Garcia VF, et al: Pneumococcal pleural empyemas in children. *Clin Infect Dis* 22:1057–63, 1996.

Diagnostic Modalities

In chest radiographs, pleural fluid is best seen on an **upright PA and lateral film or a decubitus film.** A supine film may show only a hazy lung field. With **small effusions, only blunting** of the costophrenic angle may be seen. A **subpleural effusion** may simulate an **elevated hemidiaphragm.** As the **fluid accumulates,** the hemithorax begins to opacify. **Pleural fluid** will **layer out** on a lateral decubitus film, allowing as little as 50 ml to be seen. If the opacity does not layer out, a loculated effusion, empyema, or lobar consolidation should be considered. An **ultrasound or computed tomography (CT) scan** may be useful in distinguishing consolidation from effusion and identifying loculations within the fluid.

Laboratory Studies

Thoracentesis and Pleural Fluid Analysis

Thoracentesis can be performed when there is **more than 10 mm of fluid layered on a lateral decubitus radiograph.** It should be performed if the cause of the effusion is unclear, to determine the need for drainage in a parapneumonic effusion, or if the pleural effusion is causing respiratory distress. If the **effusion is small or loculated, ultrasound or CT-guided thoracentesis** may be necessary.

Classification of Transudates Versus Exudates

Pleural fluid should be sent for **pH, LDH, and total protein** with concurrent determination of **serum LDH and total protein.** The sample for pH must be collected anaerobically in a heparinized syringe and transported promptly on ice for analysis. The **Light criteria define an effusion as an exudate** if it fulfills **at least one of the following criteria.** In adult studies, this definition is 98% sensitive and 83% specific for an exudate.

TABLE 61.2. Other Pleural Fluid Studies that May Be Helpful in the Differential Diagnosis of an Exudate

Test	Comments
White blood cell count and differential	Lymphocyte predominance in neoplastic processes, tuberculosis, chylothorax, or certain fungal infections
	Segmented neutrophil predominance in bacterial infections, connective tissue disease, pancreatitis, or pulmonary infarction
	Eosinophil count may be elevated in patients with bacterial infections, a neoplastic process, or a connective tissue disease
Red blood cell (RBC) count	RBC count > 100,000/mm: consider trauma, neoplasia, or pulmonary infarction
Microbiologic studies ▼ Gram stain and fluid culture for aerobes and anaerobes ▼ AFB smear and culture ▼ Viral culture ▼ Fungal culture	Consider the clinical context
Cytology	May reveal malignant cells
Rheumatoid factor, lupus erythematosus preparation, and antinuclear antibody levels	Useful if a collagen vascular disorder is suspected
Amylase	Elevated in pancreatitis or esophageal rupture
Triglycerides	> 110 mg/dl in chylothorax
Cholesterol	May be markedly elevated in certain inflammatory conditions, especially tuberculosis and rheumatoid arthritis

▼ Pleural fluid/serum protein ratio > 0.5
▼ Pleural fluid LDH > 200 IU/L
▼ Pleural fluid/serum LDH ratio > 0.6

Table 61.2 lists other studies that may be helpful in the differential diagnosis of an exudate.

Unexplained exudates require further work-up beyond the scope of this chapter.

▼ TREATMENT OF PLEURAL EFFUSION

In all cases, the **underlying disease** stimulating effusion formation **should be treated.** The patient's **respiratory status** should be **monitored closely.** If the effusion significantly compromises the patient's respiratory status, **therapeutic thoracentesis or chest tube placement** may be indicated.

Rarely, **pleurodesis with a sclerotic agent** (e.g., tetracycline) is used to fibrose the two pleural linings to prevent fluid reaccumulation.

The management of parapneumonic effusions has attracted much attention due to the risk of empyema, and some elements remain controversial.

▼ **An uncomplicated parapneumonic effusion** is defined as one that will resolve with systemic antibiotic therapy alone.

▼ **A complicated parapneumonic effusion** requires chest tube or surgical drainage for resolution.

Diagnostic thoracentesis in patients with an effusion ≥ 10-mm deep on a lateral decubitus film is recommended. A **pH < 7.0 or a glucose level < 40 mg/dl predicts a complicated effusion** and is an **indication for drainage.** In addition, a **positive Gram stain or culture,** or the **presence of frank pus** is **an indication for drainage.** Effusions that do not meet these criteria but have a **pH between 7.0 and 7.2 or an LDH > 1000 UI/L are borderline** and may require repeat thoracentesis. **Ultrasound and chest CT can** be used to **identify loculations. Intrapleural fibrinolytic therapy** is useful in patients with loculated pleural effusions. **Video-assisted thoracoscopic debridement (VATS) or open drainage** has been used for patients with loculated effusions or for those who do not respond to tube drainage. Some authors have advocated earlier, more universal use of VATS in complicated parapneumonic effusion; however, the indications for this procedure remain controversial. **Surgical decortication** has been used in the organized stage of empyema.

Suggested Readings

Alkrinawi S, Chernick V: Pleural infection in children. *Semin Respir Infect* 11(3):148–154, 1996.

Burgess LJ: Comparative analysis of the biochemical parameters used to distinguish between pleural transudates and exudates. *Chest* 107(6):1604–1609, 1995.

Givan DC, Eigen H: Common pleural effusions in children. *Clin Chest Med* 19(2):363–371, 1998.

Kinasewitz GT: Pleural fluid dynamics and effusions. In *Fishman's Pulmonary Diseases and Disorders,* 3rd ed. Edited by Fishman AP. New York, McGraw-Hill, 1998, pp 1389–1409.

Light RW: A new classification of parapneumonic effusion and empyema. *Chest* 108(2):299–301, 1995.

Light RW, MacGregor MI, Luchsinger PC, et al: Pleural effusions: the diagnostic separation of transudates and exudates. *Ann Intern Med* 77:507–513, 1972.

Montgomery M: Air and liquid in the pleural space. In *Kendig's Disorders of the Respiratory Tract in Children,* 6th ed. Edited by Chernick V, Boat TF. Philadelphia, WB Saunders, 1998, pp 389–403.

Rosen H, Nadkarni V, Theroux M, et al: Intrapleural streptokinase as adjunctive treatment for persistent empyema in pediatric patients. *Chest* 103:1190–1193, 1993.

Winterbauer RH: Nonmalignant pleural effusions. In *Fishman's Pulmonary Diseases and Disorders,* 3rd ed. Edited by Fishman AP. New York, McGraw-Hill, 1998, pp 1411–1427.

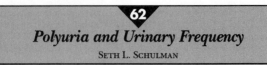

62
Polyuria and Urinary Frequency
Seth L. Schulman

▼ INTRODUCTION

Polyuria is defined as **urine output greater than 2000 ml/24 hr/1.73 m²**. It has various causes and can present during infancy, childhood, or adolescence. Polyuria must be **distinguished from increased urinary frequency unassociated with polyuria,** a common finding in children.

▼ DIFFERENTIAL DIAGNOSIS LIST

Infectious Causes

Pyelonephritis
Meningoencephalitis
Congenital cytomegalovirus and toxoplasmosis

Toxic Causes

Furosemide
Phenytoin
Demeclocycline
Amphotericin B
Vinblastine
Cisplatin
Lithium

Neoplastic Causes

Craniopharyngioma
Meningioma
Glioma
Metastasis—lymphoma, leukemia

Traumatic Causes

Severe head trauma
Hypophysectomy

Congenital or Vascular Causes

Obstructive uropathy
Cerebral hemorrhage

Metabolic or Genetic Causes

Inherited nephrogenic diabetes insipidus
Sickle cell disease (SCD)
Fanconi syndrome (e.g., cystinosis)
Polycystic kidney disease
Familial juvenile nephronophthisis
Bartter syndrome

DIDMOAD (central diabetes insipidus, diabetes mellitus, optic atrophy, deafness) syndrome
Laurence-Moon-Biedl syndrome

Psychosocial Causes

Primary polydipsia

Miscellaneous Causes

Diabetes mellitus
Idiopathic central diabetes insipidus
Hand-Schüller-Christian disease
Sarcoidosis
Sjögren syndrome
Postobstructive diuresis

Urinary Frequency

Cystitis
Neuropathic bladder
Urethritis
Hypercalciuria
Pollakiuria

▼ DIFFERENTIAL DIAGNOSIS DISCUSSION

Central Diabetes Insipidus

Etiology

Central diabetes insipidus may be **idiopathic, acquired,** or **inherited.** Approximately one-third of infants and children has the idiopathic (primary) form. Secondary causes include trauma, tumors (especially craniopharyngioma), hemorrhage, central nervous system (CNS) infection, hypoxia, and Langerhans cell histiocytosis. The autosomal dominant form of central diabetes insipidus is rare.

Clinical Features

Children present with a **sudden onset of polyuria, nocturia, and polydipsia with a predilection for cold water.** Hypernatremia and dehydration do not occur if the thirst mechanism is intact and there is ample access to water. There are no specific abnormal physical findings in primary central diabetes insipidus.

Evaluation

Laboratory studies reveal a consistently **low urine osmolality,** but in the absence of dehydration it is difficult to distinguish central diabetes insipidus from nephrogenic diabetes insipidus and psychogenic polydipsia. A **water-deprivation study** (Table 62.1) is **diagnostic** for central diabetes insipidus when the serum osmolality is increased, and the urine osmolality and the plasma vasopressin concentration are decreased. A brisk response to the administration of exogenous antidiuretic hormone is expected.

Radiographic imaging of the head is necessary to exclude secondary causes. In both primary and secondary forms, the **hyperintense signal of the posterior lobe of the pituitary** seen on T_1-weighted images on **magnetic resonance imaging (MRI)** is **absent.**

TABLE 62.1. Water-Deprivation Study: Administration, Procedures, and Interpretation

Administration

Supervision of subjects is required because dehydration and hypernatremia may develop. In addition, patients with primary polydipsia may drink surreptitiously, which interferes with the results of the study. Ideally, the study is performed in a clinical research center; A regular inpatient unit must have the appropriate personnel and equipment to adequately monitor the patient.

Procedure

1. Start the test in the early morning, after allowing the patient to drink fluids as needed overnight.
2. Enforce complete fluid restriction, and take the following measurements:
   ▼ Body weight and urine specific gravity, hourly
   ▼ Urine osmolality, serum osmolality, and serum sodium, every 2 hours
   ▼ Plasma vasopressin, at baseline, and on completion of the study
3. Stop fluid deprivation after 5% weight loss or when the serum sodium level is greater than 145 mmol/L (usually within 8 hours of initiating the test). Limit additional fluid intake to 1.5 times amount of urine passed up to this point and beyond.
4. Administer desmopressin acetate (DDAVP) intramuscularly at a dose of 0.25 ml (1 μg) if the child weighs less than 30 kg and at a dose of 0.5 ml (2 μg) if the child weighs more than 30 kg.
5. Take the following measurements:
   ▼ Total urine output, over 12 hours
   ▼ Urine specific gravity, every hour for 6 hours
   ▼ Urine osmolality, serum osmolality, and serum sodium every 2 hours for 6 hours

Interpretation

▼ A urine osmolality of greater than 750 mOsm/kg associated with a serum osmolality of greater than 295 mOsm/kg implies normal concentrating ability and primary polydipsia.

▼ A urine osmolality of less than 200 mOsm/kg in the presence of an elevated serum osmolality is consistent with diabetes insipidus. If the urine osmolality increases after desmopressin administration, the patient has central diabetes insipidus. No response indicates that the patient has nephrogenic diabetes insipidus.

Vasopressin levels may be necessary to assist in diagnosing partial central diabetes insipidus.

Treatment

Treatment consists of replacement therapy with **desmopressin acetate (DDAVP),** a synthetic analogue of vasopressin administered either intranasally or orally. The dose is adjusted to the patient's needs. Hyponatremia can develop if the patient drinks inappropriately while on therapy. **Specific treatment** is recommended **for secondary causes.**

Inherited Nephrogenic Diabetes Insipidus

Etiology

Nephrogenic diabetes insipidus is a **rare genetic disorder** characterized by **insensitivity** of the **distal nephron to arginine vasopressin.** The most common form is X-linked and associated with one of several described mutations of the vasopressin V_2 receptor. Female carriers may demonstrate partial or complete manifestations of the illness. An autosomal recessive form of the disease is caused by genetic abnormalities of the water channel protein aquaphorin 2.

Clinical Features

Infants present with **failure to thrive, dehydration, lethargy,** and **unexplained fever.** Symptoms may be severe during concomitant episodes of gastroenteritis. **Older children** have **polydipsia** and **polyuria** with **growth impairment** secondary to the preference of water over calorie-containing formula and foods. Recurrent episodes of dehydration may affect psychomotor development.

Evaluation

Laboratory studies reveal **hypernatremia** and **hypokalemia** when the infant is dehydrated. The diagnosis is **confirmed** by the presence of **hyposmolality of the urine** and the **lack of response to exogenous vasopressin** during periods of dehydration. The dehydration may need to be induced by a **water-deprivation study** (see Table 62.1). Fluids should not be restricted at home in an attempt to make the diagnosis. A **family history** of nephrogenic diabetes insipidus is often sufficient to avoid performing this study. It is **imperative to exclude medications and systemic conditions** (e.g., sickle cell anemia, tubulointerstitial diseases) that cause an acquired form of nephrogenic diabetes insipidus.

⚡ HINT Bilateral hydronephrosis may be seen on renal imaging studies that may be suspicious for obstructive uropathy.

Treatment

Treatment consists of providing **sufficient free water** to prevent complications associated with dehydration. **Restricting sodium intake** may reduce urine output. **Thiazide diuretics** decrease extravascular volume and increase proximal tubular sodium reabsorption, reducing urine output. **Amiloride** and **nonsteroidal antiinflammatory drugs,** particularly indomethacin, have also been shown to be beneficial.

Primary Polydipsia

Etiology

Primary polydipsia is **water ingestion greater than** that **necessary** to maintain water balance. It may be the result of **behavioral abnormalities** (psychogenic polydipsia or compulsive water drinking) or **physiologic abnormalities** of the hypothalamus affecting the thirst mechanism (neurogenic polydipsia).

Clinical Features

It is **difficult to distinguish primary polydipsia from diabetes insipidus.** Symptoms are similar to that seen in diabetes insipidus, although there may not be nocturia or the desire for iced water. Because excess free water is ingested, the patient should not be dehydrated.

Evaluation

Patients with primary polydipsia may have serum sodium concentrations slightly below normal. A **water-deprivation study** may be necessary to differentiate this condition from diabetes insipidus. A thorough **neurologic and**

psychologic examination is recommended before labeling primary polydipsia as psychogenic in origin.

📛 HINT In patients with primary polydipsia, the water-deprivation study may not allow maximal urinary concentrating ability secondary to "wash-out" of the medullary concentration gradient. These patients must be watched carefully during the study to avoid the possibility of surreptitious water ingestion, which will confound the results.

Treatment

Psychiatric counseling aimed at gradual weaning of water intake is recommended if it appears the polydipsia and polyuria are interfering with the patient's ability to function.

Cystitis and Urethritis

Etiology

Bacterial infection is the leading cause of cystitis in children, with **girls affected significantly more often** than boys. In prepubertal girls, urethritis is usually secondary to **chemical inflammation** (e.g., bubble bath in contact with the perineum).

Clinical Features

Frequency, rather than polyuria, is seen when the bladder or urethra are inflamed. Associated symptoms include **urgency, dysuria,** and **incontinence. Fever with flank pain** suggests the diagnosis of pyelonephritis.

Evaluation

A **urine culture** revealing **more than 100,000 colony-forming units/ml** of a single organism on a clean-catch specimen is diagnostic of cystitis. A **negative culture** suggests **urethritis,** although viral cystitis caused by adenovirus is a possibility, especially if gross hematuria is present.

Treatment

Antibiotic therapy for cystitis is based on the sensitivity of the offending organism. Urethritis can be treated with **frequent sitz baths** on baking soda and **avoidance of chemical irritants.**

Pollakiuria

Etiology

Pollakiuria, or the sudden onset of increased urinary frequency, is usually **related to stress** and is seen most commonly in children 4–6 years of age.

Clinical Features

Children with pollakiuria present with **extraordinary urinary frequency,** voiding in low volumes as often as 15 times an hour during the day. Incontinence is absent and affected children usually sleep through the night without awakening or wetting the bed.

Evaluation

Urinalysis and **urine culture** are recommended to exclude occult renal disease, diabetes mellitus, and urinary tract infection (UTI). A thorough **history**

of potential **factors leading to stress** (e.g., marital discord, recent move, family illness) should be obtained.

Treatment

Reassurance and **relaxation techniques** are usually recommended in this self-limited condition.

▼ EVALUATION OF POLYURIA AND URINARY FREQUENCY

Patient History

Key associated complaints include **polydipsia, nocturia, incontinence, enuresis, urgency,** and **dysuria.** Symptoms associated with tumors of the CNS, such as **headache** or **visual disturbances,** may be present. The patient may have a **family history** of nephrogenic diabetes insipidus. Any past **history of dehydration or UTI** should be recorded, along with any **medications** recently taken. Finally, a **social history** with emphasis on stress factors should be obtained.

Physical Examination

Clinical evidence of dehydration may be present, especially in infants, if the urine output exceeds the fluids ingested. Growth parameters suggesting **failure to thrive** are seen in patients with nephrogenic diabetes insipidus or renal insufficiency. **Ophthalmologic and neurologic examinations** must be performed to seek findings suggestive of an intracranial mass.

Laboratory Studies

▼ **Urinalysis, urine culture,** and **serum chemistries** (including a serum creatinine concentration) should be performed to exclude diabetes mellitus, most renal conditions, and UTI. A low urine specific gravity should be expected in diabetes insipidus and primary polydipsia. Hypernatremia may be noted in diabetes insipidus if dehydration is present. Hemoglobin electrophoresis should be considered if SCD is suspected.

▼ **Renal ultrasound** should be performed to exclude renal parenchymal disorders and obstructive uropathy, although some degree of hydronephrosis may be seen in high-output states.

▼ A **water-deprivation study** may be necessary to distinguish central diabetes insipidus, nephrogenic diabetes insipidus, and primary polydipsia.

▼ TREATMENT OF POLYURIA AND URINARY FREQUENCY

In general, polyuria does not require treatment prior to diagnosis except when hypernatremic dehydration is present. Patients with **diabetes insipidus** have hypernatremia on the basis of free water losses and require **replacement with low-sodium solutions** (except in the case of intravascular depletion). It is important to recognize that ongoing losses occur and typical calculations for maintenance fluids will be inappropriately low. Frequent **serum electrolyte determinations, body weight measurements, vital signs,** and **strict intake and output measurements** are necessary to judge the efficacy of treatment.

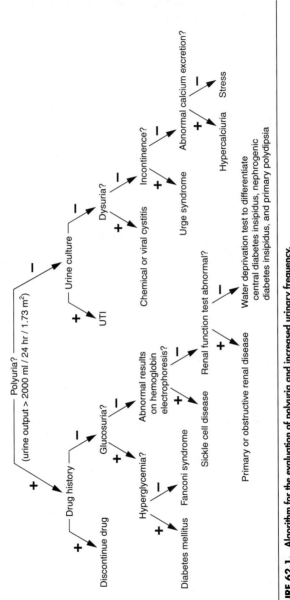

FIGURE 62.1. Algorithm for the evaluation of polyuria and increased urinary frequency.
UTI = urinary tract infection.

▼ APPROACH TO THE PATIENT WITH POLYURIA OR URINARY FREQUENCY (FIGURE 62.1)

Suggested Readings

Alon U, Warady BA, Hellerstein S: Hypercalciuria in the frequency-dysuria syndrome of childhood. *J Pediatr* 116:103, 1990.

Baylis PH, Cheetham T: Diabetes insipidus. *Arch Dis Child* 79:84, 1998.

Benchimol C: Nephrogenic diabetes insipidus. *Pediatr Rev* 17:145, 1996.

Horev Z, Cohen AH: Compulsive water drinking in infants and young children. *Clin Pediatr* 33:209, 1994.

Leung AKC, Robson WLM, Halperin ML: Polyuria in childhood. *Clin Pediatr* 30:634, 1991.

Zoubek J, Bloom DA, Sedman AB: Extraordinary urinary frequency. *Pediatrics* 85:1112, 1990.

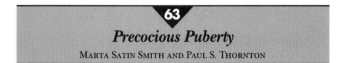

63

Precocious Puberty

MARTA SATIN SMITH AND PAUL S. THORNTON

▼ INTRODUCTION

Normal Pubertal Development

Girls

In girls, **puberty** usually begins at 10.5 to 11 years with a range of **9 to 11 years.** **Breast development (thelarche)** is usually the **first sign** of normal sexual development; however, in a small number of girls, pubic hair development may precede breast development by 6 months. **Pubic hair development (adrenarche)** usually **follows thelarche** by 6 months and **axillary hair** 12 to 18 months later. The **growth spurt occurs early** in pubertal development in girls at a mean age of 11.5 years (between Tanner stages 2 to 3 [See Chapter 2, "The Physical Examination," Table 2.6]). **Menses (menarche)** begin 18 to 24 months after thelarche and become ovulatory in most girls within 18 months. Puberty is completed within 1.5 to 6 years. Pubertal growth in girls contributes 25 cm to overall height.

Breast development and cornification of the vaginal mucosa are controlled primarily by **ovarian estrogens,** which are influenced by follicle-stimulating hormone (FSH). Pubic and axillary hair growth is stimulated primarily by **adrenal androgens,** although there may also be an ovarian contribution.

Boys

In boys, puberty usually begins at age 11.5 to 12 years with a range of **10 to 14 years. Testicular enlargement** occurs first, followed by the **development of pubic hair** approximately 6 months later. **Phallic enlargement** usually begins 12 months after testicular size begins to increase. The pubertal **growth spurt** in boys occurs between Tanner stages 3 and 4, with progression of male pubertal development occurring over 2 to 4.5 years (see Chapter 2, "The

Physical Examination," Table 2.5). The average growth during puberty is 28 cm. Onset of **spermatogenesis** occurs early in puberty with the mean age of conscious ejaculation of 13.5 years (range 12.5 to 15.5 years).

The virilizing changes seen at puberty are mainly the result of **testosterone secretion** from the testes. Growth of the penis and pubic hair are stimulated primarily by **testicular androgens;** however, **adrenal androgens** also contribute. Luteinizing hormone (LH) stimulates Leydig cell production of testosterone, whereas FSH supports spermatogenesis. It is now clear that peripheral **conversion of testosterone to estrogen** is important in bone growth and maturation in males.

Precocious Puberty

Precocious puberty is defined as the development of secondary sexual characteristics before the age of 6 years in African–American girls and 7 years in Caucasian American girls, and before the age of 9 years in boys regardless of race. Precocious puberty is classified as either **central (gonadotropin-dependent)** precocious puberty (CPP), which is caused by an elevation of FSH and LH; or **peripheral (gonadotropin-independent)** precocious puberty (PPP), which is caused by an elevation of sex steroids.

▼ DIFFERENTIAL DIAGNOSIS LIST

Central (Gonadotropin-dependent) Precocious Puberty (CPP)

Infectious Causes

Brain abscess
Meningitis—viral or bacterial
Encephalitis
Granulomatous disease
Tuberculosis, sarcoidosis, or histiocytosis

Toxic Causes

Chronic exogenous androgen or estrogen exposure (initially presenting as peripheral precocious puberty)

Brain Tumor

Glioma
Astrocytoma
Ependymoma
Hypothalamic hamartoma

Brain Injury

Head trauma
Brain surgery
Cranial irradiation
Hemorrhage and stroke

Congenital Causes

Central nervous system (CNS) malformation
Suprasellar cyst
Hydrocephalus
Idiopathic precocious puberty
Constitutional precocious puberty

Peripheral (Gonadotropin-independent) Precocious Puberty (PPP)

Toxic Causes

Exogenous estrogens—face creams, breast enlarging creams, contraceptive pill, and vaginal creams

Excess ingestion of phytoestrogens in soy products

Exogenous androgens—transdermal testosterone gel, anabolic steroid abuse

Neoplastic causes

Boys

Human chorionic gonadotropin (HCG)-secreting tumors—brain, liver choriocarcinomas

Leydig cell tumor

Virilizing adrenal tumor

Girls

Ovarian tumors

Adrenal tumors

Congenital Causes

Congenital adrenal hyperplasia (CAH)

Familial gonadotropin-independent Leydig cell maturation—testitoxicosis

McCune-Albright syndrome

Ovarian follicular cysts

▼ DIFFERENTIAL DIAGNOSIS DISCUSSION

Central (Gonadotropin-dependent) Precocious Puberty (CPP)

Etiology

CPP, or true precocious puberty, refers to sexual precocity **secondary to elevations in the gonadotropins (FSH and LH).** CPP arises from early activation of the hypothalamic-pituitary-gonadal axis. CPP is investigated five times more often in girls than in boys.

In most cases of CPP, especially in girls, **no cause is identified** (idiopathic precocious puberty). The younger the onset, the more likely an etiological factor will be found. Other cases involve various forms of **CNS pathology,** including malformations and benign or malignant tumors. **Hamartomas of the tuber cinereum** are the CNS tumors most frequently identified as causing precocious puberty. These tumors contain ectopic gonadotropin-releasing hormone (GnRH) neurosecretory cells. The pulsatile release of GnRH from these cells stimulates the pituitary gland. These hamartomas may be associated with gelastic seizures. CPP has also developed after **cranial irradiation therapy** for CNS tumors and after **head trauma.**

Clinical Features

As with children progressing through normal puberty, the first physiologic change is an increase in the amplitude and frequency of hypothalamic GnRH pulses. This causes **increased FSH and LH secretion** from the pituitary gland, **maturation of the gonads,** and **increased release of sex steroids.**

TABLE 63.1. Normal Ranges for Gonadotropin and Sex Steroid Levels: Females

	LH (mIU/ml)	FSH (mIU/ml)	Estradiol (ng/dl)	Testosterone (ng/dl)
0–1 year	0.02–7.0	0.24–14.2	0.5–5.0	< 10
Prepubertal	0.02–0.3	1.0–4.2	< 1.5	< 3–10
Tanner 2	0.02–4.7	1.0–10.8	1.0–2.4	7.0–28
Tanner 3	0.10–12.0	1.5–12.8	0.7–6.0	15–35
Tanner 4	0.4–11.7	1.5–11.7	2.1–8.5	13–32
Tanner 5	0.4–11.7	1.0–9.2	3.4–17.0	20–38
Adult	...	...	...	10–55
Follicular phase	2.0–9.0	1.8–11.2	3.0–10.0	...
Mid-cycle	18.0–49	6.0–35.0	...	...
Luteal phase	2.0–11.0	1.8–11.2	7.0–30.0	...

FSH = follicle-stimulating hormone; LH = luteinizing hormone.

Evaluation

Boys have pubertal FSH and LH levels, a pubertal response to GnRH, and a pubertal value of **testosterone. Girls** have pubertal FSH and LH levels, a pubertal response to GnRH, and a pubertal value of **estradiol** (Tables 63.1 and 63.2). The diagnosis of **CPP in boys is almost always serious** and necessitates a search for a **CNS tumor.**

Treatment

CNS tumors associated with CPP are rarely completely resectable because of their proximity to vital structures. Therefore, a **joint medical and surgical approach** is required. Usually a **biopsy** is performed and treatment is determined based on the results.

Hamartomas of the tuber cinereum are benign tumors of the hypothalamus that are usually asymptomatic, except for causing precocious puberty and gelastic seizures. Surgical treatment is not indicated for these hamartomas; treatment is directed at **medically halting the puberty.**

The treatment of choice for CPP is a **synthetic GnRH agonist,** which, when administered chronically, suppresses gonadotropin secretion and gonadal

TABLE 63.2. Normal Ranges for Gonadotropin and Sex Steroid Levels: Males

	LH (mIU/ml)	FSH (mIU/ml)	Estradiol (ng/dl)	Testosterone (ng/dl)
0–1 year	0.02–7.0	0.16–4.1	1.0–3.2	< 10
Prepubertal	0.02–0.3	0.26–3.0	< 1.5	< 3–10
Tanner 2	0.2–4.9	1.8–3.2	0.5–1.6	18–150
Tanner 3	0.2–5.0	1.2–5.8	0.5–2.5	100–320
Tanner 4	0.4–7.0	2.0–9.2	1.0–3.6	200–620
Tanner 5	0.4–7.0	2.6–11.0	1.0–3.6	350–970
Adult	1.5–9.0	2.0–9.2	0.8–3.5	350–1030

FSH = follicle-stimulating hormone; LH = leuizeing hormone.

steroid output. Several different forms of GnRH analogs are available, including long-acting forms that can be administered on a monthly basis.

Peripheral (Gonadotropin-independent) Precocious Puberty (PPP)

Etiology

The secondary sexual development in PPP results from circulating sex steroids that originate independently of gonadotropin stimulation. Possible sources of sex steroids are:

▼ The **gonads** (e.g., ovarian cysts, ovarian tumors, and testicular tumors)
▼ The **adrenal glands** (e.g., CAH, adrenal tumors)
▼ **Exogenous administration** in the form of estrogen creams, birth control pills, or anabolic steroids.

Isosexual precocity occurs when the hormonal changes are consistent with gender (e.g., excess estrogens in a female) and **heterosexual precocity** occurs when the hormonal changes are of the opposite gender (e.g., adrenal carcinoma producing androgens in a female).

PPP may develop in boys via **autonomous secretion of sex steroids** or as a result of **human chorionic gonadotropin (HCG) secretion,** which stimulates testosterone secretion from the Leydig cells. **Autonomous androgen secretion** can result from adrenal 21-hydroxylase deficiency or 11-β-hydroxylase deficiency, adrenal carcinomas, interstitial cell tumors of the testes, or premature Leydig cell maturation. **Tumors that secrete HCG** include hepatomas; hepatoblastomas; teratomas; chorioepitheliomas of the gonads, mediastinum, retroperitoneum, or pineal gland; and germinomas of the pineal gland.

PPP can develop in girls from **ovarian or adrenal estrogen secretion** or from **exogenous estrogen.** Follicular ovarian cysts, granulosa cell tumors, gonadoblastomas, lipoid tumors, and ovarian carcinomas can all secrete estrogen.

Of note, certain forms of PPP, such as poorly controlled CAH, can eventually activate the hypothalamic-pituitary-gonadal axis and therefore initiate true precocious puberty via central mechanisms.

Clinical Features

The hypothalamic-pituitary-gonadal axis has not been activated and therefore the sexual characteristics that are manifested are limited to those stimulated by the elevated sex steroid level (e.g., breast development following estrogen production). Adrenal tumors can produce excessive androgens or estrogens, resulting in **virilization** or **feminization.** Ovarian abnormalities can also produce both androgens and estrogens. The classical features of PPP in boys are **development of the penis without testicular enlargement.**

Evaluation

If sex steroid levels are elevated but gonadotropin levels are decreased, the diagnosis is likely PPP. LH cross-reads with HCG on some radioimmunoassays; therefore, **measurement of HCG** along with **LH, FSH, and testosterone** should be done to rule out an HCG-secreting tumor in boys. An **ultrasound evaluation** of the pelvis should be performed if ovarian pathology is suspected.

Treatment

Treatment of PPP is dictated by the cause. In the case of steroid-producing tumors, **surgery, chemotherapy,** or both may be indicated. McCune-Albright syndrome has been treated with **ketoconazole** and a combination of **spirono-lactone and testolactone.**

Premature Adrenarche

Etiology

Premature adrenarche, the **isolated appearance of sexual hair** before the age of 6 or 7 years in girls or the age of 9 years in boys, is the most common cause of premature pubic hair development. Premature adrenarche, which is more common in girls, is a **benign condition** that appears to be secondary to premature increased secretion of adrenal androgens or increased end organ sensitivity, or both.

Clinical Features

Affected children may have only pubic hair, or they may also have **axillary hair, acne, perspiration,** and **body odor.** There is no premature growth spurt. Girls do not have associated clitoromegaly. **Repeat observation** is the most important evaluation and diagnostic tool.

Evaluation

The need for laboratory studies is dictated by the **degree of concern** raised by the results of complete and repeated examinations, and by the **bone age.** Premature adrenarche is usually slowly progressive. Dehydroepiandrosterone sulfate (DHEAS) levels are modestly elevated in patients with premature adrenarche. Plasma levels of gonadotropin and gonadal steroids are normal. Measurements of 17-α-hydroxyprogesterone, androstenedione, and testosterone are indicated to differentiate premature adrenarche from true precocious puberty (in boys) and from adrenal tumors or adrenal hyperplasia (in boys and girls). The bone age is often mildly advanced but not significantly advanced. Beware the patient with **rapidly progressive pubic hair development and normal bone age.** This may suggest an aggressive androgen-producing tumor.

Treatment

Because there are no long-term sequelae other than progression into central puberty, **observation** is the only necessary treatment.

Premature Thelarche

Etiology

Premature thelarche refers to **isolated breast development,** which usually appears in the first 3 years of life. It is felt to be secondary to episodic formation of ovarian cysts or increased sensitivity of the breasts to estradiol.

Clinical Features

Affected children have **unilateral or bilateral** premature breast development. There are **no other signs of estrogen effect** or precocious puberty (e.g., vaginal cornification, pubic hair, or growth spurt).

Evaluation

As with premature adrenarche, **examination on a regular basis** for several months should precede any laboratory or radiologic evaluations. **Plasma levels of FSH, LH, and estradiol** should be obtained if significant progression or signs of other estrogen effects develop with repeat observations. Gonadotropin levels, estradiol levels, and bone age are usually normal. **Continued observation** is necessary because this may be the first sign of CPP or PPP.

Treatment

Because there are no long-term sequelae, **observation** is the only necessary treatment.

▼ EVALUATION OF PRECOCIOUS PUBERTY

Patient History

The following information should be sought:

▼ History of accelerated growth
▼ Behavioral changes
▼ CNS infections or trauma
▼ Use of steroid medications
▼ Family history of precocious puberty

⚡ HINT Ask specifically about the presence of estrogen- or testosterone-containing preparations in the house.

Physical Examination

▼ Breast, genital, and sexual hair development should be carefully assessed and Tanner staged.
▼ Special measuring devices such as testicular volume beads (Prader orchidometer) may be useful.
▼ Skin should be examined for acne, oiliness, and hirsutism (signs of androgen secretion), and café aux lait spots (McCune-Albright syndrome).
▼ Funduscopic and neurologic evaluations should be performed to investigate the possibility of intracranial lesions.

Laboratory Studies

Initial laboratory and radiologic evaluations should be guided by the history and physical examination findings. In general, **blood work** should include determination of LH, FSH, estradiol, testosterone, and adrenal steroid levels. If these initial studies are abnormal or equivocal, **provocative testing with synthetic GnRH** may be indicated. Prepubertal children respond to GnRH stimulation with an increase in FSH. In contrast, normal pubertal children and children with true precocious puberty have a mature LH response to exogenous GnRH administration. Normal ranges for gonadotropin and sex steroid levels are presented in Table 63.1 (girls) and Table 63.2 (boys).

Imaging Studies

The **bone age** should be determined. If indicated, **ultrasound of the ovaries and adrenal glands** should be performed. The need for additional studies, such as a **magnetic resonance imaging (MRI) scan** of the head to investigate the cranial cavity and pituitary fossa, is dictated by the results of these initial studies.

⚡ HINT Small cysts on the ovaries are not uncommon in girls who have no clinical evidence of puberty.

▼ APPROACH TO THE PATIENT

Treatment options for precocious puberty are dictated by the cause. However, while the inciting cause of the precocious pubertal development is being sought and treated, the physician must also focus on the **long-term consequences of the physical changes** that are occurring. **Short stature** is the most obvious result of early pubertal development. The advanced skeletal maturity associated with some forms of precocious puberty results in a child who initially is taller and stronger than his or her peers but who, ultimately, if the disorder is untreated, loses years of growth potential as a result of fusion of the epiphyseal growth plates.

Suggested Readings

Motzin B: Precocious puberty: diagnosis, evaluation, and management. *Pediatr Rev* 14:336, 1993.

Pescovitz OH: Precocious puberty. *Pediatr Rev* 11:229, 1990.

Wheeler MD, Styne DM: Diagnosis and management of precocious puberty. *Pediatr Clin North Am* 37:1255, 1990.

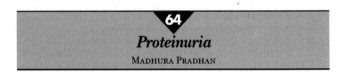

64
Proteinuria
MADHURA PRADHAN

▼ INTRODUCTION

Proteinuria, the presence of excessive protein in the urine, is a **common finding in school-aged children.** As many as 10% of children test positive for proteinuria **(1+ or higher dipstick reading)** at some time (Table 64.1). The prevalence of proteinuria increases with age and **peaks during adolescence.** Though most proteinuria is transient or intermittent, it is the most **common laboratory finding of renal disease.** The challenge is to differentiate proteinuria caused by renal disease from that associated with benign conditions. Normal urinary protein excretion in adults is < 150 mg/day whereas in children it is < 4 mg/m^2/hour (Table 64.2).

▼ DETECTION OF PROTEINURIA
Qualitative

The **dipstick measures the concentration of protein in urine.** It is impregnated with tetrabromophenol blue, which changes color in the presence of albumin when the pH is in the normal range. A urine sample is considered positive for protein if it measures $\geq 1+$ when the specific gravity of urine is < 1.015,

TABLE 64.1.   Qualitative Evaluation of Proteinuria by Dipstick

Grade	Protein Concentration (mg/dl)
Trace	10–20
1+	30
2+	100
3+	300
4+	1000–2000

or $\geq$ 2+ when the specific gravity is > 1.015. A child is said to have persistent proteinuria if the dipstick is **positive for protein** in at least **two of three random urine samples** collected at least a week apart.

Although not as convenient as dipstick analysis, a reagent called **sulfosalicylic acid detects all forms of proteinuria.** False-positive results by this method may result from radiographic contrast material, penicillins, cephalosporins, sulfonamides, and high uric acid concentrations.

✄ HINT   The following can cause false-positive results on dipstick analysis: alkaline urine (pH greater than 7.0), overlong immersion, placing the strip directly in the urine stream, cleansing of the urethral orifice with quaternary ammonium compounds prior to collecting the sample, pyuria, and bacteriuria. False-negative results can occur when the urine is too dilute (i.e., the specific gravity is less than 1.005) or when the patient excretes abnormal amounts of proteins other than albumin.

Quantitative

A timed urine collection for protein quantitation is essential to establish the degree of proteinuria. A **24-hour urine collection** can be done by asking the child to void as soon as he wakes up and discarding the specimen; then every void should be collected for the next 24 hours including the first void the next morning. In clinical practice, it is difficult to obtain timed urine collections in children. A **random urine specimen** can be analyzed for protein and creatinine concentration and the ratio of the urine protein (in milligrams) to urine creatinine (in milligrams) can be used as a measure of 24-hour urine protein. The normal ratio of urine protein to urine creatinine in children > 2 years is 0.2 and in children < 2 years is 0.5.

▼ DIFFERENTIAL DIAGNOSIS LIST
Transient Proteinuria

Fever
Dehydration

TABLE 64.2.   Quantitative Evaluation of Proteinuria by Timed 24-Hour Urine Collection

Normal	< 4mg/m^2/hour
Abnormal	4–40mg/m^2/hour
Nephrotic range	> 40mg/m^2/hour

Exercise
Cold exposure
Congestive heart failure
Seizures
Emotional stress
Epinephrine administration

Isolated Proteinuria

Orthostatic proteinuria
Persistent asymptomatic isolated proteinuria (PAIP)

Glomerular Disease

Minimal change nephrotic syndrome (MCNS)
Focal segmental glomerulosclerosis (FSGS)
Postinfectious glomerulonephritis
Membranoproliferative glomerulonephritis
Membranous nephropathy
Immunoglobulin A (IgA) nephropathy
Henoch-Schönlein purpura
Hemolytic uremic syndrome
Hereditary nephritis
Systemic lupus erythematosus (SLE)
Diabetes mellitus
Sickle cell disease (SCD)
HIV-associated nephropathy

Tubulointerstitial Disease

Reflux nephropathy
Pyelonephritis
Interstitial nephritis
Fanconi syndrome—cystinosis, tyrosinemia, Lowe syndrome
Toxins—drugs (aminoglycosides, penicillins, heavy metals)
Ischemic tubular injury
Renal hypoplasia or dysplasia
Polycystic kidney disease

▼ DIFFERENTIAL DIAGNOSIS DISCUSSION
Proteinuria Caused by Structural Abnormalities

Damage to the glomerulus or tubules can cause proteinuria. Proteinuria from glomerular insult can be in the nephrotic range (Table 64.2), whereas proteinuria from tubular injury rarely exceeds 1 g/day.

Transient Proteinuria

Transient proteinuria is **unrelated to renal disease** and resolves when the inciting factor disappears. It is rarely > 2+ on the dipstick. **Febrile proteinuria** usually appears with the onset of fever and resolves by 10–14 days. Proteinuria that occurs **after exercise** usually abates 48 hours after cessation of exercise. Transient proteinuria seen with fever, exercise, and congestive heart failure is due to hemodynamic alterations in glomerular blood flow.

Orthostatic Proteinuria

Etiology and Incidence

Orthostatic proteinuria is abnormal protein excretion that **occurs only when the patient is in an upright position.** Although the exact mechanism is unclear, orthostatic proteinuria is most likely the result of excessive glomerular filtration of protein. Orthostatic proteinuria is the most common form, accounting for **60% of all proteinuria in children.** The prevalence is even higher among **teenagers,** especially **girls.**

Orthostatic proteinuria is an incidental finding, and there are no specific clinical features.

Evaluation

The diagnosis of orthostatic proteinuria can be made if urinary protein excretion is abnormal in samples obtained while the patient is upright, but normal in samples obtained when the patient is recumbent. Total protein excretion should be less than 1 g/day. In some patients, orthostatic proteinuria is reproducible, while in others it is intermittent. There are three approaches to evaluating orthostatic proteinuria:

▼ **Dipstick analysis of first morning (recumbent) and daytime (upright) random urine samples.** Negative or trace protein in the first morning sample with a 1+ or greater protein in the daytime urine sample is suggestive of orthostatic proteinuria.

▼ **Quantitative evaluation of proteinuria in a split collection.** Urine samples may be collected at timed intervals while recumbent as well as while ambulating, and evaluated quantitatively for protein excretion (see Table 64.2). The timed urine samples should be collected by asking the child to void and discarding the urine just prior to going to bed. Collect the void into a container marked "recumbent" immediately on arising. Then collect all the urine during the day including the specimen voided just prior to going to bed in a separate container labeled " ambulatory." In orthostatic proteinuria, the amount of protein in the ambulatory collection should be 2 to 4 times that of the recumbent collection.

▼ **Calculation of the urine protein to urine creatinine ratio.** The urine protein to urine creatinine ratio is calculated on first morning and upright random urine samples. A normal urine protein to urine creatinine ratio is less than 0.2 in children older than 2 years and less than 0.5 in children younger than 2 years.

Management

The prognosis for orthostatic proteinuria is thought to be very good.

▼ **Development in young children.** Follow-up for as long as 50 years has shown a benign course among patients who developed orthostatic proteinuria as young adults.

▼ **Development in children and adolescents.** There is a paucity of long-term studies involving patients who developed orthostatic proteinuria as children and adolescents. Therefore, children with orthostatic proteinuria should be followed with first morning urinalysis and blood pressure evaluations as part of their yearly routine well visit.

Persistent Asymptomatic Isolated Proteinuria (PAIP)

Etiology

PAIP is defined as proteinuria **detected in more than 80% of the urine spec-imens taken,** including recumbent samples, in an **otherwise healthy child,** which persists for 3 months. The prevalence in school aged children is 6%. It is usually < 2 g/day and is never associated with edema. Numerous studies have revealed that children with PAIP have normal histology or mild nonspe-cific glomerular abnormalities. Other studies have reported divergent results with a significant number of patients having glomerular abnormalities such as focal sclerosis. Children with PIAP form a heterogeneous group, and in the absence of large prospective studies, the prognosis of PAIP should be viewed with caution.

Nephrotic Syndrome

Nephrotic syndrome is defined by the presence of proteinuria, edema, hy-percholesterolemia, and hypoalbuminemia.

Etiology

Nephrotic syndrome can be **primary** (isolated to the kidney) or **secondary** (part of a systemic disease, such as SLE). Glomerular diseases that can cause primary nephrotic syndrome include MCNS (77%), FSGS (10%), mem-branoproliferative glomerulonephritis (5%), diffuse mesangial proliferation (3%), crescentic glomerulonephritis (3%), and membranous nephropathy (2%).

Clinical Features

Edema is the cardinal finding in nephrotic syndrome. One of the most com-mon manifestations is periorbital edema on awakening, which is sometimes mistaken for an allergic reaction. The **edema increases over time,** and the child may develop ascites, pleural effusion, and labial or scrotal edema.

Clinical features that favor a diagnosis of MCNS are **male gender,** age **younger than 6 years** at onset of disease, **absence of hypertension,** and only a **small degree of hematuria.**

Evaluation

Evaluation entails a **urinalysis,** a **serum albumin level,** and a **serum choles-terol level.** Nephrotic syndrome is characterized by proteinuria greater than 40 mg/m^2/hour, a serum albumin level of less than 2.5 g/dl, and hyperc-holesterolemia.

A biopsy is indicated for patients who:

▼ Are younger than 1 year or older than 10 years
▼ Have manifestations of nephritis [hematuria with red blood cell (RBC) casts], azotemia, hypertension
▼ Fail a 4-week course of prednisone

Treatment

More than 80% of patients with nephrotic syndrome, and approximately 95% of children with MCNS, respond favorably to **corticosteroid therapy.** Corticosteroids are generally started in a dose of 2 mg/kg/day (to a maximum dose of 80 mg/day), administered in divided doses, and tapered over 4–8 weeks, after the urine is free of protein. The taper should be gradual enough to reduce the rate of relapse, without causing side effects (e.g., growth retardation).

Approximately 80% of the children who initially respond to prednisone will **relapse.** Those who do not respond or those with frequent relapses (> 3 relapses/year) are candidates for **immunosuppressive medications,** such as cyclophosphamide or cyclosporine A.

⚡ HINT   Most children have fewer relapses as they grow older and generally do well.

▼ EVALUATION OF PROTEINURIA

Once abnormal proteinuria has been found and confirmed, a stepwise work-up can be initiated.

Phase I Work-Up

The initial work-up of proteinuria should begin with a complete history and physical examination.

The physician should elicit history of **recent infections** (streptococcal, impetigo), **urinary tract infections, oliguria/hematuria,** and **family history** of renal disease. The physical examination should be focused on looking for **hypertension** (glomerulonephritis), **edema** (nephrotic syndrome), **rash/arthritis** (vasculitis), and **short stature** (chronic renal disease). Laboratory investigations in this phase should include a **urine dipstick** (ambulatory and recumbent), a **urine analysis** including microscopic examination, and a **urine protein to creatinine ratio.**

Phase II Work-Up

Laboratory tests for serum electrolytes, creatinine, albumin, cholesterol, blood urea nitrogen, anti-streptococcal antibodies, complement levels, and antinuclear antibodies should be done. A **renal ultrasound** should be performed to look for abnormalities of size and structure in the kidney. **Timed 12-hour urine protein quantitation** should be done for recumbent and upright samples to look for orthostatic proteinuria and a **24-hour urinary protein level** should be obtained.

Phase III Work-Up

If the initial work-up suggests the presence of an underlying renal disease, a **referral to a pediatric nephrologist** should be made. A referral should be made in the following situations:

▼ Persistent fixed, i.e., nonorthostatic, proteinuria
▼ Family history of glomerulonephritis
▼ Systemic complaints (e.g., fever, rash, arthralgias)
▼ Hypertension

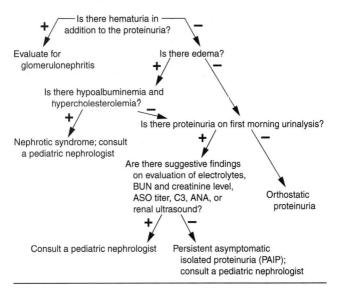

FIGURE 64.1. Approach to the patient with proteinuria.
ANA = antinuclear antibody; *ASO* = antistreptolysin O; *BUN* = blood urea nitrogen; *C3* = third component of complement.

▼ Edema
▼ Cutaneous vasculitis or purpura
▼ Hematuria
▼ Abnormal renal function
▼ Abnormal ultrasound
▼ Increased parental anxiety

The nephrologist may perform a renal biopsy to define the etiology of proteinuria in some of these situations.

Most cases of proteinuria in children can be managed by a primary care physician at times in consultation with a pediatric nephrologist. **Long-term follow-up** is important, since prognosis in some of the conditions is not well defined.

▼ APPROACH TO THE PATIENT (FIGURE 64.1)

Suggested Readings

Ettenger RB: The evaluation of the child with proteinuria. *Pediatr Ann* 23(9):486–494, 1994.

Roy S: Proteinuria *Pediatr Ann* 25(5):277–278, 281–282, 1996.

Yoshikawa N, Kitagawa K, Ohta K, et al: Asymptomatic constant isolated proteinuria in children. *J Pediatr* 119(3):375–379, 1991.

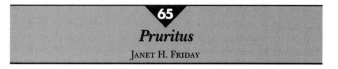

Pruritus
JANET H. FRIDAY

▼ INTRODUCTION

Pruritus, simply defined, means "itching." Pruritus that is **persistent and severe** requires further investigation. Pruritus usually has a primary **dermatologic** cause, but may also be **drug-induced** or caused by **systemic disease.**

▼ DIFFERENTIAL DIAGNOSIS LIST

Infectious Causes

Varicella
Enterovirus
Pinworms
Scabies
Pediculosis
Trichinosis
Hookworms

Toxic Causes

Scombroid ingestion
Opiates
Barbiturates
Aminophylline
Aspirin
Erythromycin
Griseofulvin
Isoniazid
Phenothiazines
Vitamin A

Neoplastic Causes

Malignancy

Traumatic Causes

Overbathing, dry heat, harsh detergents
Healing wounds
Irritant-mediated contact dermatitis
Ultraviolet or chemical burns
Insect bites
Coelenterata envenomation
Foreign body (cactus spines or fiberglass)

Congenital or Vascular Causes

Congenital ectodermal dysplasia
Erythropoietic protoporphyria

Urticaria pigmentosa
Mastocytosis
Neurofibromatosis

Metabolic or Genetic Causes

Hypothyroidism or hyperthyroidism
Diabetes mellitus
Hypercalcemia
Hyperparathyroidism

Inflammatory Causes

Atopic dermatitis
Contact dermatitis, allergen mediated
Urticaria
Systemic lupus erythematosus (SLE)
Juvenile rheumatoid arthritis (JRA)

Psychosocial Causes

Neurogenic pruritus

Miscellaneous Causes

Uremia
Cholestasis
Iron-deficiency anemia
Polycythemia
Pityriasis rosea
Psoriasis
Seborrheic dermatitis
Acropustulosis of infancy
Lichen planus
Pregnancy
Nummular eczema

▼ DIFFERENTIAL DIAGNOSIS DISCUSSION

Any skin condition comprising exudation, lichenification, and pruritus falls under the broad category of eczema. Two common forms of eczema, atopic dermatitis and contact dermatitis, are considered, and other common causes of pruritus are discussed.

Atopic Dermatitis

Etiology

Although it is one of the **most common causes of pruritus** in children, this condition is **poorly understood.** Characterized by **inflammatory hyperreactivity,** the disease is currently believed to be caused by aberrancies in T-cell function, with immunoglobulin E overproduction and cell-mediated immune dysfunction.

Clinical Features and Evaluation

Most children with atopic dermatitis have a **family history of atopic disease** (asthma, hay fever, or atopic dermatitis). Many children also have or later develop **asthma or hay fever.** The rash usually appears in susceptible patients during the first year of life, and involves the **face, neck, and trunk.** Distribution in older children is typically in **flexor creases of the elbows and knees.** The eruption consists of **erythematous, poorly demarcated patches,** and **initially is exudative, later forming crusts.** There may be **associated papules or vesicles.** With the **scratching** that ensues, the lesions become **thickened or lichenified,** and may develop a **surface scale. Pigmentation changes** are common complications. Atopic dermatitis has a **chronic, recurrent, or recalcitrant nature.**

⚕ HINT It may be difficult to differentiate seborrheic dermatitis from atopic dermatitis in infants. Classically, seborrheic dermatitis appears in the first 2 months of life, whereas atopic dermatitis may appear later. The scale of seborrhea is yellow and greasy, and is often seen behind the ears. The diagnosis of atopic dermatitis may be delayed until repeated outbreaks occur.

Treatment

Treatment focuses on **moisturizing the skin, avoiding overdrying, and eliminating possible irritants.** Increasing hydration by means of **bathing followed by application of a hydrophobic barrier** is essential. A **topical steroid,** such as 1% hydrocortisone cream, is used initially to control flares. Severe disease may require treatment with **fluorinated steroid creams or systemic steroids.** Such cases are best handled in **consultation with a pediatric dermatologist,** because complications of growth impairment need to be considered. The patient with severe atopic dermatitis is at risk for **secondary skin infections** with staphylococci, extensive primary herpes (eczema herpeticum), and varicella zoster infection.

Contact Dermatitis

Etiology

Contact dermatitis can be mediated by irritants or allergens.

▼ **Primary irritant dermatitis** is a direct response of the skin to an irritant. The most common irritants are soaps, bubble baths (may cause severe vaginal pruritus in prepubertal girls), saliva, urine, feces, perspiration, citrus juice, chemicals (creosote, acids), and wool.

▼ **Allergic contact dermatitis** requires reexposure to the allergen and is characterized by a delayed hypersensitivity reaction. The most common allergens implicated include poison ivy, poison oak, and poison sumac (rhus dermatitis) (Figure 65.1); jewelry (nickel); cosmetics (causing eyelid involvement) and nail polish; topical medications [neomycin, thimerosal, calamine, para-aminobenzoic acid (PABA)]; shoe materials (rubber, tanning agents, dyes); and clothing materials (elastic or latex compounds).

Clinical Features and Evaluation

In either case, the **rash is the key to diagnosis,** being **most prominent in the areas of direct approximation to the trigger.** It may appear as erythematous papules, vesicles, bullae, or patches.

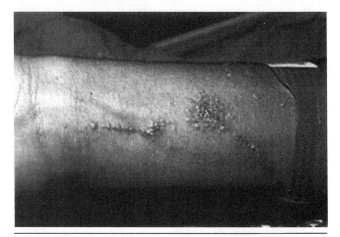

FIGURE 65.1. Rhus dermatitis (poison ivy), an example of allergic contact dermatitis.
(Reprinted with permission from Avery ME, First LR: *Pediatric Medicine*, 2nd ed. Baltimore, Williams & Wilkins, 1994.)

Treatment

The cornerstone of treatment is **removal of the offending agent.** A short course of **topical steroids** may help speed recovery. **Failure to respond** to these measures **indicates possible misdiagnosis.**

Xerosis

Etiology

Xerosis refers to **dryness of the skin,** and may be the diagnosis of exclusion in common pruritus. Children of any age may be affected.

Clinical Features and Evaluation

The rash often has a **fine, flaky, white, diffuse scale,** which may be **excoriated from scratching.** The **lower legs** are commonly involved. The **hands** may also be afflicted in older children, especially when exposed to frequent handwashing or dishwashing. The condition is **made worse by dry heat, frequent bathing in hot water, and wool fabrics.**

Treatment

Treatment with **emollients** and **cessation of causative behaviors** are effective.

Scabies

Etiology

Scabies is caused by an **infestation with the mite** *Sarcoptes scabiei.* The mites burrow into the stratum corneum and deposit eggs and feces, which cause the itching.

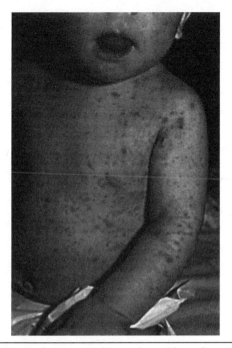

FIGURE 65.2. Erythematous papules, pustules, vesicles, and crusted lesions of scabies.
(Reprinted with permission from Avery ME, First LR: *Pediatric Medicine*, 2nd ed. Baltimore, Williams & Wilkins, 1994.)

Clinical Features

Lesions may be **papules, pustules, or vesicles** (Figure 65.2). Fewer than 15% of patients have the classic "S"-shaped burrows. The **rash distribution on infants** (neck, face, scalp, axilla, and groin) **differs from that of older children** (wrists, axilla, interdigital webs, intragluteal web, and beltline).

Evaluation

Skin scrapings from an unscratched burrow in immersion oil under 10x magnification should reveal the female mite, her eggs, and her feces.

Treatment

Treatment with **permethrin 5% cream** has replaced γ-benzene-hexachloride because of concerns about the latter's toxic effects in young children. The permethrin cream is applied to the **entire body** and left on **for 12 hours.** This treatment may be repeated in 2 weeks if necessary. Because the **infestation is highly contagious,** household contacts should also be treated. **Bedding and** clothing may harbor the mites and should be **laundered;** the dryer heat will kill the remaining animals.

Varicella

Etiology

Varicella is caused by **primary infection with varicella zoster virus,** usually from droplet contact with a primarily infected individual. It is contagious from several days before the outbreak of lesions until all of the lesions are crusted over. Children who have received the varicella vaccine may exhibit milder symptoms.

Clinical Features

The rash is characterized by a **progression of lesions from erythematous macules, to papules, to fluid-filled vesicles, to crusted lesions.** Crops of lesions appear on the **face, trunk, and scalp,** with minimal involvement of the distal extremities. The **mucous membranes** are often involved; commonly, superficial ulcerations appear on the oral mucosae after the vesicles rupture. The clinician should always look for lesions in the **scalp, mouth, and vaginal areas.** Classically, lesions in various stages of evolution are simultaneously present. **Fever and malaise** may accompany the rash.

Treatment

Treatment is **supportive,** including attempts to **alleviate the itching** and **avoidance of secondary bacterial infections. Antiviral agents** (e.g., acyclovir) are effective only in shortening the course of illness **if given within 24 hours** of the onset of lesions.

▓ HINT   Aspirin use in patients with varicella has been associated with Reye syndrome and is contraindicated. Immunocompromised hosts and neonates warrant special precautions and consultation with infectious disease specialists.

Drug Reaction Pruritus

Etiology

Although many medications have been known to cause pruritus, in an otherwise ill patient, **iatrogenic effects** may be **difficult to separate from the disease** process. The pruritus may be caused by **drug-induced intrahepatic cholestasis** (from erythromycin, oral contraceptives, anabolic steroids, phenothiazines) or **mast cell degranulation** (from codeine, aspirin, penicillin).

Treatment

If clinically feasible, a **trial period** during which the **patient is off medication** should be attempted. Relief of pruritus should occur **within several days if it is histamine mediated,** but can take **several weeks to resolve if it is caused by cholestasis.**

Urticaria

Etiology

This classic pruritic rash is a manifestation of **immediate hypersensitivity reaction,** which may or may not be allergen mediated. The most common triggers are **foods** (nuts, berries, shellfish, dairy products), **plants, viral** infections (enterovirus, hepatitis), **group A streptococci, and drug reactions** (codeine, aspirin, penicillin). Intravenous injection of **radiopaque contrast material or blood products** may cause **severe reactions.** Less commonly, the trigger may be **cold, heat, tactile stimuli, or sunlight.**

Clinical Features and Evaluation

Diagnosis is on a clinical basis. The classic appearance of urticaria is a **rash of erythematous raised, often evanescent, wheals** scattered over the body.

Treatment

Treatment may begin with **subcutaneous injection of epinephrine,** which usually clears the rash temporarily. Signs of **systemic progression** such as **laryngospasm, wheezing, and hypotension** warrant **more aggressive treatment. Antihistamines** are commonly prescribed to help alleviate itching, and should be continued for 7–10 days. Attempts should be made to **identify and remove the trigger,** although often none can be found. The patient should be counseled that the rash may persist for days to weeks.

▼ EVALUATION OF PRURITUS

Patient History

Key complaints are the presence of rash, fever, or both. Answers to the following questions should be sought:

- ▼ Are there any new or unusual exposures?
- ▼ What is the patient's drug history?
- ▼ Are any household contacts also suffering from similar symptoms?
- ▼ What is the patient's past medical history, including renal and hepatic disorders, atopic disease, psychiatric disorders, and autoimmune diseases?

Physical Examination

Physical examination findings that may point to the diagnosis include wheezing, oral lesions, organomegaly, ascites, and any abnormal skin findings. The pattern of distribution should be noted.

Laboratory Studies and Diagnostic Modalities

Appropriate laboratory studies and diagnostic modalities may include:

- ▼ CBC
- ▼ Blood urea nitrogen and creatinine levels
- ▼ Liver function tests
- ▼ ß-Human chorionic gonadotropin level
- ▼ Chest radiograph
- ▼ Skin biopsy
- ▼ Microscopic examination of skin scrapings
- ▼ Chest radiograph

▼ TREATMENT OF PRURITUS

If **urticaria** is present, the patient should be **urgently assessed for airway compromise, breathing, and circulation,** because **airway edema and shock**

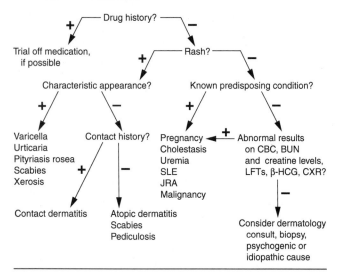

FIGURE 65.3. Evaluation of a patient with pruritus.
If the diagnosis remains elusive, refer the patient to a dermatologist. *β-HCG* =
β-human chorionic gonadotropin; *BUN* = blood urea nitrogen; *CBC* = complete
blood count; *CXR* = chest radiograph; *JRA* = juvenile rheumatoid arthritis; *LFTs*
= liver function tests; *SLE* = systemic lupus erythematosus.

can rapidly progress. If the rash is thought to be urticarial, a **rapid improvement after subcutaneous epinephrine administration** confirms this suspicion.
Treatment with **intravenous antihistamines and steroids** is indicated if any
systemic signs or symptoms are present.

▾ APPROACH TO THE PATIENT (FIGURE 65.3)

Suggested Readings

Angel TA, Nigro J, Levy ML: Infestations in the pediatric patient. *Pediatr
  Dermatol* 47:4, 2000.
Frieden IJ, Resnick SD: Childhood exanthems, old and new. *Pediatr Clin North
  Am* 38:859, 1991.
Hanifin JM: Atopic dermatitis in infants and children. *Pediatr Clin North Am*
  38:763, 1991.
Hurwitz S: *Clinical Pediatric Dermatology: A Textbook of Skin Disorders of Childhood
  and Adolescence,* 2nd ed. Philadelphia, WB Saunders, 1993.
Kristal L, Klein PA: Atopic dermatitis in infants and children. An update.
  Pediatr Dermatol 47:4, 2000.
Raimer SS: New and emerging therapies in pediatric dermatology. *Dermatol
  Clin* 18:1, 2000.

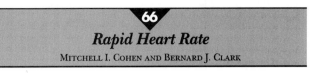

Rapid Heart Rate
MITCHELL I. COHEN AND BERNARD J. CLARK

▼ INTRODUCTION

Rapid heart rate (tachycardia) can be defined as a **ventricular rate in excess of the age-related normal range.** The upper limits of normal are approximately as given in Table 66.1.

- ▼ **Sinus tachycardia** is caused by abnormalities of the sinus node (or normal sinus node responses to physiologic alterations).
- ▼ **Supraventricular tachycardia (SVT)** is caused by abnormalities originating above the ventricle.
- ▼ **Ventricular tachycardia (VT)** is caused by abnormalities originating below the bundle of His.

▼ DIFFERENTIAL DIAGNOSIS LIST

Sinus Tachycardia

Noncardiac Causes

Exercise
Fever
Anemia
Hyperthyroidism
Excessive catecholamines–stress, pheochromocytoma
Arteriovenous malformation (AVM)
Drugs–therapeutic, illicit
Seizures

Cardiac Causes

Congestive heart failure
Myocardial dysfunction
Congenital heart disease
Cardiac tamponade
Sick sinus syndrome

Supraventricular Tachycardia (SVT)

Abnormal (Nonsinus) Focus of Automaticity

Automatic (ectopic) atrial tachycardia
Multifocal atrial tachycardia
Junctional ectopic tachycardia

Accessory Route of Electrical Conduction

Atrial flutter
Atrioventricular nodal re-entrant tachycardia
Atrioventricular reciprocating tachycardia
Permanent junctional reciprocating tachycardia

TABLE 66.1. Upper Limit of Normal for Heart Rate

Age (Years)	Upper Limit of Normal for Heart Rate (beats/min)
< 1	180
1–3	150
4–6	130
7–10	110
> 10	100

Ventricular Rhythm Disturbance

Ventricular tachycardia (VT)
Ventricular fibrillation
Accelerated idioventricular rhythm
Torsades de pointes–long QT syndrome, electrolyte disturbance, drug toxicity
Structural heart defects

▼ DIFFERENTIAL DIAGNOSIS DISCUSSION
Sinus Tachycardia

Etiology

Sinus tachycardia occurs when the **normal pacemaker, the sinoatrial cells, responds either normally or abnormally to an alteration in physiologic conditions.** Sinus tachycardia occurs as a normal response to increased physiologic demands (e.g., exercise, fever, anemia) and as a normal response to certain pathological changes (e.g., hyperthyroidism, pheochromocytoma, AVM). Various medications and drugs of abuse can elevate the resting sinus rate (Table 66.2), especially decongestants, caffeine, and β-adrenergic

TABLE 66.2. Drugs Associated with Rapid Heart Rates

Prescription drugs
β-adrenergic agonists (e.g., albuterol)
Methylxanthines (e.g., theophylline)
Tricyclic antidepressants (e.g., imipramine)
Nonsedating histamines (e.g., terfenadine)

Over-the-counter drugs
Decongestants (e.g., pseudoephedrine)
Diet aids (phenylpropanolamine)
Inhaled bronchodilators (e.g., albuterol)
Caffeine-containing products

Drugs of abuse
Nicotine
Cocaine
Amphetamines
Alcohol
Marijuana
LSD
Phencyclidine
Amyl nitrate

agonists. The normal physiologic response to increased metabolic demands is to **increase cardiac output,** either by **increasing the stroke volume or the heart rate (or both).** During infancy, the heart is less able to increase stroke volume; therefore, the cardiac output is primarily augmented by an increase in heart rate.

▼ **Cardiac causes** for sinus tachycardia include any condition that depresses myocardial function (e.g., myocarditis, pericarditis, endocarditis).
▼ **Noninfectious causes** include congestive heart failure from large left-to-right shunts ($\dot{Q}p:\dot{Q}s > 2:1$), atrioventricular valve regurgitation, or left ventricular outflow tract obstruction (aortic stenosis or coarctation of the aorta).
▼ **The sinus node may be injured by certain surgeries** (e.g., Mustard, Senning, or Fontan operations), resulting in sick sinus syndrome (tachycardia–bradycardia syndrome).

Clinical Features

Patients with sinus tachycardia may be asymptomatic or minimally symptomatic with complaints of **palpitations, chest pain, dyspnea, or lightheadedness.** Rarely, a patient presents with cool extremities as a result of a low cardiac output. Symptoms often **depend on the age of the patient and the duration of the tachycardia.**

Evaluation

A **12-lead electrocardiogram (ECG)** should be obtained to determine the correct P-wave axis. During sinus tachycardia, the P-wave axis is $0°–90°$ and the QRS complex is narrow, unless there is a pre-existing intraventricular conduction delay (e.g., bundle branch block). There is typically a "warm-up and cool-down" period that lasts a few minutes.

A **complete blood cell count, a glucose level, thyroid tests, and 24-hour urine catecholamine studies** may be indicated. Often, **observing the patient** on a monitor for a short period of time helps make the diagnosis.

Treatment

Treatment of nonphysiologic sinus tachycardia is geared toward **correction of the underlying abnormality,** such as infection, anemia, or hyperthyroidism.

Supraventricular Tachycardia (SVT)

⚄ HINT There are generally two epidemiological SVT peaks: infancy and adolescence.

Etiology

Although SVT occurs in anatomically normal hearts, it is usually the result of either an **abnormal focus of automaticity** or an **accessory route of electrical conduction** to the ventricles.

▼ **Ectopic atrial tachycardia** is an automatic tachycardia identified on an ECG by an abnormal P-wave axis or different morphological P wave. It can be difficult to distinguish ectopic atrial tachycardia from sinus tachycardia when the ectopic focus is in the high right atrium (near the sinus node) and has a normal P-wave axis. The tachycardia typically has a "warm-up and cool-down" phase.

▼ **Atrial flutter** is caused by one or more re-entrant circuits within the atrium and does not require the atrioventricular node or ventricle to sustain itself. Atrial flutter is frequently seen in patients after the Mustard/Senning operation for D-transposition of the great arteries or following the Fontan operation for single ventricle heart disease.

▼ **Atrioventricular nodal re-entrant tachycardia** is most common in adolescents and young adults.

▼ **Atrioventricular reciprocating tachycardia** is the most common type of SVT seen in children. It is caused by an abnormal accessory pathway that bypasses normal atrioventricular node conduction. There are generally two types—an accessory pathway that allows antegrade conduction to the ventricle, bypassing the normal atrioventricular node (Wolff-Parkinson-White syndrome), or an accessory pathway that allows only retrograde conduction and is "concealed" on the resting ECG. Wolff-Parkinson-White syndrome is often seen in patients with Ebstein anomaly of the tricuspid valve. In a significant number of infants with Wolff-Parkinson-White syndrome, the condition resolves without treatment within the first few years of life.

Clinical Features

Patients with SVT may be minimally symptomatic, complaining of **palpitations, chest pain, dyspnea, or lightheadedness.** Symptoms often depend on the **age of the patient** and **the duration of the tachycardia.** Patients who have been in SVT for **more than 24–48 hours** may have **cool extremities and pallor,** suggesting low cardiac output. Patients with **Wolff-Parkinson-White syndrome** may have **atrial fibrillation** with rapid conduction down an accessory pathway, resulting in **ventricular fibrillation and sudden death.**

On admission, the patient's **heart rate, blood pressure, and intravascular status** should be assessed. A **12-lead ECG and rhythm strip** should be obtained. It is important to be able to answer the following questions [**Is the RR interval regular? Can P waves be identified, and if so, what is the relationship to the QRS complex? How does this ECG differ from the patient's baseline ECG? If P waves cannot be seen, a transesophageal recording may be helpful to identify P waves and their association with ventricular beats.**]

▼ **Automatic (ectopic) atrial tachycardia.** The P wave morphology, the PR interval, or both may be different from the baseline sinus rhythm. The atrial rate is usually 100–240 beats/min and atrioventricular block can occur during the tachycardia.

▼ **Atrial flutter.** In general, the rate in atrial flutter is 150–400 beats/min, with the ventricular rate being a multiple of the atrial rate, based on variable atrioventricular block. Classic "saw-toothed" flutter waves are typically seen in the inferior leads (II, III, and aVF) in children with structurally normal hearts. This may not be apparent in children after the Fontan operation, in which the flutter cycle lengths are longer.

▼ **Wolff-Parkinson-White syndrome** appears on the resting ECG as a short PR interval accompanied by a "delta wave" (i.e., slurring of the initial component of the QRS complex, as a result of ventricular pre-excitation).

▓ **HINT** If the patient complains of palpitations, but no documented rhythm disturbance is seen on the 12-lead ECG, 24-hour ambulatory Holter monitoring, transtelephonic recordings, or exercise testing may be helpful.

Treatment

Acute conversion of SVT is indicated for all initial events, symptomatic episodes, and whenever the patient shows signs of hemodynamic compromise.

▼ **Vagal maneuvers.** Mainstays of nondrug therapy include performing a Valsalva maneuver, standing the patient on his head, or inducing the diving reflex by placing ice on the patient's face.

▼ **Adenosine.** Adenosine causes a profound but short-lived increase in the atrioventricular nodal refractory period. Adenosine may be given as a rapid intravenous bolus (50–300 μg/kg, to a maximum dose of 12 mg) while a 12-lead ECG is continuously running.

▼ **Direct current (DC) cardioversion.** If the patient is hemodynamically compromised, synchronized DC cardioversion (0.5–1 joules/kg) is the most effective means of terminating SVT.

▼ **Transesophageal or transvenous overdrive atrial pacing** can also be effective in acute situations. These procedures should be attempted only by an experienced cardiologist.

▼ **Verapamil** should be avoided as acute treatment of SVT in children younger than 3 years because of its vasodilating and negative inotropic effects. In older children it may be used, but intravenous calcium chloride and isoproterenol should be readily available.

▓ **HINT** Adenosine or vagal maneuvers may be therapeutic as well as diagnostic, in that flutter waves or ventricular pre-excitation can occasionally be seen in the first few post-tachycardia beats as the atrioventricular node is blocked.

Treatment of **chronic SVT** (e.g., atrioventricular reciprocating tachycardia, atrioventricular nodal re-entrant tachycardia) entails the use of **agents that alter refractoriness** of an integral component of the circuit.

▼ **Digoxin** is given initially for atrioventricular nodal re-entrant tachycardia caused by a concealed accessory pathway. The risk of increasing antegrade conduction through an accessory pathway makes the use of this drug in patients with Wolff-Parkinson-White syndrome controversial.

▼ **β Blockers** (e.g., propranolol, atenolol, nadolol) should be the first-line agent in patients with pre-excitation syndromes. Side effects of the beta-blockers include fatigue, bronchospasm, hypoglycemia, and/or exercise intolerance.

▼ **Procainamide, flecainide, sotalol, and amiodarone** are alternative second-line agents in the treatment of SVT. Careful attention to myocardial performance, proarrhythmia, and hepatic and thyroid dysfunction should be carefully monitored.

▼ **Radiofrequency catheter ablation** can be performed safely in children (> 4 years old) who have SVT refractory to single-line medications, or side effects associated with medications (e.g., increased bronchospasm in a patient with asthma who is being treated with a β-blocker). Patients with potentially rapidly conducting accessory pathways should be considered for an ablation, even in the absence of a history of SVT.

Ventricular Tachycardia (VT)

Etiology

A premature ventricular contraction (PVC) is defined as a **single ventricular beat that arises earlier than the sinus beat with a full compensatory pause.** A **consecutive pair** of PVCs is a **couplet; three or more PVCs** are defined as **VT.** PVCs may be further classified as **monomorphic or polymorphic** and occur in either a **bigeminal, trigeminal, or quadrigeminal pattern.**

▼ **Isolated finding.** VT can be an isolated finding in children with otherwise normal hearts and is usually monomorphic and suppressed with exercise.
▼ **Structural heart defects.** VT can be associated with structural heart defects (Table 66.3) and is often inducible with exercise and other catecholamine stimulation.
▼ **Torsades de pointes ("twisting of the point")** is a variant of polymorphic VT in which the QRS morphology changes over time. Torsades de pointes can be associated with any of the long QT forms (Table 66.4).
▼ **Ventricular fibrillation** is rare in the pediatric population and is characterized by rapid, bizarre, chaotic QRS complexes without any effective cardiac

---

TABLE 66.3. Structural Heart Disease Associated with Tachycardia

Defect	Type of Tachycardia
Congenital heart disease	
Mitral valve prolapse	SVT, VT
Aortic valve stenosis or regurgitation	VT
Ebstein anomaly of the tricuspid valve	SVT (WPW) commonly, VT less commonly
Tetralogy of Fallot	VT
Mustard/Senning repair of D-TGA	SVT (particularly atrial flutter)
Fontan repair of single ventricle	SVT (particularly atrial flutter)
Cardiomyopathy	
Hypertrophic cardiomyopathy	SVT, VT
Dilated cardiomyopathy	SVT, VT
Arrhythmogenic right ventricular dysplasia	VT (monomorphic, left bundle branch block)
Miscellaneous causes	
Eisenmenger complex (pulmonary vascular disease and pulmonary hypertension)	VT
Cardiac tumor (atrial myxoma, rhabdomyosarcoma)	SVT, VT (depending on tumor site)

D-TGA = D-transposition of the great arteries; SVT = supraventricular tachycardia; VT = ventricular tachycardia; WPW = Wolff-Parkinson-White syndrome.

TABLE 66.4. Causes of Prolonged QT Interval

Congenital
  Hereditary
    Jervell-Lange-Nielsen syndrome: long QT interval, stress-induced syncope, congenital nerve deafness, autosomal recessive inheritance
    Romano-Ward syndrome: long QT interval, stress-induced syncope, autosomal dominant inheritance (usually incomplete penetrance)
    Brugada syndrome
    Right ventricular dysplasia
  Sporadic
Acquired
  Electrolyte abnormalities
    Hypocalcemia
    Hypomagnesemia
  Metabolic disturbances
    Malnutrition
    Liquid protein diets
  Drugs
    Phenothiazines (e.g., haloperidol)
    Tricyclic antidepressants (e.g., imipramine)
    Nonsedating antihistamines (e.g., terfenadine)
    Class Ia antiarrhythmic agents (e.g., quinidine)
    Class III antiarrhythmic agents (e.g., amiodarone)
  CNS trauma
  Cardiac abnormalities
    Ischemia
    Mitral valve prolapse
    Myocarditis
  Intraventricular conduction abnormalities
    Bundle branch blocks

CNS = central nervous system.

output. Ventricular fibrillation may be seen in children with the long QT syndrome or cardiomyopathy, after cardiac surgery, or rarely in association with atrial fibrillation and antegrade accessory pathway conduction (Wolff-Parkinson-White syndrome).

Clinical Features

Symptoms generally depend on the **age of the patient** and **the rate and duration of the VT.** Patients may present with **simple palpitations, signs of low cardiac output, shock, or "sudden death."**

Evaluation

A complete history and physical examination should be performed, with particular attention to the patient's **vital signs** and any underlying structural heart disease. Always determine the **corrected QT interval** and take a detailed **family history** regarding **sudden death, history of congenital heart disease, and deafness** (some syndromes are associated with long QT and deafness).

A **12-lead ECG** should be obtained to determine QRS duration, morphology, axis, and ventriculoatrial relationship. If a **prior ECG** is available, the **two should be compared.** A tachycardia originating below the bundle of His typically has a wide QRS complex, with a different QRS axis from that seen in patients in sinus rhythm. Atrioventricular dissociation may be present. The ventricular rate is typically 100–350 beats/min. Accelerated idioventricular rhythm ("slow VT") has the same ECG characteristics as VT, with a slower rate (80–120 beats/min).

If the 12-lead ECG reveals only single monomorphic PVCs, **ambulatory Holter recordings or transtelephonic monitors** may help determine if the patient is having VT. An **exercise stress test** in older children and adolescents can determine the response to exercise; idiopathic VT is usually suppressed with exercise.

Consultation with a **cardiologist** is indicated for all patients suspected of having ventricular arrhythmias.

Treatment

Treatment for VT, like that for SVT, is **based on the underlying mechanism.**

▼ **Asymptomatic VT.** In patients who have structurally normal hearts, normal QT intervals, and asymptomatic slow VT suppressed by exercise, no treatment may be indicated. These patients should be followed periodically with noninvasive monitoring.

▼ **Acute, symptomatic VT.** Therapy with lidocaine (1 mg/kg administered as an intravenous push, followed by an infusion at a rate of 20–50 μg/kg/min, assuming normal renal function) is indicated for these patients. If the patient is known to have long QT syndrome (or clinical suspicion is strong for this disorder), intravenous magnesium sulfate (30–50 mg/kg for children, 1–2 g for adults) can be given over 1 minute. Lidocaine and phenytoin may also be used. Overdrive transvenous pacing may also be needed. Amiodarone and other medicines known to prolong the QT interval should be avoided.

▼ **VT with hemodynamic compromise.** If the patient has hemodynamically compromising VT, synchronized cardioversion with 1–2 joules/kg (adult: 100–400 joules) should be used, and cardiopulmonary resuscitation should be initiated. Treatment of ventricular fibrillation is emergent electrical asynchronous defibrillation and initiation of advanced cardiac life support.

▼ **Chronic, symptomatic VT.** Chronic treatment of patients with long QT syndrome is with β-blockers, the only medication demonstrated to decrease the mortality rate associated with this syndrome. Patients with structural heart disease, or symptomatic or exercise-induced VT, are generally treated after an electrophysiology study. Medications typically used, alone or in combination, include mexiletine, phenytoin, β-blockers, and amiodarone. Radiofrequency ablation can also be performed and some patients may warrant implantation of an internal cardiac defibrillator.

Suggested Readings

Ackerman MJ: The long QT syndrome. *Pediatr Rev* 19(7):232–238, 1998.

Deal BJ, Miller SM, Scagliotti D, et al: Ventricular tachycardia in a young population without overt heart disease. *Circulation* 73:1111, 1986.

Garson A Jr, Gillette PC, McNamara DG: Supraventricular tachycardia in children: clinical features, response to treatment, and long-term follow-up in 217 patients. *J Pediatr* 91:875, 1981.

Perry JC, Garson A: Supraventricular tachycardia due to Wolff-Parkinson-

White syndrome in children: early disappearance and late recurrence. *J Am Coll Cardiol* 16:1215, 1990.

Pfammatter JP, Paul T: Idiopathic ventricular tachycardia in infancy and childhood: a multicenter study on clinical profile and outcome. Working Group on Dysrhythmias and Electrophysiology of the Association for European Pediatric Cardiology. *J Am Coll Cardiol* 33(7):2067–2072, 1999.

Vetter VL, Horowitz LN: Electrophysiology residua and sequelae of surgery for congenital heart defects. *Am J Cardiol* 50:588, 1982.

Yabek SM: Ventricular arrhythmias in children with an apparently normal heart. *J Pediatr* 119:1, 1991.

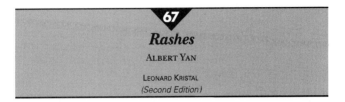

67

Rashes

ALBERT YAN

LEONARD KRISTAL
(Second Edition)

▼ DIFFERENTIAL DIAGNOSIS LIST

Rash Accompanied by a Fever

Bacterial Causes

Scarlet fever
Staphylococcal scalded skin syndrome
Toxic shock syndrome
Acute meningococcemia
Rocky Mountain spotted fever
Periorbital or buccal cellulitis

Viral Causes

Lyme disease
Varicella-zoster virus or herpes zoster virus
Roseola
Erythema infectiosum
Measles
Enteroviruses—e.g., hand-foot-mouth disease
Rubella

Miscellaneous Causes

Juvenile rheumatoid arthritis (JRA)
Kawasaki disease

Rash in a Neonate

Erythema toxicum neonatorum
Transient neonatal pustular melanosis
Miliaria
Candidiasis
Acropustulosis of infancy
Seborrheic dermatitis
Neonatal acne

Eczematous Dermatitis

Atopic dermatitis
Contact dermatitis
Nummular eczema
Asteatotic eczema
Id reaction

Papulosquamous Disease

Psoriasis
Seborrheic dermatitis
Lichen planus
Pityriasis rosea
Exfoliative dermatitis
Tinea capitis, corporis, faciei, and pedis
Tinea versicolor
Secondary syphilis
Pityriasis lichenoides et varioliformis acuta
Acrodermatitis enteropathica

Vesiculobullous Disease

Rhus dermatitis (poison ivy)
Contact dermatitis
Erythema multiforme
Insect bite or papular urticaria
Herpes zoster
Herpes simplex
Varicella
Urticaria pigmentosa

Papular Eruptions

Scabies
Papular acrodermatitis of childhood (Gianotti-Crosti syndrome)
Papular urticaria
Warts
Molluscum contagiosum

▼ DIFFERENTIAL DIAGNOSIS DISCUSSION

Scarlet Fever

Etiology

Scarlet fever is caused by **group A β-hemolytic *Streptococcus*.**

Clinical Features

Illness begins with **fever and pharyngitis** followed in 24–48 hours by an **enanthem and exanthem.**

The **face appears flushed, except for circumoral pallor.** The **tongue** initially has a **white coating (white strawberry tongue)** that is **gone by the fourth day,** revealing a very **erythematous tongue** with **prominent papillae (red strawberry tongue).** Cervical and submandibular **lymphadenopathy** are noted.

The **rash** appears as a **diffuse erythema;** small, fine papules give it a **sandpaper-like quality.** The rash **begins on the neck** and **spreads rapidly to**

the trunk and extremities. It is **accentuated** in the **intertriginous areas** (i.e., the axillae and antecubital, inguinal, and popliteal creases), and the **palms and soles are spared.** The rash resolves in 4–5 days with **fine peeling of the skin.** Peeling **begins on the face,** spreading to the **trunk and extremities.** On the **hands and feet, peeling in large sheets** may occur.

> ▓ **HINT** Petechiae may occur on the soft palate and uvula, or in streaks in the intertriginous areas (Pastia's lines).

Evaluation

Diagnosis is by **culture of a pharyngeal swab. Antistreptolysin O (ASO) titers** or a **streptozyme test** may also be used.

Treatment

Treatment of choice is with **penicillin, amoxicillin, or a first-generation cephalosporin.** Erythromycin can be used in penicillin-allergic patients.

Staphylococcal Scalded Skin Syndrome

Etiology

Staphylococcal scalded skin syndrome is caused by an **epidermolytic toxin, exfoliatin,** which is **produced by** *Staphylococcus aureus.*

Clinical Features

Staphylococcal scalded skin syndrome occurs in children **younger than 5 years.** The illness begins with **fever and irritability after conjunctivitis, rhinitis, or an upper respiratory tract infection.** The skin first becomes **erythematous** and then **tender to the touch.** The eruption usually begins around the **nose and mouth** and **spreads to the trunk.** The rash is most **prominent in the flexures,** and can involve the hands and feet. After 1–2 days, the **skin develops bullae** and begins **peeling in sheets.** After 2 days, the involved **skin surfaces become crusted** and then begin to **develop scaling,** which lasts up to 5 days.

Evaluation

S. aureus can often be isolated by **bacterial culture of the nose, nasopharynx, throat, conjunctiva, or perianal area.**

> ▓ **HINT** This illness is sometimes confused with toxic epidermal necrolysis (TEN), another disorder in which the skin may peel in sheets. The diagnosis can be made easily by examining newly desquamating skin under a microscope—in staphylococcal scalded skin syndrome, the split occurs below the stratum corneum in the granular layer, whereas in TEN, the split is found at the base of the epidermis.

Treatment

Treatment is with a **penicillinase-resistant antibiotic.**

Meningococcemia

Etiology

Meningococcemia is caused by *Neisseria meningitidis.*

Clinical Evaluation

The illness begins with symptoms of a **mild upper respiratory tract infection,** followed by **fever, malaise, headache, and the development of a petechial eruption on the skin and mucous membranes.** In addition, patients can have **erythematous macules, papules, and urticarial lesions.** In severe cases, the purpura can involve **large areas that eventually necrose.**

Many patients develop **meningitis, disseminated intravascular coagulation, and hypotension.**

✄ HINT Always think of meningococcemia when a patient presents with fever and petechiae.

Evaluation

Cultures of blood and cerebrospinal fluid are indicated. The organism can sometimes be recovered from a small petechial lesion if a **biopsy of the lesion** is performed and cultured. A **Gram stain** of a scraped petechiae may reveal organisms.

Treatment

Initial treatment is with a **broad-spectrum antibiotic;** once the diagnosis is confirmed, the patient can be treated with **penicillin, ceftriaxone, or cefotaxime.**

Rocky Mountain Spotted Fever

Etiology

Rocky Mountain spotted fever is caused by *Rickettsia rickettsii*, which is transmitted by **ticks.**

Clinical Features

After a **prodrome** characterized by **headache, malaise, photophobia, and joint and muscle pain,** the patient develops a **fever** followed on the **fourth day** by a **rash.**

The rash begins on the **wrists and ankles as small erythematous macules** that eventually become **petechial or purpuric.** The rash then **spreads to the trunk** and within 2 days is **generalized,** with involvement of the **palms and soles.**

Other findings may include **generalized edema** (especially affecting the periorbital area in children), **severe muscle tenderness, photophobia, and hyponatremia.**

✄ HINT Consider Rocky Mountain spotted fever in any patient with fever and a petechial eruption involving the palms and soles.

Evaluation

Diagnosis is with the **Weil-Felix test,** which detects antibodies that develop against specific *Proteus* antigens. **Direct immunofluorescence of a skin lesion biopsy specimen** is useful for confirming a clinical diagnosis, but is not widely available.

Treatment

The treatment of choice for all patients is a **tetracycline derivative.** In children **younger than 8** years, **chloramphenicol** can be considered as an alternative.

Varicella (Chicken Pox)

Varicella is discussed in Chapter 65, "Pruritus."

Kawasaki Disease

Etiology

The cause of Kawasaki disease is **unknown.**

Clinical Features

The **rash** can have many different forms, including **generalized erythema, scarlatiniform lesions, erythema multiforme lesions, and pustular lesions.** The **lips** are usually **bright red** with some **crusting,** and the patient may have a **strawberry tongue.** The patient must present with five of the following six criteria to make the diagnosis of Kawasaki disease:

- ▼ Fever lasting 5 days or more
- ▼ Bilateral nonpurulent conjunctivitis
- ▼ Erythema and crusting of the lips
- ▼ Edema or erythema of the palms and soles with subsequent desquamation
- ▼ Rash
- ▼ Cervical adenopathy

⚫ HINT An important cutaneous finding is that of fine desquamation of the perineal area early in the course of the disease.

Evaluation

Thrombocytosis is present by the second week of illness. An **echocardiogram** should be performed to look for coronary artery aneurysmal dilatation.

Treatment

Treatment is with **intravenous gamma globulin and aspirin.**

Erythema Toxicum Neonatorum

Etiology and Clinical Features

The cause of erythema toxicum neonatorum is **unknown.** Affected infants are healthy appearing, except for the development of an **eruption within 3–4 days of birth.** The eruption is characterized by **erythematous macules, papules, and/or pustules** and may occur **anywhere on the body except for the palms and soles.** There may be **few or several hundred lesions.**

Clinical Evaluation

A **smear** of a pustule reveals **clusters of eosinophils;** Gram staining is negative for bacteria. As many as 15% of patients have **peripheral eosinophilia.**

Treatment

No treatment is needed. The eruption generally resolves by the time the patient reaches 2 weeks of age.

Transient Neonatal Pustular Melanosis

Etiology and Clinical Features

The cause of transient neonatal pustular melanosis is **unknown.** This condition is more commonly seen in **African-American infants** and is characterized by **pustules, vesicles, and hyperpigmented macules** that are **present at birth.** Pustules **rupture,** leaving a **fine, white collarette of scale.** The eruption **resolves within several days,** most of the time **leaving pigmented macules.** The eruption can appear **anywhere on the body, including the palms and soles.** A **smear** of the pustules shows neutrophils.

Evaluation and Treatment

Gram stain, a Tzanck preparation, and potassium hydroxide preparation are negative. No treatment is needed.

Miliaria

Etiology

An **eruption,** characterized by **small, nonfollicular, erythematous papules,** is caused by **sweat retention in eccrine ducts.** The rash is most commonly seen in the **intertriginous or flexor regions** of the body, but can appear anywhere. There is no evidence of infection. Treatment entails **avoidance of excessive heat and humidity.**

Infantile Seborrheic Dermatitis

Etiology

The cause is **unknown,** but may be related to **maternal hormonal stimulation.**

Clinical Features

The eruption often begins during the **first 12 weeks of life** with **scaling of the scalp,** sometimes associated with **erythema ("cradle cap");** the eruption generally **clears by the age of 1 year.** The eruption is characterized by **greasy, yellow scales** associated with **patches of erythema, fissuring, and occasional oozing** on the **scalp, face, ears, trunk, and intertriginous areas.**

✂ HINT Pruritus is not associated with this condition.

Treatment

Parents should be advised to **gently loosen the scale while shampooing.** A **low-potency topical corticosteroid** (i.e., hydrocortisone) may be applied to acutely inflamed areas.

Neonatal Acne

The cause is **unknown,** but the condition is probably related to **stimulation of sebaceous glands** by maternal and infant **androgens.** Neonatal acne is **more commonly seen in boys,** and has been reported in as many as 20% of newborns. **Closed comedones (whiteheads) are most common, but open** comedones, inflammatory papules, and pustules may also be noted. **No treatment** is necessary for most patients; patients with **moderate to severe cases** should be **referred to a pediatric dermatologist.**

Dermatitis

Atopic dermatitis and contact dermatitis are discussed in Chapter 65, "Pruritus."

Nummular Eczema

The cause of nummular eczema is **unknown,** although it tends to be a manifestation of **dry skin and ichthyosis.** The **rash** is characterized by **coin-shaped lesions** with **vesicles and papules that enlarge by confluence** or peripheral extension. Lesions are treated with **mid-potency topical steroids.**

⚡ HINT Lesions may be confused with impetigo or tinea corporis.

Psoriasis

Etiology

The cause is **unknown,** although there is some evidence that there is a **genetic** component. An **immune defect** may be a primary or secondary factor.

Clinical Features

Psoriasis is characterized by **thick, silvery scaled, erythematous plaques** located **symmetrically** on the **elbows, knees, extensor surfaces of the wrist, genitalia, and scalp.** Children usually present with **guttate (teardrop-like) plaques on the trunk.** Patients can also present with **large plaques, pustular plaques, or as an erythroderma,** whereby most of the body's skin is erythematous and scaling. **Nail changes include pitting** on some or all of the fingers **and onycholysis** (i.e., separation of the nail plate from the nail bed).

Evaluation

Psoriasis is a **clinical diagnosis,** but if there is doubt, a **biopsy** may be beneficial.

Treatment

Midpotency topical steroids, tar preparations, and **antiseborrheic shampoos** are used. Patients with severe cases may require **ultraviolet light therapy** or **systemic medication. Referral to a pediatric dermatologist** is recommended for all patients with psoriasis, except those with very mild cases.

Lichen Planus

Etiology and Clinical Features

Lichen planus is a dermatologic disorder with lesions characterized by the **"five Ps"—pruritic, polygonal, purple, planar, papules** located on the **flexor surfaces, genitalia, mucous membranes, scalp, and nails.** The cause is **unknown.** The disease can eventually lead to **scarring of the scalp and nails.**

Evaluation

A **biopsy** confirms the diagnosis when the clinical lesions do not conform to the classic description.

> **✂ HINT** When mineral oil is placed on individual lesions, the surface appears to have a white network of lines known as Wickham's striae.

Treatment

Initial treatment is with **mid- to high-strength topical steroids;** these patients are best managed by a **dermatologist.**

Seborrheic Dermatitis

Etiology

The cause is **unknown,** although there appears to be a relation to the yeast *Pityrosporum ovale.* In addition, there may be a **hormonal component** to the eruption because it usually appears at the time of or after the onset of puberty.

Clinical Features

Typically, **scalp scaling** is present and may be associated with **erythema and pruritus.** In addition, **erythematous, scaly plaques** may be present **behind the ears, on the forehead and eyebrows, and in the nasolabial folds.** The eruption can occasionally be seen in the **presternal area, axillae, and inguinal folds.**

> **✂ HINT** Seborrheic dermatitis is not seen in patients between the ages of 1 year and puberty. In patients in this age group, one must always think of the possibility of tinea capitis.

Treatment

Treatment entails **frequent shampooing with antidandruff shampoo** and the application of **low-potency topical steroid solutions.**

Pityriasis Rosea

Etiology and Clinical Features

Pityriasis rosea is an **acute, self-limited eruption.** The cause is **unknown.** Most cases start with a **single, large, oval, scaling plaque** known as a **herald patch.** Within 1 week of the initial lesion, crops of **small, pink, finely scaled plaques** develop on the **trunk.** These lesions have a tendency to follow **skin cleavage lines,** creating a **"Christmas tree" pattern.** The rash usually **spares the face, except in children,** where facial involvement is common. The eruption may be associated with **moderate pruritus.**

> **✂ HINT** The eruption of secondary syphilis can mimic pityriasis rosea and should be considered in sexually active adolescents.

Treatment

Topical antipruritics can help alleviate the itching.

Scabies

Scabies is discussed in Chapter 65, "Pruritus."

Papular Acrodermatitis of Childhood (Gianotti-Crosti Syndrome)

Etiology

Papular acrodermatitis of childhood is **associated with many viruses,** most commonly **Epstein-Barr virus in the United States.** In Europe, there is a strong association with nonicteric hepatitis B infection.

Clinical Features

The patient presents with **skin-colored to erythematous flat-topped papules** that are found on the **face, extremities, and buttocks,** with the trunk usually spared. **Pruritus** is sometimes associated with the eruption. **Hepatomegaly and lymphadenopathy** are occasionally present.

Evaluation and Treatment

Liver function tests may be abnormal in those patients with hepatomegaly. Usually, there is no need to do any laboratory tests because the diagnosis can usually be made clinically and the eruption is **benign and self-limiting,** usually **resolving in 3–6 weeks.**

Papular Urticaria

Etiology and Clinical Features

Papular urticaria, caused by **hypersensitivity to insect bites,** is characterized by **intensely pruritic wheals** (5–10 mm in diameter) **and papules** that contain a **central punctum.** Many times, the central punctum cannot be seen secondary to excoriation.

Lesions can be seen on any part of the body, but are typically seen on exposed areas such as **the extremities, head, neck, and shoulders.** The eruption can **persist for months** and lesions can become **secondarily infected.** Extremely sensitive patients can develop **bullous lesions.** Fully resolved lesions tend to have **temporary hyperpigmentation.**

⚡ HINT Always consider an insect bite reaction when a patient presents with grouped urticarial papules that occur only on exposed areas.

Evaluation

The **history and physical examination** are diagnostic.

Treatment

In patients with prolonged episodes, it is important to find out **what is biting the patient** and where it is coming from. **Pets** should be **treated for infestations.** Secondarily infected lesions should be treated with the appropriate **antibiotics.**

▼ EVALUATION OF RASH

Patient History

It is important to obtain information regarding **how the rash has evolved.** If the rash is extensive, a **complete drug and immunization history** should be obtained.

Physical Examination

When evaluating the pediatric patient with a rash, it is important to consider the presence or absence of **fever,** the **morphology** of the eruption, and its **distribution.** A complete examination of the **skin, hair, nails, and mucous membranes** should be performed.

▼ TREATMENT OF RASH

Table 67.1 summarizes commonly used topical corticosteroids, but is not all-inclusive.

TABLE 67.1. Topical Corticosteroids

Class	Generic Name	Brand Name	Formulation
1: highest potency	Clobetasol propionate 0.05%	Temovate	Cream, ointment
	Betamethasone dipropionate 0.05%	Diprolene	Cream, ointment
	Diflorasone diacetate 0.05%	Psorcon	Ointment
2: high-potency	Fluocinonide 0.05%	Lidex	Cream, ointment, gel
	Desoximetasone 0.25%	Topicort	Cream, ointment
3: mid- to high-potency	Triamcinolone acetonide 0.5%	Aristocort Kenalog	Cream, ointment Cream, ointment
	Mometasone furoate 0.1%	Elocon	Ointment
	Betamethasone valerate 0.1%	Valisone	Ointment
4: mid-potency	Triamcinolone acetonide 0.1%	Aristocort Kenalog	Ointment Ointment
	Mometasone furoate 0.1%	Elocon	Cream
	Fluocinolone acetonide 0.025%	Synalar	Ointment Cream
	Desoximetasone 0.05%	Topicort LP	Cream
5: low- to mid-potency	Alclometasone dipropionate 0.05%	Aclovate	Cream, ointment
	Betamethasone valerate 0.1%	Valisone	Cream, lotion
	Fluocinolone acetonide 0.025%	Synalar	Cream
	Hydrocortisone valerate 0.2%	Westcort	Cream, ointment
6: low-potency	Triamcinolone acetonide 0.025%	Aristocort	Cream
	Desonide 0.05%	Desowen	Cream
	Fluocinolone acetonide 0.01%	Synalar	Cream, lotion
7: lowest potency	Hydrocortisone 1% Hydrocortisone 2.5%	Numerous over-the-counter preparations	Cream

Suggested Readings

Hanifin JM: Atopic dermatitis in infants and children. *Pediatr Clin North Am* 38(4):763–809, 1991.

Johr RH, Schachner LA: Neonatal dermatologic challenges. *Pediatr Rev* 18(3):86–94, 1997.

Lobato MN, Vugia DJ, Friday IJ: Tinea capitis in California children. *Pediatrics* 99:551–554, 1997.

Winston M, Shalita A: Acne vulgaris: pathogenesis and treatment. *Pediatr Clin North Am* 38(4):889–904, 1991.

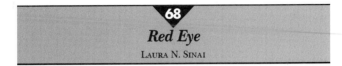

68

Red Eye

LAURA N. SINAI

▼ INTRODUCTION

Red eye may refer to **erythema of the ocular adnexa, conjunctiva, sclera, or cornea,** or **inflammation of deeper structures.**

▼ DIFFERENTIAL DIAGNOSIS LIST

Ocular Adnexa

Infectious Causes

Hordeolum and chalazion
Dacryocystitis
Molluscum contagiosum
Blepharitis
Phthiriasis (louse)
Frontal sinus infection or other sinusitis
Periostitis of orbital bones
Orbital cellulitis, periorbital cellulitis
Dental abscess

Neoplastic Causes

Neuroblastoma
Leukemia
Neurofibroma

Traumatic Causes

Insect bites
Basilar skull fracture
Trauma to eyelid or nose

Miscellaneous Causes

Frequent eye rubbing
Cavernous sinus thrombosis
Prolonged crying

Contact dermatitis
Seborrhea

Conjunctiva

Infectious Causes

Bacteria
Viruses
Fungi
Protozoans
Helminths—onchocerciasis (river blindness)

Toxic Causes

Atropine, scopolamine
Irritants—makeup, smoke, smog, chemicals, contact lenses, caterpillar hair, wind, ultraviolet light, tobacco

Neoplastic Causes

Orbital tumors—retinoblastoma

Traumatic Causes

Foreign body
Entropion, ectropion
Child abuse
Blunt or penetrating trauma
Traumatic glaucoma
Subconjunctival hemorrhage

Immunologic Causes

Allergic/inflammatory conjunctivitis
Keratoconjunctivitis sicca and other dry eye disorders
Nasal inflammation
Sjögren syndrome and other collagen vascular diseases
Kawasaki syndrome
Stevens-Johnson syndrome
Inflammatory bowel disease
Juvenile rheumatoid arthritis (JRA)
Grave's disease

Miscellaneous Causes

Bone marrow transplant
Ectodermal dysplasia
Subconjunctival hemorrhage (secondary to severe cough, bacteremia, blood dyscrasia, or vomiting)

Cornea

Infectious Causes

Keratitis
Syphilis

Traumatic Causes

Contact lenses
Corneal ulcer

Corneal abrasion
Chemical irritant

Uveal Tract

Iridocyclitis
Reiter syndrome

Sclera

Episcleritis
Scleritis
Collagen vascular disease

Pupil

Hyphema
Globe
Glaucoma

▼ DIFFERENTIAL DIAGNOSIS DISCUSSION
Neonatal Conjunctivitis

Etiology

Neonatal conjunctivitis is most often **secondary to infection or chemical irritation.**

▼ **Infection.** Causes of infectious conjunctivitis in the neonate include sexually transmitted and nonsexually transmitted organisms. Sexually transmitted agents, in order of decreasing frequency, are *Chlamydia trachomatis, Neisseria gonorrhoeae,* and herpes simplex virus (HSV), usually type 2. *Staphylococcus aureus* is the most common nonsexually transmitted infectious pathogen. Other bacterial causes include enteric gram-negative rods.

▼ **Chemical irritation.** Silver nitrate is the most common cause of neonatal chemical conjunctivitis, although other antibiotics used for prophylaxis can also cause conjunctivitis.

Clinical Features

Conjunctivitis that presents in the **first 24 hours of life** is most likely **secondary to chemical irritation,** unless there was prolonged rupture of membranes before delivery.

▼ **Gonococcal conjunctivitis,** which presents 2–6 days after birth, is an acute to hyperacute infection that causes edema of the eyelids and conjunctiva (chemosis), local pain, and a copious purulent discharge. Swelling and discharge can be so extensive that the orbit is difficult to view. Often there is a palpable preauricular node, a finding otherwise uncommon in bacterial conjunctivitis.

▼ **Chlamydial conjunctivitis** has a slightly later onset than gonococcal conjunctivitis, but can be symptomatic as early as 4–5 days after birth. Modest purulent drainage and mild to moderate inflammation are seen. As with gonococcal conjunctivitis, the preauricular lymph node may be tender.

▼ **Herpes simplex conjunctivitis** is associated with clusters of vesicles on the face, eyelids, and mucous membranes.

▓ HINT Chlamydial conjunctivitis is, in general, markedly less acute and impressive than gonococcal conjunctivitis.

▓ HINT Chlamydial pneumonitis occurs in as many as one-third of infants with chlamydial conjunctivitis.

Evaluation

Bacterial culture, including **chocolate agar or Thayer-Martin plates,** and **Gram stain of the purulent material** should be obtained. In up to 95% of cases of gonococcal conjunctivitis, gram-negative intracellular diplococci are identified by Gram stain.

Chlamydia **culture and a rapid assay** should be obtained on **conjunctival scrapings** (not purulent material). In patients with suspected herpes simplex conjunctivitis, conjunctival scrapings reveal mononuclear cells and giant multinucleated epithelial cells.

Treatment

▼ **Chlamydial conjunctivitis.** Hospitalization is not necessary. Treatment consists of 14 days of oral erythromycin combined with topical erythromycin.
▼ **Gonococcal conjunctivitis.** Hospitalization and consultation with an ophthalmologist is required. The eye should be irrigated every 1–2 hours to reduce bacterial load and local irritation. Improperly treated gonococcal conjunctivitis can quickly damage vision. Intravenous antibiotic therapy for 7 days is indicated. Cefotaxime or ceftriaxone are appropriate until sensitivities are known.
▼ **Herpes simplex conjunctivitis.** Patients must be followed by an ophthalmologist to minimize the chance of permanent scarring and damage to vision.

Infectious Conjunctivitis (Outside the Neonatal Period)

Etiology

The most common bacterial cause of conjunctivitis is *S. aureus,* which affects all age groups. *Haemophilus influenzae* and *Streptococcus pneumoniae* are common causes of conjunctivitis in **young children.** Adolescents can also present with **gonococcal** conjunctivitis **secondary to sexual contact.**

Epidemic keratoconjunctivitis, the name given to rapidly spreading viral conjunctivitis, most often occurs secondary to adenoviral infection. **HSV, types 1 and 2,** and **varicella-zoster virus** are more serious causes of viral conjunctivitis; these organisms are associated with **corneal destruction** (keratitis) and **loss of vision.** Herpes simplex keratitis is the most common infectious cause of corneal blindness in developed countries.

Protozoal infections, specifically *Acanthamoeba,* are seen almost **exclusively in contact lens wearers.**

▓ HINT Contact lens wearers are more susceptible to virulent gram-negative infections and unusual fungal infections of the conjunctiva.

Clinical Features (Table 68.1)

The clinical signs and symptoms of **bacterial** conjunctivitis include **tearing, purulent discharge, conjunctival hyperemia, and foreign body sensation.** The eyelids are often **crusted closed** on arising in the **morning.** *H. influenzae* and *S. pneumoniae* conjunctival infections are often associated with **subconjunctival hemorrhage.** Infection is often **bilateral.**

The physical findings of **nonherpetic viral** conjunctivitis include a **serous or lightly purulent discharge, minimal to moderate eyelid swelling, a unilateral or bilateral presentation, and occasional systemic symptoms** (e.g., malaise, fever, or sore throat). **Profuse tearing** is often present. Viral conjunctivitis is much more likely than bacterial infection to be associated with **tender preauricular adenopathy.**

⚡ HINT Subconjunctival hemorrhage may point to adenoviral conjunctivitis.

In patients with **herpetic viral** conjunctivitis, the **initial HSV infection** is clinically **indistinguishable from other causes of viral conjunctivitis,** with the exception that it is almost always **unilateral.** Herpetic recurrences are unilateral in 96% of patients, are often **corneal** (keratitis), and produce the classic **dendritic lesion of the cornea best seen with fluorescein.**

Evaluation

Culture is necessary only **if an unusual or serious pathogen** is suspected. Although recovery of the offending organism is difficult once antibiotic therapy has been initiated, cultures are also recommended **if treatment failure occurs.** Culture recovery of HSV is successful in only 70% of patients with herpetic conjunctivitis.

TABLE 68.1. Differentiation of Conjunctivitis (Outside the Neonatal Period)

Clinical Findings	Viral	Bacterial	Chlamydial	Allergic
Itching	Minimal	Minimal	Minimal	Severe
Hyperemia	Generalized	Generalized	Generalized	Generalized
Tearing	Profuse	Moderate	Moderate	Moderate
Exudation	Minimal	Profuse	Profuse	Minimal
Preauricular node	Common	Uncommon*	Inclusion conjunct	None
Stained scraping	Monocytes	Bacteria, PMNs	PMNs, plasma cells	Eosinophils
Sore throat/ fever?	Occasionally	Occasionally	Never	Never

* Except in gonococcal conjunctivitis.

Modified with permission from Schwab I, Dawson C: Conjunctiva. In *General Ophthalmology*, 14th ed. Edited by Vaughan D, Ashbury T, Riordan-Eva P. Norwalk, CT, Appleton & Lange, 1995, p 98.

PMN = polymorphonuclear cells.

Treatment

Viral and bacterial conjunctivitis are **self-resolving** illnesses **except for herpes simplex** conjunctivitis and conjunctivitis caused by **varicella zoster virus.** Because it is **impossible to clinically differentiate viral and bacterial** conjunctivitis with certainty, **nonherpetic viral** conjunctivitis is **treated in the same fashion as bacterial** conjunctivitis. Treatment involves instillation of **antibiotic drops and periodic removal of eye discharge with warm, wet washclothes.** Improvement usually occurs within 3–4 days. Without treatment, bacterial conjunctivitis usually resolves within 2 weeks. In the event of **treatment failure,** a **second antibiotic** with a significantly **different spectrum** from the first antibiotic should be prescribed.

Any child with a **prior history of herpetic conjunctivitis** who presents with red eye should be assumed to have **recurrent herpes infection** and must be **referred to an ophthalmologist urgently. Steroid use** in all types of conjunctivitis is best **left to an ophthalmologist** because **serious harm** can result **if steroids** are inadvertently **prescribed for a patient with herpetic conjunctivitis.**

Allergic Conjunctivitis

Etiology

Common environmental allergens (e.g., animal dander, dust, molds, grass, pollens) can cause allergic conjunctivitis. **Antibiotic drops and facial creams or lotions** have also been implicated.

Clinical Features

The hallmark of allergic conjunctivitis is **pruritus.** There can be significant **erythema and swelling of the eyelids,** most often in a **bilateral** distribution. These symptoms can be confused with those of periorbital or orbital cellulitis; however, a **lack of tenderness** and the **absence of systemic symptoms** make cellulitis unlikely. **Conjunctival hyperemia** is **diffuse. Discharge** is **moderate** in volume and **clear.** Adenopathy is not found.

The **onset of symptoms** can be **abrupt,** after acute exposure to the offending agent, **or chronic,** with repeated or continuous exposure. Symptoms may show a **seasonal variation,** commonly **worsening in the spring. Rhinitis and other allergic symptoms** may also be present.

Treatment

Treatment depends on the age of the child and the subjective symptoms. **Erythema alone does not warrant intervention. Cold compresses** are effective for short-term relief of pruritus. **Topical vasoconstrictors and antihistamines** are the first-line medications if treatment is undertaken. If unsuccessful, **topical steroids** may be required. **Systemic antihistamines** and **nasal steroids** often provide relief.

Chalazia and Hordeola

Etiology

A chalazion is a **chronic inflammatory lipogranuloma of the meibomian gland** resulting from obstruction of the gland duct. **Secondary infection** is common. An infected chalazion is sometimes referred to as an **internal hordeolum.**

An **external hordeolum (stye)** is a **purulent,** usually **staphylococcal, infection of the follicle of an eyelash** or its associated **sebaceous or sweat gland.**

Clinical Features and Evaluation

Uninfected chalazia are characterized by **gradual, painless swelling** in the body of the **eyelid.** Chalazia that become **secondarily infected** usually **point and drain on the inside of the eyelid** (the conjunctival side).

Hordeola present with **swelling, induration, and purulent drainage** at or near the margin of the eyelid. Hordeola tend to **point and drain outward.** Hordeola often occur in **groups,** following the spread of infection from one follicle to another.

Both chalazia and hordeola may be **unilateral or bilateral.** The child with either a hordeolum or an infected chalazion is **afebrile and appears otherwise well.**

Treatment

Small, uninfected chalazia may **resolve spontaneously. Large chalazia** must be **surgically removed. Infected** chalazia require **medical management.**

Hordeola and infected chalazia are treated identically. **Warm to hot compresses** should be applied to the affected eye for **20 minutes, four times per day,** to encourage spontaneous drainage of the purulent collections. Some advocate daily **cleaning of the lid margins, using baby shampoo and water on a washcloth** rubbed on the lid margin with the eyes held shut. **Topical antibiotic ointment or drops** should be instilled daily. Attention to **general hygiene** keeps recurrences to a minimum.

Corneal Abrasion

Etiology

Corneal abrasions result from **traumatic removal of part of the corneal epithelium.**

Clinical Features

The signs and symptoms seen with corneal abrasion often mimic those of infectious conjunctivitis—**diffuse injection of the conjunctiva, watery discharge, pain,** and, often, **decreased visual acuity.** The main difference is found in the history—**trauma,** even if apparently minor, **immediately precedes the onset of symptoms** in patients with corneal abrasion.

Evaluation

Patients presenting with **red eye** and any **history of trauma** should have a **fluorescein examination of the eye** to rule out an abrasion. The eye should be carefully examined to **exclude** the possibility of a **retained foreign body** or a **deeper injury.** This includes performing a **maneuver to flip the upper lid and inspect the inner surface.** If the **pain** persists for **more than 24 hours** after the initial trauma, **referral to an ophthalmologist** should be made.

Treatment

The primary goal of treatment is to **prevent further injury. Foreign bodies** should be **removed by irrigation** with sterile saline solution. If this is ineffective, an **ophthalmologist** should be **consulted** for removal. After careful evaluation, a **sterile light-pressure dressing** should be placed over the eye for **approximately 24 hours.** Many authors also recommend **topical antibiotic eyedrops.** The eye should be **examined daily** until fully healed.

⚇ HINT Topical anesthetics should never be given to a patient for repeated home instillation after corneal injury. Their use delays healing, masks damage, and can lead to permanent corneal scarring.

Orbital and Periorbital Cellulitis

Etiology

Periorbital cellulitis refers to **infection of the tissues anterior to the globe.** Infection occurs either via **hematogenous spread or local trauma.** In the past, hematogenously spread disease was most often caused by *H. influenzae,* but *S. pneumoniae* and other organisms are becoming more prevalent as a result of the success of the universal *H. influenzae* type B vaccination. In patients with a **history of local trauma,** *S. aureus* and *Streptococcus* are the most common pathogens.

Orbital cellulitis most commonly results from **direct spread of infection from the sinuses.** The infectious process in orbital cellulitis involves the **retrobulbar tissues,** including the **ocular muscles, orbital fat, and bone.**

Clinical Features

Periorbital cellulitis is a unilateral disease that presents with **significant swelling, induration, tenderness, and erythema of the eyelids** and a variable amount of **purulent discharge. Fever** is common.

Orbital cellulitis presents with a clinical picture **similar to** that of **periorbital** cellulitis. In addition, orbital cellulitis is characterized by a **decreased range of motion of ocular muscles, proptosis, changes in vision, and papilledema.**

Evaluation

Children with periorbital or orbital cellulitis may be **bacteremic,** and **blood cultures** should be obtained. **Computed tomography** (CT) should be used whenever **orbital** cellulitis is considered. **Some clinicians perform CT scans** on all patients with **periorbital** cellulitis to detect subtle cases of orbital cellulitis.

Treatment

Hospitalization and the intravenous administration of antibiotics is indicated for patients with periorbital or orbital cellulitis. **Oxacillin and chloramphenicol or ceftriaxone** are appropriate antibiotic choices. **Surgical drainage** may be required in the case of orbital cellulitis.

Patients with **orbital** cellulitis should be seen by an **ophthalmologist** because orbital cellulitis carries **a significant risk for damage to the visual axis**—specifically, **optic neuritis with atrophy. Significant extraocular complications** are also associated with orbital cellulitis, including **cavernous sinus thrombosis, meningitis, and brain abscess.**

Suggested Readings

Block SL, Hedrick J, Tyler R, et al: Increasing bacterial resistance in pediatric acute conjunctivitis (1997–1998). *Antimicrob Agents Chemother* 44(6):1650–1654, 2000.

King RA: Common ocular signs and symptoms in childhood. *Pediatr Clin North Am* 40:753, 1993.

Leibowitz HM: The red eye. *N Engl J Med* 3;343(5):345–351, 2000.

Limberg M: A review of bacterial keratitis and bacterial conjunctivitis. *Am J Ophthalmol* 112:2s–9S, 1991.

Roy, FH: *Ocular Differential Diagnosis*, 6th ed. Baltimore, Williams & Wilkins, 1996.

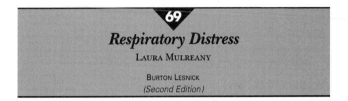

69

Respiratory Distress

LAURA MULREANY

BURTON LESNICK
(Second Edition)

▼ INTRODUCTION

Respiratory distress may be defined as **increased work of breathing** that causes the patient to have a **sense of altered well-being.** Symptoms may include shortness of breath, chest tightness, chest pain, cough, and even mental status changes in later stages.

▼ DIFFERENTIAL DIAGNOSIS LIST

Infectious Causes

Peritonsillar abscess
Retropharyngeal abscess
Epiglottitis
Croup (Viral laryngotracheobronchitis)
Bacterial tracheitis
Bronchiolitis
Pertussis
Pneumonia

Structural Lesions

Vocal cord paralysis
Subglottic stenosis
Laryngomalacia
Tracheomalacia
Bronchomalacia
Lobar emphysema
Bronchogenic cyst
Vascular ring, other aberrant vessels
Mediastinal or other intrathoracic mass (cystic hygroma, teratoma, cystic adenomatoid malformation, neuroblastoma, diaphragmatic hernia or eventration)

Toxic Causes

Carbon monoxide poisoning
Methemoglobinemia

Neoplastic Causes

Hemangioma
Papilloma
Brain stem tumor

Traumatic Causes

Foreign body aspiration
Aspiration due to gastroesophageal reflux disease
Pneumothorax

Metabolic or Genetic Causes

Metabolic acidosis
Cystic fibrosis

Psychosocial Causes

Psychogenic hyperventilation

Neuromuscular Disorders

Respiratory muscle weakness, myopathy
Duchenne muscular dystrophy
Spinal muscle atrophy
Prune-belly syndrome
Werdnig-Hoffmann disease

Miscellaneous Causes

Anaphylaxis
Asthma
Atelectasis
Pleural disease (effusion, empyema)
Pulmonary hemorrhage
Pulmonary edema
Pulmonary embolism
Sickle cell crisis—acute chest syndrome
Vocal cord dysfunction

▼ DIFFERENTIAL DIAGNOSIS DISCUSSION

Infectious Causes

Infections causing respiratory distress may be **bacterial or viral,** and may **affect any part of the respiratory tract.** Some syndromes are more common in different age groups, aiding in the diagnosis. In addition to the symptoms of respiratory distress mentioned earlier, the patient may have **congestion** or a **runny nose** or a variety of constitutional symptoms such as **fever, malaise, poor appetite, or body aches.** The causative agent may be identified by cultures of the nasopharynx, pharynx, or sputum.

Epiglottitis

Etiology

Infection of the epiglottis is most commonly caused by *Haemophilus influenzae,* type B, and results in **rapid swelling and airway compromise,** creating a **medical emergency.** Fortunately, near universal use of the *H. influenzae,* type B vaccine has dramatically reduced the incidence of this disease.

Clinical Features

Epiglottitis is most common in children **between the ages of 3 and 6** years who have not been vaccinated against *H. influenzae,* type B. Symptoms develop over several hours and include **high fever, dysphasia, drooling, inspiratory stridor, and holding the head in an upright "sniffing" position,** with the neck extended and the jaw protruding.

Evaluation

When the history is suggestive, **the child should not be excessively disturbed.** Attempts to directly visualize the pharynx may result in **complete occlusion** of the airway and **respiratory arrest.** Vaccination status of a patient with suspected epiglottitis must be assessed, although a positive history of vaccination does not rule out the possibility of epiglottitis. A **lateral neck radiograph** should be obtained **in the presence of a physician and nursing staff** who are prepared to perform **immediate intubation or tracheostomy.** A **characteristic "thumb-print" epiglottis** (the epiglottis is swollen) is diagnostic.

A blood culture drawn after an airway has been established may help determine the causative bacteria.

Treatment

The **most experienced staff** available should **establish an artificial airway under controlled circumstances.** When intubation of the trachea cannot be accomplished, **tracheostomy** is indicated. **Broad-spectrum antibiotics** are then administered **intravenously.**

Croup

Etiology

Most cases of croup are caused by **parainfluenza virus. Edema of the larynx, trachea, and bronchi** results in increased airway resistance. Rarely, airway obstruction is so severe that cardiopulmonary arrest ensues.

Clinical Features

Patients are usually **younger than 3 years old,** although the presence of typical symptoms in the first few months of life should prompt evaluation for congenital anomalies. Patients with mild cases may demonstrate a **bark-like cough, nasal congestion, and fever.** Typically, a mild cough with intermittent stridor **progresses to continuous stridor, especially at night.** Many patients improve after exposure to humidified air or cool night air.

Evaluation

Critical airway narrowing is denoted by severe retractions, inspiratory stridor, and decreased air entry on physical examination. In patients with severe airway obstruction, **cyanosis and weakness** may be noted. **Cyanosis, tachycardia, and mental status changes** accompany hypoxia. **Lateral and**

anterior–posterior neck radiographs can help differentiate croup from epiglottitis. A characteristic **"steeple sign"** is often seen in the subglottic airway in croup, and the epiglottis is normal. **Arterial blood gas analysis** can help to determine the adequacy of air exchange.

Treatment

An **artificial airway** should be established for patients with impending respiratory failure. Therapeutic strategies include the following:

▼ **Humidified oxygen.** Cool, humidified oxygen is the best treatment for patients with mild to moderate cases of croup.
▼ **Racemic epinephrine.** Patients with severe cases may benefit from the inhalation of racemic epinephrine. These patients may need to be hospitalized to observe for rebound effects, which may occur 30–60 minutes after the administration of racemic epinephrine.
▼ **Intravenous fluids.** Fluids are helpful to maintain adequate hydration in patients with severe tachypnea.
▼ **Steroids.** The use of steroids in treating croup is controversial; however, if administered early, steroids may be beneficial in patients with severe symptoms.
▼ **Antibiotics.** Unless a secondary bacterial infection is suspected, antibiotics are not indicated.

Bronchiolitis

Etiology

Viruses [e.g., respiratory syncytial virus (RSV), parainfluenza viruses, and adenoviruses] infect the **lining of the small airways (bronchioles),** resulting in **mucosal edema and intraluminal accumulation of mucus and cellular debris.** Infants **younger than 2 years old** are predominantly affected because the small caliber of their airways predisposes them to the development of increased airway resistance with even mild airway narrowing.

Clinical Features

A **prodrome of nasal congestion and coryza** of several days' duration is usual. A **fever and anorexia** may be present, particularly in young infants with severe nasal congestion who may have difficulty feeding. Often, another family member will have a mild upper respiratory tract infection. **Respiratory distress** usually **develops gradually** and is characterized by a worsening cough and wheezing. Typically, the **symptoms are worse at night.**

Evaluation

On physical examination, infants are usually **tachypneic,** with a respiratory rate of 60–80 breaths/min. The **expiratory phase is usually prolonged** and **diffuse wheezing** is often present. **Breath sounds** may be diminished in severe cases. **Severe retractions and the use of accessory muscles** are common. Lung hyperinflation and depression of the diaphragm typically result in a **palpable liver and spleen.** A **chest radiograph** shows hyperinflation, peribronchial thickening, and, in many patients, subsegmental atelectasis. A **nasopharyngeal swab** or washing for RSV may be helpful in confirming the diagnosis.

Treatment

Supportive care entails administration of **humidified oxygen** and positioning of the infant with the **head and neck slightly elevated.** Frequent **nasal suctioning** is often helpful. **Intravenous fluids** are useful in maintaining hydration in the presence of tachypnea and decreased oral intake. **Nebulized albuterol** may benefit some patients, and **nebulized racemic epinephrine** has also been tried with some success in a limited number of patients with reactive airway disease. **Sedatives should not be used,** and steroids and antibiotics are generally not helpful. In infants with a severe course, or those with underlying cardiac or pulmonary disease, **ribavirin** may have a role in treating bronchiolitis caused by RSV.

✄ HINT Young infants and infants with a history of premature birth (with or without associated lung disease) or chronic heart or lung disease, are at greater risk for apnea and poor outcome. A vaccine (Palivizumab) is available for patients who meet high-risk criteria.

Pertussis

Etiology

The classic causative organism is *Bordetella pertussis,* but *Bordetella parapertussis* and adenovirus infection can also cause pertussis, which is characterized by **necrosis** and desquamation of the superficial epithelium of the pharynx. Children **younger than 2 months** are most at risk, even if immunized.

Clinical Features

▼ **A catarrhal stage,** consisting of symptoms of an upper respiratory tract infection, lasts 1–2 weeks.

▼ **A paroxysmal stage** follows and is characterized by a distinctive, repeated, staccato cough that occurs during a single expiration, often emptying the lungs of all their vital capacity. In the following inspiration, a "whoop" sound is produced as the edematous, narrowed glottis oscillates between the open and closed position, causing the column of inspired air to vibrate. Whoops are not always present. Patients are usually well between paroxysmal attacks.

▼ **During the convalescent stage,** the frequency of paroxysms gradually decreases, although the cough often persists for several months (called the "100-day cough"). With repeated coughing, facial redness or cyanosis and neck vein distention may occur. Post-tussive emesis is common. Petechiae of the head and neck and conjunctival hemorrhages may develop after severe coughing. Infants may develop respiratory distress, apnea, or both.

Evaluation

During the early paroxysmal phase, a **complete blood cell count** reveals lymphocytosis. **Chest radiographs** may show perihilar infiltrates and subsegmental atelectasis. **Fluorescent antibody staining** can be performed on pharyngeal swabs to detect *B. pertussis.* A positive culture is necessary to confirm the diagnosis.

Treatment

Erythromycin can help reduce the spread of infection but will not shorten the disease once it has progressed to the paroxysmal phase. Supportive care consists of maintaining adequate **hydration,** administering **supplemental oxygen** for patients with respiratory distress, and **suctioning nasal secretions** in infants. **Inhaled bronchodilators** may help reduce coughing paroxysms. Cough suppressants are generally not helpful.

Structural Lesions

Structural lesions may occur at any point along the respiratory system and may cause respiratory symptoms any time from the early neonatal period onward. The symptoms may worsen in the face of an intercurrent acute respiratory illness such as a viral infection or asthma exacerbation. Treatment for lesions may involve **observation, medical therapy, or surgical intervention.**

Laryngomalacia, Tracheomalacia, Bronchomalacia

Etiology

Weakened or softened underlying cartilaginous and/or muscular infrastructure of the airway results in **collapse of the airway** and **luminal narrowing.** The process may be **primary or secondary,** often due to insults such as prolonged mechanical ventilation in the premature newborn or recurrent aspiration from gastroesophageal reflux disease.

Clinical Features

The patient may demonstrate **stridor if the lesion is extrathoracic** or **wheezing if the lesion is intrathoracic.** The wheeze is often homophonous and vibratory. The symptoms may be accentuated during crying or agitation, or during an intercurrent acute respiratory illness.

Evaluation

The history and physical examination are often highly suggestive of the diagnosis. Confirmation requires visualization by **endoscopy.**

Treatment

Since airway collapsibility improves with increasing age, malacia usually **resolves spontaneously by 15 to 18 months of age.** Intercurrent acute illnesses should be managed accordingly and causative diseases, such as reflux, should be treated appropriately. In severe cases, **positive airway pressure** (either noninvasively or invasively through a tracheostomy) or **surgical procedures** may be needed.

Traumatic Causes

Foreign Bodies

Etiology

Foreign bodies may be **inhaled into the airway,** or they may get **caught in the esophagus** and externally compress the trachea. Foreign body aspiration is more common in toddlers and infants, who tend to put objects in their mouths. Parents may even recall the exact time of the start of symptoms.

Clinical Features

If the object is **in the esophagus, drooling, dysphagia, and anorexia** may accompany **respiratory distress.** Respiratory symptoms may be **acute or chronic,** with a history of **chronic cough** unresponsive to other treatments.

Evaluation

A **monophonic wheeze or absent breath sounds on one side** may be noted on chest examination.

Chest and neck radiographs with lateral views may be helpful in identifying the location of an object. **Inspiratory and expiratory lateral decubitus films** may denote an area of hyperinflation.

Arterial blood gas analysis (to establish the adequacy of gas exchange) is indicated when the patient is in severe distress.

Treatment

▼ **If the child is calm with good air exchange, removal of the foreign body should take place under controlled circumstances** because manipulation may change the position of the object, inducing more severe obstruction.

▼ **If the child is in significant distress, back blows and chest thrusts** may be performed as per the standard technique for cardiopulmonary resuscitation. **Emergency tracheostomy** may be necessary.

Aspiration Due to Gastroesophageal Reflux Disease (GER)

Etiology

GER may cause respiratory symptoms from **large bolus aspiration, recurrent microaspiration, or reflex laryngospasm or bronchospasm.** Patients with underlying neurologic disorders are at increased risk for aspiration.

Clinical Features

Patients may or may not have a history of **overt reflux with vomiting followed by coughing or choking.** Some patients may simply have **recurrent cough (especially at night), frequent stomachaches, heartburn or chest pain, or sour burps.** With aspiration pneumonitis, significant **respiratory distress and hypoxemia** may occur as well as **fever.**

Evaluation

GER is diagnosed by **radionucleotide scan** (milk scan) **or pH probe.** To ensure the absence of an anatomic abnormality causing the reflux, an **upper gastrointestinal series** is often performed prior to the initiation of therapy. After aspiration, a **chest radiograph** may show a consolidation in the affected area.

Treatment

Aspiration pneumonitis requires **antibiotic therapy,** usually intravenous antibiotics until fever and significant respiratory symptoms have resolved. GER is treated usually with a combination of **prokinetic agent and an H_2 blocker or proton pump inhibitor.** In severe reflux that does not respond to medical therapy, **surgical treatment** (fundoplication) may be necessary.

Pneumothorax

Etiology

Trauma to the chest, foreign body aspiration (with a ball–valve effect), **severe underlying pulmonary disease, or idiopathic bulla formation** may result in the entry of air into the potential space between the parietal and visceral pleurae, impairing the ability of the chest wall to adequately inflate the lung parenchyma on the affected side. Patients with connective tissue diseases (e.g., Marfan syndrome) may be at **increased risk for pneumothorax.** Often, the precipitating event is a **Valsalva maneuver,** which causes a transient elevation of intrathoracic pressure. **Commercial air travel** in pressurized cabins and **scuba diving** are also risk factors.

Tension pneumothorax (a life-threatening event that results from the rapid filling of the pleural space by gas under pressure) can **distort the vascular flow** via compression and **cause rapid death.** Patients undergoing positive-pressure mechanical ventilation are at risk for tension pneumothorax.

Clinical Features

Symptoms are usually **abrupt in onset** and consist of **pleuritic chest pain, tachypnea, and hypoxemia.** With large pneumothoraces, **cough and cyanosis** may be seen as well.

The degree of distress is related to the size of the pneumothorax, usually described as a percentage of the thoracic volume on the affected side. Small pneumothoraces may be asymptomatic.

Evaluation

A **history** of trauma, underlying lung disease, or past pneumothoraces from bullae should be elicited. **Chest examination** demonstrates **decreased breath sounds** on the affected side and **tympany** to percussion. **Heart tones may be shifted** toward the affected side (as a result of lung collapse) or away from the affected side (in patients with tension pneumothorax). **Transillumination of the chest** is helpful in demonstrating pneumothorax. **Chest radiographs** should be done in the expiratory phase to accentuate areas of hyperlucency. **Arterial blood gas analysis** may help establish the degree of ventilatory compromise.

Treatment

Tension pneumothorax is a **medical emergency. Thoracentesis** should be attempted by placing a needle at the second anterior intercostal space at the midclavicular line. Care must be taken not to puncture the underlying lung. For large pneumothoraces, **tube thoracostomy** may be necessary to drain the air until the visceral pleura can repair itself. Occasionally, in patients with recurrent pneumothoraces, **sclerosing the pleura by chemical or physical means** to the internal chest wall is necessary to allow the lung to remain re-expanded. **Supplemental oxygen** should be given to hypoxemic patients. Inhalation of **100% oxygen can displace the nitrogen** in the gas that forms the pneumothorax. Because oxygen is more readily absorbed by the body, displacement of nitrogen with oxygen can hasten resolution of the pneumothorax.

Neuromuscular Disorders

Etiology

Respiratory muscle weakness accompanies skeletal muscle weakness. This weakness results in failure of the respiratory pump that functions in ventilation. Patients with neuromuscular diseases also may have a **weak cough** resulting in impaired airway clearance that may cause recurrent infections or atelectasis. In the face of an acute respiratory illness, these patients are at risk for significant respiratory decompensation and failure.

Clinical Features

The patient may demonstrate **shallow, rapid respiratory pattern and a weak cough.** With worsening respiratory failure, **morning headaches** and **poor sleep quality** may be present. **Hypoxemia and respiratory distress** may accompany an acute illness.

Evaluation

Pulmonary function testing, including spirometry, lung volumes, and maximal respiratory pressures, should be measured on a regular basis to follow the patient's trend. **End tidal carbon dioxide level** may indicate worsening ventilatory failure. **Overnight polysomnography** is used to evaluate sleep pattern, respiratory events, and oxygenation and ventilation during sleep.

Treatment

Aggressive airway clearance, on a regular basis as well as during an acute illness, is a mainstay of therapy. **Early recognition** of impending respiratory failure should be followed by early **initiation of nocturnal noninvasive ventilation.** Some patients progress to needing invasive chronic mechanical ventilation via **tracheostomy.**

Miscellaneous Causes

Asthma

The triggers for asthma are discussed in Chapter 23, "Cough." This discussion focuses on asthma as a cause of respiratory distress and impending respiratory failure.

Clinical Features

Important differential diagnoses include **anaphylaxis and foreign body aspiration.** A thorough history should be taken, including the **duration, frequency, and severity of attacks;** the **medications** the patient uses acutely and chronically, as well as any used during this particular exacerbation; **peak flows** (if the patient keeps a log); and the **family history.** On physical examination, the **expiratory phase is prolonged. Breath sounds are often tubular or decreased** at the bases. **Heterophonous wheezing** is usually appreciated diffusely, but it may be absent when air exchange is severely affected.

Evaluation

A **pulsus paradoxus** may be measured. If the patient is severely affected, **arterial blood gases** should be ordered to assess oxygenation and carbon dioxide elimination. Normal values are given in Table 69.1. **Pulse oximetry**

TABLE 69.1. Normal Blood Gas Values from the Children's Hospital of Philadelphia Blood Gas Laboratory

Parameter	Age of Patient	Normal Value
pH	1 day	7.29–7.45
	3–24 months	7.34–7.46
	> 7 years	7.37–7.41
P_{CO_2}	1 day	27–40 mm Hg
	3–24 months	26–42 mm Hg
	> 7 years	34–40 mm Hg
PO_2	1 day	37–97 mm Hg
	3–24 months	88–103 mm Hg
	> 7 years	88–103 mm Hg
Base excess	1 day	> 8–(−2)
	3–24 months	−7–0
	> 7 years	−4–(+2)
HCO_3	1 day	19 mmol/L
	3–24 months	16/24 mmol/L
	> 7 years	22–27 mmol/L
O_2 saturation	· · ·	94%–99%
Venous pH	· · ·	7.32–7.42
Venous CO_2		25–47 mm Hg
Venous O_2		25–47 mm Hg

CO_2 = carbon dioxide; HCO_3 = bicarbonate; O_2 = oxygen; P_{CO_2} = carbon dioxide tension; PO_2 = oxygen tension.

is useful for determining oxygenation status but should not be substituted for arterial blood gas analysis in severely compromised patients. **Spirometry** may be helpful in patients with mild to moderate symptoms.

▰ **HINT** A near-normal carbon dioxide tension in the presence of significant tachypnea heralds impending respiratory failure.

Treatment

▼ **Oxygen** should be administered to all patients with evidence of hypoxemia.
▼ **Bronchodilation.** Patients with mild symptoms may improve with the inhalation of a nebulized beta agonist, such as albuterol. The continuous use of nebulized albuterol (administered at a rate of 5–10 mg/hr) in severely affected patients with impending respiratory failure is often necessary. Care must be taken to monitor for hypokalemia, a side effect of high-dose albuterol therapy. Intravenous bronchodilators, such as terbutaline, may also be considered.

▼ **Fluids and steroids.** Patients with severe symptoms may benefit from intravenous fluids. Intravenous or oral steroids (usually methylprednisolone sodium succinate, 1–2 mg/kg every 6 hours) are vitally important in the management of an asthma exacerbation to treat the inflammation.

▼ **Aminophylline.** The intravenous administration of aminophylline may be helpful in some patients, but constant cardiac monitoring is indicated.

Atelectasis

Etiology

Partial or complete collapse of normally aerated pulmonary parenchyma can result from an **intraluminal obstruction, extrinsic compression of the airway, or decreased respiratory muscle strength.** Loss of gas-exchanging regions of the lung may lead to **ventilation/perfusion mismatching** and **respiratory distress.**

Atelectasis is common in **postoperative patients** with impaired respiratory drive or muscle strength, **patients with infection or bronchospasm** leading to airway plugging, and **patients with alterations in the normal airway structure** as a result of congenital lesions, bronchopulmonary dysplasia, or recurrent aspiration.

Evaluation

Breath sounds are usually decreased in the affected area. Anterior–posterior and lateral **chest radiographs** help delineate the affected region. Volume loss results in displacement of fissures toward the area of atelectasis.

Treatment

Definitive treatment entails eliminating the pathological process that is responsible for the atelectasis. **Chest physiotherapy** and **postural drainage** combined with **bronchodilator therapy** can help reexpand atelectatic areas. In refractory cases, **bronchoscopy** may help to remove a particularly tenacious mucus plug. **Supplemental oxygen** is indicated for patients with hypoxemia. In the postoperative period, **early incentive spirometry, early ambulation, and good pain control** are helpful in preventing atelectasis.

Vocal Cord Dysfunction

Etiology

Vocal cord dysfunction, an **asthma-like syndrome** that is unresponsive to typical bronchodilator therapy, often develops as a somatic manifestation of **psychosocial stress** in preadolescents and adolescents.

Clinical Features

The **associated cough and respiratory distress are real** and are a result of paradoxical vocal cord movement.

Evaluation

An attempt should be made to **identify significant psychosocial stressors** in the patient's life.

On physical examination, **wheezing is absent,** or a monophonic wheeze is heard on auscultation of the neck. **Flow–volume loops** performed as part of pulmonary function testing may show **flattening of the inspiratory curve.**

Flexible laryngoscopy can identify paradoxical vocal cord movement.

Treatment

Psychological counseling to relieve the antecedent stressor is appropriate. Many patients with vocal cord dysfunction have **real asthma;** for these patients asthma therapy is indicated, in addition to counseling.

▼ APPROACH TO THE PATIENT

On physical examination, one may note **tachypnea, tachycardia, decreased oxyhemoglobin saturation, positioning with the neck hyperextended, cyanosis, nasal flaring, retractions or accessory muscle use, grunting, wheezing, or stridor.** Helpful diagnostic studies include **arterial blood gas, radiographic studies** (chest radiograph, chest computed tomography scan, upper airway films, fluoroscopy, barium swallow, bronchogram, pulmonary arteriogram, ventilation perfusion scan), **endoscopy, and pulmonary function testing.** Hallmarks of therapy include **maintaining airway patency, oxygenation, and circulation** first and foremost. Continuing care may involve a variety of medical treatments, including **bronchodilators, anti-inflammatories, airway clearance, antimicrobials, analgesia, and** even **mechanical ventilation.** Surgical procedures, such as **thoracentesis** or **lung biopsy,** may be necessary for diagnosis or treatment. The underlying cause of respiratory distress should be sought and treated, if possible. Untreated respiratory distress may advance to respiratory failure, in which oxygenation and ventilation are impaired.

Suggested Readings

Ausejo M, Saenz A, Pham B, et al: Glucocorticoids for croup. *Cochrane Database Syst Rev* (2):CD001955, 2000.

Cressman WR, Myer CM: Diagnosis and management of croup and epiglottitis. *Pediatr Clin North Am* 41:265, 1994.

Klassen TP: Croup. A current perspective. *Pediatr Clin North Am* 46(6):1167–1178, 1999.

Nafstad P, Magnus P, Jaakkola JJ: Early respiratory infections and childhood asthma. *Pediatrics* 106(3):E38, 2000.

Panitch HB: Bronchiolitis in infants. *Curr Opin Pediatr* 13(3):256–260, 2001.

Shapiro GG: Childhood asthma: update. *Pediatr Rev* 13:403, 1992.

Stempel DA, Redding GJ: Management of acute asthma. *Pediatr Clin North Am* 39:1311, 1992.

Werner HA: Status asthmaticus in children: a review. *Chest* 119(6):1913–1929, 2001.

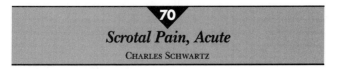

70
Scrotal Pain, Acute
CHARLES SCHWARTZ

▼ INTRODUCTION

When evaluating a patient with acute scrotal pain, **testicular torsion** should be considered **the diagnosis until proven otherwise.** This complaint must be **evaluated in person;** telephone consultation for such symptoms is dangerous because valuable time may be wasted, leading to testicular loss. Approximately 25% of males presenting with acute scrotal pain to a hospital emergency department will prove to have testicular torsion. This represents a **surgical emergency** because **testicular viability is compromised beyond 8 hours** of warm ischemia time. Therefore, patients presenting with this complaint must be given high priority in an acute care setting.

Another inherent danger in evaluating this complaint is the definition of "acute," because the patient's time frame is often different from that of the clinician. **Adolescent patients are especially at risk** because the **symptoms are often denied** for some time before treatment is sought. This may account for the fact that the salvage rate is lowest in this age group. It is also important that the clinician not be led astray by a **history of trauma** since this history **can mask a serious testicular problem.**

▼ DIFFERENTIAL DIAGNOSIS LIST

Testicular torsion
Torsion of the appendix testis
Epididymitis
Hernia/hydrocele
Trauma
Varicocele
Tumor
Bites and stings
Henoch-Schönlein purpura
Mumps orchitis
Vasculitis
Ureteral colic (referred pain)

▼ DIFFERENTIAL DIAGNOSIS DISCUSSION
Common Causes

Of the entities shown in the differential diagnostic list, 95% will fall into one of the top four categories. In one study, almost 70% of all cases of acute scrotal pain were classified as either being a testicular torsion or torsion of the appendix testis.

Testicular Torsion

Testicular torsion results from a **complete twist of the testis on its vascular pedicle.** The **resulting ischemia** produces **pain** that can be **constant** or, at times, **colicky** in nature. The **sudden onset of pain** is often accompanied by **nausea and vomiting.** The testis in question **is pulled up high in the scrotum** (secondary to the twists in the spermatic cord). In the majority of cases, **no cremasteric reflex** can be elicited. A strong 2–4 cm testicular excursion during a cremasteric reflex usually rules out acute testicular torsion, though this sign is less reliable in delayed presentations. Because the cremasteric reflex is not always present, especially in older males, **absence of a cremasteric reflex does not invoke a diagnosis** of testicular torsion.

Testicular torsion is felt to occur **secondary to a congenital anatomic malpositioning of the testis,** termed the **bell-clapper deformity.** A normal testis and its blood supply are attached to the tunica vaginalis posteriorly. However, with the bell-clapper deformity, **no such posterior attachment exists to anchor the testis** and prevent it from twisting completely around its blood supply. Establishing this **diagnosis early on is crucial,** for the situation presents a **surgical emergency;** the longer the delay in diagnosis, the lower the chances for testicular salvage.

Torsion of the Appendix Testis

Torsion of the appendix testis results when this tiny **müllerian remnant twists around its base, and ischemia results.** The typical presentation is characterized by a **gradual onset of pain,** and patients often note significant **scrotal swelling** and **erythema** secondary to a **reactive hydrocele.** The appetite is unaffected and nausea and vomiting are rare. It is often possible to elicit a **strong cremasteric reflex,** which greatly aids in distinguishing this condition from torsion of the testis. If the patient presents early on, **point tenderness** is noted **on the upper outer pole.** Some patients will have a **blue dot on the scrotum.** Once the diagnosis is established, treatment consists of **nonsteroidal anti-inflammatories and rest.** Over a 1-week period, 90%–95% of these patients will improve with no need for further treatment. In about 5%–10% of cases, the **appendix will torse intermittently,** and **surgical excision of the appendix testis** will be warranted.

Epididymitis

This diagnosis is **extremely rare in the prepubertal boy.** A true bacterial epididymitis in a prepubertal boy is usually secondary to a urethral stricture or posterior urethral valve. In the adolescent male, the usual causes of bacterial epididymitis are **chlamydia or gonorrhea.** However, at times the adolescent male may present with a **normal urinalysis and a tender and inflamed epididymis.** Often these patients will present **following a period of heavy physical exertion** such as weight lifting. It is felt that **reflux of sterile urine via the prostatic ducts under pressure** sets up an **inflammation** within the epididymis. Regardless of etiology, the diagnosis of epididymitis is established by the history and physical findings. The **onset of pain is slow,** and the **appetite is preserved.** A history of **urethral discharge and/or dysuria** may be noted. The physical examination demonstrates a **nontender testis,** with a **large and very tender epididymis palpable posteriorly.**

Hernia/Hydrocele

Patients may present with an acute herniation that produces **significant pain.** This is because the hernia sac represents an extension of the peritoneal cavity, which, when suddenly distended, can cause pain. The findings of an **enlarged** scrotum that transilluminates in conjunction with a **thickened inguinal bulge** provide evidence for a **patent processus vaginalis.** This allows for **peritoneal fluid to roll down and pool within the scrotum.** The **testis will not be tender** in this setting. On occasion the patent processus vaginalis expands from a **small tunnel** that only allows for **passage of fluid to a much larger diameter** that enables **bowel or omentum to herniate** into the sac. Presence of bowel or omentum will produce a **thicker spermatic cord.** On occasion the bowel or omentum will become **inflamed,** causing pain, and becoming more difficult to reduce. At this point **surgical consultation** is required.

▼ EVALUATION OF ACUTE SCROTAL PAIN

Despite technological advances in Doppler sonography, the vast majority of patients presenting with scrotal pain may be accurately diagnosed with a **complete history and physical examination,** especially when patients present early in the course of their symptoms. **After 8–12 hours of inflammation,** it becomes much more difficult to distinguish the individual scrotal contents, and it is in this setting that **Doppler sonography** becomes especially useful. The summary of the diagnostic features for acute scrotal pain is shown in Table 70.1.

Patient History

The history provides valuable clues to the cause of acute scrotal pain. Answers to the following specific questions should be sought:

▼ Has the patient ever experienced pain like this before? Often patients with torsion have had several episodes of intermittent torsion preceding the current presentation.

TABLE 70.1. Diagnostic Features of Acute Scrotal Pain

	Testicular Torsion	Torsed Appendix	Epididymitis	Hernia/ Hydrocele
History				
Sudden onset	+	+/−	−	+/−
Nausea/vomiting	+	−	−	−
Altered gait	−	+	−	−
Prior episodes	+	−	+/−	+
Physical Exam				
High riding	+	−	−	−
Transilluminates	−	+/−	−	+
Cremasteric reflex	−	+	+	+/−
Laboratory				
Urine dipstick	−	−	+/−	−
CBC	−	−	+/−	−
Radiology				
Doppler flow	−	+	+	+
Radionuclide perfusion	−	+	+	+

▼ Was the onset sharp and acute in onset, or slow and gradual? Patients with testicular torsion may be able to note the time of day when the pain began. In some instances, the pain awakens the patient from sleep.

▼ Has there been nausea or vomiting? The presence of these symptoms is often seen with testicular torsion. In contrast, boys presenting with a torsed appendix testis will often be hungry.

▼ Is the patient having difficulty finding a position of comfort? In testicular torsion, parents will describe their child as restless and writhing. Patients with a torsed appendix testis will prefer to lie still, and parents may describe a change in their child's gait while walking. This wide-based gait (cowboy gait) produces less parietal irritation of the inflamed tunica vaginalis and tunica albuginea.

Physical Examination

Observation of the patient provides useful clues. The patient who is in **obvious pain and writhing** at times has a higher **likelihood of having testicular torsion.** In contrast, the **patient with a torsed appendix testis** will prefer to **lie still.** The **appearance of the scrotum** is also helpful, for if one testis is **high riding,** this clue favors **testicular torsion.** This is because the torsed testis has a shorter spermatic cord because of the twisting that has produced the ischemia. A major component of the physical examination is the eliciting of the **cremasteric reflexes.** A brisk stroking of the inner thigh should result in a rise in the testis that is prominent (at least 2 cm). Such a brisk cremasteric reflex **will not be seen in cases of testicular torsion** in which the twisted cord precludes such movement.

▨ HINT A high-riding testis and absent cremasteric reflex are strong signs suggesting that testicular torsion is present.

An effort should be made to **distinguish pain within the testis from pain in the epididymis or an inflamed appendix testis.** With a **gentle touch** it is often possible to isolate the **localized point tenderness** associated with an early torsed appendix testis, which will always be located on the **upper outer pole.** If the examiner's large fingers diminish such accuracy, the **use of a pencil eraser** can be helpful in locating the **exact point of discomfort.** Doppler stethoscopes were recommended in the past to diagnose torsion, but false-positive and false-negative results have rendered this test ineffective. However, the sound of the Doppler and the distraction it provides make it useful while probing for point tenderness.

Finally, it is important to note that **manual detorsion of a torsed testis** can be **diagnostic** as well as **temporarily therapeutic.** Early on in the course of testicular torsion, the testis can be rotated laterally in a series of 180° flips. Since 80% of all torsions occur with a medial rotation of the testes, detorsion should **first be tried with a lateral rotation.** Once the critical turns have been reached, the **relief of pain is instantaneous.** If the pain subsides, this can be diagnostic. If access to the operating room or surgical subspecialist is limited, manual detorsion can be a valuable maneuver. However, the patient must be **explored as soon as possible,** for **retorsion** may occur, and despite relief of symptoms, there may still be a **residual twist** in the cord producing venous stasis.

Laboratory Studies

A **urine dipstick test** should be performed to assist in the work-up of epididymitis, and this is **especially important in adolescent males.** If a urethral discharge is present, swabs should be sent for **gonorrheal cultures** as well as **chlamydia** screening. A CBC is rarely helpful in establishing the diagnosis or altering therapy.

Imaging Studies

Scrotal pain lasting **longer than 12 hours** is often associated with **significant inflammation and edema** that renders the physical examination less accurate. The **exquisite point tenderness** seen with a torsed appendix testis **becomes less prominent as a reactive hydrocele forms,** and the **tunica vaginalis and albuginea become inflamed.** Surprisingly, many teenagers have stoically dealt with their pain and the physical examination reveals only mild discomfort with palpation.

In this kind of setting, **Doppler ultrasound** has become the imaging modality of choice. This noninvasive test is readily available, and provides a quick answer as to whether or not blood flow is present within the testis itself. This **spatial localization of blood flow is crucial** because the hand-held Doppler stethoscope often picks up arterial flow within the scrotal wall. The spatial localization of flow (or lack thereof) makes Doppler sonography far more accurate. The role of **nuclear scintography** has faded since procuring of isotope during off-peak hours can be a rate-limiting step. As such this test takes longer to perform in the scenario of a diagnosis in which time is of the essence. In some institutions, this may still remain the diagnostic test of choice, and it remains an accepted and valid measure of testicular perfusion.

As accurate as such technology might be, it is **critical to remember that the image is but one moment in time.** Cases in which flow was present at one time, and subsequent exploration demonstrated testicular torsion have been reported. This serves as a reminder that **intermittent testicular torsion** is a real phenomenon, and on occasion urologists will recommend **surgical correction even in the presence of blood flow,** based on the **history alone.**

Surgery

When there is doubt about the diagnosis of testicular torsion it is prudent to perform **exploratory surgery.** If a surgical team is 100% accurate in their diagnosis of the acute scrotum, they are missing the occasional case of torsion. It is **never wrong to operate and establish an exact diagnosis** of the acute scrotum by ruling out torsion. While it is true that Doppler sonography has made negative exploratory surgery more rare, the fact remains that the study is not perfect. **Testes may torse and detorse** to a point **allowing for arterial inflow at the time of the actual study.** The best way to establish the diagnosis is by examining the patient at the time of symptom occurrence. However, occasionally physicians are asked to assess the patient who has pain of short duration without classic symptoms. This patient may have **intermittent torsion,** and could benefit from elective orchiopexies. Such patients should still be **referred for urologic evaluation** and are advised to **keep a diary** of such episodes, noting their **frequency, degree of pain, and duration.**

Suggested Readings

Barada JH, Weingarten JL, Cromie WJ: Testicular salvage and age related delay in the presentation of testicular torsion. *J Urol* 142:746–747, 1989.

Cattolica EV: Preoperative manual detorsion of the torsed spermatic cord. *J Urol* 133:803–804, 1985.

Cronan KM, Zderic SA: Manual detorsion of the testes. Edited by Henretig FM, King C. In *Textbook of Pediatric Emergency Procedures.* Baltimore, Williams & Wilkins, 1991, pp 1003–1006

Rabinowitz R: The importance of the cremasteric reflex in acute scrotal swelling in children. *J Urol* 132:89–91, 1984.

Siegel A, Snyder H, Duckett JW: Related epididymitis in infants and boys: underlying urogenital anomalies and efficacy of imaging modalities. *J Urol* 133:1100–1103, 1987.

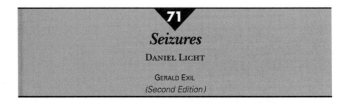

71

Seizures

DANIEL LICHT

GERALD EXIL
(Second Edition)

▼ INTRODUCTION

A seizure is a sudden attack characterized by **altered behavior, consciousness, sensation, or autonomic function.**

Seizures may be **epileptic** or **nonepileptic.** Epileptic seizures result from excessive firing of neurons in the cerebral cortex (excitation) or from hypersynchronization (inhibition). The differences between epileptic and nonepileptic seizures are summarized in Table 71.1. Seizure classification is given in Table 71.2.

▼ DIFFERENTIAL DIAGNOSIS LIST

Infectious Causes

Meningitis—viral, bacterial, fungal, tubercular
Encephalitis—viral or bacterial
Cat-scratch disease
Tick-borne disorders—e.g., Eastern equine encephalitis, LaCrosse encephalitis, Rocky Mountain spotted fever

Inflammatory Causes

Vasculitis—collagen vascular diseases, systemic lupus erythematosus
Rasmussen encephalitis
Lupus cerebritis

Toxic Causes

Lead poisoning
Drug overdose—cocaine, heroin

TABLE 71.1. Epileptic Versus Nonepileptic Seizures

Is the Event:	Epileptic	Nonepileptic
Detectable on EEG?	Often	Never
Stereotyped?	Usually	Never
Responsive to anticonvulsants?	Often	Never
Precipitated by emotional factors?	Never	Often
Reproducible on request?	Never	Sometimes
Characterized by tongue-biting and bladder incontinence?	Common	Rare

EEG = electroencephalogram.

Neoplastic Causes

Primary central nervous system (CNS) neoplasia
Metastatic neoplasia

Congenital Causes

Cerebral Dysgenesis

Holoprosencephaly
Lissencephaly
Polymicrogyria
Pachygyria
Schizencephaly
Neuronal heterotopias

Intrauterine Insults

Infection
Toxin exposure
Hypoxic—ischemic encephalopathy (HIE)

TABLE 71.2. Seizure Classification

Generalized
  Primary generalized
    Grand mal (tonic, clonic, tonic–clonic)
    Myoclonic
    Atonic
  Absence
    Typical
    Atypical
    Juvenile
Partial
    Simple (with motor, sensory, or autonomic manifestations)
    Complex
    Simple or complex partial with secondary generalization
Mixed
Unclassified

Vascular Disorders

Arteriovenous malformation (AVM)
Aneurysm
Intracranial hemorrhage
Intraventricular hemorrhage
Stroke

Metabolic Causes

Inborn Errors of Metabolism

Urea cycle disorders
Aminoacidopathies
Organic acidurias
Mitochondrial encephalopathies
Storage diseases
Vitamin B_6 deficiency
Nonketotic hyperglycinemia

Transient Metabolic Derangement

Hyponatremia
Hypocalcemia
Hypomagnesemia
Hypokalemia
Hypoglycemia

Genetic Disorders

Inherited epilepsy
Chromosomopathies

Miscellaneous Causes

Idiopathic
Neurodegenerative disorders
Cerebral palsy (CP)

▼ DIFFERENTIAL DIAGNOSIS DISCUSSION
Febrile Seizures

Etiology and Incidence

A febrile seizure is a **provoked, generalized seizure** that occurs in the setting of an **acute febrile illness** in an otherwise healthy child. Febrile seizures occur in 2%–4% of children and are most common in children between the ages of 3 months and 6 years, with a peak incidence in 2-year-old children.

Clinical Features

Febrile seizures are classified as **simple** or **complex.** In order to be classified as complex, the seizure must **last longer than 15 minutes, recur within 24 hours, or show focality** (manifested as a partial onset or Todd paralysis).

One-third of patients who have a febrile seizure have **recurrent febrile seizures** with subsequent febrile illnesses. Children who experience a febrile seizure before the age of 1 year or who have a first-degree relative with a history of febrile seizures are more likely to have recurrent febrile seizures.

Of children with febrile seizures, 3%–6% develop epilepsy. Risk factors for the development of epilepsy following a febrile seizure include a preexisting structural brain abnormality, a family history of epilepsy, and complex (i.e., prolonged, focal, or repetitive) febrile seizures.

Evaluation

With simple febrile seizures, **observation and reassurance** is the rule. When clinically indicated, underlying sepsis, meningitis, or encephalitis must be excluded. An **interictal electroencephalogram** (EEG) is usually **normal** in patients with simple febrile seizures, but postictal slowing is common if the study is performed immediately after the event.

Neuroimaging [magnetic resonance imaging (MRI) or **computed tomography** (CT)] and **electroencephalography** are recommended for patients with **complex febrile seizures.**

Treatment

Treatment is directed toward **preventing recurrent febrile seizures.** It cannot prevent the later development of epilepsy.

▼ **Acetaminophen and sponge baths** are indicated to control fever.
▼ **Phenobarbital.** Daily administration of phenobarbital may be considered for patients with recurrent or complex febrile seizures, and for patients at high risk for the development of epilepsy (e.g., those with CP, a structural brain lesion, febrile status epilepticus, or a very abnormal EEG). A maintenance dose of phenobarbital (3–5 mg/kg/day, in two divided doses) is given to maintain a serum level of 15–30 μg/ml.
▼ **Valproic acid** may be used if there is a contraindication for the use of phenobarbital. Caution must be used in the administration of valproic acid in children under the age of 2 years because there is a risk of fulminant liver failure in this age group. The maintenance dose of valproic acid is 15–30 mg/kg/day, in two or three divided doses, depending on the formulation, to maintain a serum level of 65–100 μg/ml.
▼ **Rectal diazepam** administered prophylactically at fever onset has proven to be effective in some cases; it is now available in a gel formulation. The dosage is 0.5 mg/kg for patients 2–5 years of age; 0.3 mg/kg for patients 6–11 years of age; and 0.2 mg/kg for patients older than 12 years.

Absence Seizures

Typical (Benign Childhood) Absence Seizures

Typical (benign childhood) absence seizures, also known as **pyknolepsy or petit mal,** usually occur after the age of 4 years, with the peak age of onset between the ages of 5 and 7 years. Events can be **provoked by hyperventilation.**

A chief complaint of **daydreaming** and **poor attention span** is common. Frequent, **brief staring spells** (usually lasting less than 10 seconds) are occasionally associated with **eye blinking and minor automatisms.** The **patient is not aware** of the event.

The neurologic examination is usually normal. Imaging studies do not reveal a structural brain abnormality. Characteristically, the **EEG** shows generalized **high-voltage, three-cycles-per-second spikes,** and **wave discharges with immediate return** to the previous baseline background.

Treatment options include the following:

▼ **Ethosuximide** (10–30 mg/kg/day in two divided doses to maintain a serum level of 40–100 mg/ml) is the drug of choice.
▼ **Valproic acid** is also effective and should be considered when there are coexisting generalized tonic–clonic seizures or when ethosuximide monotherapy fails.
▼ **Lamotrigine.** Recent data support the efficacy of lamotrigine (2–10 mg/kg/day in two divided doses).

Atypical Absence Seizures

Atypical absence seizures are seen in patients with **Lennox-Gastaut syndrome.** The **EEG** is characterized by **slow spike–wave discharges** at 2.5 Hz/sec or less. **Prolonged absences, atonic seizures** (drop attacks), and **tonic seizures** constitute the major components of this mixed seizure disorder. These patients often have **refractory epilepsy** and **mental retardation** and typically require polytherapy.

Juvenile Absence Seizures

Typically starting in early adolescence, **staring spells are less frequent and more prolonged** (often lasting longer than 10 seconds) than the staring spells of typical (benign childhood) absence seizures. There is an increased frequency of associated **generalized tonic–clonic seizures on awakening.** Some patients are **photosensitive.** Patients with juvenile absence seizures are at **major risk for nonconvulsive status epilepticus.**

The EEG shows generalized spike slow-wave discharges at 4–5 Hz/sec; occasionally generalized polyspike discharges are also seen.

Valproic acid is the drug of choice. The initial dose is 15 mg/kg/day, increased by 5–10 mg/kg/day at 1-week intervals to a maximum dose of 60 mg/kg/day. The goal is to maintain a level of 50–100 μg/ml.

Juvenile Myoclonic Epilepsy

Juvenile myoclonic epilepsy is an epileptic syndrome that manifests during adolescence. Patients have a benign neurologic examination and no findings on imaging studies. Patients report **myoclonic jerks on awakening** without alteration of consciousness. Associated **generalized tonic–clonic seizures** and **absence seizures** are common. **Valproic acid** is the drug of choice.

Neonatal Seizures

Etiology

Causes of neonatal seizures include HIE; subdural, intraventricular, and subarachnoid bleeds; cerebral dysgenesis; infections (congenital, acquired); transient metabolic disturbances; inborn errors of metabolism; familial seizures; and idiopathic seizures. Most seizures (70%–80%) that present in the neonatal period are **provoked seizures** (i.e., reactive to a physiologic or chemical derangement).

Clinical Features

Seizures can be **generalized tonic, clonic, or myoclonic.** More subtle findings include **lip smacking, tongue thrusting, eye blinking, eye rolling, staring, autonomic changes** (increased or decreased blood pressure), **apnea, bicycling or rowing movements,** or simply a **change in alertness.**

Evaluation

The evaluation of a neonate with seizures is twofold. First, the clinician must be certain that the infant has actually experienced a seizure. Then, he must initiate a search for the underlying cause.

Making the **diagnosis of seizures** on the basis of only clinical findings **can be difficult, especially in premature infants.** Some normal behaviors are often mistaken for epileptic seizures (Table 71.3). In addition, many seizures are subtle and overlooked, especially in depressed infants or those treated with neuromuscular blocking agents.

Video EEG is the best diagnostic tool in cases of subtle seizures. It improves the diagnostic accuracy by simultaneously matching the behavior event with the ictal pattern. An **interictal EEG** is valuable for predicting the neurologic outcome. For example, a burst suppression pattern on the EEG is frequently associated with a poor outcome. To avoid misdiagnosis, the EEG must be **interpreted by an electroencephalographer** who is skilled in reading **neonatal EEGs.** Certain artifacts, such as patting, ventilator, pulse, and extracorporeal membrane oxygenation, can be mistakenly interpreted as seizures by an inexperienced reader.

✍ HINT   A normal interictal EEG does not necessarily rule out seizure.

A diligent search for the cause of the seizure is important because, usually, the seizures can be **resolved by treating the cause** (e.g., an infection or transient metabolic disorder).

▼ **Suspected inborn error of metabolism.** Serum amino acids, a urine organic acid screen, and serum ammonia levels may be appropriate. Vitamin B_6 deficiency is diagnosed by EEG monitoring of the patient's response to a 50- to 100-mg single intravenous dose of pyridoxine.

TABLE 71.3.   Conditions Commonly Mistaken for Epileptic Seizures

Neonates
- REM sleep behaviors (eye rolling, leg jerking)
- Apnea or bradycardia
- Arching to stimuli
- Hyperexplexia

Children
- Psychogenic seizure
- Paroxysmal vertigo
- Breath-holding spell
- Syncope
- Sleep disorder (night terror)
- Movement disorder

Adolescents
- Psychogenic seizure
- Convulsive syncope
- Drug withdrawal

REM = rapid eye movement.

▼ **Suspected infection.** A lumbar puncture should be performed when sepsis or meningitis is suspected or whenever the cause of the seizures is uncertain.

Treatment

In many cases, definitive treatment entails **treating the underlying illness.** A **phenobarbital bolus** (20 mg/kg, administered intravenously), followed by a **maintenance dose** of 3–5 mg/kg/day in two divided doses (to maintain a serum level of at least 20 mg/ml) constitutes acute therapy. Adverse effects of phenobarbital include cardiorespiratory depression and sedation. **Phenytoin** can be used when phenobarbital is contraindicated (e.g., in patients with intracranial hemorrhage). Both medications should be used with **great caution in patients with myocardial insufficiency.**

Status Epilepticus

Clinical Features

Status epilepticus is classically defined as **prolonged seizures that last over 30 minutes, or recurrent epileptic seizures** during which the **patient does not regain consciousness within a 30-minute period.** However, **any seizure that lasts greater than 5 minutes is abnormally long** and is a **medical emergency.** Neuronal loss has been documented in both animal and clinical studies of status epilepticus lasting over 1 hour. New, permanent neurologic deficits have been reported in children after prolonged seizures. Status epilepticus can be classified as **convulsive** or **nonconvulsive.**

🖋 HINT Nonconvulsive status epilepticus can only be diagnosed by electroencephalography and must be suspected in any patient with an acute change in mental status.

Treatment

The mortality rate associated with status epilepticus has decreased in the past decade owing to more aggressive therapeutic approaches. The success of treatment depends on **prompt recognition** of status epilepticus and appropriate **administration of antiepileptic drugs.** There are many protocols for treatment of status epilepticus. The following is a typical approach:

▼ **ABCs (airway, breathing, circulation)** should be established by protecting the airway and ensuring that the patient is breathing. Vital signs, including the blood pressure, must be monitored. Oxygen should be administered via a nasal cannula or mask, and an intravenous line should be placed.
▼ **Continuous EEG monitoring** should be established, if possible.
▼ **History and physical examination.** A brief history is concomitantly obtained from witnesses (e.g., emergency medical system personnel, family members), and a neurologic examination is performed to rule out acute paralysis, increased intracranial pressure, and herniation.
▼ **Laboratory studies.** Blood should be drawn for immediate assessment of magnesium, calcium, blood urea nitrogen, and creatinine levels; arterial blood gas analysis; a toxicology screen to determine anticonvulsant medication levels; a complete blood cell count with differential; and culture (if appropriate).

▼ **Termination of the seizure.** Lorazepam (0.05–0.1 mg/kg intravenously) and diazepam (0.2–0.5 mg/kg intravenously) are rapidly effective benzodiazepines. Side effects include decreased blood pressure and respiratory depression; the clinician should be prepared to initiate bag-valve-mask ventilation and intubation. Phenobarbital is administered as a loading dose of 20 mg/kg intravenously over 20 minutes (i.e., at a rate of less than 100 mg/min) to obtain a serum level of at least 20 mg/ml. Side effects can include cardiorespiratory depression and sedation.

▼ **Treatment of persistent seizure.** If the seizure persists, the patient must be intubated, and an EEG should be performed. Administration of lorazepam (0.1. mg/kg, to a maximum dose of 0.5 mg/kg) may be repeated, and additional phenobarbital may be given to a total dose of 40 mg/kg. If the seizure still persists, a second anticonvulsant (e.g., phenytoin, 15–20 mg/kg as an intravenous bolus) may be administered. Side effects can include cardiac arrhythmias.

▼ **Treatment of refractory status epilepticus.** After 60 minutes of aggressive treatment, persistent seizures are classified as refractory status epilepticus. The patient should be admitted to the intensive care unit and induction of a barbiturate coma must be considered. Three to four hours after treatment is initiated, antiepileptic drug levels should be checked and additional doses administered as needed to maintain therapeutic levels.

Infantile Spasms (West Syndrome)

Infantile spasms (West syndrome) is an age-specific epileptic encephalopathy that most commonly affects infants **between the ages of 3 and 9 months.** West syndrome is classified as **symptomatic** (when there is an **identifiable cause**) and **cryptogenic** (when the **cause is unknown**). With prompt and adequate therapy, at least **50% of patients with cryptogenic** West syndrome have **some degree of neurologic sequelae,** whereas neurologic abnormalities are seen in **over 90% of patients with symptomatic** West syndrome.

Etiology

Certain risk factors have been linked to the development of infantile spasms. **Prenatal risk factors** include cerebral dysgenesis; hypoxia; and toxoplasmosis, other, rubella, cytomegalovirus, and herpes simplex virus (TORCH) infection. Perinatal risk factors include HIE, trauma, intracranial hemorrhage, and infections. **Postnatal risk factors** include meningitis, Down syndrome, tuberous sclerosis, Sturge-Weber syndrome, some genetic disorders, and some metabolic diseases such as phenylketonuria.

Clinical Features

The triad of **spasms** (i.e., the sudden flexion and extension of the arms and trunk), **hypsarrhythmia on EEG** (high voltage, disorganized chaotic slowing, mixed with multifocal spikes and sharp waves), **and developmental arrest or regression** characterize West syndrome. Spasms can be single but usually occur in **clusters during sleep–wake transition.**

Evaluation

An **EEG** (including **sleep and wakefulness**) must be performed to identify the pathognomonic hypsarrhythmic patterns. Clinical spasms may be correlated with a decremental response on the EEG.

TABLE 71.4. Proposed Protocol for ACTH Administration

Dose	Rate	Route	Duration (Weeks)
100 U/m²/day	Daily	IM	2
50 U/m²/day	Daily	IM	2
50 U/m²/day	Every other day	IM	1
20 U/m²/day	Every other day	IM	1

ACTH gel — 40 U/ml.
ACTH = adrenocorticotropic hormone; IM = intramuscularly.

Metabolic studies and MRI are essential to determine the underlying cause. Newer diagnostic techniques, such as **positron emission tomography (PET)** and **single photon emission computed tomography,** allow more cases of symptomatic West syndrome to be identified.

Treatment

Adrenocorticotropic hormone (ACTH) is the drug of choice for the treatment of infantile spasms. There is no universally accepted protocol for the initiation, maintenance, and duration of treatment, but a suggested approach is detailed in Table 71.4. The **initial phase of treatment** must take place in an **inpatient** setting. Because of the numerous **side effects** associated with the use of ACTH, certain tests are recommended before initiating treatment, including a **purified protein derivative test, stool guaiac test, serum electrolyte and glucose levels,** and assessment of **weight and blood pressure.** During ACTH therapy, **periodic reassessment** of these areas is advised, and the patient should be observed for **opportunistic infections. A follow-up EEG** should be obtained in 2 or 3 weeks to monitor the response to therapy.

Topiramate, valproic acid, and **clonazepam** have also been used in the treatment of infantile spasm, with a somewhat lower rate of success. There is a higher risk for **hepatotoxicity** from **valproic acid** in infants, and **liver function** should be carefully monitored. When prescribing valproic acid to infants, some clinicians also prescribe carnitine and selenium supplements.

Vigabatrin has been reported to be effective in some patients with infantile spasm, and may be the treatment of choice in patients with **tuberous sclerosis.**

Although infantile spasm has been classified as a generalized epilepsy, in some cases there is an obvious focal quality. There have been recent reports of infantile spasms resolving after **focal cortical resection** of an epileptic focus that was identified using PET.

▼ EVALUATION OF SEIZURES
Patient History and Physical Examination

The **history** and **physical examination** are two of the most important components of the evaluation of seizures in infants and children. A structured interview, oriented toward elucidating possible causes, helps guide further examination and laboratory studies, and allows **differentiation of epileptic and nonepileptic mechanisms** in many cases. Factors that influence the prognosis (e.g., a family history of epilepsy, the presence of an underlying CNS disorder) must be explored as well.

▼ **Was the event preceded by an aura?** A generalized seizure preceded by an aura is classified as a secondary generalized seizure (rather than a primary generalized seizure); classification has major implications in terms of the differential diagnosis and the choice of antiepilepsy medication. Auras can include smells, visual disturbances, visual or auditory hallucinations, tingling sensations, and unusual psychic phenomena. The aura, actually a partial seizure, points to the possible location of the epileptic focus.

▼ **What was the patient's observed behavior during the event? How long did the event last?** A detailed description of the observed behavior should be obtained. Witnesses may describe focal twitching, generalized clonic movements, tonic posture, tonic–clonic activities, tongue biting, and staring (with or without automatisms). Witnesses should be asked about the patient's state of consciousness and about bladder and bowel incontinence.

▼ **Were there any postictal phenomena?** Postictal phenomena, such as Todd palsy (postseizure weakness), confusion, fatigue, or sleep must also be described.

▼ **Was the seizure provoked?** An attempt should be made to identify possible triggers for the seizure (e.g., reaction to an illness or circumstance). This is important because brief impact seizures associated with head trauma and seizures that occur in the setting of acute hyponatremia do not require antiseizure treatment.

▼ **What is the patient's past history?** The pregnancy and birth history should be sought. Areas of note include the type of delivery, the infant's estimated gestational age, the infant's Apgar scores, and any indication of trauma, perinatal asphyxia, intraventricular hemorrhage, meningitis, cardiopulmonary arrest, or neonatal seizure. The child's growth and development and general health should be included in the history. Previous serious head injuries, a history of previous seizures, and a medication history are also important to note.

Diagnostic Modalities

Routine Scalp EEG

An **EEG** is indicated for all patients with **new-onset of seizures,** and also for patients with a known seizure disorder **when the quality of the seizures has changed.** A routine EEG can provide important information about the functional capability of the brain (e.g., background rhythms, sleep pattern), even if there is no epileptiform activity. Sleep deprivation increases the yield of abnormal studies. Findings may include the following:

▼ **Persistent focal slowing** may be seen in the setting of a structural abnormality involving that region.

▼ **Focal spikes or sharp waves** may indicate a possible seizure focus.

▼ **A diffusely slow, disorganized background** suggests encephalopathy caused by a metabolic or postanoxic process; it may also indicate a postictal state.

A routine scalp EEG has some limitations:

▼ A normal interictal EEG does not necessarily rule out an epileptic basis for the event.

▼ Rarely, an ictal EEG is normal in some patients with partial seizures.

▼ A small percentage of healthy patients have incidental epileptiform discharges on routine EEG.

Advanced EEG Techniques

Video EEG monitoring has opened a new frontier in the management of epilepsy. **Prolonged ambulatory EEG** can provide information that allows the clinician to identify epileptic seizures, subclinical seizures, and interictal epileptiform activity. More **invasive monitoring** (e.g., the placement of sphenoidal, subdural, or depth electrodes) is reserved for patients who are **candidates for surgery** to correct the epilepsy.

Neuroimaging Studies

Neuroimaging, **preferably MRI**, is warranted for all patients with **new cases of unprovoked seizure** to exclude a mass lesion, focal atrophy, cerebral dysgenesis, or AVM. **CT** is the first choice in the **emergency department** when **head trauma** is suspected.

▼ TREATMENT OF SEIZURES

▼ **Antiepileptic drugs are not indicated** for patients with an isolated, brief, provoked seizure; treatment of the underlying illness is sufficient.
▼ **Short-term use of anticonvulsants** might be considered for a patient with prolonged or multiple seizures until the patient's clinical condition is stable.
▼ **Long-term drug therapy** is standard for patients with epilepsy (recurrent unprovoked seizures). Complete seizure control with monotherapy is preferable, but some patients with severe epilepsy require polytherapy.

The following considerations must be taken into account when anticonvulsant therapy is being contemplated:

▼ Risks and benefits of treatment
▼ Seizure type
▼ Age of onset
▼ Long-term side effects
▼ Quality of life
▼ Specific epileptic syndrome

Often, the **withdrawal of antiepileptic medication** can be reasonably considered when the patient has been **seizure-free for at least 2 years** and the **EEG does not display marked seizure tendency.** The decision to withdraw medication must be made in cooperation with the patient and the patient's caregivers.

Suggested Readings

Dodson WE, Pellock JM, Bourgeois BFD: *Pediatric Epilepsy: Diagnosis and Therapy,* 2nd ed. New York, Demos Publications, 2001.

Duchowny MS: Surgery for intractable epilepsy: issues and outcome. *Pediatrics* 84:886, 1989.

Duffner PK, Baumann RJ: A synopsis of the American Academy of Pediatrics' practice parameters on the evaluation and treatment of children with febrile seizures. *Pediatr Rev* 20(8):285–287, 1999.

Freeman JM, Vining PG: Decision making and the child with afebrile seizures. *Pediatr Rev* 13:305, 1992.

Freeman JM, Vining PG: Decision making and the child with febrile seizures. *Pediatr Rev* 13:298, 1992.

Hirtz D, Ashwal S, Berg A, et al: Practice parameter: evaluating a first non-febrile seizure in children: report of the quality standards subcommittee of the American Academy of Neurology, The Child Neurology Society, and The American Epilepsy Society. *Neurology* 55(5):616–623, 2000.

Maytal J, Shinnar S, Moshe SL, et al: Low morbidity and mortality of status epilepticus in children. *Pediatrics* 83:323, 1989.

Offringa M, Moyer VA: Evidence based paediatrics: evidence based management of seizures associated with fever. *BMJ* 323(7321):1111–1114, 2001.

Painter MJ, Bergman I, Crumrine P: Neonatal seizures. *Pediatr Clin North Am* 33:91, 1986.

Shinnar S, Berg AT, Moshe SL, et al: Discontinuing antiepileptic drugs in children with epilepsy: a prospective study. *Ann Neurol* 35:534, 1994.

Verrotti A, Morresi S, Basciani F, et al: Discontinuation of anticonvulsant therapy in children with partial epilepsy. *Neurology* 55(9):1393–1395, 2000.

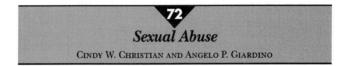

72
Sexual Abuse
CINDY W. CHRISTIAN AND ANGELO P. GIARDINO

▼ INTRODUCTION

Child sexual abuse is defined as the involvement of children in sexual activities that they cannot understand, are not developmentally prepared for, cannot give informed consent to, and that violate societal taboos. Sexual abuse is a general term that includes a broad range of activities, including **noncontact activities** (e.g., pornography, either in its production or in its viewing; inappropriate observation of the child while dressing, toileting, or bathing; and perpetrator exhibitionism directed at the child) and **contact activities**. Sexual abuse **frequently occurs over time** as the perpetrator gains the trust of the child, and can progress from noncontact to contact forms of abuse.

▼ DIFFERENTIAL DIAGNOSIS LIST

Child sexual abuse can have various presenting signs and symptoms. The following are physical signs associated with sexual abuse and the differential diagnosis for each.

Vaginal or Penile Discharge

Infectious Causes

Sexually transmitted diseases (STDs)—*Neisseria gonorrhoeae, Chlamydia trachomatis, Trichomonas vaginalis*
Group A streptococcus
Haemophilus influenzae
Staphylococcus aureus
Corynebacterium diphtheriae
Mycoplasma hominis

Gardnerella vaginalis
Shigella

Anatomic Causes

Ectopic ureter
Rectovaginal fistula
Draining pelvic abscess

Traumatic Causes

Foreign body
Chemical irritation (e.g., bubble bath)
Tight, nonporous clothing

Miscellaneous Causes

Nonspecific vulvovaginitis
Leukorrhea

Genital Bleeding

Infectious Causes

Urinary tract infection with gross hematuria
Vaginitis

Anatomic Causes

Vaginal polyp
Urethral prolapse
Vulvar hemangioma

Traumatic Causes

Straddle injuries (usually anterior lacerations)
Impaling (penetrating) injuries
Foreign body (e.g., toilet paper, small toys)

Dermatologic Causes

Lichen sclerosus et atrophicus (girls)
Balanitis xerotica obliterans (boys)

Endocrinologic Causes

Neonatal estrogen withdrawal
Precocious puberty

Neoplastic Causes

Sarcoma botryoides
Estrogen-producing tumors

Genital Inflammation or Pruritus

Infectious Causes

Nonspecific vulvovaginitis
STDs—*N. gonorrhoeae, C. trachomatis, T. vaginalis*
Pinworms
Scabies
Vaginal candidiasis
Group A streptococcal perianal cellulitis

Traumatic Causes

Poor hygiene
Poorly ventilated or tight underwear
Chemical irritation
"Sandbox" vaginitis

Dermatologic Causes

Atopic dermatitis
Contact dermatitis
Seborrhea
Diaper dermatitis
Psoriasis
Lichen sclerosus et atrophicus (girls)
Balanitis xerotica obliterans (boys)

Systemic Causes

Urticaria
Crohn disease
Kawasaki syndrome
Stevens-Johnson syndrome

Bruising

Infectious Causes

Purpura fulminans
Disseminated intravascular coagulation (DIC)

Traumatic Causes

Straddle injuries
Accidental penetrating injuries

Dermatologic Causes

Lichen sclerosus et atrophicus (girls)
Balanitis xerotica obliterans (boys)
Erythema multiforme
Mongolian spots
Vascular nevi

Hematologic Causes

Idiopathic thrombocytopenic purpura
Leukemia
Vitamin K deficiency
Coagulopathies
DIC

Metabolic Causes

Ehlers-Danlos syndrome
Osteogenesis imperfecta

Autoimmune Causes

Henoch-Schönlein purpura
Vasculitis

Anatomic Variations

Acquired

Labial agglutination
Hair thread tourniquet syndrome
Phimosis
Paraphimosis
Urethral prolapse

Congenital

Septate hymen
Cribriform hymen
Microperforate hymen
Imperforate hymen
Urethral caruncles
Vestibular bands
Median raphe
Ectopic ureterocele

▼ DIFFERENTIAL DIAGNOSIS DISCUSSION

A few diagnoses are commonly mistaken for sexual abuse and deserve comment.

Lichen Sclerosus et Atrophicus

Etiology

Lichen sclerosus et atrophicus, a **dermatologic condition,** generally affects **prepubertal and postmenopausal women** and is characterized by **thin, atrophic vulvar skin that is easily injured.** The atrophic skin typically involves the labia majora, perineum, and perianal area in an hourglass configuration. The hymen is not usually involved.

Clinical Features and Evaluation

Leukoplakia and hemorrhagic bullae may develop. Children often present with **pruritus and vaginal bleeding after minimal trauma.** The diagnosis is usually made clinically, although biopsy is sometimes required.

Treatment

Treatment is usually **symptomatic, with attention to hygiene. Hydrocortisone** can be used to relieve irritation and pruritus.

Straddle Injuries

Etiology

These common injuries to the genitalia of both boys and girls result from the **crushing of the genital tissues between the bony pelvis and a solid structure** (e.g., a bicycle bar or the arm of a chair).

The term "straddle injury" is also used to describe **accidental, penetrating trauma to the genitals.** These injuries can occur in any area of the genitalia and in girls can potentially lead to injury of the hymen. Accidental penetrating injuries to the genitals are far less common than straddle injuries and should be accompanied by a history that confirms an impaling injury.

Clinical Features

In girls, most nonpenetrating straddle injuries cause **ecchymosis and/or lacerations of the anterior vulva,** often involving the labia minora. Because of its posterior location and recessed position, the hymen is not typically involved. **In boys,** straddle injuries commonly cause **scrotal and penile lacerations or ecchymoses.** These injuries **heal quickly** and usually no treatment is needed other than **sitz baths.** Some lacerations or impaling injuries require **surgical repair,** with the patient under general anesthesia.

Vulvovaginitis

Etiology

There are many causes of vulvovaginitis in children, many of which do not relate to sexual abuse. In **adolescent females,** most cases of vulvovaginitis are caused by a **specific infectious organism.** The most common type of vulvovaginitis in **prepubertal children,** however, is **nonspecific vulvovaginitis,** which results from a combination of **anatomic, physiologic, and hygienic factors.** Vulvovaginitis may also result from **sexual abuse,** either as a result of mechanical trauma and irritation or from STDs.

Clinical Features

The **discharge** associated with nonspecific vulvovaginitis is **generally chronic, intermittent, scant to moderate,** and may or may not be seen in the introitus during the examination.

Evaluation

The laboratory evaluation of a genital discharge in a child should include **cultures for** *N. gonorrhoeae, C. trachomatis,* and *T. vaginalis,* a **general vaginal culture,** a **wet mount** for *T. vaginalis* and **"clue cells"** (vaginal epithelial cells with adherent bacteria), a **Gram stain** of the discharge, and a **potassium hydroxide preparation** for *Candida.* A **whiff test** is done by mixing a sample of the **vaginal discharge** with a **small amount of potassium hydroxide;** an **amine-like odor** is present in **bacterial vaginosis** as well as in **trichomoniasis.**

Treatment

The treatment of **nonspecific vulvovaginitis** is aimed at **modifying hygiene practices** (e.g., wiping front to back after a bowel movement; wearing loose-fitting clothing and white cotton underwear). The treatment of vulvovaginitis caused by STDs and other infectious pathogens is detailed in Chapter 73, "Sexually Transmitted Diseases."

▼ EVALUATION OF CHILD SEXUAL ABUSE

Discovery of sexual abuse is usually by one of the following mechanisms:

- ▼ The child discloses abuse.
- ▼ A third party discovers the abuse (e.g., a sibling walks in the room during an assault).
- ▼ The child presents with physical injuries.
- ▼ The child develops an STD.

Many sexually abused children **do not have physical injuries at the time of an examination,** either because the child did not sustain physical injury during the abuse or the injuries have healed. The evaluation of a patient in whom sexual abuse is suspected therefore requires **careful attention to the history, physical examination, and laboratory specimen collection** and must include **meticulous documentation** of both historical and physical findings.

Patient History

Complaints may be related to physical injuries or STDs, but, more commonly, the signs and symptoms of sexual abuse are nonspecific and are **manifestations of the psychological stress** associated with the abuse. These include **nonspecific behavioral complaints** (e.g., hypersexualized behaviors, phobias, sleep disturbances, poor school performance, runaway behaviors, truancy, aggressive behavior, symptoms and signs of depression) as well as **nonspecific physical complaints** [e.g., enuresis (secondary, day or night); encopresis; headaches; abdominal, genital, and/or rectal pain; dysuria; vaginitis; genital erythema; vaginal or penile discharge; genital and/or rectal bleeding; pregnancy]. Information related to both physical and behavioral symptoms of abuse should be explored.

In most cases, the diagnosis of child sexual abuse depends on the **history obtained from the child.** Ideally, the **interview** of the child is **conducted by a professional** familiar with the dynamics of sexual abuse, knowledgeable about child development, and comfortable with speaking to children about these issues. **Joint interviews** (with a representative from Child Protective Services and a law enforcement official) are **recommended,** although in the medical setting, this is often not possible. The child should be **interviewed with the parents absent,** because some children are hesitant to talk with a parent present, and others may be overly coached by anxious parents.

The child should be asked **nonleading questions,** although specific questions to clarify statements are, of course, necessary. It is best to start the interview with an **open-ended question** such as "Can you tell me why you were brought here today?" The interviewer should ask **developmentally appropriate questions.** For example, a young child's sense of dates and time is best approximated by references to seasons, holidays, and other important events in the child's life. Statements made by the child should be **recorded verbatim** in the medical record if possible.

It is important to try and elicit the following information:

▼ Identity of the alleged perpetrator and his or her relationship to the child
▼ The time of the last contact
▼ The reason why the child chose to disclose the incident at this time
▼ The frequency of abuse (one time versus chronic)
▼ The specific types of sexual contact included in the abuse
▼ History of perpetrator ejaculation
▼ Whether threats were made to the child by the alleged perpetrator
▼ Whether prior official reports of the abuse have been made

Physical Examination

The type of examination performed depends on the age of the child. **Adolescent girls** require a **full pelvic examination,** whereas **prepubertal children** usually require only **careful inspection of the vulva.** Common positions used for examination of prepubertal children include the supine, frog-leg position with labial traction (young girls), lithotomy position (adolescent girls), knee-chest position, and lateral decubitus position.

Few physical findings are pathognomonic of sexual abuse. Many genital findings are nonspecific, but with a history, may support the diagnosis of sexual abuse. **Definitive findings** of sexual abuse include the **finding of semen or sperm. In pregnant patients and those with STDs** or injuries **without a history of sexual activity, sexual abuse is a very likely possibility.** Further investigation is warranted for patients with **suspicious injuries or anatomic variants** (e.g., posterior angular concavities or transections of the hymen, or a dilated anus without a history of constipation). **Less serious vaginal problems** (e.g., infections, adhesions) are **common in children** and do not independently suggest sexual abuse. Perianal erythema or hyperpigmentation are examples of nonspecific changes.

The decision to complete a **"rape kit"** is **determined by clinical presentation.** Recent research suggests that forensic evidence collection can be limited to children who present for medical evaluation **within 24 hours of the last assault,** or those who have **injury or bleeding** on examination. Local crime laboratories have different protocols for collection of evidence. In general, the following evidence may be collected:

▼ **Victim's clothing.** Clothing provides the highest yield of forensic evidence in child sexual assault and should be vigorously sought. The clothing that the child was wearing at the time of the assault is collected by having the child undress while standing on a sterile sheet and placing all items into a clean paper bag. (Plastic bags should not be used because they may be airtight; the buildup of heat and moisture can degrade evidence.) Police should be notified of unwashed clothing at home that might provide forensic evidence.

▼ **Swabs for semen, sperm, acid phosphatase, and P30 analysis.** Moist secretions should be collected from the oral cavity (e.g., the pharynx, gum line), vagina, and rectum with a swab and allowed to air-dry before packaging. Swabs may also be collected from areas of the body that appear to have dried secretions, either by scraping a dry sample into a paper envelope or using a swab slightly moistened with sterile water, which is then allowed to air-dry.

▼ **Fingernail scrapings for foreign debris** should be placed into a paper envelope.

▼ **Pubic hair collection.** Collect combed pubic hairs into a paper envelope.

▼ **Foreign debris.** Any suspicious foreign debris found on the victim should be placed in a paper envelope.

▼ **Victim identification samples.** Collect a saliva sample and a blood sample from the victim to be used for identification of secretor status of the patient or for later DNA analysis.

Laboratory Studies

Laboratory evaluation is not universally required. When indicated, recommended tests to screen for STDs include the following:

▼ Culture of the cervix, vagina, or urethra; rectum; and pharynx for *N. gonorrhoeae*

▼ Culture of the cervix/vagina/urethra and rectum for *C. trachomatis*

▼ Wet preparation of vaginal secretions for *T. vaginalis*
▼ Culture of lesions for herpes simplex virus
▼ Serology for syphilis
▼ Serology for HIV, based on the prevalence of infection and suspected risk (should be repeated 3 and 6 months after last assault; obtain written consent)
▼ Gram stain and general culture of any vaginal, urethral, or anal discharge

Documentation

A **detailed medical record** is imperative to ensure that the best interests of the child are served. A well-documented medical evaluation in the medical record can serve as the basis for future discussion of the case. The physician should not rely on memory alone to reconstruct what occurred. The following hints are offered as a quick reference:

Do:

▼ Describe findings simply.
▼ Be aware of the child's developmental status.
▼ Use the child's words, defining the child's language if necessary.
▼ Ask nonleading questions.
▼ Record questions asked and specific answers given.
▼ Use diagrams and photographs to supplement the written record.

Do not:

▼ Use leading questions if at all possible.
▼ Use the terms "virginal" or "intact hymen," because these terms are imprecise and can be problematic during the legal investigation of the case.
▼ State conclusions in absolute terms; rather, describe findings and comment if they are consistent with expectations based on information known at that time.

▼ TREATMENT OF CHILD SEXUAL ABUSE

Medical treatment is guided by the **specific injuries or infections.** Hospitalization of sexually abused children is rarely required and, in general, is limited to children with severe genital trauma or systemic manifestations of STDs. Victims of sexual abuse, nonoffending parents, and perpetrators may all benefit from **therapy,** and referrals for patients should be made.

▼ APPROACH TO THE PATIENT

All cases of suspected sexual abuse must be reported to Child Protective Services (for abuse committed by a caretaker or household member), **law enforcement, or both.** Each state has laws that define child sexual abuse, and physicians should be aware of the laws operating in their state of practice. Individual institutions often have policies or guidelines regarding the evaluation of abuse, and some hospitals have a multidisciplinary team with expertise in recognizing and evaluating child abuse. Physicians who report suspected abuse "in good faith" are given immunity should a suit be brought against a physician for "false reports." **Parents should be informed of the need to report** before doing so.

Suggested Readings

Adams JA, Harper K, Knudson S, et al: Examination findings in legally confirmed child sexual abuse: it's normal to be normal. *Pediatrics* 94:310–317, 1994.

American Academy of Pediatrics: Guidelines for the evaluation of sexual abuse of children. *Pediatrics* 103:186–191, 1999.

Berenson AB, Chacko MR, Wiemann CM, et al: A case-control study of anatomic changes resulting from sexual abuse. *Am J Obstet Gynecol* 182:820–834, 2000.

Christian CW, Lavelle JM, De Jong AR, et al: Forensic evidence findings in prepubertal victims of sexual assault. *Pediatrics* 106:100–104, 2000.

Finkelhor D: *A Source Book on Child Sexual Abuse.* Beverly Hills, Thousand Oaks, CA, Sage Publications, 1986.

Giardino AP, Finkel MA, Giardino ER, et al: *A Practical Guide to the Evaluation of Sexual Abuse in the Prepubertal Child.* Thousand Oaks, CA, Sage Publications, 1992.

Kellogg ND, Parra JM, Menard S, et al: Children with anogenital symptoms and signs referred for sexual abuse evaluations. *Arch Pediatr Adolesc Med* 153:634–641, 1998.

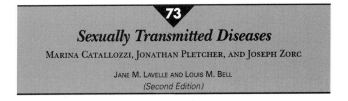

73

Sexually Transmitted Diseases

Marina Catallozzi, Jonathan Pletcher, and Joseph Zorc

Jane M. Lavelle and Louis M. Bell
(Second Edition)

▼ INTRODUCTION

Over one-third of sexually transmitted diseases (STDs) are diagnosed in patients less than 19 years of age. The rates of many STDs are **highest among adolescents** [e.g., gonorrhea in 15- to 19-year-old females, chlamydia prevalence, and human papillomavirus (HPV) infections]. Adolescents are at such high risk for STDs because of the frequency of unprotected sex, biologic susceptibility to infection, and the myriad health utilization issues that they face.

Clinical presentation can be protean, with females presenting with **vaginal discharge, abnormal vaginal bleeding, vaginal itching, dysuria, or pain** (lower abdominal, right upper quadrant, or rectal). **Males** may present with **urethral discharge, dysuria, testicular pain or swelling, or rectal pain.** Presentation can also include rash, arthralgia or arthritis, and inguinal adenopathy.

Clinicians can **educate adolescents about the risks and consequences of STDs,** and can institute **primary prevention interventions** by helping the development of healthy sexual behaviors and the avoidance of patterns of behavior that can undermine sexual health. There are limited exceptions, but, in general, adolescents in the United States can consent to the **confidential diagnosis and treatment of STDs** so that medical care for STDs can be provided to adolescents without parental consent or knowledge. Providers should respect confidentiality of adolescents and should follow policies that comply with state laws to ensure the confidentiality of STD-related services provided to adolescents.

Appropriate treatment of the patient and partner is essential.

▼ DIFFERENTIAL DIAGNOSIS LIST

Bacterial Infection

Chancroid (*Haemophilus ducreyi*)
Gonorrhea (*Neisseria gonorrhoeae*)
Granuloma inguinale (*Calymmatobacterium granulomatis*)
Lymphogranuloma venereum (*Chlamydia trachomatis*)
Shigella species
Syphilis or condyloma latum (*Treponema pallidum*)
Ureaplasma urealyticum
Vaginitis (*Gardnerella vaginalis*)

Parasitic Infection

Pubic lice (*Phthirus pubis*)
Scabies (*Sarcoptes scabiei*)

Protozoal Infection

Trichomonas vaginalis
Entamoeba histolytica
Giardiasis (*Giardia lamblia*)

Viral Infection

Cytomegalovirus infection
Hepatitis A, B, or C
Herpes simplex virus (HSV) infection
HIV
Human papillomavirus infection (genital warts, condyloma acuminatum)
Molluscum contagiosum

▼ DIFFERENTIAL DIAGNOSIS DISCUSSION
Selected Diseases that Cause Genital Lesions

Syphilis

Etiology

Syphilis is caused by the spirochete *T. pallidum.*

Clinical Features

▼ **Primary syphilis** is characterized by a painless ulcer or chancre at the site of inoculation.
▼ **Most children and adolescents present with secondary syphilis.** Most commonly, a maculopapular rash involving the palms and soles is the presenting complaint. Other symptoms include mucocutaneous lesions (condyloma lata) and systemic symptoms (e.g., adenopathy, fever, pharyngitis, malaise).

▼ **Tertiary syphilis** includes aortitis, neurologic dysfunction, and gummatous lesions of the bone, kidney, and liver.

▼ **Latent syphilis** describes disease in patients who have no symptoms of infection. Early latent syphilis refers to infection within the past year. Late latent syphilis and syphilis of unknown duration make up the remainder of this category.

Evaluation

The diagnosis of syphilis is generally made by using a **nonspecific** (non-treponemal) **antibody test** such as **Venereal Disease Research Laboratory (VDRL) test** and the **rapid plasma reagin test.** The specific tests for treponemal antibody tests, fluorescent treponemal antibody, absorbed (FTA-ABS) or the microhemagglutination–*T. pallidum* (MHA-TP) test remain positive for life; therefore, they do not denote activity. Nontreponemal tests can be quantified by **testing serial dilutions of serum. Quantification is important** because the appearance of clinical lesions correlates with a rise in titers. These titers diminish with appropriate treatment and can be used to follow response to therapy.

✂ HINT FTA-ABS or MHA-TP help differentiate infections from diseases such as lupus that produce a false-positive VDRL. However, these tests are positive in Lyme disease, which does not have a positive VDRL.

T. pallidum cannot be cultured in artificial media but **darkfield examination and direct fluorescent antibody tests** of lesion exudate or tissue are definitive ways to diagnose syphilis.

Treatment

Parenteral penicillin G is the treatment of choice for all stages of syphilis (see Table 73.1 for details).

Treatment may be complicated by an **acute febrile syndrome** known as the **Jarisch-Herxheimer reaction.** This reaction **resolves within 24 hours.**

The expected serologic response to treatment is a minimum fourfold decrease in nontreponemal test titers within 6 months.

Herpes Genitalis

Etiology

Most cases of herpes genitalis result from **herpes simplex virus-type 2 (HSV-2),** but 15% are caused by **HSV-1,** the type more commonly associated with stomatitis. These viruses account for up to 90% of all ulcerative lesions of the genitalia. As evidence of high contagiousness, as many as 90% of women exposed to infected men develop genital herpes. Transmission can occur in patients who are asymptomatic and often unaware that they are infected.

Clinical Features

Primary infection is characterized by **single or multiple vesicles** that may appear anywhere on the genitalia. These vesicles **spontaneously rupture to form shallow ulcers,** which are exquisitely **painful** but **resolve spontaneously** without scarring. Some cases of primary genital herpes are severe enough to require **hospitalization.** Mild to severe **systemic symptoms** may accompany

TABLE 73.1. Selected Sexually Transmitted Diseases (STDs)

Etiology	Disease	Diagnostic Tests	Treatment
Treponema pallidum	Syphilis[a]	Darkfield microscopy or direct fluorescent antibody Serology Nontreponemal (VDRL, RPR) Treponemal (MHA-TP, FTA-ABS)	
	Primary: chancre Secondary: rash adenopathy, fever Tertiary: cardiac, gummatous Neurosyphilis		Benzathine penicillin G, 2.4 million units IM × 1 Benzathine penicillin G, 2.4 million units IM × 1 Benzathine penicillin G, 2.4 million units IM weekly × 3 Aqueous penicillin G, 18–24 million units daily for 10–14 days
	Early latent Late latent or latent of unknown duration		Benzathine penicillin G, 2.4 million units × 1 Benzathine penicillin G, 2.4 million units IM weekly × 3
Herpes simplex virus	Herpes[b]	Culture Rapid fluorescent antibody test	
	Primary: painful genital mucosal lesions, mild systemic symptoms		Acyclovir, 400 mg PO 3 times daily or 200 mg PO 5 times daily for 7–10 days Famciclovir, 250 mg PO 3 times daily for 7–10 days Valacyclovir, 1 g PO twice daily for 7–10 days
	Secondary: less severe recurrence		Acyclovir, 200 mg PO 5 times daily or 800 mg PO twice daily for 5 days Famciclovir, 125 mg PO twice daily for 5 days Valacyclovir, 500 mg PO twice daily or 1.0 g PO once daily for 5 days
Trichomonas vaginalis	Trichomoniasis: vaginal discharge, dysuria, local irritation	Wet mount Culture	Metronidazole, 2 g PO × 1
Human papilloma virus	Condyloma acuminata (genital warts)[c]	Visual inspection	Patient applied: Podofilox, 0.5% solution or gel. Apply twice daily for 3 days then 4 days off up to 4 cycles.

Organism	Condition	Test	Treatment[a]
			Imiquimod, 5% cream. Apply 3 times weekly up to 16 weeks. Wash off after 6–10 hours.
			Provider administered:
			Cryotherapy
			Podophyllin resin 10%–25%. Apply weekly. Wash off in 1–4 hours.
			Trichloroacetic acid (TCA) or bichloroacetic acid (BCA) 80%–90%. Apply weekly.
			Surgical removal
Chlamydia trachomatis	Uncomplicated cervicitis	LCR (urethral, cervical, urine)	Azithromycin, 1 g PO × 1 OR
	Urethritis	Culture	Doxycycline, 100 mg PO twice daily for 7 days
	Epididymitis		In pregnant women:
	Proctitis		Erythromycin base, 500 mg PO 4 times daily for 7 days
	Neonatal conjunctivitis or pneumonia		Amoxicillin, 500 mg PO 3 times daily for 7 days
			Neonatal: Erythromycin, 50 mg/kg/d in 4 doses for 14 days
Neisseria gonorrhoeae	Uncomplicated cervicitis	LCR (urethral, cervical, urine)	Ceftriaxone, 125 mg IM × 1 OR
	Urethritis	Culture	Ciprofloxacin,[d] 500 mg PO × 1 OR
	Pharyngitis	Gram stain (urethral discharge)	Ofloxacin, 400 mg PO × 1 OR
	Epididymitis		Levofloxacin, 250 mg PO × 1 OR
	Proctitis		Cefixime, 400 mg PO × 1 OR
	Conjunctivitis		Ceftriaxone, 1 g IM × 1, consider eye lavage with saline
	Disseminated disease		Ceftriaxone,[e] 1 g IV q24h OR
			Cefixime, 1 g IV q8h OR
			Ciprofloxacin, 400 mg IV q12h

FTA-ABS = fluorescent treponemal antibody, absorbed (test); IM = intramuscularly; IV = intravenously; LCR = ligase chain reaction; MHA-TP = microhemagglutination-*Treponema pallidum*; PO = orally; VDRL = Venereal Disease Research Laboratory (test).

[a] All doses listed for adolescents and adults. Doses for children and alternative regimens for persons with penicillin allergies can be found in Centers for Disease Control and Prevention: Sexually Transmitted Diseases Treatment Guidelines 2002, 51 (No RR-6).

[b] Regimens for suppressive therapy for recurrent genital herpes can be found in Centers for Disease Control and Prevention: Sexually Transmitted Disease Treatment Guidelines 2002, 51 (No RR-6).

[c] Exact regimens for the treatment of external genital warts and future inflammation in treatment of cervical warts can be found in Centers for Disease Control and Prevention: Sexually Transmitted Diseases Treatment Guidelines 2002, 51 (No RR-6).

[d] Fluoroquinolones have not been recommended for persons < 18 years of age because of possible damage to articular cartilage. Because of the lack of data the CDC recommends any adult regimen for patients > 45 kg.

[e] See the 2002 CDC STD guidelines for other treatment options for disseminated gonorrhea. The parenteral regimens can be switched to oral regimens for 7 days after 24–48 hours of improvement.

the genital lesions. The mean duration of the initial episode of HSV is 12 days.

Recurrent infections, which occur in some patients, are less painful and of shorter duration, lasting 4–5 days.

Evaluation

Viral culture allows detection of the virus in 1–3 days. New vesicles are unroofed and scraped for inoculation of viral media. The yield of culture diminishes over time. **Direct fluorescent antibody tests** are available and are rapid and highly sensitive. Serologic testing is available, but is of limited value in the management of the patient.

Treatment

▼ **Management of a first episode** of genital herpes includes antiviral therapy and counseling regarding the natural history of genital herpes with particular emphasis on potential recurrent episodes, asymptomatic viral shedding, sexual transmission, risk for neonatal infection for women of childbearing age, and risk reduction. Acyclovir, famciclovir, and valacyclovir can all be used. Analgesics as well as local care (e.g., sitz baths) may offer some relief. Herpes proctitis may require higher doses of antiviral medication.

▼ **For recurrent disease,** acyclovir is most beneficial if initiated within 2 days of the onset of lesions. It may be administered as 800 mg orally twice daily for 5 days. Famciclovir and valacyclovir have also been effective in decreasing the severity and length of recurrent infection. In patients who have frequent recurrences (at least six per year) the physician may want to consider suppressive oral therapy, which requires continuous treatment with antiviral agents.

Human Papilloma Virus

Etiology

There are more than **20 types of HPV** that can infect the genital tract. Although most HPV infections are asymptomatic, types 6 and 11 are implicated with **visible genital warts** and types 16, 18, 21, 33, and 35 have been strongly **associated with cervical dysplasia.** The virus is **transmitted by direct contact.** The incubation period can be as long as 20 months. **In children, the presence of genital warts** can be secondary to **vertical transmission at birth and sexual abuse.**

✚ HINT Sexual abuse has been implicated in 50%–80% of cases of genital condyloma in the pediatric population. Any lesions discovered after the second year of life should alert the clinician to the possibility of sexual abuse.

Clinical Features

Warts can be **asymptomatic or symptomatic** and are found in a variety of locations, including the uterine cervix, vagina, urethra, anus, and extragenital areas (conjunctival, nasal, oral, laryngeal). Depending on the location and size of the warts, they can be **painful, friable, and pruritic.**

Evaluation

Identification of the characteristic lesion is diagnostic. Application of **3% acetic acid** produces a **classic acetowhite appearance.** Depending on the location and appearance, condyloma acuminatum can be confused with urethral prolapse, syphilis, vulvar tumors, and sarcoma botryoides.

Treatment

Since there are no currently available treatments that eradicate or affect the natural history of HPV infection, the primary goal of treating genital warts is the **removal of symptomatic or visible warts.** Treatment often induces wart-free periods, but does not necessarily decrease infectivity. There is no known effect of treatment on the subsequent development of cervical cancer. Without treatment, genital warts can resolve on their own, stay unchanged, or increase in both size and number.

Since none of the available treatments is superior, **treatment should be guided by the preference of the patient and the experience of the health care provider.** Medical and surgical treatments are available. Treatments include **patient-applied therapies** (e.g., podofilox and imiquimod) and **provider-administered therapies** (e.g. cryotherapy, podophyllin resin, trichloroacetic acid, interferon, and surgery). Warts on moist surfaces respond better to topical treatment. The treatment modality should be changed if a patient does not have significant improvement after three provider-administered treatments. Recurrences are most common in the first 3 months after treatment. Although the presence of genital warts is not an indication for cervical colposcopy, **regular surveillance and cytologic screening is recommended**, given the association of HPV with cervical dysplasia.

Selected Diseases that Cause Mucopurulent Discharge: Urethritis and Cervicitis

Chlamydia Trachomatis

Etiology

C. trachomatis is an intracellular organism. Prevalence rates of chlamydia genital infections are as high as 25% in sexually active individuals between 15 and 24 years of age.

Clinical Features

In females, *C. trachomatis* can cause **cervicitis, urethritis, or pelvic inflammatory disease (PID).** Although many **females** are asymptomatic or mildly symptomatic (vaginal discharge, dysuria, dyspareunia, urinary frequency) serious sequelae include **PID, ectopic pregnancy, and infertility.**

In **males,** chlamydia infection can result in **urethritis, epididymitis, proctitis, or prostatitis.** Clinical signs of epididymitis are **pain and swelling of the epididymis;** for prostatitis the patient has **pain in the testicles and scrotum;** for proctitis, the patient complains of **rectal pain** on defecation, or tenesmus.

Reiter syndrome (conjunctivitis, dermatitis, urethritis, and arthritis) or reactive arthritis can occur in males or females.

Evaluation

In females, pelvic examination is vital. The cervix can appear normal or be friable with the presence of mucopurulent discharge. Swabs from the endocervical canal can be used for ligase chain reaction (LCR) for chlamydia.

The LCR is performed by cleaning the cervix then rotating in the canal for 10 seconds to ensure that columnar epithelial cells are sampled. If blood is present or the sample is being obtained in a prepubertal girl, vaginal or cervical cultures should be obtained.

In males, first morning void or urethral swab can be sent for chlamydia LCR.

The Centers for Disease Control and Prevention does not recommend that a chlamydia test be performed after completing treatment unless there are persistent symptoms or there is suspicion for reinfection. A test of cure can be considered 3 weeks after completing treatment. Testing with nucleic acid amplification test that is done less than 3 weeks after completion of therapy may give false positive results due to detection of nonviable organisms.

Because of high reinfection rates secondary to partners not being treated and the increased risk of PID with repeat infection, women with chlamydia infections should be re-screened 3–4 months after treatment.

Treatment

Most recommended regimens include either **azithromycin or doxycycline.** Given the high coinfection rates with gonococcal infection, presumptive treatment is appropriate in patients with gonococcal infection. Many experts believe that the routine use of dual therapy has resulted in substantial decreases in the prevalence of chlamydial infection. Presumptive treatment is indicated for patients who may not return for test results. See Table 73.1 for treatment regimens.

Partners with sexual contact 60 days preceding symptoms or diagnosis should be evaluated, tested, and treated. Patients should abstain from sexual intercourse until 1 week after they and their partners have completed treatment.

Gonorrhea

Etiology

Gonorrhea is caused by a gram-negative diplococcus, *N. gonorrhoeae.* In the United States, approximately 600,000 new infections occur each year. Since gonococcal **infections in women** are often asymptomatic and **can lead to PID, tubal scarring and subsequent infertility or ectopic pregnancy** can occur.

Clinical Features

In **premenarchal females,** the **vagina** is the primary site of infection, while in **postmenarchal females** the organism can cause **endocervicitis, urethritis, bartholinitis, perihepatitis, or upper genital tract disease.** Common presentations include vaginal discharge, dysuria, labial swelling and tenderness, abnormal vaginal bleeding, or abdominal pain. Only about 50% of women with gonorrhea are symptomatic.

In **males,** *N. gonorrhoeae* infection can cause **urethritis, prostatitis, or epididymitis.**

In both **males and females** infection in **extragenital sites** includes **pharyngitis, conjunctivitis, or disseminated infection** presenting as meningitis, septic arthritis, osteomyelitis, or septic shock. Gonococcal endocarditis and pericarditis have been described but are rare. **Adolescents** commonly have **migratory arthritis or tenosynovitis.** The two patterns of arthritis are the **arthritis–dermatitis syndrome** and **monoarticular arthritis.** The arthritis–dermatitis syndrome, characterized by fever, chills, and arthritis or tenosynovitis, is accompanied by skin lesions that affect approximately 50% of patients. There are usually less than 20 lesions, which are small, tender papules or pustules on the distal extremities. The remainder of patients with gonococcal arthritis have a monoarticular arthritis affecting, in order of frequency, the knees, elbows, ankles, wrists, and small joints of the hands and feet.

Evaluation

Culture and Gram stain are the mainstays of diagnosis for gonorrhea, but the **LCR** is now available for detection of genital *N. gonorrhoeae* infection. Diagnosis of the gonococcal infection depends on the location and circumstances of the infection.

▼ **In males, a Gram stain of the urethral exudates** (revealing typical gram-negative intracellular diplococci) is sufficient for the diagnosis of gonorrhea, but, in the absence of urethral exudates, cultures or preferably LCR specimens from the **anterior urethra** should be obtained.

▼ **In female patients, the presence of blood** would necessitate testing with cultures from the endocervix. Otherwise, LCR can be used. Gram stains are not helpful in females.

▼ **In patients with gonococcal arthritis–dermatitis syndrome, blood cultures** may be positive.

▼ **In patients with gonococcal monoarticular arthritis, joint fluid culture** may be positive; blood cultures are usually negative.

Treatment

Given the **high coinfection rates of** *N. gonorrhoeae* with *C. trachomatis,* patients that are treated for gonococcal infection are also routinely treated with a regimen effective against uncomplicated genital *C. trachomatis* infection. See Table 73.1 for details of treatment.

Pelvic Inflammatory Disease

Etiology

The term PID refers to a spectrum of infections of the **upper female genital tract** including endometritis, salpingitis, tubo-ovarian abscess, and pelvic peritonitis. Although *C. trachomatis* and *N. gonorrhoeae* are the most important causative organisms of PID, it should be managed as a **polymicrobial infection** of microorganisms that are part of the **vaginal flora** (e.g., anaerobes, *G. vaginalis, H. influenzae,* enteric gram-negative rods, and *Streptococcus agalactiae*) as well as other organisms (e.g., *M. hominis* and *U. urealyticum*).

Risk factors for PID include age (typically 15–19 years of age), increased number of sexual partners, previous history of PID, sexual partner with an STD, and socioeconomic factors such as drug addiction and waywardness.

Clinical Features

The wide variety of signs and symptoms plus many asymptomatic patients make the **diagnosis of PID difficult.** Chlamydial and gonococcal disease are more likely to begin during the first half of the menstrual cycle. **Bilateral lower abdominal pain** is the most common presenting symptom. Other associated symptoms include abnormal vaginal discharge, abnormal uterine bleeding, dysuria, dyspareunia, nausea, vomiting, and fever. Because of this presentation, **other common causes of lower abdominal pain** (e.g., ectopic pregnancy, ovarian torsion, acute appendicitis, urinary tract infection, and functional pain) **must be considered and ruled out.**

Evaluation

Given the potential for **devastating sequelae if left untreated,** the diagnosis of PID should be **considered in any female of child-bearing age who has pelvic pain.** As noted earlier, history can be very helpful and information should be obtained regarding past episodes of PID (increased risk for recurrent PID) and date of last menstrual cycle. Since visualization of the pelvic structures for inflammation by laparoscope, the gold standard, is almost never practical, the diagnosis is made on clinical evidence. Most women with PID have pelvic tenderness in addition to either mucopurulent discharge or evidence of WBCs in saline preparation of vaginal fluid. Table 73.2 reviews the criteria for the diagnosis of acute PID.

Important laboratories include a **pregnancy test** (to rule out pregnancy or complications of pregnancy), **complete blood cell count with differential (CBC), erythrocyte sedimentation rate (ESR), LCR** (or cultures if the patient is having vaginal bleeding) for *N. gonorrhoeae* and *C. trachomatis,* **urinalysis, and urine culture. Blood cultures** should be obtained in septic patients. **Pelvic ultrasonography** is indicated in all adolescents with the diagnosis of PID because a tubo-ovarian abscess (TOA) may not be noted on the examination and the patient will not necessarily present any differently than a patient without a TOA. **Ultrasonography** can also help to rule out acute appendicitis and torsion. **Transvaginal sonography** will show thickened fluid-filled tubes with or without free pelvic fluid or tubo-ovarian complex in cases of PID. **Laparoscopy** is only indicated when the diagnosis of PID is uncertain or for patients with a diagnosis of PID who have recurrent abdominal pain.

Treatment

Since even mild disease can result in long-term sequelae, clinicians should have a **low threshold for making the diagnosis** and initiating treatment.

PID treatment regimens must provide empiric, **broad-spectrum coverage** of likely pathogens. Coverage should include *N. gonorrhoeae, C. trachomatis,* anaerobes, gram-negative facultative bacteria, and streptococci. Table 73.3 reviews appropriate antibiotic regimens for the treatment of PID.

The Centers for Disease Control and Prevention recommends considering **hospitalization when the diagnosis is unclear, the possibility of surgical emergencies** (e.g., appendicitis, ectopic pregnancy) **cannot be excluded, the**

TABLE 73.2. Criteria for the Diagnosis of Acute Pelvic Inflammatory Disease (PID)

Minimum criteria (initiate empiric treatment if present and no other causes):
  Uterine/adnexal tenderness
  Cervical motion tenderness
Additional criteria to support a diagnosis of PID:
  Abnormal cervical or vaginal mucopurulent discharge
  Presence of WBCs on saline microscopy of vaginal secretions
  Elevated erythrocyte sedimentation rate
  Elevated C-reactive protein
  Laboratory documentation of cervical infection with *N. gonorrhoeae* or
    C. trachomatis
  Temperature > 38° C (101° F)

TABLE 73.3.   Regimens for the Treatment of Pelvic Inflammatory Disease (PID) in Adolescents

Oral/Outpatient Regimens
  Regimen A
    Ofloxacin, 400 mg PO twice daily for 14 days
    OR
    Levofloxacin, 500 mg orally once daily for 14 days
    PLUS
    Metronidazole, 500 mg PO twice daily for 14 days
  Regimen B
    Ceftriaxone, 250 mg IM once
    OR
    Cefoxitin, 2 g IM once WITH probenecid, 1 g PO once
    OR
    Other parenteral third-generation cephalosporin (e.g., ceftizoxime or
      cefotaxime)
    PLUS
    Doxycycline, 100 mg PO twice daily for 14 days WITH or WITHOUT
      metronidazole, 500 mg orally twice daily for 14 days
Parenteral/Inpatient Regimens
  Regimen A
    Cefoxitin, 2 g IV every 6 hours
    OR
    Cefotetan, 2 g IV every 12 hours
    PLUS
    Doxycycline, 100 mg orally or IV every 12 hours
  Regimen B
    Clindamycin, 900 mg IV every 8 hours
    PLUS
    Gentamicin, 2 mg/kg IV loading dose followed by a maintenance dose of
      1.5 mg/kg every 8 hours

IM = intramuscularly; IV = intravenously; PO = orally. Adapted from Centers for Disease Control and Prevention: Sexually Transmitted Diseases Treatment Guidelines 2002. MMWR 2002, 51 (No RR-6). Published by the United States Centers for Disease Control and Prevention.

patient is pregnant, the patient has a TOA, the patient has sepsis (severe illness, nausea and vomiting, or high fever), or there is **intolerance or failure of an outpatient regimen** (after 72 hours). Since there are no data to suggest that either adolescent women or women with HIV infection benefit from hospitalization for PID treatment, clinical judgment and an assessment of the patient's compliance is recommended based on the previously described considerations.

▼ EVALUATION OF SEXUALLY TRANSMITTED DISEASES
Patient History

Important questions to ask include:

▼ Are there other common symptoms consistent with infection (e.g., presence of abnormal vaginal discharge or bleeding, dysuria, abdominal pain, genital lesions)?

▼ Is there testicular pain or swelling?
▼ What type of birth control method is used?
▼ Is there a previous history of STDs or known exposure to an infected partner?
▼ What was the beginning date of the last menstrual period?
▼ Is there a history of pregnancy or abortion?
▼ When was the last pelvic examination?

Physical Examination

In all patients, when there is concern about an STD, the **external genitalia** must be examined. In sexually active adolescent females, the **internal genitalia** should be examined as well, using a speculum. In males, the **penis, testes, scrotum, and rectum** should be examined. Vaginal or meatal discharge, skin lesions, lacerations, contusions, epididymal or testicular tenderness, or inguinal adenopathy should be noted.

HINT Avoid using lubricant for speculum insertion because the lubricant may interfere with cultures. Instead, rinse the speculum with warm water before inserting.

Laboratory Studies

▼ **Cultures or LCR** should be performed on samples from the endocervical canal and urethra or urine (for males) if chlamydia or gonorrhea is suspected.
▼ **Wet mount.** In females, a wet mount should be done if *Trichomonas* is suspected.
▼ **Gram stain** of urethral discharge can be useful in diagnosing gonococcal urethritis in males.
▼ **Blood tests.** In females with suspected upper genital tract disease, a CBC and ESR should be considered.
▼ **Urinalysis.** In males, a urinalysis should be performed.

HINT In prepubertal girls, Dacron swabs are gently inserted approximately 1 inch into the vagina and gently rotated for a few seconds to obtain a specimen for LCR or culture.

HINT In a prepubertal boy, specimens are obtained by swabbing the urinary meatus only. In postpubertal boys, the swab is inserted into the urethra a short distance [i.e., approximately 1 inch (2.5 cm)] and rotated for a few seconds. Urine testing can be used in both males and females but is not suggested for symptomatic females.

▼ TREATMENT OF SEXUALLY TRANSMITTED DISEASES
Females

Empiric therapy for gonorrhea and chlamydia should be instituted **for patients with a mucopurulent cervical or vaginal discharge** while awaiting results of cultures or LCR. Additionally, empiric therapy is warranted **if the partner** (or perpetrator, in the case of suspected sexual abuse) **has been diagnosed** with an STD. In most other patients, treatment can be deferred until the results of testing are available, provided appropriate follow-up is feasible.

Males

Empiric therapy for gonorrhea and chlamydia should be **considered in males with a urethral discharge.** In patients with dysuria or an abnormal urinalysis, further work-up for STD is warranted prior to treatment.

▼ SCREENING, PROPHYLAXIS, AND PREVENTION OF SEXUALLY TRANSMITTED DISEASES

The consideration of an STD in a sexually active adolescent or young adult can serve as an effective encounter to **initiate STD screening, prophylaxis,** and a discussion about **prevention.**

Screening

All patients diagnosed with an STD should be **screened for syphilis and offered HIV antibody testing.**

Yearly screening for chlamydia and gonorrhea by culture or LCR should be considered for all sexually active males and females.

Pap smear should be performed on all females who are sexually active or diagnosed with an STD. Pap smears should be deferred until symptoms of cervicitis resolve.

Prophylaxis

- ▼ **Hepatitis B.** Effective prophylaxis for hepatitis B can be accomplished with the hepatitis B vaccine. The vaccine should be considered in all sexually active individuals without hepatitis B or prior vaccination.
- ▼ **HIV.** There is no consensus on the use of antiretroviral medications for HIV-negative patients with sexual exposure to an HIV-infected or suspected HIV-infected individual. In certain settings, however, postexposure prophylaxis may be considered for HIV.

Prevention

Information regarding major STDs should be **provided to all adolescents and individuals diagnosed with an STD.**

Education on the correct use and on the efficacy of condoms in preventing pregnancy and STDs should be given to all patients, male and female, diagnosed with an STD or engaging in sexual activity. The **limitations of condoms should also be stated,** namely, that they may not prevent many cases of HPV and some cases of HSV.

Treatment of partners of patients with chlamydia, gonorrhea, syphilis, and trichomonas is an effective means of preventing symptomatic disease in the partner. It also minimizes the risk of reinfection in the patient and future infection of other sexual partners. **Local health departments** may pursue **contacts of cases of primary or secondary syphilis,** and this process has been effective in reducing the rate of syphilis in this country.

Suggested Readings

Braverman P: "Sexually transmitted diseases." Adolescent health update. American Academy of Pediatrics section in Adolescent Health. Vol 14, No 1, October 2001: 1–12.

Centers for Disease Control and Prevention: Sexually transmitted diseases treatment guidelines 2002. *MMWR* 2002. 51 (No RR-6); 1–80.

Drake S, Taylor S, Brown D, et al: Improving the care of patients with genital herpes. *BMJ* 921 (7201):619–623, 2000.

English A: Runaway and street youth at risk for HIV infection: legal and ethical issues in access to care. *J Adolesc Health* 12:504–510, 1991.

Gaston JSH: Immunological basis of chlamydia induced reactive arthritis. *Sex Transm Infect* 76(3):156–161, 2000.

Hurwitz S: Insect bites and parasitic infestation. In *Clinical Pediatric Dermatology*, 2nd ed. Edited by Hurwitz S. Philadelphia, WB Saunders, 1993, pp 405–426.

Ikeda MK, Jenson HB: Evaluation and treatment of congenital syphilis. *J Pediatr* 117:843–852, 1990.

McCormack WM: Pelvic inflammatory disease. *N Engl J Med* 330(2):115–119, 1994.

McIlhaney JS Jr: Sexually transmitted infection and teenage sexuality. *Am J Obstet Gynecol* 183(2):334–339, 2000.

Neinstein LS: Sexually transmitted diseases. In *Adolescent Health Care: A Practical Guide*, 3rd ed. Edited by Neinstein LS. Baltimore, Williams & Wilkins, 1996.

Reust CE: SOAP: solutions to often asked problems. Chlamydia trachomatis testing. *Arch Fam Med* 9(9):885–886, 2000.

Ross J: Pelvic inflammatory disease. *BMJ* 322(7287):658–659, 2001.

Sacks S: Genital herpes simplex virus and its treatment: focus on famciclovir. *Semin Dermatol* 15 (suppl1):32–36, 1996.

Tramont EC: Treponema pallidum (syphilis). In *Principles and Practice of Infectious Diseases*, 4th ed. Edited by Mandell GL, Douglas RG, Bennett JE. New York, Churchill Livingstone, 1995, pp 2117–2133.

Washington E, Berg AO: Preventing and managing pelvic inflammatory disease: key questions, practices, and evidence. *J Fam Pract* 43:283–293, 1996.

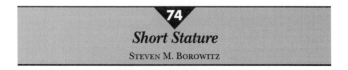

74

Short Stature

STEVEN M. BOROWITZ

▼ INTRODUCTION

Because normal linear growth is an important indicator of physical and emotional well-being during childhood, the regular assessment of growth and development is central to the care of children. Altered or abnormal linear growth may represent a normal variant or may be a sign of a serious physical or emotional illness. Regardless of which definition of short stature is used,

TABLE 74.1. Stages of Growth and Associated Growth Rates

Stage	Average Growth Rate (cm/yr)
Fetal	68
Infancy	
0–1 years	25
1–2 years	10
Childhood (2 years–puberty)	5–6
Adolescence	10

the physician must make the distinction between a normal, healthy child with short stature and a child with short stature as the result of an underlying medical condition. In general, **the more the child's height or growth rate deviates from normal, the greater the likelihood of an underlying medical condition.**

Defining Short Stature

Short stature is usually defined as a **height that is more than 2–2.5 standard deviations below the mean height for the patient's age.** Because height is a normally distributed characteristic, this purely statistical definition of short stature **identifies some normal and healthy children** with heights below an arbitrary cutoff point. Poor linear growth can also be defined as an abnormally slow rate of growth (Table 74.1) or as a height that is unexpectedly low for a child's genetic potential (Figure 74.1).

Stages of Human Growth

Human growth can easily be divided into four distinct stages (see Table 74.1):

▼ **Fetal period.** Growth is fastest during the fetal period. Fetal size largely relates to maternal genetics and maternal nutritional status during pregnancy.

▼ **Infancy.** During the first several months of infancy, maternal influences on growth diminish, and genetic factors begin to predominate. In this period, infants often cross length percentiles upward or downward, whereas after the second birthday, shifting percentiles is abnormal. Growth velocity gradually slows during this period.

▼ **Childhood.** Growth velocity remains fairly constant between 2 years of age and puberty. Childhood growth is slowest just prior to puberty.

▼ **Adolescence.** During adolescence, children experience a growth spurt; on average, girls grow 20 cm and boys grow 28 cm during this growth spurt.

$$\text{Boy's predicted height} = \frac{(\text{Father's height}) + (\text{Mother's height} + 13 \text{ cm})}{2}$$

$$\text{Girl's predicted height} = \frac{(\text{Father's height} - 13 \text{ cm}) + (\text{Mother's height})}{2}$$

FIGURE 74.1. Calculation of predicted height, based on the child's genetic potential. The 95% confidence limit is mean ± 8.5 cm.

Growth Parameters

When evaluating a child with short stature, it is often useful to compare the child's chronological age to her height age, weight age, and bone age:

▼ **Chronological age** is the child's age in years.
▼ **Bone (skeletal) age** is the age for which the child's bone maturation is at the fiftieth percentile.
▼ **Height age** is the age for which the child's height is at the fiftieth percentile.
▼ **Weight age** is the age for which the child's weight is at the fiftieth percentile.

⚒ HINT The bone age corresponds better than the chronological age to the timing of puberty and is a better indicator of estimated adult height than is the height age.

▼ DIFFERENTIAL DIAGNOSIS LIST

Variations of Normal Growth

Familial short stature
Constitutional short stature

Congenital or Vascular Causes

Intrauterine growth retardation (IUGR)

Metabolic or Genetic Causes

Chromosomal Disorders

Trisomies—8, 13, 18, 21
Turner syndrome
Noonan syndrome
Prader-Willi syndrome

Primary Bone Disease

Skeletal dysplasias—achondroplasia, osteogenesis imperfecta
Metaphyseal dysotoses
Rickets—X-linked or autosomal dominant hypophosphatemic rickets, vitamin D–resistant rickets

Inborn Errors of Metabolism

Mucopolysaccharidoses
Mucolipidoses
Glycogen storage diseases
Galactosemia

Poor Nutrition
Chronic Systemic Disorders

Cardiac Disease

Cyanotic heart disease
Chronic congestive heart failure

Pulmonary Disease

Asthma
Cystic fibrosis

Gastrointestinal Disease

Chronic malabsorption–celiac disease, cystic fibrosis, Schwachman syndrome

Inflammatory bowel disease (particularly Crohn disease)

Chronic liver disease or liver failure

Hematologic Disease

Chronic anemia

Malignancies

Immunologic Disease

AIDS and other immunodeficiency disorders

Collagen vascular diseases

Renal Disease

Chronic renal failure with uremia

Renal tubular acidosis (RTA)

Endocrinologic Disorders

Growth hormone (GH) deficiency

Glucocorticoid excess

Hypothyroidism

Excessive androgens

▼ DIFFERENTIAL DIAGNOSIS DISCUSSION
Familial Short Stature

Familial short stature (genetic short stature) is a **normal variant of growth** that largely reflects a child's genetic endowment. Familial short stature basically represents the bottom end of the spectrum of normal height.

Clinical Features

Children with familial short stature come from families with members who are short but otherwise healthy. Typically, the **heights of both parents** (and often many other family members) are 1–2 standard deviations **below the mean.** Most children with familial short stature are **short at birth** but they continue to grow at a normal rate, albeit **below the third or fifth percentile for their age.** They do not have delayed skeletal growth, and **puberty and their pubertal growth spurt occur at the usual chronological age.**

Evaluation

Physical examination and review of systems are normal, other than short stature.

This diagnosis is largely established with a careful history, review of the heights of family members, and a review of the child's growth data. The patient's **growth velocity and bone age are normal.** Any laboratory abnormalities or abnormalities on review of systems should suggest another diagnosis.

Treatment

Treatment is **expectant.** The **child and the family should be reassured** that puberty and the pubertal growth spurt will occur at the normal time and that the child's short stature will not affect his or her self-esteem, behavior, or academic performance. There are conflicting data as to whether supplemental human GH administration increases the final adult height in children with familial short stature, and there are conflicting opinions as to whether **human GH treatment** should be offered to normal short children.

Constitutional Short Stature

Constitutional short stature, another **normal variant of growth,** represents the **late end** of the normal spectrum of **pubertal and skeletal maturation.**

Clinical Features

Children with constitutional short stature generally have a **normal birth length,** but their growth **slows during the first 2 years of life** and is associated with a decline in their height percentile. Between the ages of 3 years and puberty, growth velocity is normal. Among children with constitutional short stature, **bone age is delayed.** Because the timing of puberty corresponds closely to bone age, **puberty and the pubertal growth spurt are also delayed** in these children. Final height is usually at or just below the child's ultimate predicted height.

Evaluation

There is generally a **family history of late puberty.** Physical examination and review of systems are normal, other than for the short stature. As with familial short stature, the diagnosis of constitutional short stature is largely established with a careful history, review of the heights and growth patterns of family members, and a review of the child's growth data. Unlike familial short stature, constitutional short stature is **associated with a delayed bone age.** Any other laboratory abnormalities or abnormalities on review of systems should suggest another diagnosis.

Treatment

In most cases, **reassurance** alone is adequate. In a small number of children **(usually boys),** a **short course of low-dose androgens** can be administered to ameliorate some of the emotional issues associated with delayed puberty. These agents must be **used with caution** because of their ability to **accelerate skeletal maturation.** There are no data indicating that supplemental GH administration increases final adult height among children with constitutional short stature.

HINT Variations of normal growth (familial short stature and constitutional short stature) are compared in Table 74.2.

▼ INTRAUTERINE GROWTH RETARDATION (IUGR)
Etiology

IUGR can be associated with **placental insufficiency** (i.e., severe preeclampsia, vascular diseases); **chromosomal abnormalities; intrauterine or congenital infections; or perinatal exposure to drugs, toxins, or teratogens** (Table 74.3).

Clinical Features

Although some children with IUGR demonstrate catch-up growth during the first 6 months of life, most infants who are born small for their gestational age **remain small throughout their lifetimes.**

TABLE 74.2. Variations of Normal Growth

	Familial Short Stature	Constitutional Short Stature
Growth rate	Normal	Normal
Bone age	Normal	Delayed
Timing of puberty	Appropriate for chronological age	Appropriate for bone age (delayed for chronological age)
Final adult height	Appropriate for mid-parental height	Appropriate for mid-parental height

Most chromosomal disorders result in poor growth prenatally as well as postnatally. Slow growth is a common finding among children with **trisomy 21** (Down syndrome) or **Turner syndrome** (45,XO).

More than 100 distinct skeletal dysplasias have been described, each of which is associated with various skeletal and nonskeletal abnormalities. **Nearly all children with a skeletal dysplasia grow slowly;** however, their growth is typically **"disproportionate,"** meaning the **ratio of upper body segment growth to lower body segment growth is abnormal.** As a result of this disproportionate growth, most affected children have **short limbs, short trunks, or both.**

Evaluation

The evaluation of a child with IUGR should begin with a **careful history and physical examination.** Depending on the history and physical findings, **chromosomal analysis** may be appropriate. If the ratio of the upper body

TABLE 74.3. Causes of Intrauterine Growth Retardation

Chromosomal and genetic disorders
  Skeletal dysplasia (e.g., achondroplasia, osteogenesis imperfecta)
  Chromosomal deletions
  Prader-Willi syndrome
  Russell-Silver syndrome
  Trisomies 8, 13, 18, and 21
  Turner syndrome (45,XO)
Congenital infections
  Cytomegalovirus infection
  Rubella
  Syphilis
  Toxoplasmosis
  Varicella
Drugs or toxins
  Amphetamines
  Cocaine
  Ethanol
  Heroin
  Hydantoin
  Methotrexate
  Nicotine
  Propranolol

segment to the lower body segment is abnormal, **skeletal radiographs** should be obtained.

⚡ HINT Although the classic features of Turner syndrome include short stature, primary ovarian failure, and multiple dysmorphic features (webbed neck, low posterior hairline, wide carrying angle, nail abnormalities, cardiac and renal anomalies), the spectrum of clinical abnormalities is sufficiently broad that this diagnosis should be considered in all girls with short stature of uncertain cause.

Treatment

Eighty to eighty-five percent of infants with IUGR will experience "catch-up" growth beginning in the **first 3 months after birth.** Those infants with **continued short stature at two years of age will likely remain short as adults.** As many as two-thirds of children with short stature secondary to IUGR will have evidence of **GH deficiency;** however, there are conflicting data as to whether supplemental human GH administration increases the final adult height in children with short stature due to IUGR. While girls with Turner syndrome generally are not GH deficient, current data strongly suggest that **treatment with human GH increases growth velocity and ultimate adult height.**

Poor Nutrition

⚡ HINT Because optimal linear growth requires good nutrition, malnutrition is the single most common cause of short stature.

Etiology

▼ **Malnutrition** may result from poverty, psychosocial deprivation, poor maternal–infant bonding, unusual dietary patterns or restrictions, or anorexia nervosa.

▼ **Undernutrition** may be associated with malformations, such as Pierre Robin sequence (i.e., a small mandible with relative hyperglossia) or cleft lip or palate. Children with severe cerebral palsy or profound developmental delays may have abnormal oral–motor function that makes eating difficult. Suppression of oral intake may also be caused by medications (e.g., cancer chemotherapeutic agents or stimulant medications used to treat attention deficit hyperactive disorder). Rarely, short stature may be the presenting symptom of an isolated nutritional deficiency (e.g., rickets caused by vitamin D deficiency).

Clinical Features

Among most children with short stature caused by inadequate nutrition, **weight tends to be depressed to a greater extent than height** (i.e., the weight age is less than the height age). The **bone age is usually delayed** and it generally **approximates the height age.**

Evaluation

The evaluation must include a **detailed dietary history,** which is usually best obtained by having the patient or parent keep a **record of dietary intake for 3–5 days.** This record can be analyzed for intake of total calories, protein, and deficiencies of potentially growth-limiting nutrients (i.e., sodium, potassium, iron, zinc). Numerous studies have demonstrated the inaccuracy of dietary histories obtained by parental recall.

Treatment

The treatment is **nutritional restitution.** If the child is unable to consume adequate numbers of calories, he can be fed either enterally with a **nasogastric or gastrostomy tube, or parenterally.** In children who are **chronically malnourished,** the provision of **large numbers of calories can be associated with very rapid "catch-up" growth;** with enough calories, malnourished children can attain growth velocities approaching those seen during the prenatal period.

Chronic Illness

Many chronic illnesses are associated with short stature. The specific mechanisms of impaired growth associated with chronic diseases vary but include:

▼ **A chronically poor appetite or poor oral intake** (seen with inflammatory bowel disease, chronic renal failure, and congestive heart failure)
▼ **Malabsorption of nutrients** (seen with celiac disease, cystic fibrosis, and AIDS)
▼ **Chronic acidosis** (seen with renal insufficiency, RTA, and chronic liver disease)
▼ **Poor or excessive use of nutrients** (seen with chronic inflammatory diseases and malignancies)
▼ **Medical therapy for the condition** (e.g., chronic glucocorticoid usage in asthma, inflammatory bowel disease, and nephrotic syndrome)

Clinical Features

In most cases, the underlying chronic disorder causing the short stature is readily apparent; however, in some cases, short stature may be the **presenting feature of a chronic disease.**

▼ **A small percentage of children with celiac disease** present during childhood with short stature and few or no gastrointestinal symptoms.
▼ **As many as two-thirds of children with Crohn disease** experience significant growth deceleration prior to the onset of overt gastrointestinal symptoms, and a small percentage of children with Crohn disease present with a chief complaint of poor growth.
▼ **Children with chronic renal insufficiency** may present with a chief complaint of short stature.

In most children with short stature caused by chronic illness, the **weight tends to be depressed to a greater extent than the height** (i.e., the weight age is less than the height age). **Bone age is usually delayed** and **approximates the height age.**

Evaluation

The **history** typically reveals that the child had **grown normally for a time and then the growth rate slowed,** suggesting the onset of illness. The history may reveal a clear diagnosis of a chronic illness or may include symptoms suggestive of an underlying disorder (e.g., chronic diarrhea, abdominal pain, mouth ulcers associated with Crohn disease).

Laboratory studies that screen for chronic illness [e.g., a complete blood cell count (CBC), erythrocyte sedimentation rate (ESR), serum biochemistry profile, serum albumin level, urinalysis] often provide clues to the diagnosis and may aid in guiding more definitive diagnostic studies (e.g., endoscopy, small bowel biopsy, renal biopsy).

Treatment

Therapy is directed at the **underlying disorder** (e.g., a gluten-free diet for a child with celiac disease, glucocorticoids or other antiinflammatory agents for patients with Crohn disease). In many cases, once the disease is adequately treated, the growth rate improves. Although **human GH therapy** has proven useful in improving growth velocity **following renal transplantation,** there are no data supporting the effectiveness of GH supplementation among children with inflammatory bowel disease or other chronic inflammatory disorders.

Hypothyroidism

✂ HINT Although many children with short stature are referred for endocrinologic evaluation, only a small number of children with short stature have an underlying endocrine disorder.

Etiology

Hypothyroidism, either **congenital or acquired,** is often associated with poor linear growth. **Acquired hypothyroidism** in childhood is **usually caused by autoimmune (Hashimoto) thyroiditis.** Children with Turner syndrome, Down syndrome, Klinefelter syndrome, and autoimmune diabetes mellitus are at increased risk for developing autoimmune thyroiditis.

Clinical Features

Although children with congenital hypothyroidism are usually of **normal size at birth,** they exhibit **profound growth failure during early infancy.**

The typical patient with acquired hypothyroidism is an older child or teenager with a **history of slow growth and excessive weight gain.** Girls may have **amenorrhea.** The other **"classic" symptoms** of hypothyroidism are **usually absent.**

Whatever the cause of the hypothyroidism, the associated short stature is characterized by an **increased upper body-to-lower body segment ratio** and a **profoundly delayed bone age.**

Evaluation

In the appropriate clinical setting, the diagnosis of hypothyroidism is usually established by demonstrating a **low circulating level of free thyroxine (T_4).** Most children with acquired hypothyroidism have an **elevated level of thyroid-stimulating hormone (TSH)** as well as autoantibodies directed toward the thyroid gland and thyroglobulin.

Treatment

If untreated, congenital hypothyroidism can result in coarse facial features, a large or persistent umbilical hernia, hypotonia, and mental retardation. Hypothyroidism is treated with **thyroid hormone (L-thyroxine),** usually **administered orally on a daily basis.** Overtreatment can result in signs and symptoms of hyperthyroidism as well as premature closure of the skeletal epiphyses; therefore, the **dose is adjusted based on serum levels of TSH and free T$_4$.**

Once the diagnosis has been established and treatment initiated, children can experience very **rapid "catch-up" growth.**

Growth Hormone (GH) Deficiency

Etiology

GH deficiency is a relatively **rare cause** of short stature. In most children, GH deficiency is an isolated finding **without any clear cause** (i.e., it is idiopathic). GH deficiency can also be seen with **congenital midline defects** (e.g., septooptic dysplasia) or as a consequence of **suprasellar brain tumors** (e.g., craniopharyngioma).

Clinical Features

Children with isolated GH deficiency are generally of **normal size at birth,** although they may experience **hypoglycemia and persistent jaundice** during the perinatal period. **Poor linear growth** is usually apparent **by 3 years of age.** On examination, affected children are **short with high-pitched voices, delayed dentition, and diminished muscle mass.** Patients are generally somewhat **chubby** in appearance and **look substantially younger** than their chronological age. Their **height is depressed more than their weight** (i.e., the height age is less than the weight age), and their **bone age is significantly delayed.**

Evaluation

There is **no clear consensus on the definition of GH deficiency.** The diagnosis is usually established by subnormal GH levels in response to pharmacological stimuli. Because **insulin-like growth factor-1 (IGF-1, somatomedin C) levels correlate fairly well with GH status,** serum levels of this compound are sometimes used as a screening test. The diagnosis is usually confirmed with the measurement of **serum GH in response to insulin, arginine, or L-dopa administration.** Since no single GH stimulation test has 100% sensitivity and 100% specificity, most countries have established **arbitrary cutoff points to at least two provocative GH stimulation tests.**

Once the diagnosis of GH deficiency has been established, **magnetic resonance imaging (MRI)** or **computed tomography (CT)** should be used to rule out an intracranial tumor or structural abnormality as the cause of the deficiency. It is also important to evaluate the child's **ability to secrete the other pituitary hormones.**

Treatment

Replacement with **synthetic human GH** is now the standard treatment for any form of GH deficiency. Recombinant human GH is generally administered as a **subcutaneous or intramuscular injection** up to three times each week. With replacement therapy, approximately 50% of children with isolated GH deficiency reach their expected adult height.

▼ EVALUATION OF SHORT STATURE

Patient History

In many cases, the diagnosis can be established with a careful history. The following areas should be covered:

▼ Were there any maternal illnesses?
▼ Was the fetus exposed to any drugs or toxins (e.g., alcohol, prescription medications)?
▼ What was the neonate's birth weight and height?
▼ Were there any perinatal problems, such as asphyxia (suggestive of placental insufficiency), persistent jaundice or hypoglycemia (suggestive of GH deficiency), or dysmorphic features (suggestive of chromosomal abnormalities or skeletal dysplasias)?
▼ What is the child's growth pattern? The child's growth pattern can be established by noting growth velocities over at least 6 months, and noting any changes in percentiles. It is only normal to change percentiles during the first 2 years of life and during adolescence.
▼ Are there any systemic signs or symptoms of chronic illness?
▼ Are there any gastrointestinal symptoms, such as diarrhea, abdominal pain, recurrent or persistent mouth ulcers, constipation, or vomiting?
▼ Are there any CNS symptoms, such as headaches or visual symptoms?
▼ What is the child's medication history?
▼ What is the child's dietary history?
▼ What was the timing and progress of puberty?
▼ How is the child's school performance? Are there behavioral problems?
▼ How tall are the child's parents and other family members?
▼ Was the onset of puberty delayed in other family members?

Physical Examination

▼ **Height and weight.** It is necessary to obtain accurate height and weight measurements. Current and previous measurements should be plotted on a growth chart. The height-to-weight ratio should also be determined; a weight age that is less than the height age suggests chronic illness or undernutrition, whereas a weight age that is greater than the height age suggests an endocrine disorder.
▼ **Body proportion measurements.** Accurate body proportion measurements are necessary to determine the ratio of upper body segment growth to lower body segment growth. The upper body segment is measured from the top of the head to the symphysis pubis, and the lower body segment is measured from the heel to the symphysis pubis. Normal values for the ratio of the upper body segment to the lower body segment are 1.7 at birth, 1.3 at age 3 years, and 1.0 in children older than 7 years. An abnormal ratio ("disproportionate growth") suggests skeletal dysplasia or rickets, whereas a normal ratio ("proportionate growth") suggests undernutrition, chronic disease, or an endocrine disorder as the cause of the short stature.
▼ **Arm span.** The patient's arm span can be used to evaluate growth. For the first 7 years of life, the arm span is less than the height. Between the ages of 8 and 12 years, it is equal to the height, and after 12 years, the arm span is greater than the height.
▼ **Tanner staging.** Delayed puberty may be a sign of constitutional short stature or Turner syndrome.

▼ **General examination.** A complete physical examination should be performed, searching for dysmorphic features, goiter and other signs of thyroid disease, and evidence of underlying systemic disorders (e.g., rachitic rosary or metaphyseal flaring with rickets, abdominal mass, abdominal tenderness or perianal skin tags with Crohn disease).

Laboratory Studies

The following laboratory studies are part of the screening evaluation:

▼ Complete urinalysis
▼ CBC
▼ ESR
▼ Serum electrolytes (including the total carbon dioxide value)
▼ Blood urea nitrogen (BUN) and creatinine levels
▼ Calcium, phosphate, and alkaline phosphatase levels
▼ Total protein, albumin, and prealbumin levels
▼ Free T_4 and TSH levels

Depending on the clinical diagnosis, the following studies may be indicated:

▼ Antigliadin and antiendomysial antibodies, to exclude celiac disease
▼ Sweat chloride analysis, to exclude cystic fibrosis
▼ Tissue transglutaminase antibodies to screen for celiac disease
▼ IGF-1 testing, to screen for GH deficiency

Diagnostic Modalities

Radiographic studies to determine bone age are part of the screening evaluation.

▼ **Anterior–posterior and lateral views of the knee** should be taken if the child is younger than 2 years
▼ **Anterior–posterior views of the left hand and wrist** should be obtained for children older than 2 years.

Depending on the diagnosis, additional radiographic studies may be indicated. For example, a **skeletal survey** can be used to confirm skeletal dysplasia, and an **MRI or CT scan** may be indicated if an intracranial mass or GH deficiency is suspected.

▼ APPROACH TO THE PATIENT (FIGURE 74.2)

In most cases, the cause of short stature can be established with a **careful history and physical examination.** It is crucial to determine the **child's growth pattern over time** and determine whether the growth velocity has been **normal for the child's chronological age and stage of pubertal development.**

If the child has had an abnormal growth velocity, it is useful to determine whether the growth has been **"proportional"** or **"disproportional"** (i.e., whether the ratio of the upper body segment to the lower body segment is normal). Children with **abnormal upper body-to-lower body segment ratios** are likely to have some form of **skeletal dysplasia. Radiologic assessment** is usually indicated for these patients.

In children with abnormal growth velocities but normal upper body-to-lower body segment ratios, additional evaluation is usually warranted. If the growth failure began during the perinatal period or there is a history of perinatal difficulties, some form of IUGR is likely. If the growth failure developed

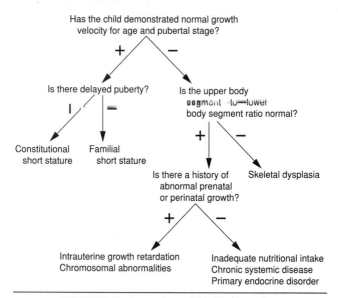

FIGURE 74.2. Approach to a child with short stature.

after the perinatal period, it is important to consider undernutrition, chronic systemic diseases, and primary endocrinologic disorders as potential sources of the short stature.

Suggested Readings

Attie KM: Genetic studies in idiopathic short stature. *Curr Opin Pediatr* 12(4):400–404, 2000.

Botero D, Lifshitz F: Intrauterine growth retardation and long-term effects on growth. *Curr Opin Pediatr* 11:340–347, 1999.

Cole TJ: A simple chart to identify non-familial short stature. *Arch Dis Child* 82(2):173–176, 2000.

Cuttler L: Evaluation of growth disorders in children. *Pediatrician* 14(3): 109–120, 1987.

Fox LA, Zeller WP: Evaluation of short stature. *Compr Ther* 21:115–121, 1995.

Guyda HF: Four decades of growth hormone therapy: what have we achieved? *J Clin Endo Metab* 84:4307–4316, 1999.

Hindmarsh PC, Brook CGD: Short stature and growth hormone deficiency. *Clin Endocrinol* 43:133–142, 1995.

Hintz RL, Attie KM, Baptista J, et al: Effect of growth hormone treatment on adult height of children with idiopathic short stature. Genentech Collaborative Group. *N Engl J Med* 340(7):502–507, 1999.

Markowitz J, Daum F: Growth impairment in pediatric inflammatory bowel disease. *Am J Gastroenterol* 89:319–326, 1994.

Pomerance HH: Growth and its assessment. *Adv Pediatr* 42:545–574, 1995.

Rimoin DL, Graham, JM: Syndromes associated with growth deficiency. *Acta Paediatr* (suppl) 349:3–10, 1989.

Rosenfield RL: Essentials of growth diagnosis. *Endocrinol Metab Clin North Am* 25:743–758, 1996.

Voss LD: Short but normal. *Arch Dis Child* 81:370–317, 1999.

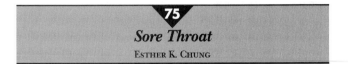

75
Sore Throat
ESTHER K. CHUNG

▼ INTRODUCTION

Sore throat is one of the most common reasons children are brought to medical attention. Most often, this complaint is part of an **upper respiratory tract infection.** Because children experience an average of 5–7 upper respiratory tract infections per year, it is essential that health care providers be familiar with the evaluation and treatment of sore throat in all ages. In addition, **misdiagnosis** or inadequate treatment of a sore throat caused by certain bacterial pathogens **can result in serious complications.**

▼ DIFFERENTIAL DIAGNOSIS LIST

Infectious Causes

Nasopharyngitis
Pharyngitis
Peritonsillar abscess or cellulitis
Retropharyngeal abscess or cellulitis
Tonsillitis
Laryngitis
Uvulitis
Epiglottitis
Laryngotracheobronchitis (croup)
Herpangina
Herpetic gingivostomatitis
Hand-foot-and-mouth disease
Cervical adenitis (referred pain)
Otitis media (referred pain)
Dental abscess (referred pain)
Scarlet fever
Kawasaki disease
Tularemia (*Francisella tularensis* infection)

Toxic Causes

Caustic or irritant ingestions—e.g., acid, lye
Inhaled irritant—e.g., tobacco smoke

Neoplastic Causes

Leukemia
Lymphoma
Rhabdomyosarcoma

Traumatic Causes

Foreign body
Intraluminal tear
Gastroesophageal reflux disease
Vocal abuse—e.g., shouting
External neck trauma—e.g., strangulation, child abuse

Congenital or Vascular Causes

Branchial cleft cyst
Thyroglossal duct cyst

Inflammatory Causes

Autoimmune disorders
Allergy
Postradiation

Psychosocial Causes

Psychogenic pain (globus hystericus)

Miscellaneous Causes

Cyclic neutropenia
Periodic fever, aphthous stomatitis, pharyngitis, cervical adenitis (PFAPA)
   syndrome
Vitamin deficiency—A, B complex, C
Dehydration
Pharyngeal irritation from breathing dry, heated air

▼ DIFFERENTIAL DIAGNOSIS DISCUSSION

Nasopharyngitis

Etiology

Most cases of nasopharyngitis, also known as the **common cold or upper respiratory tract infection,** are caused by **viral** agents. There are more than 200 serologically different causative agents, the most common being rhinoviruses, coronaviruses, parainfluenza virus, enteroviruses (coxsackievirus A and B, echovirus, polio virus), adenovirus, influenza virus A and B, respiratory syncytial virus, and group A streptococci.

Clinical Features

The clinical picture typically includes **fever, runny nose, sneezing,** and **nasal congestion** with clear or purulent nasal secretions, a **sore throat** lasting for several days, and a self-limited clinical course of 4–10 days. Streptococcal infection may present as a seromucoid rhinitis in toddlers.

Associated symptoms may include irritability, restlessness, muscle aches, cough, eye discharge, vomiting, or diarrhea, depending on the causative agent. Otitis media with effusion, laryngotracheobronchitis, or bronchiolitis may be present.

Complications are typically attributable to **bacterial superinfection** and include sinusitis, cervical adenitis, mastoiditis, peritonsillar and periorbital cellulitis, otitis media, and pneumonia.

Evaluation

The patient or parent should be asked about **associated symptoms** and about **ill contacts** at home, school, or day care. A **complete physical examination** should be performed, paying particular attention to the patient's overall **appearance** and **hydration** status.

Treatment

The treatment of nasopharyngitis consists of **bed rest,** increased intake of **fluids,** and the administration of **acetaminophen or ibuprofen** for pain and fever. Because of the **risk of Reye syndrome** with influenza infection, **aspirin should be avoided.** **Oral decongestants** (e.g., pseudoephedrine), **oral antihistamine** agents, and **phenylephrine drops** may be used for **older children.** **Saline drops** and **nasal suctioning** are appropriate for **infants** with nasal obstruction. **Humidifiers and vaporizers** may be useful to prevent drying of secretions.

Pharyngitis

Etiology

Most cases of acute pharyngitis are caused by **viruses**—most commonly, **adenoviruses.** Other viral causes include influenza viruses A and B; parainfluenza viruses 1, 2, and 3; Epstein-Barr virus (EBV); and enteroviruses. Bacterial causes include group A β-hemolytic streptococci, group C streptococci, group G streptococci, *Mycoplasma pneumoniae, Corynebacterium diphtheriae, Arcanobacterium hemolyticum, Neisseria gonorrhoeae,* and *Neisseria meningitidis.*

Clinical Features

▼ **Viral pharyngitis (caused by viruses other than EBV)** is characterized by the gradual onset of a sore throat, fever, hoarseness, and halitosis (in some patients), and an erythematous throat with or without exudate. Follicular and ulcerative lesions, mild cough, rhinorrhea, conjunctivitis, enanthem, or exanthem suggest a viral cause. Cervical adenopathy (tender or nontender) and poor intake of solid foods and decreased appetite are seen. The clinical course is self-limited and lasts 1–5 days.

▼ Although **infectious mononucleosis is rare before the age of 4 years, young children may experience pharyngitis caused by EBV.** Clinical features include fever and a sore and erythematous throat with or without exudate. Palatal petechiae, poor intake of solid foods, posterior cervical and generalized adenopathy, hepatosplenomegaly, and fatigue may be seen.

▼ **Pharyngitis caused by group A streptococci (strep throat) is uncommon in children younger than 3 years.** It may present with the sudden onset of a sore throat, a fever as high as 40°C (104°F), erythematous tonsils with or without exudate, petechiae on the soft palate, and headache. Nausea, vomiting, and stomach ache are often associated symptoms. Tender, anterior cervical adenopathy and a fine, sandpaper-like rash may be noted on physical examination. Complications include otitis media, sinusitis, peritonsillar and retropharyngeal abscesses, acute glomerulonephritis, rheumatic fever, suppurative cervical adenitis, and Lemierre syndrome.

✂ HINT Clinical findings useful in defining the cause of a sore throat are given in Table 75.1.

Evaluation

The parent should be asked about **associated symptoms** and **whether** the child has had **contact with anyone** at home or at school with a **sore throat, mononucleosis, strep throat, scarlet fever,** or **rheumatic fever.**

The **tonsils, pharynx, soft palate, skin, lymph nodes, liver,** and **spleen** should be **examined,** and the patient's overall **respiratory status** and **hydration status** should be assessed.

A **rapid strep test** should be obtained for all patients with an inflamed throat on physical examination.

Treatment

The treatment for pharyngitis of any cause includes **acetaminophen and ibuprofen** for pain and fever **(avoid aspirin),** increased **fluids,** and the administration of **nonprescription lozenges** and gargle solutions to provide temporary pain relief. **Gargling with salt water** (1/4–1/2 tsp of salt in 8 oz of warm water) and drinking warm liquids may be soothing. In severe cases, especially with infectious mononucleosis, patients may need to be **hospitalized** for intravenous hydration.

In patients with **strep throat,** the primary reason for treating with **antibiotics** is to **prevent rheumatic fever.** Antibiotic treatment has been shown to shorten the course of illness, decrease the incidence of suppurative complications, and prevent transmission to others. Penicillin V 400,000 U, 250 mg for children, and 500 mg two to three times per day for adolescents and adults, is administered orally for **10 days.** For penicillin-allergic patients, use **erythromycin** 40 mg/kg/day in two to four divided doses for 10 days. Other **macrolides** including 5 days of azithromycin, clindamycin, and the cephalosporins, are also **effective against group A streptococci.** Tetracycline, sulfonamides, and trimethoprim–sulfamethoxazole are ineffective in treating streptococcal infections. If **poor compliance** with oral medication is expected, **benzathine penicillin** G [600,000 U for children less than 60 lb

---

TABLE 75.1. Clinical Findings Useful in the Diagnosis of Streptococcal Pharyngitis

Findings that indicate likely viral pharyngitis
▼ Exposure to contacts with symptoms of upper respiratory tract infection
▼ Patient younger than 2 years
▼ Cough, runny nose, or eye discharge predominate

Findings that suggest streptococcal pharyngitis
▼ Exposure to contacts with strep throat, scarlet fever, or rheumatic fever
▼ Sore throat predominates
▼ Inflamed throat on physical examination

Findings that indicate likely streptococcal pharyngitis
▼ Palatal petechiae and tonsillar exudate
▼ Associated headache and abdominal pain
▼ Fine, sandpaper-like rash over the torso and other parts of the body

(27 kg); 1.2 million U for larger children and adults] should be administered in a single intramuscular dose (maximum dose, 1.2 million U). Following **completion of 24 hours of antibiotics,** the **patient** may **return to school or day care.** Good hand washing should be encouraged, and the patient should be counseled to **avoid sharing food and drink containers and towels.** Empiric treatment of contacts is not recommended.

For isolated bacterial **pharyngitis** that is **not caused by group A streptococcus, antibiotic treatment** is **not required,** because rheumatic fever is not a complication and the effect of treatment is unknown or minimal. Groups C and G streptococci are very sensitive to penicillin and may be treated with this medication; however, effectiveness of treatment has not been studied. Bacterial **pharyngitis caused by** *M. pneumoniae* **or** *C. pneumoniae* is often **associated with lower respiratory tract infection,** which **requires treatment.**

Herpangina

Etiology

The etiologic agents of herpangina are **viral:** nonpolio enteroviruses, coxsackieviruses A and B, and echoviruses.

Clinical Features

Herpangina affects children of all ages. The typical clinical picture includes discrete, **painful vesicular and ulcerative lesions** on the tonsillar pillars, soft palate, uvula, and posterior pharynx; **sore throat; poor appetite;** and a **fever** as high as 41°C (105.8°F). **Nausea, vomiting,** and **abdominal pain** may be present. The course is usually self-limited and resolves within **1 week.**

Evaluation

Herpangina can be **differentiated** from herpes simplex virus gingivostomatitis **by the location of the ulcerative lesions.** With **herpangina,** the **lesions** tend to be **in the posterior pharynx.** In **herpes gingivostomatitis,** the **lesions** are usually **in the anterior oropharynx. Hydration status** must be assessed.

Treatment

Herpangina should be treated with acetaminophen and ibuprofen for fever and pain. **Topical analgesics** may provide temporary relief. Some physicians prescribe a mixture of viscous lidocaine (2%), Maalox, and Benadryl elixir in equal parts. The patient should be given adequate **hydration** and **nutrition.** Severe cases, especially in young children, may require **hospitalization** for intravenous fluid administration.

Peritonsillar Cellulitis and Peritonsillar Abscess

Etiology

Peritonsillar **infections** may result from **acute tonsillar pharyngeal infection** or **obstruction and infection of Weber glands,** located in the superior pole of the tonsillar fossa. Peritonsillar **abscesses** are more commonly seen in **children older than 10 years.** Their causes are **polymicrobial,** involving either anaerobic or aerobic bacteria. The aerobic bacteria may include group A β-hemolytic streptococci, α- and γ-hemolytic streptococci, group D streptococci, coagulase-negative staphylococci, and *Haemophilus influenzae.*

Clinical Features

The clinical features of peritonsillar cellulitis or abscess include **fever, dysphagia, voice changes** (e.g., "hot potato" or muffled voice), **trismus,** and **drooling. Unilateral tonsillar or peritonsillar swelling** (usually on the superior aspect of the tonsil), **deviation of the uvula** to the contralateral side, ipsilateral cervical **adenopathy,** and trismus may be seen on physical examination.

Dehydration, upper airway obstruction, or aspiration of ruptured abscess contents may occur.

Evaluation

Peritonsillar cellulitis, which is not associated with the drainage of pus, and **parapharyngeal abscess,** which involves inflammation of the pharyngeal wall, are in the differential diagnosis for peritonsillar abscess. The patient's **respiratory status and hydration status** should be assessed. The patient should be **encouraged to speak** so the examiner can assess the quality of the voice. The **pharyngeal wall and both tonsils** should be **thoroughly inspected for asymmetric swelling and** any **uvular deviation.** Avoid using a tongue blade if epiglottitis is suspected.

Treatment

A pediatric **otolaryngologist** should be consulted to confirm the diagnosis and, possibly, to perform a **needle aspiration** of the abscess. Needle aspiration should be performed initially in older children and adolescents. The contents of the abscess need not be cultured except in children who are immunocompromised.

Penicillin VK (15–40 mg/kg/day, divided, every 6–8 hours for 10–14 days) should be started for **outpatient** management. **Aqueous penicillin G** (100,000–250,000 U/kg/day, divided, every 4–6 hours, with a maximum dose of 4.8 million U per 24 hours) should be given intravenously for **inpatient** management. If penicillin alone is not effective, a semisynthetic penicillin or clindamycin may be added. **Clindamycin** (25–40 mg/kg/day, divided, every 6–8 hours for 10–14 days) is used for patients who are **allergic to penicillin.**

Acetaminophen may be administered for fever and pain management. **Hydration** status should be carefully monitored. **Tonsillectomy** may be necessary in severe cases, in patients who are unresponsive to needle aspiration and antibiotics, and in patients with a history of recurrent peritonsillar abscesses.

Retropharyngeal Cellulitis and Retropharyngeal Abscess

Etiology

Retropharyngeal **infections** occur **in the potential space between the posterior pharyngeal wall and the prevertebral fascia.** They are believed to occur as a **complication of pharyngitis,** but may also occur **following a foreign body or penetrating injury** to the posterior pharynx, and as an **extension of vertebral osteomyelitis.** Retropharyngeal abscesses most often occur in young children. The etiologic agents are **polymicrobial,** and may include group A streptococci, anaerobic bacteria, *Staphylococcus aureus,* and *Klebsiella pneumoniae.*

Clinical Features

The clinical features of retropharyngeal cellulitis and retropharyngeal abscess include a **high fever, difficulty swallowing,** and a **severe sore throat.** The patient may **refuse to eat.**

Hyperextension of the neck; noisy, gurgling respirations or stridor; or meningismus (caused by irritation of the paravertebral ligaments) may be present. **Drooling** and **increased work of breathing** may be seen.

Complications include respiratory compromise, aspiration of the abscess contents, expansion along fascial planes to the mediastinum (resulting in mediastinitis), and erosion into major blood vessels.

Evaluation

The patient should be **assessed for drooling and difficulty breathing.** A bulge may be seen in the posterior pharyngeal wall. A **tongue blade** should be **used with caution** because the abscess may rupture if poked or digitally manipulated.

Treatment

An **otolaryngologist** should be consulted. A **semisynthetic penicillin** should be administered to cover penicillinase-producing *S. aureus*. **Clindamycin** (25–40 mg/kg/day, divided, every 6–8 hours for 10–14 days) is used for penicillin-allergic patients.

Cardiorespiratory monitoring is recommended because of the risk of airway compromise. **Acetaminophen** (with or without codeine) should be administered for pain; narcotics must be used with care because of the risk of airway obstruction.

▼ EVALUATION OF SORE THROAT

Patient History

The following aspects of the history can provide important clues to the diagnosis:

▼ Concurrent upper respiratory tract symptoms (e.g., cough, runny nose) suggest a viral etiology
▼ Thickened secretions suggest an infectious cause
▼ Similar complaints in household and other close contacts suggest an infectious etiology
▼ Seasonal variation and associated allergic symptoms suggest an allergic cause
▼ Recurrence every 3–6 weeks: consider cyclic neutropenia or PFAPA
▼ Bleeding with injections may suggest a neoplastic process
▼ Change in vocal quality suggests laryngitis, but may also be the muffled voice heard with peritonsillar and retropharyngeal abscesses
▼ Drooling or painful or difficult swallowing suggests the presence of ulcerative lesions or enlarged tissue

Physical Examination

The following should be noted on physical examination:

▼ The patient's general appearance and any signs of drooling or difficulty breathing (e.g., nasal flaring, stridor)
▼ The patient's vital signs, including temperature
▼ Mouth-breathing or change in vocal quality
▼ Tympanic membrane erythema or a middle ear effusion suggests otitis media, which often accompanies nasopharyngitis

▼ Nasal mucosal erythema may suggest an infectious or allergic process
▼ Oral vesicular eruptions suggest a viral cause (e.g., HSV, enterovirus, coxsackievirus)
▼ Symmetric tonsillar hypertrophy may be seen in nasopharyngitis and pharyngitis
▼ Unilateral tonsillar inflammation suggests peritonsillar cellulitis or abscess or the presence of a tumor
▼ Tonsillar exudates may be seen in viral and bacterial infections
▼ Palatal petechiae may be seen in strep throat and mononucleosis
▼ Lymphadenopathy in the posterior cervical triangle is seen in mononucleosis
▼ Tender anterior cervical adenopathy is typically seen in strep throat

---

▓ HINT When palpating potential abscesses, use caution. Patients may aspirate contents of ruptured abscesses.

Laboratory Studies

A **rapid strep test** should be done. This test, which requires vigorous swabbing of the tonsillar pillars and the posterior pharynx, identifies the presence or absence of **group A streptococcal carbohydrate** by specific antisera, but does not detect group C and G streptococci. Avoid swabbing the uvula, because doing so may result in dilution of the sample. The rapid strep test is **highly specific** and **sensitive.** False-negative results may occur if small numbers of streptococci are present. **Negative tests should always be confirmed by throat culture.** A positive test indicates that group A streptococci are present in the pharynx.

A **throat culture,** which is considered to be the **gold standard** for the diagnosis of strep throat, should be obtained. Untreated patients with strep throat may have positive cultures for several weeks to months. Notify the laboratory if *N. gonorrhoeae, C. diphtheriae,* or fungal infection is suspected, so that appropriate culture media is used.

A **complete blood cell count** may also be revealing. The white blood cell (WBC) count may be elevated in patients with peritonsillar abscesses, retropharyngeal abscesses, and other bacterial infections. Mild anemia and mild thrombocytopenia may be seen during viral illnesses. An **atypical lymphocytosis** making up 10%–25% of the total WBC count is suggestive of infection with EBV.

EBV titers and **monospot tests** are useful for **confirming EBV infection.**

TABLE 75.2. Symptoms Associated with Life-Threatening Causes of Sore Throat

Tachypnea
Respiratory retractions
Stridor
Drooling
Difficulty swallowing
Muffled, "hot potato" voice
Neck stiffness

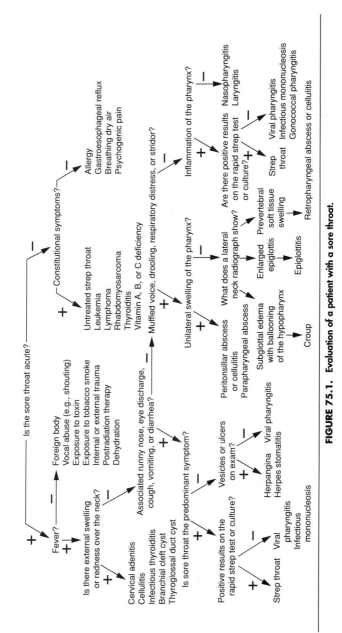

FIGURE 75.1. Evaluation of a patient with a sore throat.

Diagnostic Modalities

A **lateral neck radiograph** should be obtained when the diagnosis of a **retropharyngeal abscess** is suspected. It is useful for assessing the airway caliber, the size of the adenoids, the size of the epiglottis, and ballooning of the hypopharynx. A retropharyngeal abscess appears as widening of the soft tissues immediately anterior to vertebral bodies C1–C4. Normally, the soft tissues measure less than half the width of the adjacent vertebral body. Air in the retropharynx or loss of the normal cervical lordosis should raise suspicion of a retropharyngeal abscess.

A **computed tomography scan of the neck** with contrast may be useful in determining the **surgical treatment** of retropharyngeal abscesses. It may also help **differentiate retropharyngeal cellulitis from retropharyngeal abscess.**

▼ APPROACH TO THE PATIENT

First, **rule out life-threatening causes of sore throat** (e.g., epiglottitis, peritonsillar abscess, retropharyngeal abscess, diphtheria, severe tonsillar hypertrophy). Symptoms associated with life-threatening causes of sore throat are given in Table 75.2. **Oxygen** should be provided if **respiratory distress** is noted.

The patient should be examined for evidence of a **peritonsillar abscess or foreign body.** The use of a **tongue blade should be avoided,** as should other invasive procedures (e.g., placement of an intravenous catheter, phlebotomy) **if epiglottitis is suspected.** The patient should be immediately referred to an **anesthesiologist,** a **critical care specialist,** and an **otolaryngologist.** If a retropharyngeal abscess is suspected, a **lateral neck radiograph** should be obtained.

Figure 75.1 outlines the approach to narrowing the differential diagnosis.

Suggested Readings

American Academy of Pediatrics: Group A streptococcal infections. In *Red Book 2000: Report of the Committee on Infectious Diseases, 25th ed.* Edited by Pickering LK Elk. Grove Village, IL, American Academy of Pediatrics, 2000, pp 526–536.

Berger MS: Throat disorders. *Prim Care* 25(3):685–699, 1998.

Bisno AL: Acute pharyngitis: etiology and diagnosis. *Pediatrics* 97(6 Pt 2):949–954, 1996.

Herzon FS, Nicklaus P: Pediatric peritonsillar abscess: management guidelines. *Curr Probl Pediatr* 26:270–278, 1996.

Stewart MH, Siff JE, Cydulka RK: Evaluation of the patient with sore throat, earache, and sinusitis: an evidence based approach. *Emerg Med Clin North Am* 17(1):153–187, 1999, ix.

Thomas KT, Feder HM Jr, Lawton AR, et al: Periodic fever syndrome in children. *J Pediatr* 135(1):15–21, 1999.

Zaoutis T, Klein JD: Enterovirus infections. *Pediatr Rev* 19(6):183–191, 1998.

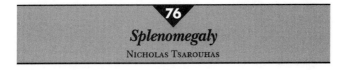

76
Splenomegaly
Nicholas Tsarouhas

▼ INTRODUCTION

Splenomegaly may be evident in benign viral infections, serious systemic infections, hematologic diseases, neoplastic conditions, and metabolic disorders. Apparent splenomegaly may be due to a normal-sized spleen being pushed down by hyperinflated lungs. The terms splenomegaly and hypersplenism are not interchangeable. **Splenomegaly refers to an enlarged spleen,** whereas **hypersplenism refers to a hyperfunctioning spleen that results in a reduction in the number of circulating blood cells.** Hypersplenism usually results in splenomegaly, but not always.

A palpable spleen tip is not necessarily pathologic. Approximately 3% of older adolescents and adults have **palpable spleens.** By adulthood, the normal spleen, which is located beneath the ninth and eleventh ribs, reaches dimensions of 12 cm long, 7 cm wide, and 3 cm thick. Careful examination of a quiet patient and thoughtful consideration of the possible underlying pathophysiology is necessary to discern the cause of splenomegaly.

✚ HINT Percussion can be used to evaluate splenic size. To delineate the lower "tip," the examiner starts in the area of tympany in the left anterior axillary line of the midabdomen and percusses upward toward the splenic dullness. The upper border is defined by starting in the left midaxillary line of the midthorax and percussing downward toward the splenic dullness.

▼ DIFFERENTIAL DIAGNOSIS LIST
Infectious Causes

Viral Infection

Benign infection
Mononucleosis [Epstein-Barr virus (EBV) infection]
Cytomegalovirus (CMV) infection
AIDS
Rubella
Herpes
Hepatitis B

Bacterial Infection

Pneumonia
Sepsis
Endocarditis
Brucellosis
Tularemia
Splenic abscess
Cat-scratch disease
Tuberculosis

Syphilis
Leptospirosis
Rocky Mountain spotted fever (RMSF)
Ehrlichiosis

Other Infections

Malaria
Toxoplasmosis
Babesiosis
Histoplasmosis
Coccidioidomycosis
Trypanosomiasis

Neoplastic Causes

Leukemia
Lymphoma
Hemangioma
Hamartoma
Metastatic disease (neuroblastoma)

Traumatic Causes

Laceration
Hematoma
Traumatic cyst

Metabolic or Genetic Causes

Lipid Metabolism Defects

Gaucher disease
Niemann-Pick disease
Gangliosidoses
Mucolipidoses
Metachromatic leukodystrophy
Wolman disease

Mucopolysaccharidoses

Hurler syndrome
Hunter syndrome

Hematologic Causes

Red Blood Cell Membrane (RBC) Defects

Hereditary spherocytosis (HS)
Hereditary elliptocytosis (HE)
Hereditary stomatocytosis

RBC Enzyme Defects

Glucose-6-phosphate dehydrogenase (G6PD) deficiency
Pyruvate kinase deficiency

Hemoglobin Defects

Sickle cell disease (SCD)
Thalassemia

Extrinsic Hemolytic Anemias

Autoimmune hemolytic anemia
Erythroblastosis fetalis

Congestive Causes

Congestive heart failure
Constrictive pericarditis
Intrinsic liver disease
Perisplenic anatomic obstructions
Splenic vein thrombosis
Splenic artery aneurysm

Miscellaneous Causes

Serum sickness
Chronic granulomatous disease
Juvenile rheumatoid arthritis (JRA)
Systemic lupus erythematosus (SLE)
Histiocytic Disorders
Langerhans cell histiocytosis
Hemophagocytic lymphohistiocytosis
Malignant histiocytic disorders
Beckwith-Wiedemann syndrome
Amyloidosis
Sarcoidosis

▼ DIFFERENTIAL DIAGNOSIS DISCUSSION

Benign Infection

Many benign infections, especially upper respiratory tract infections, can be associated with **mild, transient splenomegaly.** Adenovirus, coxsackievirus, and *Streptococcus* are commonly involved organisms.

Epstein-Barr Virus (EBV) Infection (Infectious Mononucleosis)

Infectious mononucleosis is discussed in Chapter 53, "Lymphadenopathy."

Cytomegalovirus (CMV) Infection

Epidemiology

CMV is ubiquitous, and **most people are infected with the virus by adulthood.** The source is body fluids, including blood, urine, breast milk, saliva, and feces. Transmission of CMV is both horizontal **(person to person)** and vertical **(mother to child).** CMV is the most common congenital viral infection.

Clinical Features

CMV infection manifests itself differently in different hosts:

▼ In **neonates**, intrauterine growth retardation (IUGR), microcephaly, jaundice, hepatosplenomegaly, a petechial or purpuric rash, chorioretinitis, and neurologic symptoms may be seen.
▼ In **immunocompetent children or adults**, infection is most commonly asymptomatic; however, patients may develop fever, malaise, anorexia, pharyngitis, headache, myalgia, abdominal pain, and hepatosplenomegaly.

▼ In **immunocompromised children and adults,** retinitis, pneumonitis, and enteritis are the primary manifestations.

Evaluation

Diagnosis is best made by **viral isolation** of the organism in cell culture of body fluids (or organs). **Serologic studies** are also available. A **computed tomography (CT) scan of the head** may demonstrate intracerebral calcifications in patients with congenital CMV infection.

Treatment

The immunocompetent host recovers completely in a few weeks with **supportive treatment.** In immunocompromised patients with retinitis, therapy with **ganciclovir** has shown efficacy.

Malaria

Etiology

Malaria, an *Anopheles* mosquito-transmitted disease of the tropics and subtropics, is acquired when the host's erythrocytes are invaded by a **mosquito-borne parasite** of the genus *Plasmodium.* Four species of *Plasmodium* cause malaria: *P. falciparum, P. vivax, P. ovale,* and *P. malariae.* The incubation period is 1–2 weeks.

Clinical Features

Although constitutional symptoms are universal, the clinical presentation of malaria is often **dictated by the infecting species.** *P. vivax* and *P. ovale,* for example, are particularly associated with hypersplenism and splenic rupture.

Evaluation

Diagnosis is confirmed by **identification of the parasite** in the blood. Special stains and smears are required for optimal yield. Thick and thin blood films should be examined.

Treatment and Prevention

Treatment entails **antimicrobial therapy** (e.g., chloroquine) and **supportive measures** (e.g., management of fluid and electrolytes, RBC transfusions). Because drug resistance is common, **alternative antibiotics** (e.g., quinine, quinidine, primaquine, mefloquine, pyrimethamine-sulfadoxine, doxycycline, tetracycline, clindamycin) may be necessary.

Control of the *Anopheles* mosquito population is important for prevention of malaria. **Chemoprophylaxis** with chloroquine, mefloquine, or doxycycline is recommended for travelers to endemic areas.

Babesiosis

Etiology

Like malaria, babesiosis is a **parasitic infection** of erythrocytes that is endemic in the coastal areas of the northeastern United States. The main reservoir of *Babesia* is the **white-footed mouse,** and the organism is transmitted by the *Ixodes scapularis* tick. The incubation period is 1–9 weeks.

Clinical Features

Symptoms include fever, chills, sweats, malaise, myalgias, nausea, and vomiting. Jaundice, dark urine, and renal failure are also possible. The clinical presentations of **babesiosis and malaria are sometimes similar.**

Evaluation

Laboratory evaluation may demonstrate hemolytic anemia and elevation of liver enzymes. The diagnosis is confirmed by **blood smears** and **serologic studies.**

Treatment

Patients with moderate or severe illness are treated with **clindamycin and quinine,** or **atovaquone and azithromycin.**

Hematologic Disorders

HS, G6PD deficiency, SCD, and thalassemia are discussed in Chapter 40, "Hemolysis."

Lymphomas

Lymphomas [non-Hodgkin lymphoma (NHL) and Hodgkin disease] are discussed in Chapter 53, "Lymphadenopathy."

Trauma

Mechanisms of injury to the spleen include motor vehicle accidents, bicycle accidents, and falls. Patients may complain of **diffuse or left upper quadrant pain.** The diagnosis is confirmed by **CT scan.**

Lacerations and hematomas are usually conservatively managed with **observation** and **supportive therapy.** Rarely, **surgical splenectomy** is necessary in patients with lacerations or hematomas. In rare cases, traumatic cysts are managed with aspiration, sclerosing, and surgery.

Gaucher Disease

Etiology

A **deficiency of β-glucosidase** leads to the pathologic accumulation of glucocerebroside in the reticuloendothelial system.

Clinical Features

Gaucher disease is categorized into three forms.

▼ **Type I, the "classic" type,** is one of the most common genetic disorders in Ashkenazi Jews. It may present at any age, but usually presents in adolescence or adulthood. Its distinguishing feature is its lack of neurologic involvement.
▼ **Type II, the infantile form,** is characterized by slow or no achievement of developmental milestones, swallowing difficulties, and opisthotonos. Its progressive neurodegenerative course culminates in death within the first 2 years of life.
▼ **Type III, the juvenile form,** presents in infancy or childhood with behavioral changes, seizures, and extrapyramidal and cerebellar signs. With all three types, **splenomegaly is universal.**

Evaluation

A **bone marrow aspirate** demonstrating Gaucher cells engorged with glucocerebroside confirms the diagnosis.

Treatment

Splenectomy has been used to manage the hematologic consequences of hypersplenism. Cerezyme (Genzyme), given every 2 weeks, has been effective in reversing the changes.

▼ EVALUATION OF SPLENOMEGALY
Patient History

The following information is important to obtain:

▼ **Does the patient have a history of a recent upper respiratory tract infection?** Benign viral infections often result in mild splenomegaly.

▼ **What is the patient's travel history?** Constitutional symptoms, in the setting of travel to a tropical area, make malaria a likely diagnosis. These same symptoms, with a history of travel to the coastal northeastern United States, suggest babesiosis.

▼ **Is there a history of tick exposure?** Ticks transmit the organisms responsible for babesiosis, RMSF, ehrlichiosis, and tularemia.

▼ **Is there a history of exposure to any animals?** Contact with cattle or other farm animals (as well as unpasteurized milk) could be the clue to brucellosis. Handling rabbits might point to tularemia as a diagnosis. Scratches from cats or kittens could lead to cat-scratch disease, while toxoplasmosis is also commonly linked to interactions with cats. Leptospirosis may be transmitted through the urine of dogs, rats, or livestock.

▼ **Is the patient immunocompromised?** An immunocompromised host with splenomegaly and constitutional symptoms may have CMV infection.

▼ **Is there a history of weight loss?** Weight loss may be seen in patients with infectious mononucleosis, CMV infection, brucellosis, ehrlichiosis, malaria, or babesiosis. Oncologic processes, especially lymphoma and leukemia, must also be considered in this setting.

▼ **What is the patient's medication history?** Splenomegaly in a patient who developed a rash in response to ampicillin therapy makes mononucleosis a likely diagnosis. In patients with G6PD deficiency, exposure to medications with oxidant properties leads to hemolysis and splenomegaly. Splenomegaly in the setting of joint complaints and rash makes a drug-induced serum sickness a likely possibility.

▼ **Is there a history of trauma?** The spleen is the most commonly injured intra-abdominal organ.

Physical Examination

Physical findings often offer important clues to the diagnosis.

▼ **Growth retardation in a microcephalic neonate** should lead to an investigation for CMV.

▼ **Exudative pharyngitis** in combination with splenomegaly suggests mononucleosis.

▼ **Rash** of the palms and soles suggests RMSF or syphilis. The rash of RMSF is usually seen first on the wrists and ankles and may be maculopapular or petechial. A maculopapular rash is characteristic with both congenital and secondary syphilis. Bullous lesions are also common in congenital syphilis. A whole body rash with "iris" or "target" lesions suggests serum sickness. JRA and SLE also have characteristic rashes.

▼ **Jaundice** may be seen with many of the infectious processes, but is more typical in the hemolytic diseases (e.g., G6PD deficiency, spherocytosis, autoimmune hemolytic anemia).

▼ **Adenopathy** in combination with splenomegaly most commonly points to mononucleosis, but lymphoma should also be considered. Axillary and cervical adenopathy are the two most common sites of lymph node enlargement in cat-scratch disease. While the examination may demonstrate evidence of feline scratches, the classic papule is usually gone by the time the node manifests.

▼ **Abdominal pain** (either diffuse or localized to the left upper quadrant) should prompt an evaluation for a traumatic cause, such as a splenic laceration or hematoma. Furthermore, one of the complications of infectious mononucleosis is splenic rupture, which can present with acute abdominal pain. The presence of fever suggests a splenic abscess.

Laboratory Studies

The following studies may be appropriate:

▼ **"Monospot."** The mononucleosis rapid slide agglutination test for heterophil antibodies is a quick test for infectious mononucleosis, but false negatives are common in children under 6 years of age.

▼ **EBV serologies.** The definitive way to diagnose both acute and past infection at any age is through the use of EBV serologies.

▼ **Complete blood count (CBC).** Atypical lymphocytosis is the hallmark finding of mononucleosis. Pancytopenia is common in sepsis, AIDS, ehrlichiosis, and oncologic processes. Thrombocytopenia is seen in RMSF and babesiosis. Evidence of a hemolytic anemia (e.g., sickled cells, target cells, schistocytes, spherocytes) should prompt consideration of the common hematologic disorders (SCD, thalassemia, G6PD deficiency, and spherocytosis), as well as certain infectious diseases (e.g., malaria, babesiosis).

▼ **Reticulocyte count.** Reticulocytosis is the confirmatory finding in hemolytic anemias.

▼ **Bilirubin level and liver enzymes.** Hyperbilirubinemia is found in both hemolytic anemias and intrinsic liver disease. An elevation in liver enzymes implicates the liver as a primary or secondary source of pathology. Common causes may be infectious, neoplastic, anatomic, metabolic, traumatic, or toxic.

▼ **Direct antibody test.** Autoimmune hemolytic anemias are usually antibody positive.

▼ **Routine blood smear.** Evidence of hemolysis is also evident on inspection of the peripheral blood smear. Additionally, infestations like malaria and babesiosis can often be readily identified on blood smears as long as the laboratory is made aware that these diseases are diagnostic possibilities.

▼ **Urinalysis (UA).** Hemoglobinuria is a common finding in hemolytic anemias. UA abnormalities are also seen with some metabolic disorders.

▼ TREATMENT OF SPLENOMEGALY

Most of the diseases presenting with splenomegaly require supportive care and observation for complications.

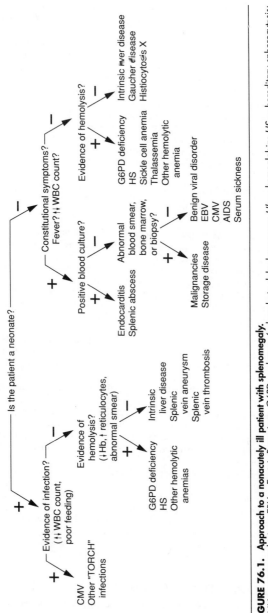

FIGURE 76.1. Approach to a nonacutely ill patient with splenomegaly.
CMV = cytomegalovirus; EBV = Epstein-Barr virus; G6PD = glucose-6-phosphate dehydrogenase; Hb = hemoglobin; HS = hereditary spherocytosis; WBC = white blood cell.

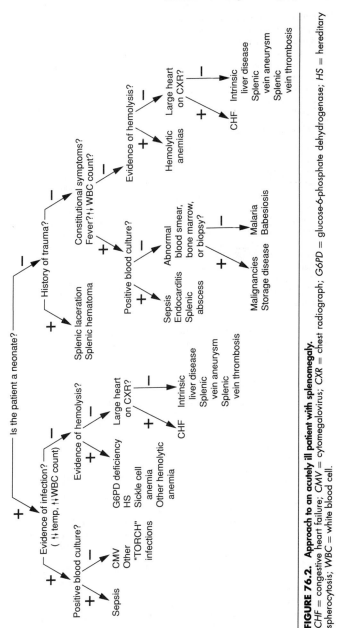

FIGURE 76.2. Approach to an acutely ill patient with splenomegaly.
CHF = congestive heart failure; CMV = cytomegalovirus; CXR = chest radiograph; G6PD = glucose-6-phosphate dehydrogenase; HS = hereditary spherocytosis; WBC = white blood cell.

▼ **Splenic rupture,** whether associated with mononucleosis or not, requires immediate surgical management.

▼ **Splenic abscess** is treated with intravenous antibiotics and sometimes surgical drainage.

▼ **Hemolytic anemias.** Patients with hemolytic anemias often require RBC transfusions until the hemolysis is either terminated or stable. Discontinuation of offending medications is indicated in patients with serum sickness and G6PD deficiency.

▼ APPROACH TO THE PATIENT

▼ **In neonates with splenomegaly,** bacterial infection should be ruled out first. If no bacterial causes are isolated, a viral cause should be aggressively pursued. If infection is deemed unlikely, a hemolytic cause should be considered. If no hemolytic disorder can be identified, anatomic abnormalities of the spleen should be investigated.

▼ **In older infants and children with splenomegaly,** trauma is the first consideration. Infection and hemolysis are the next two possibilities to be considered. If these categories are eliminated and the patient has constitutional symptoms, an oncologic process is likely; rarely, a metabolic disorder also presents in this fashion.

▼ Regardless of age, in an **acutely ill patient** with splenomegaly and cardiomegaly, congestive heart failure is a likely diagnosis. In a nonacutely ill child, serum sickness should be considered if all other possibilities are ruled out.

The approach to nonacutely ill patients with splenomegaly is given in Figure 76.1. The approach for acutely ill patients with splenomegaly is given in Figure 76.2.

Suggested Readings

American Academy of Pediatrics: Babesiosis. Brucellosis. Ehrlichiosis. Malaria. In *2000 Red Book: Report of the Committee on Infectious Diseases,* 25th ed. Edited by Pickering, LK. Elk Grove Village, IL: American Academy of Pediatrics, 2000, pp 181–182, 192–193, 234–236, 381–385.

Galanakis E, Bourantas KL, Leveidiotou S, et al: Childhood brucellosis in north-western Greece. *Eur J Pediatr* 155:1–6, 1996.

Grover SA, Barkun AN, Sackett DL: Does this patient have splenomegaly? *JAMA* 270:2218, 1993.

Khan SB, Alkan S, Pooley R: A 14-year old boy with splenomegaly. *Arch Pathol Lab Med* 124:1239–1240, 2000.

Scully RE (ed.): Case records of the Massachusetts General Hospital. Weekly clinicopathological exercises. A two-year-old boy with thrombocytopenia, leukocytosis, and hepatosplenomegaly *N Engl J Med* 330:1739–1746, 1994.

Tamayo SG, Rickman LS, Mathews WC, et al: Examiner dependence on physical diagnostic tests for the detection of splenomegaly: a prospective study with multiple observers. *J Gen Intern Med* 8:69, 1993.

Vane DW: Left upper quadrant masses in children. *Pediatr Rev* 13:25, 1992.

Woods M, Greenes D: A 16-year-old girl with epistaxis and hepatomegaly. *Curr Opin Pediatr* 7:733–739, 1995.

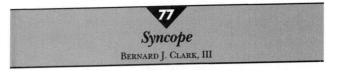

77
Syncope
BERNARD J. CLARK, III

▼ INTRODUCTION

Syncope, a common complaint in children, refers to a **loss of consciousness, usually lasting 1–2 minutes because of a transient drop in cerebral perfusion pressure.** The most common form is **vasomotor or vasovagal syncope.** In this condition, external stimuli such as pain, emotional upset, and increased vagal tone lead to slowed heart rate, peripheral vasodilatation, and decreased cerebral perfusion pressure. One-third of syncopal spells in children are accompanied by a convulsion that may last for several minutes. Infants may have pallid or cyanotic breath-holding spells that follow pain, excitement, or frustration. These spells start with a deep inspiration or expiration. Usually these spells do not have any neurologic consequences.

More serious are the rarer **syncopal spells associated with heart disease.** Specific cardiac diagnoses can also be associated with syncope. The final common pathway of all syncope is a decrease in blood perfusion to the brain.

▼ DIFFERENTIAL DIAGNOSIS LIST
Left Ventricular Outflow Tract Obstruction

Aortic stenosis
Subaortic stenosis
Hypertrophic cardiomyopathy

Arrhythmias

Ventricular tachycardia
Prolonged QT syndrome
Heart block and bradycardia

Other

Vasodepressor syncope
Primary pulmonary hypertension

▼ DIFFERENTIAL DIAGNOSIS DISCUSSION

Cardiac syncope is the result of a **sudden decrease in cardiac output, leading to decreased cerebral perfusion and a loss of consciousness.** The differential diagnosis of cardiac syncope includes left ventricular outflow tract obstruction and arrhythmia.

Left Ventricular Outflow Tract Obstruction

Anatomic causes of left ventricular outflow tract obstruction can be considered as a single cause of cardiac syncope. All of these causes **limit cardiac output, especially during exercise,** and all have as part of the physical examination a **systolic murmur with an ejection quality.** In children with a history of syncope and a significant ejection murmur, left ventricular outflow tract obstruction should be presumed and the patient referred to a **pediatric cardiologist. Chest radiograph or electrocardiogram (ECG)** may suggest left ventricular hypertrophy in these patients but both tests often can be normal. Thus **echocardiography** will be needed to make the diagnosis.

Treatment of symptomatic left ventricular outflow tract obstruction includes **balloon dilation or surgical valvotomy for aortic stenosis** and **surgical resection for subaortic resection,** which has a small but finite rate of recurrence despite successful initial resection. **Hypertrophic cardiomyopathy** can be managed by the use of **beta-receptor antagonists** such as propranolol or **calcium channel antagonists** or with **surgical resection.**

Limitations to competitive sports, especially those with isometric exercise effort such as football, wrestling, and heavy weight lifting, may be required in patients with unrepaired, and in some cases repaired, left ventricular outflow tract obstruction. Decisions regarding participation in sports should be made in consultation with a pediatric cardiologist.

Ventricular Tachycardia (VT)

Patients with VT can present with a history of **palpitation, chest pain, or syncope.** VT presents as a wide **QRS tachycardia** with a rate of **120 to 240 beats per minute.**

VT can be a **medical emergency** because this rhythm can rapidly **deteriorate into ventricular fibrillation.** For patients who appear hemodynamically stable, an attempt at **intravenous access** and **pharmacological conversion to sinus rhythm with lidocaine** should be attempted. For patients who are not hemodynamically stable or who present with mental status changes, **cardioversion** is the treatment of choice.

The underlying cause of VT is often difficult to delineate. Emergently, evaluation of VT should include **assessment and correction of electrolyte disturbances** including hypocalcemia or hypomagnesemia. In adolescents, **illegal drug abuse** such as cocaine should be assessed and tested for. A new onset of VT can be due to myocardial damage secondary to myocarditis and, thus, a **recent viral illness.** Patients who have undergone corrective **open heart surgery** for congenital heart disease, **especially tetralogy of Fallot,** are at risk for ventricular arrhythmias. Other causes of VT include **prolonged QTc, exercise-induced** VT, and **benign VT** of the newborn older child. Patients with a suspected history of VT require evaluation by a **pediatric cardiologist.**

Prolonged QT Syndrome

In patients with a **history of syncope** and a **family history of sudden death,** it is essential to rule out prolonged QTc syndrome as the cause of syncope. The QTc interval is calculated from surface ECG by measuring the **QT interval in seconds from the onset of the Q wave to the end of the T wave and dividing this interval by the square root of the R-R interval in seconds.** Thus measured, the corrected QT, or QTc, is independent of heart rate and, outside the infant period, has an **upper normal limit of 0.44 seconds.**

Children with **prolonged QTc syndrome** can have drop attacks associated with **life-threatening arrhythmias,** including VT. If a child is found to have prolonged QTc, the **entire family,** including all first-degree relatives, **should be screened,** since several inherited forms of this disease exist. Evaluation includes **12-lead ECG,** looking specifically at the QTc interval, and **Holter monitoring** to look for occult arrhythmias and measured QTc at several heart rates. Often **exercise testing** is used to calculate changes in the QTc during exercise. In normal patients, the QTc remains constant or shortens slightly during exercise. In patients with prolonged QTc, the QTc actually lengths during exercise. Other testing can include recording the QTc during an **infusion of the beta agonist, isoproterenol.**

Heart Block and Bradycardia

Symptomatic bradycardia caused by sick sinus syndrome or the onset of late, complete heart block can cause cardiac syncope. This is most commonly seen in children who have undergone **cardiac surgery.** More specifically, patients with **transposed great arteries who have undergone an atrial inversion procedure** have a high incidence of both **automatic atrial tachycardia and sick sinus syndrome.** Patients who have had a **ventricular septal defect closure** may suffer a late complication of intermittent, complete heart block. These patients are typically cared for by a cardiologist and have routine annual follow-up examinations that include **24-hour Holter monitoring** to evaluate for these arrhythmias. Other causes of bradycardia that could present as syncope include **second-degree heart block,** in which several atrial beats are not conducted to the ventricle. The cause of second-degree heart block includes **inflammatory disease** such as rheumatic fever or myocarditis.

Vasodepressor Syncope

Vasodepressor syncope is perhaps the **most common cause of cardiac syncope in childhood.** It is included here as a cardiac cause of syncope because its pathophysiology includes an **inappropriate low heart rate or slowing of the heart** at a time of **decreased filling secondary to vascular dilatation.** Often these children present **without an identifiable trigger** such as the classic fear of the sight of blood or other key environmental surroundings. The child with recurrent episodes is frequently referred for cardiac evaluation.

Cardiac evaluation will include a **12-lead EKG, echocardiogram,** and, when indicated, **tilt-table evaluation.** The last is a relatively new procedure that can allow more accurate definition of patients with significant recurrent vasodepressor syncope. The patient fasts for 4 hours and is then brought to the cardiac catheterization laboratory, where an intravenous line and blood pressure monitoring are put in place and the EKG is continuously recorded. The patient then rests supine for 1 hour. Afterward, resting catecholamine levels are drawn by intravenous methods. The patient is then tilted upright, and blood pressure and heart rate are continuously monitored. Patients are asked to report any symptoms. If the patient reports dizziness, nausea, or an altered level of consciousness, she is again placed in the supine position for a recovery period. In patients who remain asymptomatic, an infusion of isoproterenol can be initiated to further provoke symptoms. Patients with **positive tilt-table tests** (i.e., those with **vasodepressor syncope**) are encouraged to **increase their intake of fluids.** If syncope persists, treatment with a **mineralocorticoid** is begun for volume expansion.

▼ EVALUATION OF CARDIAC SYNCOPE

Patient History

In patients who present with syncope as a chief complaint, questions regarding the history should be directed toward **defining the circumstances** under which the child fainted.

▼ Were there **definable triggers** to account for the event such as crowding, heat, or an emotional trigger?
▼ Did the child have **palpitations** prior to syncope?
▼ Is there a **family history** of syncope, arrhythmias, or sudden cardiac events?

In suspected cases of vasodepressor syncope, a **detailed history of diet** is important, specifically, how much on average the child drinks in a day. Finally, if the event occurred **during exercise,** cardiac syncope should be included in the differential and an **ECG** should be performed.

Physical Examination Findings

The physical examination should be directed toward cardiac evaluation to help rule out cardiac syncope:

▼ Is there a significant systolic murmur?
▼ Are the heart tones normal?
▼ Is there a gallop rhythm suggestive of cardiac dysfunction?
▼ In younger children, is there evidence of hepatomegaly?

Laboratory Studies

It can be argued that **every child with syncope should have an ECG.** This test is readily available and reliable, and the intervals are usually calculated by computer. Thus it can help to delineate at least those children with prolonged QTc that can be life threatening. However, statistically, most of these ECGs will be normal. In the patient with a **single episode** of well-documented syncope triggered by an emotional or environmental event, **initial observation** is warranted. Further evaluation including **Holter monitoring** should be performed in any child suspected of an **arrhythmia** as a cause of syncope. This would include children with a history of palpitations, a history of an irregular heart rate when first checked following syncope, or in children with syncope while active. Any patient with **syncope and a significant murmur** should have an **echocardiogram.**

▼ APPROACH TO THE PATIENT

The **most common cause** of syncope in children is either **noncardiac or vasomotor syncope.** Children with symptoms consistent with vasodepressor syncope do not need further evaluation unless syncope is recurrent. In patients without symptoms consistent with noncardiac or vasomotor syncope, an **ECG** should be performed **to assess the QTc.** If an arrhythmia is thought to be responsible for a syncopal episode, then **Holter monitoring** is necessary to attempt to document ventricular arrhythmias as the potential cause. Children with **recurrent syncope and a positive family history of sudden death** should have an evaluation by a **pediatric cardiologist.** Finally, in a patient with syncope, especially if it occurs **during exercise,** or in a child with a **significant organic murmur,** evaluation by a **pediatric cardiologist** is indicated and an **echocardiogram** should be performed.

Suggested Readings

Cadman CS: Medical therapy of neurocardiogenic syncope. *Cardiol Clin* 19(2):203–213, v, 2001.
Fenton AM, Hammill SC, Rea RF, et al: Vasovagal syncope. *Ann Intern Med* 133(9):714–725, 2000.

Lewis DA, Dhala A: Syncope in the pediatric patient. The cardiologist's perspective. *Pediatr Clin North Am* 46(2):205–219, 1999.

Low PA: Update on the evaluation, pathogenesis, and management of neurogenic orthostatic hypotension: introduction. *Neurology* 45(4 suppl 5):S4–5, 1995.

McLeod KA: Dysautonomia and neurocardiogenic syncope. *Curr Opin Cardiol* 16(2):92–96, 2001.

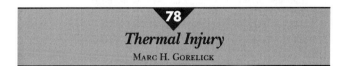

78
Thermal Injury
Marc H. Gorelick

▼ INTRODUCTION

Thermal injury in children can involve not only the **skin,** but also the **respiratory, circulatory, immune,** and **central nervous systems.** Successful treatment of the child with thermal injury requires comprehensive assessment and management. Management of burn injury is dictated by the **assessment of its severity,** which is determined by the mechanism, depth, and extent of injury.

▼ DIFFERENTIAL DIAGNOSIS LIST

Thermal causes—direct flame burns, contact burns, scald burns
Chemical causes
Electrical causes
Radiation

▼ DIFFERENTIAL DIAGNOSIS DISCUSSION
Thermal Burns

Thermal burns are the **most common type of burns** affecting children. They may result from contact with **hot liquids** (scalds), **hot surfaces,** or **flames.** Scald burns tend to be more extensive but more superficial than contact burns. Flame injuries are most often associated with inhalation injuries.

Chemical Burns

Chemical burns are caused by contact with **corrosive substances.** Contact with **acids** causes **coagulation necrosis,** whereas contact with **alkali** causes **liquefaction necrosis.** Alkali burns are typically deeper and more severe than acid burns. Chemical burns require **extensive irrigation** with water or saline to remove the corrosive agent and prevent further injury.

Electrical Burns

Electrical injury results from contact with a source of electrical current, or from arcing of current near the body.

Electrical injury typically produces a **depressed entry wound,** and an **exit wound** that appears "blown out." With high-voltage currents (> 1000 V), the extent of the underlying deep tissue damage is typically far in excess of that suggested by the appearance of the cutaneous burn. Both low- and high-voltage currents can cause **cardiac arrhythmias,** even in the absence of visible burns.

Patients exposed to significant electrical current should have an **electrocardiogram (ECG)** to monitor for arrhythmia.

Radiation Burns

The most common type of radiation burn in children is **sunburn.** Sunburn is typically **first degree,** or, rarely, **superficial second degree.**

▼ EVALUATION OF THERMAL INJURY
Patient History

The following information should be ascertained during the history:

▼ The mechanism of injury
▼ The duration of exposure
▼ If the cause of injury was fire, whether the fire occurred in a closed space
▼ Whether the patient has a history of loss of consciousness
▼ The patient's tetanus immunization status

Physical Examination

🛠 HINT Always consider the possibility of an intentionally inflicted injury. The following features may be cause for concern: inconsistent or implausible explanation (remember to relate the reported mechanism with the developmental age of the child); the presence of other abuse risk factors; burns to typically protected areas (e.g., the dorsum of the hand or back of the neck); burns in a "stocking-glove" distribution, particularly in the absence of splash marks; burns to the buttocks or genitalia; or multiple cigarette burns.

Burns are classified according to their **depth and extent** (Table 78.1). Depth of injury is assessed on the basis of the clinical findings and is classified

TABLE 78.1. Classification of Burns		
Type of Burn	Affected Skin Layer	Appearance
First degree	Epidermis	Erythema, hypersensitivity
Second degree		
Superficial	Upper (papillary) dermis	Erythema, blistering intact hairs, exquisite pain
Deep	Deep (reticular) dermis	Skin may be white or mottled and nonblanching, or blistered and moist; pain may or may not be present; hairs easily pulled
Third degree	Entire dermis	Dry, white, or charred skin; leathery appearance, painless, no hair
Fourth degree	Subcutaneous tissue	Same as third degree; may have exposed muscle and bone

TABLE 78.2. "Rule of Nines"

Body Part	Percent of BSA		
	Infant	Child	Adolescent/Adult
Head	18%	13%	9%
Anterior trunk	18%	18%	18%
Posterior trunk	18%	18%	18%
Upper extremity (each)	9%	9%	9%
Lower extremity (each)	14%	16%	18%
Genitalia	1%	1%	1%

For small burns, a rough estimate of the affected BSA can be made by comparing the burn with the size of the child's palm (which represents approximately 1% of the BSA).
BSA = body surface area.

as **superficial** (first degree), **partial thickness** (superficial second degree), or **full thickness** (deep second degree, third degree, and fourth degree). Initially, the percentage of body surface area (BSA) involved with partial- and full-thickness burns should be estimated using the **"rule of nines"** (Table 78.2). After the patient has been stabilized, a more detailed assessment of the extent of burns is made using a modified **Lund and Browder chart.**

The patient should be assessed for signs of **inhalation injury** (Table 78.3). Significant inhalation injury may exist in the absence of any surface burns; therefore, a high index of suspicion should be maintained in the face of a suggestive history (e.g., fire in a closed space).

HINT The presence of signs of pulmonary injury early in the course is a poor prognostic indicator.

HINT Frank shock is uncommon in the first 30–60 minutes after a burn. Its presence should prompt a search for other causes of shock (e.g., abdominal trauma with occult blood loss, spinal cord injury).

TABLE 78.3. Signs of Inhalation Injury

Pulmonary	CNS	Skin
Tachypnea	Confusion	Facial burns
Stridor	Dizziness	Singed nasal hairs
Hoarseness	Headache	Cyanosis
Rales	Hallucinations	Cherry-red color
Wheezing	Restlessness	
Cough	Coma	
Retractions	Seizures	
Nasal flaring		
Carbonaceous sputum		

CNS = central nervous system.

Laboratory Studies

For children with minor burns, no laboratory studies are routinely needed. The following may be helpful in specific circumstances:

▼ **Arterial blood gases.** Arterial blood gas measurements must be interpreted with caution; normal arterial blood gases are not reassuring in the presence of clinical findings. The arterial oxygen tension (Pao_2) and the calculated oxygen saturation are unaffected, even by significant carbon monoxide (CO) poisoning. Metabolic acidosis in a patient with inhalation injury suggests the possibility of cyanide toxicity.

▼ **Carboxyhemoglobin level.** An elevated carboxyhemoglobin level helps in making the diagnosis of CO poisoning, but a normal level does not exclude it, especially if there is a delay in measuring the level.

▼ **Blood work.** A complete blood count (CBC) and blood type and cross-match may be indicated for patients with concomitant trauma or extensive burns.

▼ **Serum creatine kinase.** A serum creatine kinase level should be obtained for patients with electrical injury to assess the extent of deep tissue injury and rhabdomyolysis.

Diagnostic Modalities

A chest radiograph is not helpful in the initial assessment of smoke inhalation, because findings are usually delayed by 24–36 hours. Diagnosis should be based on **clinical assessment.**

▼ TREATMENT OF THERMAL INJURY

The appropriate treatment depends on the severity of the injury. The American Burn Association classifies burns as **major** (requires burn center referral), **moderate** (requires inpatient treatment), or **minor** (requires outpatient treatment). The American Burn Association criteria for burn severity and disposition are given in Table 78.4.

Emergency Management of Major Burns

▼ **First, an airway must be secured.** Concomitant trauma is common in burn patients, and cervical spine immobilization should be maintained if injury is suspected. Because rapid edema formation can make airway management difficult, intubation should be considered early in patients with evidence of significant thermal injury to the upper airway.

▼ **Hyperbaric oxygen therapy** should be considered if any of the following are present: a carboxyhemoglobin level greater than 30%, neurologic symptoms (confusion and disorientation, focal deficit, history of loss of consciousness), or cardiac disturbance.

▼ Consider **presumptive therapy with sodium thiosulfate** (25% solution), 1.65 ml/kg given intravenously over 30–60 minutes, to counteract cyanide toxicity.

▼ **Burns covering a large surface area cause substantial fluid losses and shifts, necessitating special fluid management,** with smaller children requiring relatively greater amounts of fluid (Figure 78.1). The amounts given in Figure 78.1 are totals for the first 24 hours: 50% of the total volume is administered over the first 8 hours after the occurrence of the burn, and the remaining 50% is administered over the subsequent 16 hours.

TABLE 78.4. Burn Severity and Disposition (American Burn Association Criteria)

Major burns: burn center referral
Partial-thickness burns affecting more than 20% of the BSA
Full-thickness burns affecting more than 10% of the BSA
Burns involving the face, eyes, ears, hands, feet, and perineum that may result in functional or cosmetic impairment
Associated inhalation injury
Electrical injury
Burns complicated by underlying illness or major trauma

Moderate burns: inpatient treatment
Partial-thickness burns affecting 10%–20% of the BSA
Full-thickness burns affecting 2%–10% of the BSA

Minor burns: outpatient treatment
Partial-thickness burns affecting less than 10% of the BSA
Full-thickness burns affecting less than 2% of the BSA (may still require surgical referral)

BSA = body surface area.

▼ **Adjunctive care** of the patient with major burns includes the removal of all clothing from the burn areas. Adherent molten material (e.g., tar, metal) should be cooled but left in place. All burns should be irrigated with water or saline solution. Chemical burns require copious irrigation (15–30 minutes) with water; a small child may be placed in a sink for this purpose. Following irrigation, the burns should be covered with saline-soaked gauze, or a dry sterile sheet if the burns are extensive.

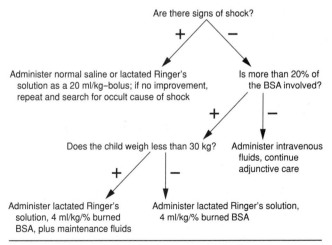

FIGURE 78.1. Fluid replacement in a patient with major burns.
BSA = body surface area.

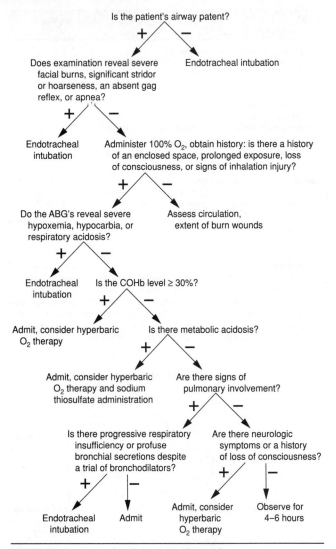

Is the patient's airway patent?

+ / **−**

(+) Does examination reveal severe facial burns, significant stridor or hoarseness, an absent gag reflex, or apnea?

(−) Endotracheal intubation

+ / **−**

(+) Endotracheal intubation

(−) Administer 100% O_2, obtain history: is there a history of an enclosed space, prolonged exposure, loss of consciousness, or signs of inhalation injury?

+ / **−**

(+) Do the ABG's reveal severe hypoxemia, hypocarbia, or respiratory acidosis?

(−) Assess circulation, extent of burn wounds

+ / **−**

(+) Endotracheal intubation

(−) Is the COHb level ≥ 30%?

+ / **−**

(+) Admit, consider hyperbaric O_2 therapy

(−) Is there metabolic acidosis?

+ / **−**

(+) Admit, consider hyperbaric O_2 therapy and sodium thiosulfate administration

(−) Are there signs of pulmonary involvement?

+ / **−**

(+) Is there progressive respiratory insufficiency or profuse bronchial secretions despite a trial of bronchodilators?

(−) Are there neurologic symptoms or a history of loss of consciousness?

+ / **−**

(+) Endotracheal intubation

(−) Admit

+ / **−**

(+) Admit, consider hyperbaric O_2 therapy

(−) Observe for 4–6 hours

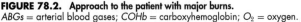

FIGURE 78.2. Approach to the patient with major burns.
ABGs = arterial blood gases; *COHb* = carboxyhemoglobin; O_2 = oxygen.

▼ **Analgesics** (e.g., morphine 0.05–0.1 mg/kg intravenously, meperidine 1 mg/kg intravenously) should be administered early. Tetanus immunoprophylaxis should be administered as needed. Steroids and prophylactic antibiotics should be avoided. Nasogastric decompression and placement of an indwelling bladder catheter are needed for seriously injured patients.

▼ **Definitive wound management** should be undertaken only in consultation with the burn surgeon who will assume care of the child.

Emergency Management of Minor Burns

▼ **An open dressing** should be applied to small burns or burns in hard-to-dress areas. Burns should be washed with mild soap and water, and an antibacterial ointment (e.g., bacitracin polymyxin B) should be applied. No covering is needed. The wound should be washed at home and ointment reapplied 2–3 times daily until healed.

▼ **A closed dressing** is used for most burns in children. The clothing should be removed from the area, and the burn should be irrigated with water or saline solution. Chemical burns should be irrigated for 15–30 minutes. Analgesia (oral acetaminophen with codeine for small burns, intravenous morphine or meperidine for larger burns) should be provided, and then the burn should be washed again with mild soap and water and rinsed with saline solution. Loose or clearly nonviable tissue should be débrided with forceps. Intact blisters should be left undisturbed; ruptured bullae should be unroofed and débrided.

▼ Several **gauze dressings** are available, either plain or treated (e.g., Adaptic, Xeroform, Vaseline, Aquaphor). Silver sulfadiazine (1%) cream is applied to the wound surface or to the underside of the dressing, in a layer approximately 2–3 mm thick. Silver sulfadiazine should not be used for facial burns. The entire wound surface is covered with the dressing, and then an outer absorbent dressing or roller gauze is applied.

▼ If the child has a second- or third-degree burn and her tetanus immunization status is not up to date, **tetanus immunoprophylaxis** should be administered.

The burn should be rechecked in 24–48 hours to assess for healing and signs of infection. Home dressing changes should be performed once or twice daily until healed, usually for 10-14 days. An analgesic (e.g., acetaminophen with codeine) should be provided for the first few days.

⚡ HINT Consider hospitalization or referral when there are concerns about loss of function (e.g., burns over the hands or joints), cosmetic results (e.g., large facial burns), or the risk of poor compliance with the treatment regimen. Final results are largely dependent on meticulous burn care.

▼ APPROACH TO THE PATIENT (FIGURE 78.2)

Suggested Readings

Baxter CR, Waeckerle JF: Emergency treatment of burn injury. *Ann Emerg Med* 17:1305–1315, 1988.

Finkelstein JL, Schwartz SB, Madden MR, et al: Pediatric burns: an overview. *Pediatr Clin North Am* 39:1145–1163, 1992.

Monafo WW: Initial management of burns. *New Engl J Med* 335:1581–1586, 1996.

Schonfeld N: Outpatient management of burns in children. *Pediatr Emerg Care* 6:249–253, 1990.

Thom SR: Smoke inhalation. *Emerg Med Clin North Am* 7:371–387, 1989.

Tibble PM, Perrotta PL: Treatment of carbon monoxide poisoning: a critical review of human outcome studies comparing normobaric oxygen with hyperbaric oxygen. *Ann Emerg Med* 24:269–276, 1994.

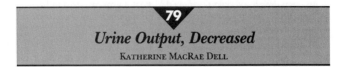

79

Urine Output, Decreased

KATHERINE MACRAE DELL

▼ INTRODUCTION

Decreased urine output can be caused by either a **decrease in urine production (oliguria)** or an **obstruction to urinary flow.** Oliguria is defined as a urine output of less than 0.5 ml/kg/hr in a child or adolescent and less than 1.0 ml/kg/hr in a neonate. Decreased urine output may result from prerenal, renal, or postrenal factors. Oliguria may occur as the result of an **acute process** or an **acute exacerbation** of an unrecognized chronic renal disease.

▼ DIFFERENTIAL DIAGNOSIS LIST

Prerenal Etiologies

Decreased Intravascular Volume

Dehydration
Hemorrhage
Inadequate fluid intake
Sepsis (with capillary leak)
Hypoalbuminemia

Ineffective Cardiac Output

Congestive heart failure
Sepsis (with hypotension)

Intrarenal Etiologies

Glomerular Causes

Primary glomerulonephritis (GN) [e.g., acute postinfectious, membranoproliferative]
Secondary GN associated with systemic disease (e.g., lupus nephritis)

Tubulointerstitial

Acute tubular necrosis (ATN)
Prolonged prerenal azotemia or ischemia
Medications
Toxins

Pigment deposition—myoglobin or hemoglobin
Acute interstitial nephritis (drugs, infections)

Vascular

Hemolytic-uremic syndrome
Renal venous or arterial thrombosis

Postrenal Etiologies

Congenital or Anatomic

Congenital obstructive uropathies (e.g., posterior urethral valves)
Urinary stone
Trauma
Abdominal mass

Functional

Acute urinary retention
Neurogenic bladder

▼ DIFFERENTIAL DIAGNOSIS DISCUSSION
Dehydration

Dehydration is the **most common cause** of **oliguria** in the pediatric population. The causes, clinical features, and evaluation are discussed in detail in
Chapter 25, "Dehydration." Treatment is directed toward restoring intravascular volume. If dehydration is mild, **oral rehydration** may be attempted. If
the patient cannot tolerate oral fluids, or if the dehydration is more severe,
initial **fluid resuscitation with normal saline** should be performed, followed
by oral or intravenous rehydration. In most patients, urine output improves
within a few hours when these simple measures are used.

⚡ HINT   If intravascular volume has been restored and minimal or no urine
output is observed, other diagnoses should be considered, such as ATN. Continuing to administer fluid to an oliguric patient who is euvolemic will be of no benefit
and could precipitate volume overload.

Acute Postinfectious Glomerulonephritis

See Chapter 39, "Hematuria."

Acute Tubular Necrosis (ATN)

Etiology

ATN is the **final common pathway of a number of renal insults,** including
prolonged prerenal ischemia, sepsis, toxicity, and **pigment deposition.** ATN
is a relatively common occurrence in severely ill patients in intensive care
units (ICUs); these patients often have multiple causes for the ATN (e.g.,
sepsis with hypotension plus aminoglycoside therapy).

Clinical Features

ATN traditionally has three phases:

▼ **Oliguric phase.** The oliguric phase may last days or even weeks. The
hallmarks of this phase are decreased urine output and loss of renal

concentrating ability, resulting in an elevated urine sodium level and a decreased urine specific gravity. Hypertension may be present, as with other forms of acute renal failure.

▼ **Diuretic phase.** In the diuretic phase, urine output increases dramatically; urine sodium and water losses may be significant.

▼ **Recovery phase.** In the recovery phase, urine output returns to a normal rate and concentrating ability returns.

Evaluation

The evaluation of patients with ATN is twofold: **assessing the clinical status** (including the volume and electrolyte status) and **determining the underlying cause,** which may not be immediately apparent.

▼ **Pertinent questions** focus on prior medication use (especially antimicrobials such as aminoglycosides and amphotericin B), recent radiocontrast dye studies, and toxin exposures (such as lead). Patients with hemoglobinuria or myoglobinuria may have a history of trauma, muscle pain, or pallor. Because prolonged ischemia from any prerenal cause can result in ATN, patients should be queried about recent gastrointestinal or blood losses.

▼ **Urinalysis** in patients with ATN typically shows a low specific gravity and variable degrees of hematuria or proteinuria. The urine sodium level in the oliguric phase is usually elevated (> 40 mEq/L). Specific tests as directed by the history (e.g., antibiotic levels, and serum creatine kinase levels) may also be indicated.

Treatment

Treatment of ATN is similar to that of other causes of acute renal failure. A significant number of patients with ATN, especially those with life-threatening conditions such as septic shock, require **dialysis.** ATN is not rapidly reversible, because tubular damage has occurred. However, a significant number of pediatric patients, even those with prolonged oliguria, may recover all or partial renal function.

Hemolytic-Uremic Syndrome

Hemolytic-uremic syndrome is a syndrome of **microangiopathic hemolytic anemia, thrombocytopenia,** and **renal failure.** There are two main categories: **diarrheal-associated** (D+ or "typical") and **nondiarrheal-associated** (D− or "atypical"). Most cases of hemolytic-uremic syndrome fall into the first category.

Etiology

D+ hemolytic-uremic syndrome results from infection with Shiga-toxin-producing *Escherichia coli,* usually the strain O157:H7. Other infectious agents have also been implicated in this form of hemolytic-uremic syndrome, including *Salmonella* and *Shigella* species. Infection usually results from **ingestion of contaminated foods,** especially ground beef, or from **person-to-person contact.**

Clinical Features

Patients with D+ hemolytic-uremic syndrome present with a **history of diarrhea, often bloody. Oliguria** often becomes evident as the diarrhea subsides. Patients also develop **pallor,** and occasionally a **petechial rash. Hypertension** is common.

Hemolytic-uremic syndrome can affect organs other than the kidney and gastrointestinal tract. Patients may have associated **central nervous system (CNS) symptoms** (e.g., irritability, lethargy, and coma), **pancreatic dysfunction** (resulting in hyperglycemia), and **cardiomyopathy** (resulting in congestive heart failure).

⚄ HINT With the advent of improved supportive care for patients with renal failure, CNS complications have become the leading cause of mortality in patients with hemolytic-uremic syndrome.

Evaluation

Evaluation of hemolytic-uremic syndrome includes a careful **history** to determine exposure to contaminated foods or ill contacts.

Physical examination is directed toward **assessing volume status** as well as **neurologic status.**

Laboratory tests include serum electrolytes, blood urea nitrogen (BUN) and creatinine levels, a glucose level, liver function tests and pancreatic enzyme measurements, urinalysis, and a complete blood count (CBC) with careful examination of the smear for evidence of schistocytes and fragmented red blood cells (RBCs). Proteinuria, hematuria, and cellular casts are common urinalysis findings.

Treatment

Treatment of D+ hemolytic-uremic syndrome is **largely supportive.** Establishing the diagnosis early in the course of disease is essential to avoid complications (e.g., volume overload). As with other forms of renal failure, specific treatments for electrolyte abnormalities may be required. **Transfusions of packed RBCs** are given only if the hemoglobin level is less than 6 g/dl. **Platelet transfusions** should be avoided unless active bleeding is present. As many as 50% of patients with hemolytic-uremic syndrome require **dialysis. Consultation with a pediatric nephrologist** early in the course of disease is strongly advised.

Posterior Urethral Valves

Etiology

Posterior urethral valves is the **most common cause of obstructive uropathy in infant boys.** The condition is caused by an **abnormality in urethral development** that results in the formation of mucosal folds, which act as valves, obstructing the outflow of urine.

Clinical Features

Patients usually present in the **first year of life** with **oliguria, poor intermittent urinary stream,** and a **distended bladder.** With the widespread use of screening antenatal ultrasounds, a significant number of patients are now identified **in utero,** by the finding of **bilateral hydronephrosis** with or without oligohydramnios. **Older patients** occasionally present with **urinary tract infection** (UTI) and a history of **poor urinary stream. A urinary concentrating defect is common** in this disorder, resulting in renal water and salt wasting. Patients with a history of severe oligohydramnios may have **pulmonary hypoplasia** and **respiratory distress.**

Evaluation

Specific evaluation of suspected posterior urethral valves includes a **renal ultrasound** to confirm obstruction and hydronephrosis, and a **voiding cystourethrogram. Serum electrolytes** and **creatinine** should also be measured. A serum creatinine level obtained within the first 24 hours of birth is not useful, because it largely reflects maternal renal function.

Urinalysis and **urine culture** should be obtained to assess for UTI.

Treatment

A **pediatric urologist** should be consulted if posterior urethral valves is suspected. Initial treatment consists of placement of a **Foley catheter** to facilitate bladder drainage. Following bladder decompression, it is important to **monitor serum electrolytes and volume status closely.** Because of renal concentrating defects and a postobstructive diuresis, hyper- or hyponatremia, hyperkalemia, and metabolic acidosis may ensue. Once the electrolyte abnormalities are normalized, definitive **valve ablation** can be performed (often in the first week of life). Despite surgical correction of the obstruction, patients with PUV are at **risk for progression to chronic renal failure.** Therefore, **referral to a pediatric nephrologist** is recommended for patients with evidence of renal insufficiency or metabolic acidosis.

▼ EVALUATION OF DECREASED URINE OUTPUT
Patient History

The history should be directed toward assessing the onset and severity of the oliguria, as well as determining possible causes:

▼ Fluid intake and losses (e.g., diarrhea, vomiting, and blood loss) should be quantified, if possible.
▼ Symptoms such as tiring with feeds, pallor, cyanosis, and difficulty with exertion are suggestive of underlying cardiac disease.
▼ Specific questions should be asked about toxin exposures (such as lead and mercury) and recent medication use [such as nonsteroidal antiinflammatory agents (NSAIDs)].
▼ Macroscopic hematuria suggests the presence of a UTI or glomerulonephritis.
▼ Flank pain is often present in patients with pyelonephritis, interstitial nephritis, renal calculi, or renal vein thrombosis.
▼ Questions directed at eliciting information about specific causes (e.g., a history of recent skin or pharyngeal infection or exposure to undercooked meat) are useful. In any patient with acute renal failure, it is important to assess for symptoms of chronic renal disease, such as a history of poor growth, recent weight loss, polyuria, or fatigue.

Physical Examination

Physical examination findings vary depending on the underlying cause:

▼ Dry mucous membranes, sunken eyes, poor skin turgor, and tachycardia suggest dehydration.
▼ Hypotension and poor perfusion are seen in patients with septic shock or cardiac dysfunction.
▼ A third heart sound (S_3) cardiac gallop may be noted if significant volume overload is present.

▼ Edema and hypertension are common in patients with acute renal failure secondary to glomerular disease.
▼ Joint symptoms and rashes may be present in patients with SLE or vasculitic diseases.
▼ Patients with rhabdomyolysis have diffuse muscle tenderness, especially in the larger muscle groups of the legs and arms.
▼ Abdominal masses may signal an obstructing malignancy.

✄ HINT   A very distended, obstructed bladder may be mistaken for an abdominal mass.

Laboratory Studies

Initial laboratory studies in any patient with oliguria include the following:

▼ A **serum electrolyte panel** and **BUN** and **creatinine levels** should be obtained first. If abnormal renal function is noted, calcium, phosphorus, and uric acid should also be assayed. A BUN:creatinine ratio of greater that 20 is suggestive of prerenal disease.
▼ A **urinalysis** with microscopy is obligatory.
▼ A **CBC** is indicated in almost all instances of acute renal failure except in certain cases, such as medication-induced acute urinary retention.
▼ **Urine sodium level and fractional excretion of sodium.** Measuring the urine sodium level is useful in helping to determine whether the disorder is prerenal or renal in origin. A urine sodium level less than 20 mEq/L suggests a prerenal cause, whereas one greater than 40 mEq/L suggests an intrinsic cause. Intermediate values of urine sodium are not diagnostic. Alternatively, a formal calculation of the fractional excretion of sodium (FENa) can be made:

$$\text{FENa} = (\text{Urine sodium /Plasma sodium}) \times (\text{Plasma creatinine/Urine creatinine}) \times 100$$

A FENa < 1% suggests a prerenal cause and values > 1% suggest an intrinsic cause. Of note, urinary sodium and FENa are not reliable for diagnostic purposes if diuretics have been administered in the previous 24 hours.
▼ **Additional laboratory studies** are ordered according to the suspected cause of the renal failure, and include laboratory investigation for past or current infection, drug levels, urine myoglobin, or serum creatine phosphokinase levels (if rhabdomyolysis suspected). Complement levels (C3, C4) and serologies, including antinuclear antibodies (ANA) and antineutrophil cytoplasmic antibodies (ANCA), should be considered in all patients with suspected glomerulonephritis.

Diagnostic Modalities

A **renal ultrasound** is indicated in all cases of suspected obstruction and most cases of acute renal failure (especially if unexplained). Additional **radiographic studies** are indicated based on the suspected cause of the acute renal failure. A **renal biopsy** may be necessary to diagnose certain forms of glomerulonephritis and for patients with unexplained renal failure.

▼ TREATMENT OF DECREASED URINE OUTPUT

The initial treatment for acute renal failure from any cause is directed toward the potentially life-threatening complications of volume depletion or overload, electrolyte imbalances, and hypertension.

▼ **Volume depletion is treated with normal saline,** 20 ml/kg administered as an intravenous bolus over 20–30 minutes and repeated as needed until the patient is euvolemic. Packed RBC transfusions or cardiac inotropic agents are given if the clinical situation dictates.

▼ **Patients unresponsive to fluid administration may be given a diuretic challenge.** Intravenous furosemide (2–4 mg/kg/dose) is given as a one-time dose. If a response is seen, the dose may be repeated every 4–6 hours. If no response is seen, additional doses are of no benefit and may cause ototoxic and nephrotoxic side effects.

▼ **Patients with persistent oliguria should be fluid restricted** to insensible losses (25%–30% of maintenance requirements given as 5%–10% dextrose in water) plus urine output (replaced cc for cc with 1/4–1/2 normal saline).

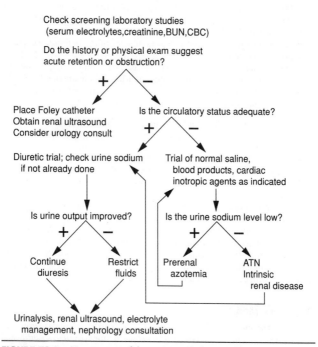

FIGURE 79.1. Management of the patient with decreased urine output. *ATN* = acute tubular necrosis; *BUN* = blood urea nitrogen; *CBC* = complete blood cell count.

▼ **Specific therapies for electrolyte disturbances** are outlined in Chapter 32, "Electrolyte Disturbances."

▼ APPROACH TO THE PATIENT (FIGURE 79.1)

Suggested Readings

Dinneen MD, Duffy PG: Posterior urethral valves. *Br J Urol* 78:275–281, 1996.

Flynn J: Causes, management approaches, and outcome of acute renal failure in children. *Curr Opin Pediatr* 10:184–189, 1998.

Gouyon JB, Guignard JP: Management of acute renal failure in newborns. *Pediatr Nephrol* 14:1037–1044, 2000.

Kaplan BS, Meyers KE, Schulman SL: The pathogenesis and treatment of hemolytic uremic syndrome. *J Am Soc Nephrol* 9:1126–1133, 1998.

Klahr S, Miller SB: Acute oliguria. *N Engl J Med* 338:671–675, 1998.

Peter JR, Steinhardt GF: Acute urinary retention in children. *Pediatr Emerg Care* 9:205–207, 1993.

Simckes AM, Spitzer A: Poststreptococcal acute glomerulonephritis. *Pediatr Rev* 16:278–279, 1995.

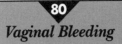

80
Vaginal Bleeding
COURTNEY SCHREIBER

MATTHEW F. RHOA AND LAURA HOLLAND
(Second Edition)

▼ DIFFERENTIAL DIAGNOSIS LIST

Premenarchal Patients

Infectious Causes

Infectious vulvovaginitis
Genital herpes
Condyloma acuminatum

Toxic Causes

Exogenous estrogens

Neoplastic Causes

Sarcoma botryoides
Adenocarcinoma of the cervix or vagina
Estrogen production from an ovarian cyst or neoplasm
Hemangioma

Traumatic Causes

Sexual abuse
Foreign body

Congenital or Vascular Causes

Urethral prolapse

Miscellaneous Causes

Vulvar skin disorders
Neonatal withdrawal bleeding
Precocious puberty
McCune-Albright syndrome

Postmenarchal Patients

Infectious Causes

Infectious vulvovaginitis
Cervicitis
Pelvic inflammatory disease

Neoplastic Causes

Benign and malignant tumors of the genital tract

Traumatic Causes

Sexual abuse
Foreign body (rare)

Metabolic or Genetic Causes

Hyper- or hypothyroidism
Hyperprolactinemia

Gynecologic Causes

Dysfunctional uterine bleeding
Abortion—threatened, incomplete, complete, or missed
Ectopic pregnancy
Polycystic ovarian disease

Hematologic Causes

Idiopathic thrombocytopenic purpura
von Willebrand disease (vWD)

Miscellaneous Causes

Chronic systemic illness—e.g., liver disease, connective tissue disorder

▼ DIFFERENTIAL DIAGNOSIS DISCUSSION
Vulvovaginitis

Vulvovaginitis is discussed in detail in Chapter 81, "Vaginal Discharge (Vulvovaginitis)." Bleeding, when present, is usually **minimal,** although a **blood-tinged discharge** is common in severe cases. *Shigella* and group A β-hemolytic streptococci are the most common causes of a bloody vaginal discharge associated with vulvovaginitis.

Foreign Body

Foreign bodies placed into the vagina account for 5% of gynecologic visits in childhood. Most children **will not remember or admit** to placing an object in the vagina. The incidence is highest in children between the ages of 2 and 4 years. **Rolled toilet tissue** is one of the most common findings.

Clinical Features

The child presents with a history of a **foul-smelling, often bloody, vaginal discharge.** The vaginal bleeding is usually **bright red, scant, and intermittent.** A strong odor may be the most bothersome symptom.

Evaluation

On physical examination, the vagina is **erythematous** and a **foul-smelling discharge** is present. A **large foreign body may be easily palpated on rectal examination.** Smaller items (e.g., toilet tissue) may not be discerned.

Radiographic studies are of little use because most foreign bodies are not radiopaque.

Treatment

Vaginoscopy is essential for diagnosis and removal. Small items can be removed with **saline irrigation. General anesthesia** is frequently required for **removal of larger objects. Antibiotic therapy** is recommended before removing foreign bodies that may have been **in place for 1 week or longer.**

Trauma

Incidence and Etiology

Genital trauma is a **serious** and common cause of vaginal bleeding. The incidence is highest in children between the ages of 4 and 12 years. Most genital trauma results from a **straddle injury** (e.g., a child landing on the center bar of a bicycle), but **sexual abuse, accidental penetration, sudden abduction** of the lower extremities, and **pelvic fractures** must also be considered.

Clinical Features and Evaluation

▼ **In patients with straddle injuries** (a type of blunt trauma), a small ecchymotic area or a large vulvar hematoma may be noted. Hematomas are tender, tense, and rounded swellings that may enlarge if bleeding continues. Lacerations of the hymen or vagina are rare in association with straddle injuries and should alert the physician to other possible sources of trauma.

▼ **Accidental penetration with pens and other small objects** is common in 2- to 4-year-olds. Lacerations can be superficial or deep and can extend to the peritoneal cavity. Isolated injuries to the hymen alone are rare, and careful examination of the vagina is mandatory.

▼ **Lacerations of the vagina can also occur as a result of sudden abduction of the legs,** as in gymnastics or water-skiing. These injuries can be difficult to distinguish from injuries sustained secondary to sexual abuse. The paucity of other injuries helps distinguish these injuries from sexual abuse.

▼ **In patients with pelvic fractures,** injuries to the urinary system are more common than are vaginal lacerations. However, in complex fractures, lacerations of the vagina can be extensive, accounting for a significant loss of blood. A thorough examination is mandatory, including evaluation of the urinary system and rectum.

If bleeding is noted from the vagina, vaginoscopy with anesthesia is mandatory to isolate the source.

Treatment

▼ **Superficial abrasions and lacerations** of the vulva, if not actively bleeding, may be cleaned and left to heal.

▼ **Small vulvar hematomas** that are not expanding may be managed conservatively with ice packs and pressure.

▼ **Large or expanding hematomas** should be managed surgically with evacuation and ligation of bleeding vessels. Perioperative antibiotics are required.

Neonatal Withdrawal Bleeding

Withdrawal of maternal estrogen after delivery causes **physiologic bleeding** in a small percentage of **newborns.** The bleeding is limited and usually **resolves within 1 week.** The parents may notice an increased, blood-tinged discharge. **No treatment** is necessary unless bleeding persists for **longer than 10 days.** At that point, a thorough examination should be performed.

Vulvar Hemangiomas

Etiology

Bleeding can result following trauma to a vulvar hemangioma. Vulvar hemangiomas are common and generally **disappear as the child ages.**

Clinical Features

Patients usually present with **painless bleeding** and a **history of vulvar hemangiomas.** The bleeding is usually self-limited; however, heavy bleeding can be seen with cavernous hemangiomas. Careful examination of the external genitalia identifies the source of bleeding. Vaginoscopy is not required if bleeding is limited to the external genitalia.

Treatment

When bleeding does not respond to **pressure, surgical ligation** may be required.

Vulvar Skin Disorders

Most vulvar skin conditions involve the labia majora and labia minora and do not extend to the vagina or perianal area. **Seborrhea, psoriasis, and eczema** are the most common diagnoses. These lesions tend to be **pruritic.** The constant **scratching with subsequent infection** can lead to a bloody discharge similar to that seen in vaginitis.

Urethral Prolapse

Etiology

Prolapse is thought to result from **increased abdominal pressure,** which could be caused by coughing or constipation. Some are predisposed to prolapse secondary to a weakness of collagen.

Clinical Features

A **small, hemorrhagic, friable mass surrounding the urethra** is the most common presentation. The bleeding associated with prolapse of the urethra is usually **painless** (because the urethra and vagina are so close in proximity, urethral bleeding may be thought to be from the vagina). The average age at diagnosis is 5 years.

The lesion can easily be **confused with condyloma acuminatum.** If the diagnosis is in question, **3% acetic acid** may be applied; condyloma acuminatum has an **acetowhite appearance.**

Treatment

If voiding is not inhibited, **local therapy** (i.e., with topical estrogen and sitz baths) may be all that is needed. The prolapse usually **resolves after 4 weeks** of therapy.

If **urine retention or necrosis** is present, **surgical removal and catheterization** are necessary.

Dysfunctional Uterine Bleeding

Dysfunctional uterine bleeding is defined as **any abnormal bleeding** from the uterus that is **not caused by structural abnormalities.** The average menstrual cycle has a mean interval of 28 days, with a mean duration of 4 days. The average blood loss is 30 ml/cycle, with an upper normal limit of 80 ml. A **menstrual cycle with an interval of 21 days or less and a duration of longer than 7 days or blood loss of more than 80 ml is abnormal.**

Etiology

Anovulation, most commonly caused by an **immature hypothalamic–pituitary axis,** is responsible for more than 75% of cases of dysfunctional uterine bleeding. Without ovulation, and the resulting formation of the corpus luteum, there is no cyclic or monthly production of progesterone. The cyclic production and withdrawal of progesterone results in a normal period. Anovulation causes continuous estrogenic stimulation of the endometrium, resulting in a thick, unstable endometrium that sheds irregularly. Hypothalamic–pituitary axis immaturity can last for as many as **18 months after menarche.** McDonough and Ganett found that 55%–82% of cycles in adolescents between menarche and 2 years after menarche were anovulatory. These percentages decreased with time.

Anovulation may also be caused by **hyperthyroidism, hypothyroidism, hyperadrenalism, hyperprolactinemia, diabetes mellitus, polycystic ovarian syndrome, chronic systemic illness, substance abuse, eating disorders, physical or emotional stress, and excessive exercise.**

Clinical Features

The patient may present with 4 or 5 months of **amenorrhea, followed by an episode of heavy bleeding** or completely irregular bleeding. Anovulatory bleeding is usually **painless.**

Evaluation

Dysfunctional uterine bleeding is a **diagnosis of exclusion.** Organic lesions, pregnancy, and coagulation disorders must be ruled out. The history and physical examination should emphasize the **common and life-threatening conditions** in the differential, with **coagulation defects** and **complications of pregnancy** leading the list. In patients with **severe bleeding, vWD should be considered.**

Studies helpful in the diagnosis include **serum thyroid-stimulating hormone, prolactin, follicle-stimulating hormone, luteinizing hormone, testosterone, dehydroepiandrosterone, and 17-hydroxyprogesterone levels.**

TABLE 80.1. Treatment of Dysfunctional Uterine Bleeding

Mild dysfunctional uterine bleeding
Reassurance
Menstrual calendar
Oral contraceptives if sexually active

Severe or recurrent dysfunctional uterine bleeding without anemia
Medroxyprogesterone acetate, 10 mg for 10 days each month
Oral contraceptives if sexually active

Acute anovulatory bleeding in a stable patient
Oral contraceptives (50 μg; one pill every 6 hours until bleeding stops)
After bleeding stops, taper oral contraceptives:
    One pill every 8 hours for 3 days
    Then one pill every 12 hours for 3 days
    Then one pill every day to complete 21 days
    Continue on oral contraceptives for 3–6 months

Acute or heavy bleeding associated with anemia or hypotension
Hospitalization
Transfusion if unstable
IV-conjugated estrogen (25 mg every 4–6 hours) until bleeding stops
Begin cyclic progestational-dominant oral contraceptive (e.g., Lo-Ovral, Ovral):
    One pill every 6 hours for 3 days
    Then one pill every 8 hours for 3 days
    Then one pill every 12 hours for 2 weeks
    Continue on oral contraceptives for 2 months after week of withdrawal

---

IV = intravenously.

Treatment

Management of dysfunctional uterine bleeding in an adolescent **depends on the severity** of the bleeding, with the emphasis placed on stopping the bleeding and preventing recurrent episodes (Table 80.1).

▼ **Patients with mild bleeding** (i.e., bleeding at 20- to 60-day intervals without anemia) should be advised that the situation usually resolves after 1–2 years with maturation of the hypothalamic–pituitary axis and subsequent ovulation. If the patient has mild dysfunctional uterine bleeding and desires some form of contraception, a low-dose oral contraceptive may be prescribed that will provide the added benefit of regular menstrual cycles.

▼ **For patients with severe or recurrent dysfunctional uterine bleeding associated with anemia,** hormonal therapy is indicated. If the patient is sexually active, low-dose oral contraceptives are the most appropriate treatment. **OCPs are appropriate first-line treatment even if the patient is not sexually active.** Otherwise, medroxyprogesterone acetate can be administered (see Table 80.1). A normal menstrual period will occur 3–5 days after discontinuation of the medroxyprogesterone. Therapy should be continued for 6–8 months, and then discontinued. Most patients have spontaneous maturation of the hypothalamus–pituitary axis with onset of regular menses after cessation of therapy. If patients continue to have irregular bleeding after stopping therapy, other causes of anovulation should be considered, including thyroid disorders, hyperprolactinemia, excessive exercise, dieting, and polycystic ovarian syndrome.

▼ **An acute episode of bleeding in a stable patient** may be treated with a 50-μg combined oral contraceptive (see Table 80.1). If the bleeding does not stop within 5 days, another cause for the bleeding, such as a coagulation disorder, must be considered. When the bleeding slows, the pills may be tapered as described in Table 80.1. The patient should be maintained on the pills for at least 3 months, or longer if sexually active.

▼ **Patients who have undergone heavy bleeding leading to hypovolemia or anemia** should be hospitalized for therapy and coagulation studies. Intravenous conjugated estrogens are given every 4–6 hours until the bleeding stops, usually 24–48 hours after initiating therapy. Once the bleeding has stopped, the patient may be started on oral contraceptives (see Table 80.1). Dilatation and curettage is to be avoided in adolescents; however, when medical therapy fails, it may be necessary for diagnostic purposes. Along with dilatation and curettage, hysteroscopy may be helpful in making a diagnosis.

Pregnancy

Bleeding **in early pregnancy is common.** In most cases, it is scant and has little clinical significance. However, bleeding may be a sign of **ectopic pregnancy, which is life threatening.** Therefore, **pregnancy must be ruled out in all adolescent patients with bleeding,** regardless of the history. Figure 80.1

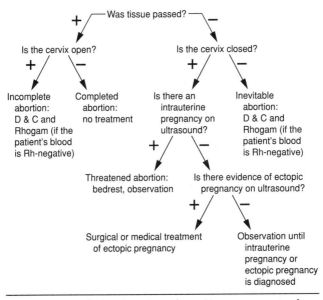

FIGURE 80.1. Evaluation of a patient with a positive pregnancy test and vaginal bleeding.
D & C = dilatation and curettage.

illustrates the approach to a patient with a positive pregnancy test and vaginal bleeding. A **gynecologic consultation is mandatory** in patients who have bleeding in pregnancy.

▼ EVALUATION OF VAGINAL BLEEDING
Patient History

The history is always helpful when evaluating children with vaginal bleeding. The physician must be aware, however, that much **information may be intentionally withheld** by both the patient and the parent. Children generally will not provide information regarding foreign bodies, manipulation, or sexual abuse. Likewise, parents will not often admit to sexual abuse. Whenever a child presents with vaginal bleeding, regardless of the history, other **indications of abuse must be sought** (see Chapter 72, "Sexual Abuse").

Physical Examination

A careful and thorough physical and gynecologic examination is mandatory. Consultation with a **pediatric gynecologist** is essential.

▼ APPROACH TO THE PATIENT

Figure 80.2 depicts the approach to a premenarchal girl with vaginal bleeding.

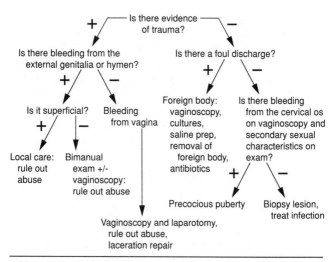

FIGURE 80.2. Evaluation of a premenarchal girl with vaginal bleeding.

Suggested Readings

Altcheck A: Common problems in pediatric gynecology. *Compr Ther* 10:19, 1984.

Altchek A: Dysfunctional uterine bleeding in the adolescent. In *The Patient;* Vol 18. 1993, p 45.

Behrman RE, Kliegman RM, Nelson WE, et al: *Nelson Textbook of Pediatrics,* 14th ed. Philadelphia, WB Saunders, 1992.

Carpenter SE, Rock JA: *Pediatric and Adolescent Gynecology.* Philadelphia, Lippincott-Raven, 1992.

Emans JH, Goldstein DP: *Pediatric and Adolescent Gynecology.* Boston, Little, Brown, 1990.

Grossman M, Dieckmann RA: *Pediatric Emergency Medicine.* Philadelphia, JB Lippincott, 1991.

Hertweck SP: Dysfunctional uterine bleeding. *Obstet Gynecol Clin North Am* 19:129, 1992.

Reece RM: *Manual of Emergency Pediatrics.* Philadelphia, WB Saunders, 1992.

Taber BZ: *Manual of Gynecologic and Obstetric Emergencies,* 2nd ed. Philadelphia, WB Saunders, 1984.

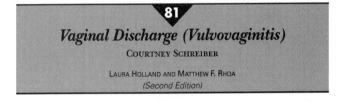

81
Vaginal Discharge (Vulvovaginitis)
COURTNEY SCHREIBER

LAURA HOLLAND AND MATTHEW F. RHOA
(Second Edition)

▼ INTRODUCTION

Vulvovaginitis, a common problem for both pediatric and adolescent patients, is an entity consisting of **vaginal and vulvar irritation** associated with **vaginal discharge.** A **lack of estrogen,** which protects and toughens the skin in the genital region, renders **premenarchal girls particularly susceptible** to vulvovaginitis. **Poor hygiene,** a common problem in young girls, also contributes to the problem. Some causes of vulvovaginitis are more prevalent in adolescents (e.g., *Candida* vulvovaginitis).

▼ DIFFERENTIAL DIAGNOSIS LIST
Infectious Causes
Bacterial Infection
Neisseria gonorrhoeae, Neisseria meningitidis
Chlamydia trachomatis
Group A β-hemolytic streptococci
Shigella flexneri
Staphylococcus aureus
Gardnerella vaginalis
Streptococcus pneumoniae

Yersinia enterocolitica
Haemophilus influenzae

Fungal Infection

Candida albicans

Parasitic Infection

Trichomonas vaginalis
Enterobius vermicularis (pinworm)

Viral Infection

Herpes simplex virus
Human papillomavirus

Neoplastic Causes

Tumor
Sarcoma botryoides

Traumatic Causes

Sexual abuse
Local irritants—bubble bath, harsh soaps, tight-fitting clothes, nylon underwear, allergy to laundry detergent or fabric softener

Congenital or Vascular Causes

Hemangioma
Ectopic ureter

Metabolic or Genetic Causes

Diabetes mellitus

Psychosocial Causes

Compulsive masturbation

Miscellaneous Causes

Systemic illness—roseola, varicella, scarlet fever, Stevens-Johnson syndrome, Kawasaki syndrome
Dermatologic disorder—seborrhea, eczema, psoriasis, lichen sclerosis et atrophicus
Nonspecific vulvovaginitis
Foreign body
Physiologic discharge of the newborn
Physiologic leukorrhea of the adolescent
Urethral prolapse
Draining pelvic abscess

▼ DIFFERENTIAL DIAGNOSIS DISCUSSION
Nonspecific Vulvovaginitis
Etiology

Nonspecific vulvovaginitis accounts for 25%–70% of all cases of pediatric vulvovaginitis and is caused by an **alteration in the vaginal flora.** The most common cause of this alteration is **poor perineal hygiene.** In adults, causes of nonspecific vulvovaginitis include antibiotic therapy and diabetes.

Clinical Features

Nonspecific vulvovaginitis is characterized by **vaginal discharge, odor, vulvar and vaginal irritation, and dysuria.**

Evaluation

The history should include the following questions:

▼ After a bowel movement or urination, does the child wipe her perineum from back to front?
▼ Does the child urinate with her knees together?
▼ Is the child exposed to local irritants such as harsh soaps, bubble bath, and shampoos?
▼ Does she wash her hair in the bathtub?
▼ Is the child's laundry washed with hypoallergenic soap?
▼ Is fabric softener (a possible local irritant) used?
▼ Does the child wear tight clothes (e.g., tights and leotards)?
▼ Does the child wear white cotton underwear and use white, unscented toilet paper?

Physical examination usually reveals **vulvar erythema and inflammation.** Often, a **vaginal discharge** is present.

A **saline smear** reveals **WBCs and bacteria.** A **potassium hydroxide (KOH) smear** reveals **no evidence of mycotic infection.** If local measures fail, cultures should be sent; in patients with nonspecific vulvovaginitis, the **culture reveals normal vaginal flora.** *N. gonorrhoeae* and *C. trachomatis* assays are routinely taken and the results are **negative.**

Treatment

Application of **1% hydrocortisone cream, A & D ointment, or Desitin cream** may be soothing. Patients may also take **sitz baths three times a day** (Aveeno oatmeal or baking soda may be added to the bath). The vulva should be **gently patted dry** or may be dried using a **hair dryer on the cool setting.**

If symptoms do not improve with local measures and a **predominant organism** is present on vaginal culture, an **appropriate antibiotic** can be prescribed. If no predominant organism is identified by culture, and vulvovaginitis does not respond to local measures, **empiric antibiotic** treatment may be tried (e.g., amoxicillin, 20–40 mg/kg/day orally for 7–10 days; or amoxicillin–clavulanate 20–40 mg/kg/day orally for 7–10 days; or cephalexin, 25–50 mg/kg/day orally for 7–10 days).

Prevention entails **improved perineal hygiene,** including correct voiding and wiping technique and **avoidance of bubble baths, harsh soaps, and tight clothes.** The child should wear **white cotton underwear.**

Candida Vulvovaginitis

Etiology

The usual cause of this infection is *C. albicans.* The disorder is **more common in adolescents** than in prepubescent girls.

▼ **Predisposing factors in prepubescent girls** include diabetes mellitus, recent antibiotic or steroid use, and immunosuppression.

▼ **In adolescents,** predisposing factors include diabetes mellitus, recent antibiotic use, pregnancy, use of oral contraceptives, tight-fitting clothes, immunosuppression, and steroid use.

Clinical Features and Evaluation

▼ **In prepubescent girls,** vulvar erythema, perianal erythema, and, often, excoriations, are visible.

▼ **In adolescent patients,** inflammation is often present, and white satellite candidal plaques are sometimes noted. A thick "cottage cheese" discharge is often present and may be associated with vulvar pruritus. A KOH smear reveals hyphae and budding yeast.

Treatment

▼ **In prepubescent girls** an antifungal cream (e.g., miconazole, clotrimazole, nystatin) should be applied to the external genitalia. If this is not successful, intravaginal nystatin liquid or gentle insertion of a vaginal suppository that has been cut in half may be prescribed. A topical steroid cream may be used to alleviate the inflammation.

▼ **Adolescents** should be treated with an antifungal medication (e.g., miconazole or terconazole) given as a cream or vaginal suppositories for a 3- to 7-day course. Oral fluconazole is available in a one-time dose.

Physiologic Leukorrhea

Etiology and Clinical Features

Physiologic leukorrhea, caused by **desquamation of epithelial cells under the influence of estrogen,** is classically described as **white, mucoid, and without odor.** It is seen in **newborns** (secondary to maternal estrogens) **and adolescents.** Sometimes it is noted months prior to the first menses.

Evaluation and Treatment

Physical examination reveals **copious white, mucoid vaginal secretions without an odor. Saline and KOH preparations reveal epithelial cells,** but no yeast, *Trichomonas*, or WBCs. **No treatment** is necessary. An adolescent may find that a panty shield is useful.

Lichen Sclerosis

Etiology and Clinical Features

The cause of lichen sclerosis, which is characterized by **vulvar pruritus and irritation,** is **unknown.** Patients sometimes complain of **constipation** (secondary to tenesmus), **dysuria, and vaginal discharge.** Chronic ulcerations and inflammation may result in areas of **ecchymosis** and **secondary infection** of the vulva.

Evaluation

The diagnosis is generally made by the classic appearance of **whitened papules and plaques on the vulva and perineum** in a characteristic **"figure eight"** or **"hourglass" distribution.** In some patients, this disorder may be difficult to distinguish from vitiligo. A **vulvar biopsy** may be necessary.

Treatment

The patient should be **referred to a dermatologist or gynecologist familiar with this condition.** Instruction in **improving perineal hygiene, use of ointments** (e.g., A & D ointment, Desitin), and **avoidance of harsh soaps** is appropriate. **Topical steroid creams** may be of benefit.

Trichomoniasis

Etiology

This infection is caused by *T. vaginalis,* **a protozoan.** Premenarchal girls are generally resistant to this organism because of their lack of estrogen.

Clinical Features

Some patients are **asymptomatic,** but the classic complaint is of a **gray, yellow, or green foul-smelling vaginal discharge.** The patient may note **postcoital spotting.**

Evaluation

Vulvar erythema and excoriations may be seen on physical examination. A **"strawberry red" cervix** is classically described but rarely seen. A **saline preparation** often reveals the **flagellated protozoa** as well as a **heavy polymorphonuclear infiltrate.** Some centers report greater detection of this organism by **culture** than wet smear.

Because trichomoniasis is generally a sexually transmitted disease, the patient should be **tested for gonorrhea and chlamydia** and should be **counseled about testing for HIV and syphilis.**

Treatment

Children infected with *T. vaginalis* should be **referred to agencies** familiar with evaluating children who have been **sexually abused.**

Gonorrhea

N. gonorrhoeae infection is discussed in Chapter 73, "Sexually Transmitted Diseases."

Chlamydia

C. trachomatis infection is discussed in Chapter 73, "Sexually Transmitted Diseases."

Bacterial Vaginosis (Nonspecific Vaginitis)

Etiology

Bacterial vaginosis results from the **overgrowth of anaerobic bacteria;** *G. vaginalis* has also been implicated. The significance of *G. vaginalis* infection or bacterial vaginosis in children is uncertain, but one should consider the **possibility of sexual abuse.**

Clinical Features

The patient may complain of a **vaginal discharge or a "fishy" odor after coitus,** and a **gray or yellow, homogeneous discharge** is noted on physical examination.

Evaluation

Adolescent and adult patients must have three of the following four criteria to make the diagnosis:

▼ Homogeneous discharge
▼ Clue cells seen on a saline preparation
▼ A positive "whiff" test (a fishy odor is noted when discharge is mixed with KOH on a slide)
▼ Vaginal secretions with a pH greater than or equal to 4.5

Treatment

In menarchal adolescents, treatment of bacterial vaginosis is with **metronidazole** (500 mg twice daily for 7 days), **metronidazole vaginal gel 75%** (applied intravaginally twice daily for 5 days), **clindamycin** (300 mg twice daily for 7 days), or **ampicillin** (500 mg four times daily for 7–14 days).

Foreign Body

Vaginal foreign bodies are discussed in Chapter 80, "Vaginal Bleeding."

Enterobius Vermicularis Infestation (Pinworms)

Clinical Features

A typical history includes **perianal and vulvar itching,** especially at night.

Evaluation

Perianal excoriations and an **erythematous vulvar area** are seen on physical examination. **Parents** should be **asked to examine the child's anus at night using a flashlight;** it may be possible to see the worms. **Cellophane tape applied to the child's anus in the morning may** reveal **characteristic eggs.**

Treatment

Pinworm infestation is treated with **one dose of mebendazole** (100 mg), **repeated in 2 weeks.** Consideration should be given to **treating family members.**

Shigella Vulvovaginitis

Etiology

S. flexneri is most often responsible for this inflammation, which is **rare in children.**

Clinical Features and Evaluation

A **mucopurulent vaginal discharge** is seen; it is **bloody** in 40%–50% of patients. Fewer than 25% of patients have associated **diarrhea. Vaginal culture** reveals the organism.

Treatment

The infection is treated with **trimethoprim** (8 mg/kg/day) and **sulfamethoxazole** (40 mg/kg/day), twice daily for 7 days.

Group A β-Hemolytic Streptococcal Infection

Group A β-hemolytic streptococci can cause vulvovaginitis that may be associated with a **bloody vaginal discharge.** The vulvovaginitis typically develops **7–10 days after an upper respiratory tract infection or sore throat.** Diagnosis is via **vaginal culture.** Treatment is with penicillin VK, 125–250 mg four times daily for 10 days.

▼ EVALUATION OF VAGINAL DISCHARGE
Physical Examination

A **pelvic examination must be done slowly,** and the physician should tell the child that he will not hurt her. The physician must be prepared to **abandon the examination if it is too painful or traumatic for the child.** The examination should be tailored to the severity of the child's symptoms; **severe symptoms require a more thorough examination.**

The child may be positioned in the **"frog leg" position,** the **lithotomy position** (with the aid of stirrups), or the knee–chest position. The **knee–chest** position often causes gaping of the hymen, allowing visualization of the vagina and the cervix.

The physician should **start by examining the external genitalia,** paying particular attention to the presence or absence of genital lesions and vulvar inflammation. **Having the patient cough may elicit vaginal discharge.**

A **rectoabdominal examination** is useful for detecting an **intravaginal foreign body or a pelvic mass,** and for expressing **vaginal discharge.**

The **hymen should be examined** for signs of trauma or tears and the **presence of a perforation.** If a hymenal opening cannot be visualized, placing **gentle traction on the labia majora while depressing the perineum** generally causes the hymenal opening to open, enabling visualization of the lower vagina.

Visualization of the **upper vagina and cervix in a premenarchal girl** can be accomplished by using one of the following methods:

▼ Placing the child in the knee–chest position
▼ Using a pediatric otoscope, cystoscope, or vaginoscope after applying a local anesthetic (e.g., 2% viscous lidocaine) to the vulva and hymen
▼ Using a narrow vaginal speculum

✄ HINT When vulvovaginitis is recurrent or bloody, vaginoscopy is required to rule out a foreign body or tumor.

Laboratory Studies
Microscopic Examination

If **vaginal discharge** is present, microscopic examination of the discharge is indicated. In a **child,** a **moistened calgi swab** is used to obtain the sample; in an adolescent, a cotton swab is used. Care should be taken to **avoid touching the hymen,** which can cause discomfort. The slides are prepared as follows:

▼ **Saline (wet) preparation.** Touch the swab to a small amount of saline solution on a glass slide, and cover the slide with a glass cover slip. Examine the slide under a microscope for the presence of *T. vaginalis*, bacteria, WBCs, RBCs, and clue cells.
▼ **KOH preparation.** Touch the swab to a small amount of 10% KOH on a glass slide. Cover the slide with a glass cover slip and examine it under a microscope for hyphae and budding yeast.

Culture

In some circumstances, it may be appropriate to obtain the following cultures:

▼ **Vaginal culture.** A vaginal culture may identify a predominant pathological organism in premenarchal girls with nonspecific vulvovaginitis. Vaginal culture is not useful in menstruating patients.

▼ ***N. gonorrhoeae* culture.** The specimen should be obtained from the endocervical canal (in postmenarchal girls) or from the vagina (in prepubescent girls). A rectal swab increases the chance that the organism will be detected.

▼ ***C. trachomatis* culture.** Several chlamydial assays are available. The specimen should be obtained from the endocervical canal (in postmenarchal girls) or from the vagina (in prepubescent girls).

Suggested Readings

Carpenter SE, Rock JA: *Pediatric and Adolescent Gynecology.* Philadelphia, Lippincott-Raven, 1992.

Emans JH, Goldstein DP: *Pediatric and Adolescent Gynecology.* Boston, Little, Brown, 1990.

Shapiro RA, Schubert CJ, Siegel RM: *Neisseria gonorrhea* infections in girls younger than 12 years of age evaluated for vaginitis. *Pediatrics* 104(6):e72, 1999.

Sweet RL, Gibbs RS: *Infectious Disease of the Female Genital Tract,* 3rd ed. Baltimore, Williams & Wilkins, 1995.

Taber BZ: *Manual of Gynecologic and Obstetric Emergencies,* 2nd ed. Philadelphia, WB Saunders, 1984.

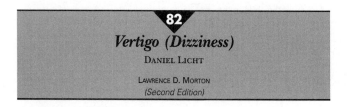

82

Vertigo (Dizziness)

DANIEL LICHT

LAWRENCE D. MORTON
(Second Edition)

▼ INTRODUCTION

Dizziness is caused by a **distortion in spatial orientation.** The primary sensory modalities of vision, vestibular function, joint position, sense (touch–pressure), and hearing are normally rapidly integrated by the central nervous system (CNS) into a composite sensation, keeping one aware of the body's position in space. Incorrect or insufficient sensory information or an error in integration of the perceptions produces distorted orientation, which in turn causes dizziness.

Vertigo is a sensation of spinning or rotation. Milder forms may be described as producing a rocking sensation or vague lightheadedness. Usually, vertigo is of sudden onset, and is associated with loss of balance, nausea, and nystagmus. The sensation can be terrifying to small children.

Vertigo can be caused by a disorder of the CNS or peripheral nerve dysfunction of the vestibular system.

▼ DIFFERENTIAL DIAGNOSIS LIST

Vertigo—peripheral or central
Faintness, giddiness, or lightheadedness
Disequilibrium

▼ DIFFERENTIAL DIAGNOSIS DISCUSSION

Historical points to document include the **course** (acute versus recurrent versus chronic), **precipitating events** (position change, trauma, infection), association with **alteration of hearing** (tinnitus or hearing impairment), **drug exposure, cardiovascular disease, and family history of migraine.**

Peripheral Vertigo

Etiology and Clinical Features

Historical points that help localize peripheral vertigo are improvement with visual fixation or holding head still, accompanying hearing complaints and absence of other complaints referable to cranial nerve dysfunction (difficulty swallowing, double vision, drooling).

▼ **Vestibular neuronitis.** Peripheral vertigo is most commonly seen in patients with vestibular neuronitis, which can occur several days after an upper respiratory tract infection. Vestibular neuronitis is a self-limited, postinfectious neuropathy, and symptoms generally resolve in 7–14 days.
▼ **Benign positional vertigo** is a rare disorder in children. These patients experience vertigo only with a change in head position. Symptoms are usually recurrent, with each attack lasting several weeks.
▼ **Ménière disease** is rare in children. It is characterized by recurring bouts of tinnitus, vertigo, and hearing loss.
▼ **Acute suppurative labyrinthitis** is caused by extension of otitis media or mastoiditis. Chronic otitis media can lead to the development of cholesteatoma, which in turn can cause labyrinth damage.
▼ **Medications,** especially aminoglycosides, can produce vertigo as a result of toxic damage to the peripheral vestibular apparatus.
▼ **Head trauma** may be followed by persistent vertigo, possibly because of dislocation of the otoliths from the macula.

Treatment

Treatment of peripheral vertigo is symptomatic. Administration of **meclizine and diazepam or oxazepam** may provide relief in children; adolescents may use **transdermal scopolamine. Trimethobenzamide hydrochloride and phenothiazines** can be used to treat nausea and vomiting. **Antibiotics** are used to treat acute suppurative labyrinthitis.

Central Vertigo

Etiology and Clinical Features

Historical points that help localize central vertigo are complaints referable to other cranial nerve dysfunction (double vision, difficulty swallowing, drooling, abnormal facial sensation), improvement with visual fixation removed (closing eyes), and lack of improvement with holding the head still.

▼ **Migraines** can occur in older children and adolescents, with episodes lasting minutes to hours. These episodes are usually associated with a strong family history.

▼ **Seizures.** Vertigo may be the only manifestation of seizures, although generally there is some alteration in consciousness. Often, careful questioning reveals confusional attacks and automatisms or other symptoms of partial complex seizures.

▼ **Other causes.** Other rare causes of central vertigo include stroke (lateral medullary syndrome of Wallenberg, with accompanying Horner syndrome) cerebellopontine angle tumors, neurofibromatosis and white matter disease (e.g., multiple sclerosis).

Treatment

In patients with frequent spells migraine prophylaxis can be used (i.e., cyproheptadine). In patients with other types of central vertigo (e.g., seizure disorder), treatment focuses on management of the underlying cause.

Faintness, Giddiness, or Lightheadedness

Symptoms of faintness, giddiness, or lightheadedness include **dimness of vision, "roaring" in the ears, and diaphoresis** with recovery on assuming the recumbent position. If symptoms are of **short duration and sudden onset,** the symptoms are most likely of **cardiovascular origin.** If symptoms persist, one must consider **hypoglycemia, hyperventilation, or a mood disturbance** (e.g., depression, anxiety).

Disequilibrium

Disequilibrium is **loss of balance** without an abnormal sensation in the head. Disequilibrium can be caused by cerebellar, peripheral nervous system, or bilateral vestibular lesions.

▼ EVALUATION OF VERTIGO (DIZZINESS)

Patient History

An effort should be made to clarify the type of dizziness by asking the following questions:

▼ Was the onset of symptoms acute, recurrent, or chronic?

▼ Were there any precipitating events (e.g., changes in position, motion, trauma, infection)?

▼ Are there any associated symptoms? Hearing loss, ear pain, or tinnitus suggest inner ear or eighth cranial nerve dysfunction, whereas nausea and vomiting indicate a peripheral vestibular apparatus disorder.

▼ Is there a history of cardiovascular disease, drug exposure, or a family history of migraine or ataxia?

Physical Examination

▼ **Ear examination.** Emphasis should be placed on the ear examination. One should look for perforations, infection, hemorrhage, or mass lesions. Blowing air into the external ear canal produces vertigo in patients with a fistula of the round or oval window of the labyrinth.

▼ **Neurologic examination.** The neurologic examination should focus on vestibular and cerebellar function. The presence of nystagmus, changes in visual fixation, hearing loss, or other evidence of cranial nerve dysfunction should be noted. In addition, evidence of decreased sensation or mild hemiparesis may indicate an underlying structural lesion.

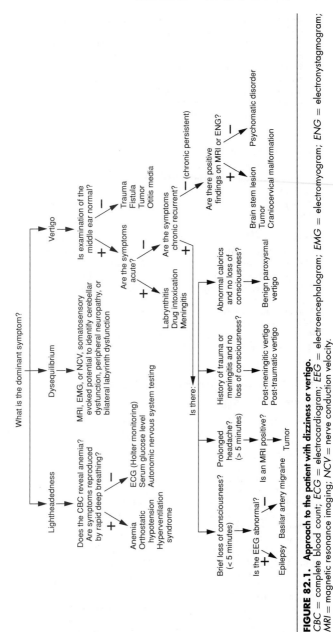

FIGURE 82.1. Approach to the patient with dizziness or vertigo.
CBC = complete blood count; ECG = electrocardiogram; EEG = electroencephalogram; EMG = electromyogram; ENG = electronystagmogram; MRI = magnetic resonance imaging; NCV = nerve conduction velocity.

▼ **Valsalva maneuver.** The patient should be asked to squat for 30 seconds, and then to stand up and strain against a closed glottis. The examiner should note whether this maneuver provokes symptoms (which would suggest a vasovagal cause, such as syncope or near fainting).

▼ **Rapid deep breathing.** Reproduction of symptoms via rapid deep breathing or within 3 minutes suggests hyperventilation syndrome.

▼ **Nylan-Hallpike maneuver.** The examiner guides the patient's head backward from a seated position so that it is hanging 45° to one side. Vertigo with nystagmus indicates benign positional vertigo.

Laboratory Studies

Laboratory testing is guided by the presenting signs and symptoms. A **complete blood cell count and electrolyte analysis,** including glucose, blood urea nitrogen, and creatinine levels, may be obtained. **Anemia** may cause presyncopal lightheadedness. **Renal failure, hyperglycemia, and hypoglycemia** have also been associated with vertigo.

Diagnostic Modalities

▼ **Magnetic resonance imaging** is indicated if there is prolonged vertigo or additional neurologic signs. One should look for evidence of a tumor or of hemorrhage into the cerebellum, brain stem, or labyrinth.

▼ **Electroencephalography** is indicated when vertigo is associated with alterations of consciousness.

▼ **Audiography** is indicated when there is evidence of hearing loss, ear pain, or tinnitus.

▼ **Electronystagmography** allows one to distinguish central vertigo from peripheral vertigo.

▼ APPROACH TO THE PATIENT (FIGURE 82.1)

Suggested Readings

Adams RD, Victor M: Deafness, dizziness, and disorders of equilibrium. In *Principles of Neurology,* 4th ed. Edited by Adams RD, Victor M. New York, McGraw-Hill, 1989, pp 226–246.

Drachman DA, Hart CW: An approach to the dizzy patient. *Neurology* 22:323–334, 1972.

Drigo P, Carli G, Laverda AM: Benign paroxysmal vertigo of childhood. *Brain Dev* 23(1):38–41, 2001.

Dunn DW: Dizziness: when is it vertigo? *Contemp Pediatr* 67:88, 1987.

Eviatar L, Eviatar A: Vertigo in children: differential diagnosis and treatment. *Pediatrics* 59(6):833–838, 1977.

Fenichel GM: *Clinical Pediatric Neurology—A Signs and Symptoms Approach,* 4th ed. Philadelphia, WB Saunders, 2001, pp 347–351.

Golz A, Netzer A, Angel-Yeger B, et al: Effects of middle ear effusion on the vestibular system in children. *Otolaryngol Head Neck Surg* 119(6):695–699, 1998.

Russell G, Abu-Arafeh I: Paroxysmal vertigo in children—an epidemiological study. *Int J Pediatr Otorhinolaryngol* 49 (suppl 1):S105–107, 1999.

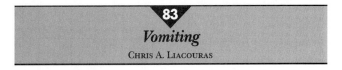

83
Vomiting
CHRIS A. LIACOURAS

▼ INTRODUCTION

Vomiting is the expulsion of stomach contents through the mouth. In children, vomiting is one of the **most common presenting symptoms of upper gastrointestinal disease.** The degree of emesis can vary from forceful, projectile vomiting to effortless regurgitation, to unseen rumination.

▼ DIFFERENTIAL DIAGNOSIS LIST
Infectious Causes

Sepsis
Meningitis
Urinary tract infection
Parasitic infection—giardiasis, ascariasis
Helicobacter pylori gastritis
Otitis media
Gastroenteritis—viral, bacterial
Hepatitis A, B, or C
Bordetella pertussis infection
Pneumonia
Sinusitis
Streptoccocal pharyngitis

Toxic Causes

Drugs—aspirin, ipecac, theophylline, digoxin, opiates, anticonvulsants, barbiturates
Metals—iron, lead
Caustic ingestions
Alcohol

Neoplastic Causes

Intracranial mass lesions

Traumatic Causes

Duodenal hematoma
Pancreatic trauma

Congenital, Anatomic, or Vascular Causes

Esophageal stricture, web, ring, or atresia
Hypertrophic pyloric stenosis
Gastric web or duplication
Duodenal atresia
Malrotation
Intestinal duplication
Hirschsprung disease

Imperforate anus
Superior mesenteric artery syndrome

Metabolic or Genetic Causes

Galactosemia
Fructose intolerance
Hereditary fructose intolerance
Other inborn errors of metabolism—amino acid or organic acid disorders, urea cycle defects, fatty acid oxidation disorders
Diabetes
Adrenal insufficiency

Inflammatory Causes

Cholecystitis or cholelithiasis
Eosinophilic enteritis
Appendicitis
Necrotizing enterocolitis
Peritonitis
Celiac disease
Peptic ulcer
Pancreatitis

Psychosocial Causes

Rumination
Bulimia
Psychogenic vomiting
"Cyclic vomiting" syndrome
Overfeeding

Gastrointestinal Causes

Gastroesophageal reflux disease (GRD)
Eosinophilic esophagitis
Achalasia
Pseudoobstruction
Obstruction—intussusception, volvulus, incarcerated hernia
Foreign body
Gastric and intestinal bezoars

Miscellaneous Causes

Pregnancy
Central nervous system (CNS) disorders—hydrocephalus, pseudotumor cerebri, migraine, motion sickness, seizure
Renal disorders—ureteropelvic junction obstruction, obstructive uropathy, nephrolithiasis, glomerulonephritis, renal tubular acidosis

▼ DIFFERENTIAL DIAGNOSIS DISCUSSION

Helicobacter pylori Infection

In older children and adults, *H. pylori* (a gram-negative, urease-producing bacterium) is the **major cause of gastric and duodenal ulcers.** Although the infection rate increases with age, children are susceptible;

approximately 15% of children undergoing gastric biopsy via endoscopy are infected.

H. pylori appears to promote disease via several mechanisms: production of urease and ammonia, adhesion to the gastric mucosa, and proteolysis of gastric mucus. All of these mechanisms result in disruption of the gastric epithelium.

Clinical Features

Complaints commonly center around **epigastric abdominal pain, vomiting, heartburn,** and **regurgitation.** Hematemesis can also occur.

Evaluation

Currently, **upper endoscopy with biopsy** is the gold standard for the diagnosis of *H. pylori* infection.

Serum antibodies to *H. pylori* can be detected; however, this test carries a poor specificity because previously infected individuals may remain serum antibody positive, despite lacking clinical evidence of gastritis.

A recently developed noninvasive **urea breath test** may supplant the need for upper endoscopy.

Treatment

Many treatment strategies have been reported in the literature, but no single therapy has been shown to be 100% effective in the eradication of *H. pylori.* Currently, the recommended treatment consists of a combination of a **drug to suppress acid production** (e.g., omeprazole), **clarithromycin,** and **either metronidazole or amoxicillin.** In the past, the treatment of choice was a combination of bismuth subsalicylate and antibiotics (amoxicillin and metronidazole).

Gastroesophageal Reflux Disease (GRD)

Etiology

GRD is the movement of stomach contents into the esophagus, past the lower esophageal sphincter. It is commonly caused by a **delay in gastric emptying** or transient **relaxation of the lower esophageal sphincter.**

Clinical Features

Many **newborns manifest inconsequential regurgitation after meals;** this condition typically resolves by 3–6 months of age. In the usual presentation of GRD, frequent small mouthfuls of stomach contents are **regurgitated in an effortless manner.** No active emesis is observed. This phenomenon is frequently referred to as "spitting" or "wet burps." Other symptoms, such as **heartburn, chest or epigastric pain, dysphagia, water brash** (a sour taste in mouth), or **globus** (the sensation that something is stuck in the throat) may be present.

In more **pathologic cases,** GRD is associated with more severe symptoms, such as **recurrent wheezing or coughing, recurrent pneumonia** from aspiration, or **apparent life-threatening episodes** (ALTEs). Many times, concomitant **esophagitis** (manifested as irritability in infants) can occur. In many cases, no obvious spitting is seen, but studies clearly document gastroesophageal reflux.

Recently, an increasing number of children with symptoms of GRD have been identified with **eosinophilic esophagitis** (EE). The presentation of EE is often very similar to GRD; however, these patients fail to respond adequately to antireflux medications. The disease is caused by **food allergy** and is characterized by a severe isolated histologic esophageal eosinophilia despite aggressive acid suppression therapy.

Complications associated with GRD include **hematemesis, aspiration,** and **failure to thrive.**

Evaluation

GRD is primarily a clinical diagnosis, but several diagnostic tests can aid in the evaluation:

▼ The **24-hour pH probe** remains the gold standard for diagnosis.
▼ **Radiographic nuclear scintiscans (milk scans)** provide information regarding gastric emptying.
▼ **Contrast studies (upper gastrointestinal series)** provide information regarding the upper intestinal anatomy.
▼ **Upper endoscopy** is useful in assessing the degree of reflux and the presence of complications (e.g., esophagitis), and for reaching a definitive diagnosis in children.

Treatment

Conservative treatment includes **improved positioning** (upright and prone with head elevated 45°) after eating and while sleeping; feeding infants **thickened food;** and **eliminating spicy foods** and foods containing **caffeine** and **peppermint.**

The mainstay of medical treatment consists of **gastric acid suppression** and the use of **intestinal prokinetic agents** (e.g., metoclopramide). **Acid-blocking medications** (e.g., ranitidine, famotidine) are effective for preventing heartburn and for healing esophagitis. Omeprazole can be used for children with refractory disease. Antacids can be substituted; however, large doses must be given and the duration of action is short.

Achalasia

Etiology

Achalasia is caused by an abnormality in the smooth muscle ganglion cells of the esophagus, which produces incomplete relaxation of the lower esophageal sphincter and poor esophageal motility. The **esophagus can become extremely dilated,** serving as a **reservoir for food,** which can be **vomited hours or days after ingestion.**

Clinical Features

Achalasia rarely develops before the **teenage years** and occurs in fewer than 1 in 10,000 individuals. **Vomiting and dysphagia** are the cardinal symptoms. Patients are typically "slow" eaters and complain of food and liquids "sticking in the throat."

Choking, coughing, gagging, and **aspiration pneumonias** typically occur in **infants** and **young children** with achalasia.

Evaluation

Although the presence of an air-fluid level in the mediastinum on the chest radiograph suggests the diagnosis of achalasia, the diagnosis is usually made using an upper gastrointestinal series or esophageal manometry:

▼ An **upper gastrointestinal series** reveals a dilated esophagus with a narrow, beak-like appearance at the level of the lower esophageal sphincter.

▼ **Esophageal manometry** reveals abnormal function of the esophageal smooth muscle.

Treatment

Balloon dilatation of the lower esophageal sphincter is the usual treatment. Unfortunately, **symptoms often recur** and repeat dilatations are typically necessary. Other treatments include **esophageal myotomy** and the injection of **botulinum toxin** into the distal esophageal mucosal wall.

Hypertrophic Pyloric Stenosis

Etiology

Hypertrophic pyloric stenosis is the most common **congenital abnormality** of children. It is caused by hypertrophy and hyperplasia of the smooth muscle that surrounds the gastric pylorus. The hypertrophy causes the **mucosal** and **submucosal tissue** to **protrude into the pyloric channel.**

Clinical Features

The incidence of pyloric stenosis is approximately 1 in 1000; symptoms usually begin between 4 and 7 weeks of age.

    Progressive, forceful, nonbilious vomiting is the first sign of pyloric stenosis in infants. **Dehydration, weight loss,** and **failure to thrive** can develop. If the diagnosis is not made and the vomiting continues, infants develop a serious hypochloremic **metabolic alkalosis;** an associated **jaundice** occurs in as many as 5% of infants.

Evaluation

Physical examination may reveal a palpable "olive" in the right upper quadrant; however, in most cases, the physical examination is of no benefit. Currently, **abdominal ultrasound** (demonstrating a thickened pyloric channel muscle layer) is the diagnostic test of choice. An upper gastrointestinal series demonstrates an elongated "double-tract" of barium along the pyloric channel.

Treatment

Infants with severe dehydration and alkalosis require **fluid resuscitation.** Once the patient is stabilized, **pyloromyotomy** can be performed to correct the defect.

Malrotation

Etiology

Intestinal malrotation is **failure** of the **fetal midgut to rotate to its normal position.** The associated shortened mesenteric ligament (ligament of Treitz) may result in twisting and torsion of the intestine and its blood supply, resulting in **intestinal obstruction** and **ischemic bowel.**

Clinical Features

Most affected infants present with **signs and symptoms of intestinal obstruction,** including bile-stained emesis, abdominal pain, and borborygmi; however, the symptoms can be delayed for many years.

Older children present with **intermittent vomiting** and **abdominal pain;** rarely, malabsorption and diarrhea are seen.

Evaluation

Radiographic contrast studies of the upper gastrointestinal tract demonstrate the positioning of the ligament of Treitz. Whenever the position of this ligament is in question, contrast should be allowed to flow into the jejunum, ileum, and cecum to define the intestinal rotation.

Treatment

Surgery is indicated to prevent the complications of malrotation, which include small bowel obstruction and midgut volvulus.

Esophageal Atresia

Etiology

Esophageal atresia occurs when the **esophagus ends as a blind tube** as a result of malformation of the tracheoesophageal septum during embryologic development. Although many forms of esophageal atresia can occur, the most common include **proximal esophageal atresia with a distal tracheoesophageal fistula** (more than 80% of patients), **isolated esophageal atresia** (10% of patients), and **pure tracheoesophageal fistula** (fewer than 5% of patients).

Clinical Features

Esophageal atresia is almost always **diagnosed within hours of birth.** Most commonly, the infant **coughs, chokes,** and **vomits** all liquids immediately. Occasionally, **aspiration pneumonia** develops.

Evaluation

The condition can be diagnosed quickly by passing a **nasogastric tube;** if the tube meets resistance at 3–5 inches, esophageal atresia is suspected. A plain **chest radiograph** confirms the presence of a blind esophageal pouch. Pure tracheoesophageal fistulas (H-type) may be missed because the esophagus is intact. **Radiographic contrast studies** can be performed; however, very small amounts of a water-soluble contrast material should be used to prevent pulmonary edema and respiratory distress.

Treatment

Initial conservative therapy includes **upright positioning,** frequent **nasopharyngeal suctioning,** and **intravenous fluids.** The infant should be placed on **NPO status.**

Surgical correction is performed to reconnect the esophagus to the gastric cavity and to repair any associated fistulas. Occasionally, reconnection of the esophagus and stomach is not possible, and **colonic interposition** (i.e., using a portion of colon to connect the distal esophagus to the stomach) is required.

Patients often require long-term **antireflux medical therapy** secondary to poor esophageal motility.

Bezoar

Etiology

Bezoars are accumulations of exogenous matter in the stomach or small intestine. The various types include **trichobezoars** (hair balls), **phytobezoars** (food balls), **lactobezoars** (milk or formula in infants), and **foreign body bezoars.**

✂ HINT Although lactobezoars usually occur in infants, the other types of bezoars most commonly occur in developmentally delayed individuals between the ages of 10 and 19 years. Bezoars are often seen in institutionalized children.

Clinical Features

Children typically present with **vomiting, abdominal distention, pain, severe halitosis,** and **weight loss,** and they may have a history of **pica. Patchy baldness** is often a clue to the presence of a trichobezoar. Commonly, an **abdominal mass** can be palpated in the epigastrium or left upper quadrant.

Evaluation

Plain radiographs and **radiographic contrast studies** may demonstrate the mass; however, **upper endoscopy** is the most useful test because it may be both diagnostic and therapeutic. Children with documented bezoars should be evaluated for **pica, iron deficiency anemia,** and **lead toxicity.**

Treatment

Lactobezoars respond to **withholding oral feeding** for 48 hours. Trichobezoars require **surgical removal.** The removal of all other bezoars may be attempted **endoscopically;** however, in many cases, surgical removal is necessary.

Cholecystitis

Etiology

Cholecystitis, **inflammation of the gallbladder,** is caused by bile stasis within the gallbladder. The causes of bile stasis in children include **cholelithiasis (most common), congenital ductal anomalies, external compression of the bile duct,** and **trauma.**

Clinical Features

Typically, the history reveals **right upper quadrant pain** radiating to the back, **jaundice, rigors,** and **fever. Nausea and vomiting** occur after eating. Symptoms usually develop rapidly; however, the patient may have mild symptoms for several years.

Evaluation

Murphy sign (a palpable tender mass located between the ninth and tenth ribs) can often be appreciated.

Hyperbilirubinemia, an **elevated γ-glutamyl transpeptidase (GGTP) level,** and **leukocytosis** may suggest cholecystitis.

Although **abdominal plain radiographs** can detect the calcified stones, **abdominal ultrasound** is warranted to detect a thickened gallbladder wall, dilated ducts, or an obstructing stone. Occasionally, **cholescintigraphy** is indicated to show abnormal filling of bile into the gallbladder (the administration of cholecystokinin can help reproduce clinical symptoms).

Treatment

Conservative therapy includes hospitalization for the administration of **intravenous fluids** and **antibiotics** (for patients with a high fever or clinical deterioration), and the **cessation of eating.** In some patients with acalculous cholecystitis, conservative therapy is all that is required for the resolution of symptoms; however, in most patients (and all of those with cholelithiasis), the accepted treatment is **cholecystectomy.**

Central Nervous System (CNS) Disorder

Irritation of the brainstem vomiting center by brain tumors, congenital cysts, hydrocephalus, or infections can cause severe vomiting; a **neurologic cause should always be considered in a child with vomiting.**

The vomiting commonly occurs in the **early morning** and is associated with **headaches.** Other signs and symptoms include **changes in the child's personality, fatigue, ataxia, diplopia, nystagmus, papilledema, head tilt,** and **loss of vision.**

Ureteropelvic Junction Obstruction

Etiology

An unusual but important cause of vomiting in children is ureteropelvic junction obstruction, a morphologic **abnormality of** the **ureteropelvic junction** that causes obstruction or restriction of urinary outflow and subsequent hydronephrosis.

Clinical Features

Children frequently present with **right- or left-sided abdominal pain and vomiting.** The pain is often **intermittent,** which makes the diagnosis difficult. Occasionally, patients also have **hematuria** or signs of a **urinary tract infection (UTI).**

Evaluation

Abdominal ultrasound usually permits diagnosis; however, because the kidneys may appear normal between episodes, the ultrasound should be performed when the child is experiencing symptoms. In rare cases, an **intravenous pyelogram** is indicated.

Treatment

Surgical correction is required.

Bulimia

Etiology

A **psychogenic cause** of vomiting should be considered in adolescents, especially adolescent girls, who otherwise appear well and have no other cause for their vomiting.

Clinical Features and Evaluation

A **careful history** should be taken, looking for evidence of **anorexia, bulimia,** or **laxative and ipecac abuse.** Questions should be designed to elicit information regarding diet, eating habits, self-worth, exercise, changes in menses, purging, and medication use. The diagnostic criteria for bulimia include repeated episodes of **binge eating,** regular episodes of **self-induced vomiting,** a persistently **poor self-image** (e.g., of being overweight), and a **lack of control of eating during meals.**

The **nails, teeth, and gums** should be examined for evidence of nutritional inadequacies.

Laboratory studies may reveal electrolyte abnormalities (as a result of persistent vomiting) and provide an overview of the patient's nutritional health (e.g., albumin, calcium, phosphorus, iron stores).

An **electrocardiogram** (ECG) may be abnormal in severely affected patients.

Treatment

The **prevention of acute life-threatening complications** (e.g., dehydration, cardiac abnormalities, electrolyte disturbances) is the primary concern. Patients should be referred to a qualified **psychotherapist** who has expertise in the management of eating disorders.

▼ EVALUATION OF VOMITING

Patient History

The following questions may provide insight into the cause of the vomiting:

▼ **Does the patient have a fever?** Fever implies infection.
▼ **Does the patient have a history of pica?** Pica implies bezoar.
▼ **Does the patient complain of heartburn, globus, water brash, or epigastric pain related to meals?** Think GRD and esophagitis.
▼ **If the child is an infant, does he have an unusual odor?** Unusual odors may be a sign of a metabolic disorder.
▼ **When does the vomiting occur?** Frequent vomiting in the morning can be a sign of pregnancy or a neurologic disorder.
▼ **How old is the patient?** Some causes of vomiting are more prevalent in certain age groups (Table 83.1).
▼ **Is the vomitus bilious or bloody?** Bile-stained vomitus points to an anatomic problem (e.g., intestinal volvulus, intussusception, incarcerated hernia).

Physical Examination

The following should be noted during physical examination:

▼ **Head and neck**—abnormal teeth, reflux, bulging fontanelle, hydrocephalus
▼ **Abdomen**—right upper quadrant mass, signs of gallbladder disease, epigastric pain (suggests pancreatitis, gastritis, or esophagitis), right upper quadrant pain (suggests liver disease), borborygmi (suggests possible intestinal obstruction)
▼ **Rectum**—heme-positive stools (suggest mucosal disease)

TABLE 83.1. Common Causes of Vomiting by Age	
Infant	Anatomic obstruction, metabolic disorder, infection, GRD, overfeeding, bezoar
Toddler	Infection, medication, GRD, intussusception, foreign body, bezoar, malrotation
Child	GRD, cyclic vomiting, malrotation, infection
Adolescent	Pregnancy, bulimia, infection, ulcer, malrotation, celiac disease, pseudoobstruction, drug abuse, pancreatitis, GRD, cyclic vomiting

GRD = gastroesophageal reflux disease.

▼ **Neurologic examination**—cranial nerve abnormalities, gait abnormalities (suggest CNS disease)

Laboratory Studies

The following studies may be appropriate:

▼ **Complete blood count (CBC) with differential**—eosinophilia suggests eosinophilic enteritis or allergic disease

▼ **Erythrocyte sedimentation rate (ESR)**—an abnormal ESR suggests inflammation, possibly of the intestine

▼ **Chemistry panel**—increased alanine aminotransferase (ALT), γ-glutamyl transpeptidase (GGT), or bilirubin levels suggest gallbladder or liver disease

▼ **Amylase and lipase levels**—increased amylase or decreased pancreatic lipase levels suggest pancreatitis

▼ **Antiendomysial, antigliadin, and antibody levels**—elevation suggests celiac disease

▼ **Stool sample**—occult blood suggests intestinal mucosal disease

Diagnostic Modalities

The following diagnostic modalities may be appropriate:

▼ **Contrast radiographic studies** are integral in the diagnosis of intestinal anatomic abnormalities.

▼ **Endoscopy** may be the most important tool for the definitive diagnosis of many esophageal, gastric, and duodenal disorders.

▼ A **barium enema** identifies distal obstructions.

▼ **Abdominal ultrasound** is useful in the evaluation of liver and gallbladder disorders, pyloric stenosis, pancreatitis, and kidney disease.

▼ An **abdominal computed tomography (CT) scan** defines the anatomy of the abdominal cavity (when used with both enteral and intravenous contrast). In most patients, CT provides a more specific image than does ultrasound.

Suggested Readings

Henretig FM: Vomiting. In *Pediatric Emergency Medicine*, 3rd ed. Edited by Fleisher GR, Ludwig S. Baltimore, Williams & Wilkins, 1993, pp 506–513.

Nelson WE, Behrman RE, Kliegman RM: *Textbook of Pediatrics*, 14th ed. Philadelphia, WB Saunders, 1992.

Polin RA, Ditmar MF: *Pediatric Secrets*, 2nd ed. Philadelphia, Hanley & Belfus, 1997.

Silverman A, Roy CC: *Pediatric Clinical Gastroenterology*, 3rd ed. St Louis, Mosby, 1983.

Treem WR: *Gastrointestinal bleeding in children*. *Gastrointest Endosc* 4:75, 1994.

Walker WA, Durie PR, Hamilton JR, et al: *Pediatric Gastrointestinal Disease*, 2nd ed. Philadelphia, BC Decker, 1996.

Wyllie R, Hyams JS: *Pediatric Gastrointestinal Disease*. Philadelphia, WB Saunders, 1993.

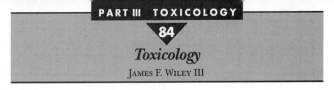

Toxicology

JAMES F. WILEY III

▼ GASTRIC DECONTAMINATION

Administration of **activated charcoal** is the preferred method of gastric decontamination. **Gastric lavage** and **syrup of ipecac** play a much lesser role in the management of the poisoned patient but may still be of benefit in selected patients.

Activated Charcoal

Indications and Contraindications

Activated charcoal is indicated for all ingestions unless specifically contraindicated. **Contraindications** include the following:

- ▼ Compromised, unprotected airway (aspiration risk)
- ▼ Gastrointestinal bleeding or perforation
- ▼ Caustic ingestions (charcoal impedes endoscopic visualization)
- ▼ Aliphatic hydrocarbon ingestion (may promote vomiting and aspiration)

HINT Not all substances bind to activated charcoal (Table 84.1).

Administration

The **dose is 1 g/kg, up to 100 g total** of activated charcoal, alone in **children < 6 years** or **premixed with 1 g/kg of 35% sorbitol in older patients.** Mixing the charcoal with **flavored syrups** and putting it in a covered cup with a straw facilitates oral administration. **Nasogastric intubation** is required in patients with altered mental status and in alert but uncooperative patients.

Complications

Complications of activated charcoal use include **vomiting** and **aspiration, constipation or obstipation, desorption of poison** from charcoal and **late absorption** in patients with delayed gastrointestinal motility (e.g., those taking drugs with anticholinergic properties). **Death** has occurred in a child who aspirated activated charcoal mixed with a magnesium cathartic.

Whole Bowel Irrigation

Whole bowel irrigation involves **copious irrigation of the gastrointestinal tract,** via nasogastric tube, to force the poisons rapidly through the bowel before significant absorption can occur. The solution used, polyethylene glycol 3500 MW iso-osmotic bowel solution **(GoLYTELY),** causes no significant fluid or electrolyte loss in the gut.

Indications and Contraindications

Potential indications, to date, have been limited to **agents that do not adsorb well to charcoal** or that have the potential for absorption distally in the gastrointestinal tract, such as **iron, heavy metals, lithium,** and **sustained-release products** (e.g., many antiarrhythmics, theophylline). Other drugs may be amenable to whole bowel irrigation as an adjunct to activated charcoal administration. In addition, whole bowel irrigation is used to **treat body packers**

TABLE 84.1. Agents with Limited or Uncertain Binding to Activated Charcoal

Iron	Caustics*
Lithium	NaOH
Heavy metals	KOH
Arsenic	HCl
Mercury	H_2SO_4
Lead	Low-molecular-weight compounds
Thallium	Cyanide
Alcohols	Pesticides
Methanol	Organophosphates
Ethanol	Carbamates
Isopropanol	
Ethylene glycol	
Hydrocarbons	
Kerosene	
Gasoline	
Mineral seal oil	

* Administration of activated charcoal may also impede further management.

(people who ingest large numbers of packets of cocaine or heroin wrapped in latex condoms). Whole bowel irrigation is **contraindicated in patients with evidence of ileus or bowel perforation.**

Administration

GoLYTELY is administered at a dose of **500 ml/hr in young children** and at a dose of **up to 2 L/hr in adolescents and adults,** usually via nasogastric tube. The **endpoint** for stopping whole bowel irrigation is a **clear rectal effluent** and **recovery from poisoning.**

Complications

The major complications reported from whole bowel irrigation are **vomiting** and **abdominal pain.**

Gastric Lavage

Gastric lavage removes 10%–25% of ingested toxin when performed within 30–60 minutes of ingestion.

Indications and Contraindications

Gastric lavage may **not be useful more than 1 hour after ingestion** unless the ingested poison delays gastric emptying. It has been shown to improve outcome in patients who are comatose and receive gastric lavage **within 60 minutes.** In other patients, the potential risks of gastric lavage must be weighed heavily against its benefit.

Gastric lavage should be reserved for the **critically ill poisoning patient** or a patient who is likely to undergo rapid decompensation. In addition, **patients who ingest large amounts of a strong acid** (e.g., toilet bowl cleaner) should receive gastric lavage via a small, flexible nasogastric tube. **Patients who ingest liquid medicines** may benefit from nasogastric lavage if it is performed within 30–60 minutes.

Gastric lavage **should not be performed in patients with airway compromise before endotracheal intubation.** Other **contraindications** include the ingestion of caustic alkaline substances or small amounts of **acids or hydro-carbons, abnormal esophageal anatomy,** and **bleeding diatheses.**

Administration

Gastric lavage requires the placement of a **large-bore** (24–36 French) **orogastric tube** followed by **repeated infusion and withdrawal** of room temperature **normal saline** in 50- to 200-ml aliquots. Before lavage, one must **ensure a protected airway:** position the patient on the left side with the head below the feet, and determine correct gastric tube position.

Complications

Complications include **vomiting** with pulmonary aspiration, **gastric or esophageal perforation, hypopharyngeal and airway trauma with bleeding, laryngospasm,** and **accidental tracheal intubation** with inadvertent pulmonary lavage.

Syrup of Ipecac

Syrup of ipecac, derived from the ipecacuanha plant, causes vomiting by **direct gastric irritation** and through a direct central effect at the chemotactic trigger zone in the medulla. Up to 93% of patients who receive ipecac vomit within 30–60 minutes.

Indications and Contraindications

Indications are now limited to **ingestion of toxic plant material** and to **home decontamination** on the advice of a physician or poison control specialist.

Contraindications consist of **altered mental status** (lethargy, coma, seizures—either existing or impending) and ingestion of **caustic substances, aliphatic hydrocarbons,** or **drugs with a high likelihood of rapid serious effects** (e.g., cyclic antidepressants, antiarrhythmics, clonidine, isoniazid, lithium, alcohol). In addition, **patients who have already spontaneously vomited** will not receive any further benefit from syrup of ipecac administration.

Administration

Dose is based on age: for children age **6 months–1 year,** give **10 ml** (2 teaspoons); **1–12 years, 15 ml** (1 tablespoon); and **older than 12 years, 30 ml** (2 tablespoons). Give the **child 10 ml/kg of water,** up to 240 ml (8 ounces), after administering the syrup of ipecac. Repeat the dose if no vomiting occurs within 30 minutes.

Complications

Complications include **excessive vomiting, Mallory-Weiss tears, pneumomediastinum,** and **delayed delivery** of activated charcoal. Chronic use of syrup of ipecac or inadvertent administration of the much more concentrated extract of ipecac has caused myocardial and neuromuscular toxicity.

Cathartics

Indications and Contraindications

Cathartics have **no demonstrated efficacy** in poisoning treatment. Coadministration of cathartic with activated charcoal in patients over 12 years of age may prevent obstipation. Cathartics are **contraindicated** in patients with **bowel perforation, ileus,** or **diarrhea.**

Administration

Cathartics should only be given as a **single dose** when administered with activated charcoal; **multiple doses** of cathartics should be **avoided except as outlined in the section on elimination enhancement.** Sorbitol 35% is the preferred agent because it has a rapid onset of catharsis. The **dose of sorbitol 35% is 1 g/kg** (3 ml/kg).

Complications

Complications include **electrolyte imbalance** and **dehydration.** Sorbitol also increases the likelihood of **vomiting** when given with activated charcoal. **Death** has occurred in several patients who received 4–6 doses of sorbitol over 24 hours.

▼ ELIMINATION ENHANCEMENT

Extracorporeal clearance of toxin can be achieved by administering multiple-dose activated charcoal, or by alkaline diuresis, hemodialysis, or charcoal hemoperfusion.

Multiple-Dose Activated Charcoal

Multiple doses of activated charcoal **increase the clearance of theophylline, carbamazepine, phenytoin, phenobarbital,** and some **cyclic antidepressants.** The dose is **1 g/kg with cathartic initially, followed by 0.5–1 g/kg of activated charcoal without cathartic every 4 hours** until the patient has nontoxic blood levels, has shown clinical improvement, and has passed charcoal-laden stool.

Alkaline Diuresis

Alkaline diuresis can **enhance the excretion of weak acids,** especially **salicylates** and **phenobarbital** (but not other barbiturates). This procedure promotes conversion of these drugs to their ionized form within the proximal renal tubule and prevents distal tubular resorption (ion trapping). **Sodium bicarbonate** is given **intravenously** until a urine pH of greater than 7.0 is achieved. Care must be taken to **avoid fluid overload, hypernatremia, hypokalemia, hypocalcemia,** and **hypomagnesemia** during alkaline diuresis.

Hemodialysis

Hemodialysis can **remove toxins with low molecular weight** (200 daltons), **low plasma protein binding,** and **low tissue binding** as expressed by the volume of distribution:

$$Vd \ (L/kg) = \text{Dose absorbed } (mg/kg) / \text{Plasma concentration } (mg/L)$$

Hemodialysis is most effective for drugs with a Vd of less than 1 L/kg (Table 84.2).

Charcoal Hemoperfusion

Charcoal hemoperfusion **diverts the patient's circulation** through a filter where the toxin binds to an activated charcoal cartridge. Charcoal hemoperfusion is technically more difficult and less available than hemodialysis. Table 84.3 summarizes toxins removed by charcoal hemoperfusion.

✄ HINT Fewer than 1% of all pediatric poisoning patients require hemodialysis or charcoal hemoperfusion.

TABLE 84.2.   Toxins Removed by Hemodialysis

Toxin	Measured Level Suggestive of Need for Hemodialysis*
Acetaminophen	> 100 μg/ml in conjunction with antidote
Arsenic	Only with coexistent renal failure
Bromide	> 150 mg/dl and severe symptoms
Chloral hydrate	250 mg/L
Ethanol	500 mg/dl
Ethylene glycol**	25 mg/dl
Isopropanol	400 mg/dl
Lithium	4 mEq/L in acute overdose
	As needed for severe symptoms in chronic overdose
Methanol	25 mg/dl
Salicylates	100–120 mg/dl in acute overdose
	60–800 mg/dl in chronic overdose

* The decision to perform hemodialysis should be based on physical findings as well as drug levels. A repeat measure should be obtained when the drug level is elevated to ensure that a laboratory error has not occurred. In addition, units of measurement should be checked before instituting hemodialysis.

** Administration of fomepizole may allow for management of higher levels of ethylene glycol without hemodialysis.

▼ APPROACH TO THE POISONED PATIENT
Stabilization

Airway, breathing, circulation, and disability (ABCD) must be assessed in order, and compromise in any of these areas requires prompt attention. Complete exposure of the patient occurs as part of the rapid assessment. **Vital**

TABLE 84.3.   Toxins Removed by Charcoal Hemoperfusion

Toxin	Measured Level Suggestive of Need for Charcoal Hemoperfusion*
Amitriptyline	Based on signs and symptoms
Chloral hydrate	250 mg/dl
Digitoxin	50 ng/ml with antidotal therapy
Digoxin	15 ng/ml with antidotal therapy
Ethchlorvynol	150 μg/ml
Glutethimide	40 mg/L
Methaqualone	40 μg/ml
Nortriptyline	Based on signs and symptoms
Pentobarbital	50 mg/L
Phenobarbital	100 mg/L
Theophylline**	100 μg/ml in acute overdose
	60 μg/ml in chronic overdose

* The decision to perform hemoperfusion should be based on physical findings as well as drug levels. A repeat measure should be obtained when the drug level is elevated to ensure that a laboratory error has not occurred. In addition, units of measurement should be checked before instituting hemodialysis.

** Hemodialysis may also be employed for serious theophylline poisoning.

signs, including a **rectal temperature,** and **continuous monitoring of the heart rate, respiratory rate,** and **blood pressure** should be initiated. **Supplemental oxygen** in an inspired concentration of 100% should be administered.

Administration of Substrates and Antidotes

Dextrose and Thiamine

The **glucose level** should be determined in any poisoned child with a depressed level of consciousness, using a rapid reagent strip. Hypoglycemia suggests certain ingestants (Table 84.4) and requires correction with **0.5–1 g/kg dextrose** administered as an **intravenous bolus followed by a 6–8 mg/kg/min dextrose infusion. Thiamine (100 mg** intramuscularly or intravenously) should precede dextrose infusion in a patient who is suspected to be **alcoholic.**

▨ HINT Hypoglycemia is the one metabolic abnormality that can cause focal neurologic findings.

Naloxone

Naloxone (**2 mg** intravenously, intramuscularly, or via endotracheal tube) **reverses coma caused by opiates.** It may also help some patients who have ingested clonidine. It should be given to **any child** with a **depressed level of consciousness** because it has **few adverse effects** in this setting and may prevent the need for aggressive intervention, such as endotracheal intubation. Response to naloxone occurs within 1–2 minutes of administration. After 30 minutes, the naloxone has worn off and resedation may occur. **Repeated naloxone administration or continuous intravenous naloxone infusion** is often required to prevent further depressed mental status.

▨ HINT Children who have ingested codeine, dextromethorphan, propoxyphene, pentazocine, butorphanol, synthetic fentanyl derivatives, LAAM (long-acting acetyl morphine) or methadone may require up to 10 mg of naloxone to fully reverse the narcotic effects.

Flumazenil

Flumazenil is a benzodiazepine antagonist that has **reversed lethargy and coma** in adult benzodiazepine overdose patients. Flumazenil **may cause seizures** in a patient who has also ingested cyclic antidepressants or in a patient with a seizure disorder controlled by benzodiazepines, and it **may cause cardiac arrhythmias** in a poisoned patient who has also ingested chloral hydrate. Other side effects include **vomiting** and **anxiety.** Flumazenil

---

TABLE 84.4. Agents Causing Hypoglycemia in Overdosed Children

Ethanol
Salicylates
Oral hypoglycemic agents
Propranolol
Insulin

administration **may help differentiate benzodiazepine overdose from other causes of coma** in children.

Given its potential risks, flumazenil should **only be given to children with severe symptoms** of benzodiazepine ingestion and **only if no signs of significant cyclic antidepressant overdose** are present and **only if the patient does not have a seizure disorder.** The currently recommended dose is **0.01 mg/kg over 1 minute up to 0.5 mg per dose** and a **total maximum** amount of drug administered of **1 mg.** Response occurs within 1 minute in most cases. Resedation may occur.

Physostigmine

Physostigmine, a cholinesterase inhibitor, **reverses the central anticholinergic effects of severe agitation and seizures** caused by **antihistamines** (e.g., diphenhydramine, doxylamine, scopolamine), **certain plants** (jimson weed, deadly nightshade, henbane), **antiparkinsonian medications, dilating eyedrops, and skeletal muscle relaxants.** Physostigmine administration has **preceded asystole and death in patients who ingested cyclic antidepressants** and should be **avoided in these patients and in patients with asthma, gastrointestinal obstruction, or genitourinary obstruction.** The dose of physostigmine for children is **0.5–1 mg,** given **intravenously,** slowly over 5 minutes, with **atropine immediately available** for administration should **cholinergic symptoms** develop. Response to physostigmine occurs within minutes, and beneficial effects may persist longer than expected based on physostigmine's half-life of 60 minutes.

> ▨ **HINT** Given the risks of physostigmine, it should be **reserved for patients with a clear central anticholinergic syndrome who display hyperthermia, seizures, or severe agitation** and only if there is no evidence of cyclic antidepressant toxicity.

Pyridoxine (Vitamin B₆)

Pyridoxine **stops seizures caused by ingestion of isoniazid** by reversing γ-aminobutyric acid (GABA) depletion. The dose is **3–5 g** or the **equivalent dose of isoniazid** ingested. This dose is much larger than the therapeutic dose and requires the administration of multiple vials of pyridoxine.

> ▨ **HINT** If you anticipate that it will be necessary to reverse seizures from an isoniazid ingestion, call the pharmacy and inform them so that they can obtain an adequate supply of pyridoxine.

Antidotes

Table 84.5 lists the most commonly used antidotes. Those who are unfamiliar with the use of antidotes should consult with a regional poison control center or medical toxicologist before attempting administration.

> ▨ **HINT** Antidotes help in approximately 3% of poisonings.

Decontamination

Gastric decontamination should be carried out as described in the previous section. External decontamination of the patient requires **removal of any**

TABLE 84.5. Common Poisons and Antidotes

Poison	Antidote	Administration
Acetaminophen	N-Acetylcysteine	Loading dose 140 mg/kg, then 17 doses at 70 mg/kg/dose. Dilute 20% solution to 5%–10% with juice or soda to improve palatability.
Anticholinergics	Physostigmine	See text
Benzodiazepines	Flumazenil	See text
β-Adrenergic antagonists	Glucagon	See text
Calcium channel blockers	Glucagon Calcium gluconate 10%	0.3–0.6 ml/kg (8–16 mEq calcium/kg)
Carbon monoxide	Hyperbaric oxygen Sodium thiosulfate 25%*	See Cyanide
Cyanide	Sodium nitrate 3%	Dose depends on hemoglobin (see cyanide antidote kit package insert). Do not exceed recommended dosage. Do not give to patients suffering from concomitant carbon monoxide exposure.
	Sodium thiosulfate 25%	Dose depends on hemoglobin (see cyanide antidote kit package insert).
Digitalis	Digitalis Fab fragments	Calculate dose based on level or dose ingested or 10 vials if acute overdose, 5 vials if chronic overdose.
Ethylene glycol	Ethanol	0.6 g/kg load over 1 hour followed by 100 mg/kg/hr infusion
	OR	
	Fomepizole	15 mg/kg loading dose, then 10 mg/kg every 12 hours for 4 doses followed by 15 mg/kg every 12 hours until ethylene glycol level < 25 mg/dL. Give fomepizole every 4 hours during hemodialysis.
	Pyridoxine	2 mg/kg Thiamine 0.5 mg/kg
Methanol	Ethanol as for ethylene glycol	50–100 mg over 6 hours
	OR	
	Fomepizole as for ethylene glycol	
	Folate	
Iron	Deferoxamine	5–15 mg/kg/hr IV infusion
Isoniazid	Pyridoxine	3–5 gm IV or dose equal to grams of isoniazid ingested

Continued

TABLE 84.5. Common Poisons and Antidotes (continued)

Poison	Antidote	Administration
Lead	Lead level 45–69 μg/dl	
	Dimercaptosuccinic acid	10 mg/kg PO three times daily for 5 days, then twice daily for 14 days (may be useful at lower levels)
	Or	
	Calcium NaEDTA	50–75 mg/kg/day divided, every 6 hours either IM or by slow IV infusion (IV use not FDA approved)
	Lead level ≥ 70 μg/dl	
	Calcium NaEDTA	Administer as described above
	And	
	British antilewisite (BAL)	3–5 mg/kg IM every 4 hours for 5 days
	d-Penicillamine	10 mg/kg/day for 1 week increasing to 30 mg/kg/day as tolerated, only if unacceptable adverse reactions to dimercaptosuccinic acid or calcium NaEDTA
Methemoglobinemia	Methylene blue 1%	1–2 mg/kg (0.1–0.2 ml/kg)
Opiates	Naloxone	2 mg IV, ETT, IM, repeat as needed
Organophosphates	Atropine	0.1–0.5 mg/kg initial dose with additional doses as needed to counteract bronchorrhea
	Pralidoxime	25–50 mg/kg (up to 1 g); for severe cases, consider 10–15 mg/kg/hr infusion
Phenothiazines (dystonia)	Diphenhydramine	1–2 mg/kg IM or IV
	Benztropine	1–2 mg/kg IM or IV

ETT = endotracheal tube; FDA = Food and Drug Administration; IM = intramuscularly; IV = intravenously; NaEDTA = sodium ethylenediaminetetraacetic acid; PO = orally.

* Consider for possible cyanide inhalation if the patient suffers from smoke inhalation.

clothing and **copious irrigation** of the skin and eyes with room-temperature, normal saline solution.

✄ HINT   External decontamination of some poisoned patients (e.g., those who have ingested pesticide) may place health care providers at risk. Universal precautions should be used.

Supportive Care

The patient's clinical course is altered by administration of specific antidotes in only 3% of toxic exposures. **Good outcome** for the remainder of patients

TABLE 84.6. Common Toxidromes in Children

Agent		Toxidrome
Opiates	VS:	Hypothermia, bradypnea, bradycardia, hypotension
	CNS:	Flaccid coma
	Pupils:	Miotic to pinpoint
	Other:	Extraocular paralysis, delayed GI motility
Sedatives	VS:	Hypothermia, bradypnea, bradycardia, hypotension
	CNS:	Coma, often prolonged or cyclical; nystagmus
	Pupils:	Miotic (early barbiturate)
		Dilated (late barbiturate, glutethimide)
	Other:	Delayed GI motility
Ethanol	VS:	Hypothermia, bradypnea, bradycardia
	CNS:	Coma, nystagmus
	Pupils:	Miotic
	Skin:	Flushed
	Odor:	Sickly sweet breath odor
	Other:	Hypoglycemia, increased osmolal gap
Anticholinergic agents	VS:	Hyperthermia, tachycardia, hypertension
	CNS:	Agitation, delirium, seizures
	Pupils:	Mydriatic
	Skin:	Flushed, dry, warm
	Other:	Decreased GI motility, urine retention, cardiac tachyarrhythmias
Sympathomimetic agents	VS:	Hyperthermia, tachycardia, hypertension (bradycardia if pure α-adrenergic)
	CNS:	Agitation, delirium, seizures
	Pupils:	Mydriatic
	Skin:	Diaphoretic, cool and clammy
	Other:	Increased GI motility, piloerection
Cholinergic agents	VS:	Bradycardia or tachycardia, hypotension, tachypnea with bronchospasm
	CNS:	Coma, seizures
	Pupils:	Miotic
	Skin:	Diaphoretic
	Other:	Muscle fasciculation, weakness, paralysis, salivation, lacrimation, vomiting, urinary and fecal incontinence
Serotonin syndrome	VS:	Hyperpyrexia, tachycardia, hypertension
	CNS:	Agitation, coma
	Pupils:	Mydriatic
	Skin:	Diaphoretic
	Other:	Lower extremity rigidity, myoclonus, hyperreflexia

Toxidromes represent a collection of clinical findings often associated with poisoning by a specific class of drugs. However, a poisoned child may not display all physical findings commonly associated with a specific drug or may have findings not usually associated with a specific drug. Toxidromes by themselves cannot be used to exclude or confirm ingestion of a particular drug.

CNS = central nervous system; GI = gastrointestinal; VS = vascular system. (Adapted from Henretig FM, Shannon M: Toxicologic Emergencies. In *Textbook of Pediatric Emergency Medicine,* 3rd ed. Baltimore, Williams & Wilkins, 1993, p 750 and Mofenson HC, Greensher J: The unknown poison. *Pediatrics* 54: 446, 1974.)

depends on adherence to **general principles of toxicology** and good general medical care, primarily **rapid assessment and intervention** to maintain **airway, breathing, and evaluation.**

⚄ HINT Institution of supportive care is most important to the successful resuscitation of the poisoned patient.

Identification of the Toxin

Presumptive Diagnosis

Presumptive diagnosis of the type of agent causing poison symptoms can **guide treatment until** a **definitive diagnosis** is made. Many times the exact toxin is known from the outset by the history. However, with very ill children, the first history is often not the best, and one must **look for specific clues** on physical examination. **Combinations of physical findings ("toxidromes") indicate specific classes of drugs** with effects on vital signs, pupillary response, neurologic status, breath and body odors, and skin changes (Tables 84.6 and 84.7). Tables 84.8 through 84.14 list representative poisons by clinical effect.

TABLE 84.7. Common Causes of Toxidromes in Children

Opiates
  Cough syrups (dextromethorphan)
  Codeine
  Propoxyphene
  Methadone (child of a heroin addict)
Sedatives
  Benzodiazepines
  Barbiturates
  Glutethimide
  Meprobamate
Anticholinergic agents
  Antihistamines
  Antidepressant drugs*
  Antipsychotic drugs*
  Plants (jimsonweed, *Amanita muscaria* mushrooms, henbane, *Atropa belladonna*)
  Skeletal muscle relaxants (cyclobenzaprine)
Sympathomimetic agents
  Decongestants (pure α-adrenergic drugs)
  Cocaine
  Amphetamines
Cholinergic agents
  Pesticides (organophosphate, carbamate)
  Mushrooms
Serotonin syndrome
  Serotonin specific reuptake inhibitors
  Monoamine oxidase inhibitors

---

* Drug effects may not be primarily anticholinergic.

TABLE 84.8. Poisons Causing Respiratory Depression or Apnea

Antipsychotic agents
Carbamate pesticides
Chlorinated hydrocarbons
  Trichloroethylene
  1,1,1 trichloroethane
Clonidine
Coral snake envenomation
Cyclic antidepressants
Ethanol (especially when combined with sedative/hypnotics)
Exotic snake envenomation
  Cobras
  Sea snakes
  Mambas
Mojave rattlesnake envenomation
Narcotics
Nicotine
Organophosphate pesticides
Sedative/hypnotics

✄ HINT The history and physical examination can provide valuable clues to the possible ingestant even when the patient does not display all the components of a toxidrome.

Bedside Tests

Bedside tests give additional information as to the poison ingested but **require definitive laboratory studies** for confirmation. **Rapid glucose reagent stick** detects the presence of hypoglycemia (see Table 84.4 for a list of the common toxic causes of hypoglycemia in children).

TABLE 84.9. Poisons Causing Tachycardia

Tachycardia and hypertension
  Amphetamines
  Antihistamines
  Cocaine
  LSD/PCP
Tachycardia and hypotension
  β_2-adrenergic agonists
  Albuterol
  Terbutaline
  Carbon monoxide
  Cyclic antidepressants
  Hydralazine
  Iron
  Phenothiazines
  Theophylline
  Any agent causing vomiting, diarrhea, or hemorrhage

LSD = lysergic acid diethylamide; PCP = phencyclidine hydrochloride.

TABLE 84.10. Poisons Causing Bradycardia

Bradycardia and hypertension
  α-Adrenergic agonists
    Phenylpropanolamine
    Ephedrine
  Clonidine
  Ergotamine
Bradycardia and hypotension
  $α_1$-Adrenergic antagonists
    Phentolamine
    Prazosin
  $α_1$-Adrenergic agonists
    Clonidine
    Tetrahydrozoline
  β-Adrenergic antagonists
    Propranolol
    Atenolol
    Metoprolol
  Calcium channel blockers
  Digitalis-containing drugs and plants
  Narcotics
  Organophosphate pesticides
  Sedatives/hypnotics

▼ **Ferric chloride 10%** (2–3 drops) turns 1 ml of urine purple in the presence of salicylates. Positive results require a quantitative serum salicylate level.

▼ The **ketone square on the urine dipstick** turns purple in the presence of acetoacetic acid (nitroprusside reaction). Urinary ketones are commonly seen after ingestion of salicylates and isopropanol.

▼ A **chocolate brown or persistent dark color of venous blood** that is exposed to air on a piece of filter paper suggests methemoglobinemia.

Laboratory Studies

Initial studies in symptomatic poisoned patients include **arterial blood gases, electrolytes** with calculation of the anion gap (Table 84.14), **serum glucose, blood urea nitrogen (BUN) and creatinine levels,** and **serum osmolarity** by the freezing point depression method with calculation of the osmolar gap:

$$\text{Osmolar gap} = \text{Measured osmolarity} \\ - [(2 \times \text{Na}) + \text{BUN}/2.8 + \text{Glucose}/18]$$

Normally, the osmolar gap is < 10 mOsm. An **elevated osmolar gap suggests** the presence of **alcohols** (e.g., ethanol, methanol, isopropanol, ethylene glycol).

✄ HINT A normal osmolar gap does not rule out the potential for serious ethylene glycol poisoning.

TABLE 84.11. Poisons Causing Cardiac Arrhythmias

Atrioventricular block
  Astemizole
  β-Adrenergic antagonists
  Calcium channel blockers
  Clonidine
  Cyclic antidepressants
  Digitalis-containing drugs and plants
Ventricular tachycardia
  Amphetamines
  Carbamazepine
  Chloral hydrate
  Chlorinated hydrocarbons
  Cocaine
  Cyclic antidepressants
  Digitalis-containing drugs or plants
  Phenothiazines (especially thioridazine)
  Theophylline
  Type Ia antiarrhythmic agents
    Quinidine
    Procainamide
  Type Ic antiarrhythmic agents
    Flecainide
    Encainide
Torsades de pointes (multifocal ventricular tachycardia)
  Amantadine
  Cyclic antidepressants
  Lithium
  Nonsedating antihistamines
    Astemizole
    Terfenadine
  Quinidine
  Phenothiazines
  Sotalol

A **discrepancy between cooximetry** (the direct measure of oxygen saturation) **and calculated oxygen saturation** (oxygen saturation reported on an unspecified arterial blood gas analysis) **suggests** the presence of abnormal hemoglobins, most commonly **carboxyhemoglobin or methemoglobin.**

Specific drug levels are useful when the poison shows a dose-dependent toxicity, when treatment with an antidote is contemplated, or when a specific intervention, such as extracorporeal removal, is helpful (Table 84.15).

The **comprehensive drug screen ("tox screen") has limited usefulness** in the management of the poisoned child (Table 84.16). **False-positive** and **false-negative drug screens** can lead to misinterpretation of the patient's signs and symptoms. **Toxicologic screening may be warranted to confirm the diagnosis of poisoning** as opposed to other conditions such as central nervous system (CNS) infection or trauma, **or if intentional ingestion or child abuse is suspected.**

TABLE 84.12. Poisons Causing Coma

Coma with miosis
   Barbiturates and other sedatives/hypnotics
   Bromide
   Chloral hydrate
   Clonidine
   Ethanol
   Narcotics
   Organophosphates
   PCP
   Phenothiazines
   Tetrahydrozoline
Coma with mydriasis
   Atropine/diphenoxylate
   Carbon monoxide
   Cyanide
   Cyclic antidepressants
   Glutethimide
   LSD

LSD = lysergic acid diethylamide; PCP = phencyclidine hydrochloride.

TABLE 84.13. Poisons Causing Seizures

Amoxapine
Amphetamines
Anticonvulsants
   Phenytoin
   Carbamazepine
Antihistamines and anticholinergic drugs or plants
Camphor
Carbon monoxide
Chlorinated hydrocarbons
Cocaine
Cyanide
Cyclic antidepressants
Isoniazid
Lead
Lidocaine
Meperidine
PCP
Phenothiazines
Phenylpropanolamine
Propoxyphene
Propranolol
Theophylline

PCP = phencyclidine hydrochloride.

TABLE 84.14. Poisons Causing an Abnormal Anion Gap

Increased anion gap with metabolic acidosis
  Carbon monoxide*
  Cyanide
  Ethanol*
  Ethylene glycol*
  Iron*
  Isoniazid
  Methanol*
  Salicylates*
  Theophylline*
Decreased anion gap
  Bromide.
  Lithium*
  Hypermagnesemia*
  Hypercalcemia*

Anion gap $= Na^+ - (Cl^- + CO_2^-)$

* Specific levels rapidly available.

▓ **HINT** Results of comprehensive drug screens typically take 6–24 hours and rarely change immediate management of the patient.

▓ **HINT** Testing in the poisoned patient should progress from less specific to more specific, with emphasis on clearly identifying the presence of toxins that require antidotes or other specific procedures to prevent morbidity or mortality.

Diagnostic Modalities

A 12-lead electrocardiogram (ECG) is an important adjunct in identifying seriously poisoned children. Strict attention should be paid to rhythm, QRS interval, and QT interval. Prolongation of the QRS interval (i.e., longer than 0.10 msec) or the QT interval indicates an increased risk of ventricular arrhythmias.

▼ **An abdominal radiograph** allows detection of some toxic agents (e.g., iron, calcium salts, potassium salts, heavy metals, chlorinated hydrocarbons).

▓ **HINT** The absence of radiopaque pills or fragments does not rule out the possibility of ingestion if the film is taken after the substance (e.g., iron) has been absorbed.

▼ **Ultrasound of the stomach** can detect the presence of pills and could be helpful for determining the usefulness of gastric emptying in selected patients. However, ultrasound is currently not available in many hospitals on an emergency basis for this indication.

TABLE 84.15. Helpful Specific Drug Levels

Drug	Time to Peak Blood Level (Hours Postingestion)	Potential Intervention
Acetaminophen	4	N-Acetylcysteine administration
Carbamazepine	2–4*†	. . .
Carboxyhemoglobin	Immediate	Hyperbaric oxygen therapy
Digoxin	2–4	Fab (digoxin antibody) fragment
Ethanol	½–1†	. . .
Ethylene glycol	½–1	Ethanol infusion OR fomepizole and hemodialysis
Iron	2–4	Deferoxamine administration
Isopropanol	½–1†	. . .
Lead	5 weeks*	Chelation and environmental abatement
Lithium	2–4	Hemodialysis
Methanol	½–1	Ethanol infusion OR fomepizole and hemodialysis
Methemoglobinemia	Immediate	Methylene blue administration
Phenobarbital	2–4	Alkaline diuresis, multiple-dose activated charcoal
Phenytoin	1–2*	Multiple-dose activated charcoal
Salicylates	6–12*	Alkaline diuresis, multiple-dose activated charcoal, hemodialysis
Theophylline	1–36*	Multiple-dose activated charcoal, whole-bowel irrigation, charcoal hemoperfusion, hemodialysis

(Adapted from Weisman RS, Howland MA, Verebey K: The toxicology laboratory. In *Goldfrank's Toxicologic Emergencies*, 5th ed. Edited by Goldfrank LR, Flomenbaum NE, Lewin NA, et al. East Norwalk, CT, Appleton & Lange, 1994, p 105.)

* Repeated measurement of levels is necessary because of significant variation in time to reach to peak level.

† The peak level is predictive of toxicity and clinical course.

TABLE 84.16. Poisons Not Detected on the Comprehensive Drug Screen

β-Adrenergic antagonists
Calcium channel blockers
Carbon monoxide
Clonidine
Cyanide
Iron
LSD (lysergic acid diethylamide)
Many benzodiazepines (alprazolam, midazolam, lorazepam)
Most plants and mushrooms

LSD = lysergic acid diethylamide.

Suggested Readings

American Academy of Clinical Toxicology; European association of poisons centres and clinical toxicologists. Position Statement: Ipecac syrup, gastric lavage, single-dose activated charcoal, cathartics and whole bowel irrigation. *J Toxicol Clin Toxicol* 35:699–761, 1997.

Ellenhorn MJ, Barceloux DG: *Medical Toxicology: Diagnosis and Treatment of Human Poisoning.* New York, Elsevier, 1988.

Goldfrank LR, Flomenbaum NE, Lewin NA, et al: *Goldfrank's Toxicologic Emergencies,* 6th ed. Stamford, CT, Appleton & Lange, 1998.

Haddad LM, Winchester JF: *Clinical Management of Poisoning and Drug Overdose,* 3rd ed. Philadelphia, WB Saunders, 1997.

Henretig FM, Shannon M: Toxicologic emergencies. In *Textbook of Pediatric Emergency Medicine,* 4th ed. Edited by Fleisher GR, Ludwig S. Baltimore, Lippincott Williams & Wilkins, 2000, pp 887–942.

Kulig K: Initial management of ingestions of toxic substances. *N Engl J Med* 326:1677, 1992.

Olson KR (ed): *Poisoning & Drug Overdose,* 3rd ed. Stamford, CT, Appleton & Lange, 1999.

Wiley JF: Novel therapies for ethylene glycol intoxication. *Curr Opin Pediatr* 11:269–273, 1999.

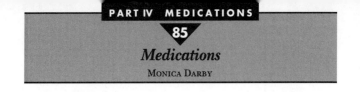

Medications

MONICA DARBY

TABLE 85.1. Medications

Drug	Dose	Dosage Forms
Acetaminophen (Feverall, Panadol, Tempra, Tylenol)	*Orally or rectally:* Children: 10–15 mg/kg repeated every 4–6 hours, up to 5 doses daily. Adults: 325–650 mg every 4–6 hours or 1 g t.i.d. or q.i.d. Do not exceed 4 g/day.	Drops: 100 mg/mL Suspension: 160 mg/5 mL Suppositories: 120 mg, 325 mg, 650 mg Tablets: 160 mg, 325 mg, 500 mg Tablets, chewable: 80 mg Also available in combination with codeine; see codeine monograph.
Acetazolamide (Diamox)	*Orally or IV:* Children and adults: 8–30 mg/kg/day in 4 divided doses. Do not exceed 1 g/day. *Altitude sickness (adults):* 250 mg every 8–12 hours beginning 24–48 hours before ascent and continuing for at least 48 hours after arrival.	Injection: 500 mg Tablets: 250 mg
Acetylcysteine (Mucomyst, Mucosil)	*Acetaminophen poisoning:* 140 mg/kg PO followed by 70 mg/kg for 17 doses administered every 4 hours until acetaminophen levels are nontoxic. Usually administered as a 5% solution diluted in juice or soda. *Inhalation* (administer 10% solution undiluted): Infants: 2–4 mL repeated t.i.d. or q.i.d. Children and adolescents: 6–10 mL repeated t.i.d. or q.i.d.	Solution for inhalation: 10% or 20% in 10-mL and 30-mL vials

Acyclovir (Zovirax)

Oral doses for children and adults:
Varicella zoster (chickenpox): 80 mg/kg/day in 4 divided doses for 5 days. Do not exceed 800 mg/dose (3,200 mg/day).
Herpes simplex virus:
Children: 1,200 mg/m^2/day in 4–5 divided doses.
Adults: 200 mg every 4 hours while awake (5 doses daily). Chronic suppressive therapy at a dose of 400 mg b.i.d. may be used for up to 1 year or longer.

IV doses for children and adults:
Neonatal HSV encephalitis: 30 mg/kg/day in 3 divided doses for 10–14 days.
HSV encephalitis: 1,500 mg/m^2/day in 3 divided doses for at least 10 days and up to 21 days.
Other HSV infections: 750 mg/m^2/day in 3 divided doses for 7 days.
Varicella zoster infections: 1,500 mg/m^2/day in 3 divided doses for 7 days.
Topically: apply ointment every 3 hours up to 6 times daily for 7 days. Use a disposable finger cot or glove when applying the ointment to avoid transmission of the virus.
Dosage may need to be adjusted in patients with renal dysfunction.

Capsules: 200 mg
Injection: 500-mg, 1-g vials
Ointment: 5%, 15 g
Suspension: 200 mg/5 mL

Adenosine (Adenocard)

IV (given via rapid push followed by a saline flush):
Children: 0.1 mg/kg initially, followed by doses increasing in 0.05 mg/kg increments every

Injection: 3 mg/mL (2-mL vial)

Continued

TABLE 85.1. Medications (continued)

Drug	Dose	Dosage Forms
Adenosine (Adenocard) (continued)	2 minutes to a maximum dose of 0.35 mg/kg or 12 mg/dose. Adults: 6 mg followed by 12 mg with a repeat dose of 12 mg, if needed.	
Albumin, human (Albuminar, Albutein, Plasbumin)	IV (as a 5% solution for hypovolemic patients or 25% for fluid- or sodium-restricted patients): Children: 0.5–1 g/kg infused over 2–4 hours. May repeat to a maximum of 6 g/kg/day. Adults: 25 g infused over 2–4 hours. Usually not to exceed 125 g/day.	Injection: 5% (50 mL, 250 mL, 5.30 mL); 25% (20 mL, 50 mL, 100 mL)
Albuterol (Proventil, Ventolin)	Oral: Age 2–<6: 0.3–0.6 mg/kg/day in 3 divided doses to a maximum of 12 mg/day. Age ≥6–≤12: 6–8 mg/day in 3–4 divided doses to a maximum of 24 mg/day. Over age 12: 6–16 mg/day in 3–4 divided doses to a maximum of 32 mg/day. Inhalation: Metered-dose inhaler: Under age 12: 1–2 inhalations q.i.d. Over age 12: 1–2 inhalations up to 6 times a day. Nebulization: 0.01–0.05 mL/kg usually repeated every 4–6 hours, but may be administered more frequently in severely ill patients under controlled conditions.	Aerosol: 90 μg/actuation Solution for inhalation: 0.5% Syrup: 10 mg/5 mL Tablets: 2 mg, 4 mg Tablets, extended release: 4 mg ε mg

Allopurinol (Zyloprim)	*Orally:* Under age 6: 150 mg/day in 3 divided doses. Age 6–10: 300 mg/day in 2 or 3 divided doses. Over age 10: 600–800 mg/day in 2 or 3 divided doses. Note: The metabolism of mercaptopurine and azathioprine is decreased by allopurinol. Decrease dose of mercaptopurine or azathioprine by 75%.	Tablets: 100 mg, 300 mg
Alprostadil (Prostin VR Pediatric)	A continuous infusion beginning at a dose of 0.05–0.1 μg/kg/min. Dosage may be adjusted downward or gradually upward based on the patient's response. Usual dosage range is 0.01–0.4 μg/kg/min.	Injection: 500 μg/mL (1-mL ampule)
Aluminum acetate (Domeboro, Burow's Solution)	*Topically:* as a wet dressing or soak 2–4 times daily for 30 minutes at a time. Usual concentrations are 1:10, 1:20, or 1:40. Ear: 4–6 drops in the ear at first every 2–3 hours, then every 4–6 hours until itching or burning subsides.	Powder (packets): 1 packet/pint of water = 1:40 dilution Solution otic, 1:10 dilution with 2% acetic acid
Aluminum and magnesium hydroxides (Maalox, Maalox Plus, Mylanta)	Children: 5–10 mL 4–6 times daily or more frequently. Adults: 15–30 mL 4–6 times daily or more frequently.	Suspension: aluminum hydroxide 225 mg and magnesium hydroxide 200 mg/5 mL Suspension with simethicone: as above with simethicone 25 mg/5 mL
Amantadine (Symmetrel)	*Orally* for prophylaxis or treatment of influenza A: Children 1–9 years of age: 5–9 mg/kg/day in 2 divided doses. Children 10 years of age and adults: 200 mg daily in 1 or 2 divided doses.	Solution: 50 mg/5 mL Capsules: 100 mg

Continued

TABLE 85.1. Medications (continued)

Drug	Dose	Dosage Forms

Amikacin (Amikin)	IV (dose should be based on ideal body weight):
	Neonates:
	  0–4 weeks, <1,200 g: 7.5 mg/kg/dose every
	    18–24 hours.
	  ≤7 days of age:
	    1,200–2,000 g: 7.5 mg/kg/dose every
	      12–18 hours.
	    >2,000 g: 10 mg/kg/dose every 12 hours.
	  Over 7 days of age:
	    1,200–2,000 g: 7.5 mg/kg/dose every 8–12
	      hours.
	    >2,000 g: 10 mg/kg/dose every 8 hours.
	Infants and children: 15–22.5 mg/kg/day in 3 divided
	  doses daily. The dose for the treatment of
	  nontuberculous mycobacterial infections is
	  15–30 mg/kg/day in 2 divided doses, to a
	  maximum of 1.5 g/day as part of a multiple-drug
	  regimen.
	Adults: 15 mg/kg/day in 2–3 divided doses.
	Dosage adjustment is required in patients with renal
	  dysfunction.
		Injection: 50 mg/mL, 250 mg/mL

Aminocaproic acid (Amicar)	IV:
	Children: 100 mg/kg over the first hour followed by
	  an infusion of 33.3 mg/kg/hr to a maximum
	  daily dose of 30 g.
		Injection: 250 mg/mL (20-mL vial)
		Solution: 1.25 g/5 mL (16-oz bottle)
		Tablets: 500 mg

Continued

Older children and adults: 4–5 g over the first hour followed by an infusion of 1 g/hr for 8 hours or until control is achieved.
Orally: doses are the same or alternatively, 100 mg/kg may be administered every 4–6 hours to a maximum of 5 g/dose.

Amiodarone (Cordarone)

Orally:
Children (use body surface area for children age 1 year or under): loading dose of 10–15 mg/kg/day or 600–800 mg/1.73 m² /day in 1–2 divided doses for 4–14 days or until adequate control of arrhythmia is achieved or prominent adverse effects occur. Then reduce dosage to 5 mg/kg/day or 200–400 mg/1.73 m² /day as a single dose for several weeks. A further dose reduction to 2.5 mg/kg/day should be attempted if the arrhythmia does not recur.
Adults: loading dose of 800–1,600 mg/day in 1–2 divided doses for 1–3 weeks, followed by dose of 600–800 mg/day in 1–2 divided doses for 1 month. Maintenance dose usually 400 mg/day, but may be lower for supraventricular arrhythmias.

IV:
Children (only limited information is available): initial loading dose of 5 mg/kg over 1 hour followed by a continuous infusion of 5 μg/kg/min has been used. The continuous infusion dosage may be increased to 10 μg/kg/min and then to 15 μg/kg/min until the desired effect is achieved.

Injection: 50 mg/mL
Tablets: 200 mg

TABLE 85.1. Medications (continued)

Drug	Dose	Dosage Forms
Amiodarone (Cordarone) (*continued*)	Adults: loading dose of 150 mg administered over 10 minutes (15 mg/min) followed by 360 mg over 6 hours at a rate of 1 mg/min, followed by the maintenance dose of 540 mg over 18 hours at a rate of 0.5 mg/min. If necessary, maintenance infusion of 0.5 mg/min may be continued past the initial 24 hours. Additional bolus doses of 150 mg may be administered over 10 minutes for breakthrough arrhythmias.	
Amitriptyline (Elavil, Endep)	*Orally:* *Chronic pain:* 0.1 mg/kg/day at bedtime initially, advancing to 0.5–2 mg/kg/day over a 2–3 week period. *Depression:* 1 mg/kg/day to start, advancing to a maximum of 5 mg/kg or 100 mg, whichever is less. Adolescents and adults: 25–50 mg at bedtime or in divided doses, increasing daily doses by 25 mg to a maximum of 100 mg/day for adolescents and 300 mg for adults. Dosage should be decreased to the lowest effective dose after symptom control has been reached.	Tablets: 10 mg, 25 mg, 50 mg. 75 mg, 100 mg, 150 mg

Amoxicillin (Amoxil, Polymox, Trimox, Wymox)

Orally:
Children ≤20 kg: 20 mg/kg/day in 3 divided doses for urinary tract infections. 40 mg/kg/day in 3 divided doses for otitis media, upper respiratory infection, or skin infections. Acute otitis media due to highly resistant strains of *S. pneumoniae* may require doses of 80–90 mg/kg/day in 3 divided doses.

Children >20 kg and adults: 750 mg/day in 3 divided doses for urinary tract infections or 1,500 mg/day in 3 divided doses for otitis media, upper respiratory infections, or skin infections. Maximum daily dose is 3 g.

Endocarditis prophylaxis: 50 mg/kg (up to 2 g) 1 hour before procedure

Capsules: 250 mg, 500 mg
Drops: 50 mg/mL
Suspension: 125 mg/5 mL, 250 mg/5 mL
Tablets, chewable: 125 mg, 250 mg

Amoxicillin and clavulanic acid (Augmentin)

Orally (based on the amoxicillin component):
20–40 mg/kg/day in 3 divided doses to a maximum of 1.5 g/day, or 25–45 mg/kg/day in 2 divided doses to a maximum of 1.75 g/day using the b.i.d. formulation of the drug.
Use the higher doses for respiratory tract infections and otitis media.

Suspension: amoxicillin 125 mg and clavulanic acid 31.25 mg/5 mL; b.i.d. formulation—amoxicillin 200 mg and clavulanic acid 28.5 mg/5 mL; amoxicillin 250 mg and clavulanic acid 62.5 mg/5 mL; b.i.d. formulation—amoxicillin 400 mg and clavulanic acid 57 mg/5 mL
Tablets: amoxicillin 250 mg and clavulanic acid 125 mg; amoxicillin 500 mg and clavulanic acid 125 mg; b.i.d. formulation—amoxicillin 875 mg and clavulanic acid 125 mg
Tablets, chewable: amoxicillin 125 mg and clavulanic acid 31.25 mg; b.i.d. formulation—amoxicillin 200 mg and clavulanic acid 28.5 mg;

Continued

TABLE 85.1. Medications (continued)

Drug	Dose	Dosage Forms
Amoxicillin and clavulanic acid (Augmentin) [continued]		amoxicillin 250 mg and clavulanic acid 62.5 mg; b.i.d. formulation—amoxicillin 400 mg and clavulanic acid 57 mg
Amphotericin B (Fungizone)	*IV* (infusion over 2–8 hours): *Test dose* (infusion over 30 minutes) < 10 kg: 0.1 mg in 1 mL D$_5$W. ≥ 10 kg: 1 mg in 10 mL D$_5$W. *Therapeutic dose:* begin with 0.25–0.5 mg/kg immediately following test dose. Doses may be doubled on each subsequent day to a maximum of 1 mg/kg as the patient tolerates. Once therapy is established, alternate day doses at a maximum of 1.5 mg/kg/day may be used. Bladder irrigations of 15–50 mg daily in 1 L of sterile water instilled over 24 hours have been used to treat bladder infections.	Injection: 50-mg vial
Amphotericin B, cholesteryl (Amphotec)	*IV* (infusion at a rate of 1 mg/kg/hr): Children and adults: 3–4 mg/kg/day as a single infusion. Doses of 6 mg/kg/day have been used to treat invasive *Candida* or *Cryptococcus* infections. Admix with 5% dextrose injection to a final concentration of about 0.6 mg/mL for administration over 3–4 hours. In patients who tolerate the longer infusion time well, the time can be shortened to 2 hours.	Injection: 50-mg vial

Continued

Amphotericin B, liposomal complex (Abelcet)	IV (infusion over 2 hours): Children and adults: 5 mg/kg/day in a single infusion. Admix with 5% dextrose to a final concentration of 1 mg/mL. A final concentration of 2 mg/mL may be used for pediatric patients or patients requiring fluid restriction.	Suspension for injection: 5 mg/mL

Ampicillin (Omnipen, Polycillin, Principen, Totacillin)	IV:
	Meningitis:
	Neonates under age 7 days:
	  <2,000 g: 100 mg/kg/day in 2 divided doses.
	  ≥2,000 g: 150 mg/kg/day in 3 divided doses.
	Neonates over age 7 days:
	  <1,200 g: 100 mg/kg/day in 2 divided doses.
	  1,200–2,000 g: 150 mg/kg/day in 3 divided doses.
	  >2,000 g: 200 mg/kg/day in 4 divided doses.
	Infants and children: 150–300 mg/kg/day in 4–6 divided doses to a maximum of 12 g/d.
	Adults: 150–200 mg/kg/day in 6–8 divided doses to a maximum total daily dose of 14 g.
	Moderate infections:
	Neonates under age 7 days:
	  <2,000 g: 50 mg/kg/day in 2 divided doses.
	  >2,000 g: 75 mg/kg/day in 3 divided doses.
	Neonates over age 7 days:
	  <1,200 g: 50 mg/kg/day in 2 divided doses.
	  1,200–2,000 g: 75 mg/kg/day in 3 divided doses.
	  >2,000 g: 100 mg/kg/day in 4 divided doses.
		Capsules: 250 mg, 500 mg
		Injection: 125-mg, 250-mg, 500-mg, 1-g, 2-g vials
		Suspension: 125 mg/5 mL, 250 mg/5 mL, 500 mg/5 mL

TABLE 85.1. Medications (continued)

Drug	Dose	Dosage Forms
Ampicillin (Omnipen, Polycillin, Principen, Totacillin) (continued)	Infants, children, and adults: 50–100 mg/kg/day in 4–6 divided doses to a maximum total dose of 12 g/day. *Orally (mild to moderate infections):* Children <20 kg: 50–75 mg/kg/day in 4 divided doses. Do not exceed adult doses for the same degree of infection. Children >20 kg and adults: 1–2 daily (250–500 mg/dose) in 4 divided doses.	
Ampicillin and sulbactam sodium (Unasyn)	*IV:* Infants and children: 150 mg/kg/day (100 mg ampicillin + 50 mg sulbactam) in 3–4 divided doses. Adults: 1.5–3 g (1–2 g ampicillin + 0.5–1 g sulbactam) given every 6 hours.	Injection: 1.5 g (1 g ampicillin + 0.5 g sulbactam), 3 g (2 g ampicillin + 1 g sulbactam)
Amrinone (Inocor)	*IV:* a bolus dose of 0.75 mg/kg administered over 2–3 minutes is followed by a maintenance infusion of 3–5 µg/kg/min for neonates or 5–10 µg/kg/min for infants, children, or adults. The bolus doses may be repeated at 30-minute intervals to a total of 3 mg/kg. Total daily dose should not exceed 10 mg/kg.	Injection: 5 mg/mL

Aspirin (Anacin, Ascriptin, Bufferin, Easprin, Ecotrin)	*Orally or rectally:* *Analgesic, antipyretic:* Children: 10–15 mg/kg every 4–6 hours. Adults: 325–1,000 mg every 4–6 hours, up to 4 g/day. *Antiinflammatory:* Children ≤25 kg: 60–90 mg/kg/day in 3–4 divided doses initially, with a usual range of 80–100 mg/kg/day. Monitor serum levels. Children >25 kg and adults: 2.4–3.6 g/day in 4 divided doses. Maximum total daily dose usually should not exceed 5.4 g. *Kawasaki syndrome:* 100 mg/kg/day in 4 divided doses until fever resolves; then 3–8 mg/kg once daily for 6–10 weeks after onset of the disease, or longer.	Suppositories: 300 mg, 325 mg, 600 mg, 650 mg Tablets: 325 mg, 500 mg, 650 mg Tablets, chewable: 81 mg Tablets, extended release: 165 mg, 325 mg, 500 mg, 650 mg, 975 mg Also available in buffered formulation, enteric-coated tablets, and chewing gum.
Atenolol (Tenormin)	*Orally:* Children: initially 0.8–1 mg/kg/day in a single dose. Dosage may be increased to 1.5 mg/kg/day or a maximum of 2 mg/kg/day if necessary. Adults: initially 25–50 mg/day, increasing to 50–100 mg/day as needed. The maximum dose for hypertension is 100 mg; for angina, 200 mg.	Tablets: 25 mg, 50 mg, 100 mg
Atropine sulfate	*Preoperative orally or IM:* 0.02 mg/kg to a maximum dose of about 1 mg. *Bradycardia:* 0.02 mg/kg with a minimum dose of 0.1 mg and a maximum dose of 0.5 mg in children, 1 mg in adolescents, and 2 mg in adults. *Ophthalmic:* 1–2 drops of 0.5–1% solution in the eye.	Injection: 0.3 mg/mL, 0.4 mg/mL, 0.5 mg/mL, 0.8 mg/mL, 1 mg/mL Ointment, ophthalmic: 0.5%, 1% Solution, ophthalmic: 0.5%, 1%, 2%

Continued

TABLE 85.1. Medications (continued)

Drug	Dose	Dosage Forms
Attapulgite (Kaopectate)	*Orally* (dose after each loose bowel movement, up to 7 times a day): Age 3–5: 7.5 mL or 1 tablet. Age 6–12: 15 mL or 2 tablets. Over age 12: 30 mL or 4 tablets.	Suspension: 600 mg/15 mL Tablets, chewable: 300 mg
Azathioprine (Imuran)	*IV or orally:* Children and adults: initially 3–5 mg/kg/day as a single dose. Maintenance doses are usually 1–3 mg/kg/day. Note: Metabolism of azathioprine is decreased by allopurinol; decrease dose of azathioprine by 75%.	Injection: 100-mg vial Tablets: 50 mg
Azelastine (Astelin)	*Intranasal metered dose spray:* 12 years of age and adults: 2 sprays in each nostril twice daily	Solution, nasal: 137 μg/metered spray
Azithromycin (Zithromax)	*Orally:* *Otitis media* (6 months of age and older): 10 mg/kg (to a maximum of 500 mg) on the first day followed by 5 mg/kg/day (to a maximum of 250 mg) for 4 days. *Pharyngitis/tonsillitis:* 2 years of age and older: 12 mg/kg/day (to a maximum of 500 mg) for 5 days. Adults: 500 mg on the first day followed by 250 mg/day for 4 days.	Capsules: 250 mg Suspension: 100 mg/5 mL, 200 mg/5 mL, 1-g packet

	Uncomplicated chlamydia infection: 1 g as a single dose for patients >8 years of age weighing at least 45 kg. *Gonorrhea:* 2 g for patients weighing at least 45 kg *Chancroid:* 20 mg/kg to a maximum dose of 1 g	
Aztreonam (Azactam)	*IV or IM:* Children over age 1 month: 60–100 mg/kg/day in 3–4 divided doses. Doses of up to 200 mg/kg/day have been used in severe infections. Maximum total daily dose is 8 g. Adults: 1–2 g every 6–8 hours, depending on the severity of the infection. Dose adjustment is necessary in renal impairment.	Injection: 500-mg, 1-g, 2-g vials
Bacitracin; bacitracin and polymyxin B (Polysporin); bacitracin, neomycin, and polymyxin B (Neosporin)	*Topically:* apply to affected area 1–3 times daily. *Ophthalmic:* apply to eyes every 3–4 hours.	Ointment, ophthalmic (all three): 3.5-g tube Ointment, topical (all three): 15-g, 30-g tubes
Beclomethasone dipropionate (Beclovent, Beconase, Vancenase, Vanceril)	*Intranasal:* Age 6–12: 1 inhalation in each nostril t.i.d. Over age 12 and adults 1 inhalation in each nostril b.i.d. or q.i.d. or 2 inhalations in each nostril b.i.d. *Intranasal aqueous formulation:* Children ≥6 years of age and adults: 1–2 sprays in each nostril b.i.d. Vancenase AQ 84 μg: 1–2 sprays in each nostril daily.	Intranasal aerosol spray: 42 μg/spray Intranasal nasal suspension spray pump: 42 μg/spray Intranasal nasal suspension spray pump double strength: 84 μg/spray Oral inhalation aerosol: 42 μg/spray Oral inhalation aerosol double strength: 84 μg/spray

Continued

TABLE 85.1. Medications (continued)

Drug	Dose	Dosage Forms
Beclomethasone dipropionate (Beclovent, Beconase, Vancenase, Vanceril) [continued]	*Oral inhalation:* Age 6–12: 1–2 inhalations t.i.d. or q.i.d. or 2–4 inhalations b.i.d. Do not exceed 10 inhalations/day. Over age 12 and adults: 2 inhalations t.i.d. or q.i.d. not to exceed 20 inhalations/day. Vanceril 84 μg Double Strength: use 1/2 the doses recommended above.	
Betamethasone (Diprolene, Diprosone, Maxivate, Uticort, Valisone)	Apply a thin film to the skin 1–3 times daily. Avoid application to the face, groin, or axillae.	Benzoate (Uticort): 0.025% cream, lotion, gel Dipropionate, augmented (Diprolene): 0.05% cream, lotion, gel, ointment Dipropionate (Diprosone): 0.05% cream, lotion, ointment, 0.1% aerosol Dipropionate with clotrimazole antifungal [Lotrisone] Valerate (Valisone): 0.01% cream, lotion, ointment
Bethanechol (Urecholine)	*Orally: Gastroesophageal reflux:* Children: 0.1–0.2 mg/kg given at least 30 minutes before a meal. Up to 4 doses/day may be given. Adults: 10–50 mg up to q.i.d. *Urinary retention:* Children: 0.6 mg/kg/day in 3–4 divided doses. Adults: 10–50 mg/dose up to q.i.d.	Tablets: 25 mg

Continued

Bisacodyl (Dulcolax)	*Orally (higher doses for evacuation, lower for laxation):* Age 3–12: 5–10 mg as a single dose. Over age 12: 5–15 mg as a single dose. Tablets are enteric coated and must not be chewed or crushed. *Rectally:* Under age 2: 5 mg/day as a single dose. Age 2–11: 5–10 mg/day as a single dose. Age 12 or over: 10 mg/day as a single dose.	Suppositories: 5 mg, 10 mg Tablets, enteric coated: 5 mg
Brompheniramine (Dimetane)	*Orally:* <6 years of age: 0.125 mg/kg/dose 4 times a day to a maximum of 8 mg/day. 6–12 years of age: 2–4 mg given 3–4 times a day to a maximum of 16 mg/day. Over age 12: 4–8 mg every 4–6 hours to a maximum of 24 mg/day. Extended-release tablets may be given as 8 mg b.i.d. or t.i.d. or 12 mg b.i.d.	Elixir: 2 mg/5 mL Tablet: 4 mg, 8 mg, 12 mg Tablets, extended release: 8 mg, 12 mg
Budesonide (Rhinocort)	*Intranasal metered dose spray:* Children ≥6 years of age and adults: 8 sprays (4 sprays in each nostril) as a single dose in the morning or as 2 divided doses. Dosage may be decreased to the lowest number of sprays that controls symptoms.	Aerosol, nasal: 50 µg/actuation

TABLE 85.1. Medications (continued)

Drug	Dose	Dosage Forms
Bumetanide (Bumex)	*Orally or IV:* Neonates: 0.01–0.05 mg/kg/dose every 24–48 hours. Infants and children: 0.015–0.1 mg/kg/dose every 6–24 hours to a maximum of 10 mg/day. Adults: 0.5–1 mg/dose IV or 0.5–2 mg/dose orally once or twice daily to a maximum of 10 mg/day.	Injection: 0.25 mg/mL Tablets: 0.5 mg, 1 mg, 2 mg
Caffeine	*Orally or IV:* *Loading dose:* 10 mg/kg caffeine base. If theophylline has been administered within the previous 3 days, a modified dose (50–75% of loading dose) may be given. *Maintenance:* 2.5 mg/kg caffeine base 24 hours after the loading dose. Dosage may be adjusted based on the patient's response and the results of serum level monitoring. Do not use caffeine and sodium benzoate injection in neonates.	Injection: 10 mg/mL Solution: 10 mg/mL
Calcitriol (Calcijex, Rocaltrol)	Individualize to maintain normal serum calcium levels. *Orally:* *Hypocalcemia in premature infants:* 1 µg/day for 5 days.	Capsules: 0.25 µg, 0.5 µg Injection: 1 µg/mL, 2 µg/mL (1-mL ampules) Solution: 1 µg/mL

Renal failure:
Children 0.25–2 μg/day (hemodialysis) or 0.014–0.041 μg/kg/day (no hemodialysis).
Adults: 0.25–1 μg/day.
IV:
Hypocalcemia in premature infants: 0.05 μg/kg/day for 4 days.
Renal failure:
Children: 0.01–0.05 μg/kg 3 times weekly (hemodialysis).
Adults: 0.5–3 μg 3 times weekly (hemodialysis).

Calcium salts

See dosage forms for calcium content of various salts. Dosage should be adjusted based on the desired response and serum calcium levels.
IV (gluconate or chloride salts):
Cardiac resuscitation:
Calcium gluconate:
Children: 60–100 mg/kg/dose to a maximum of 3 g.
Adults: 500 mg–1 g/dose.
Calcium chloride:
Children: 20 mg/kg/dose to a maximum of 1 g.
Adults: 2–4 mg/kg/dose to a maximum of 1 g.
Hypocalcemia (usually the gluconate salt):
Neonates: 200–800 mg/kg/day, usually as a continuous infusion.
Infants and children: 200–500 mg/kg/day as a continuous infusion or in 4 divided doses.
Adults: 2–15 g/day as a continuous infusion or in divided doses.

Calcium acetate = 25% Ca = 250 mg Ca per 1 g Ca acetate
Calcium carbonate = 40% Ca = 400 mg Ca per 1 g Ca carbonate
Calcium chloride = 27% Ca = 270 mg Ca per 1 g Ca chloride
Calcium citrate = 21% Ca = 210 mg Ca per 1 g Ca citrate
Calcium glubionate = 6.5% Ca = 65 mg Ca per 1 g Ca glubionate
Calcium gluconate = 9% Ca = 90 mg Ca per 1 g Ca gluconate
Calcium lactate = 13% Ca = 130 mg Ca per 1 g Ca lactate
Injection:
Chloride salt: 1 g (100 mg/mL) = 27 mg Ca/mL
Gluconate salt: 1 g (100 mg/mL) = 9 mg Ca/mL
Suspension: carbonate salt: 1.25 g/5 mL = 500 mg Ca/5 mL

Continued

TABLE 85.1. Medications (continued)

Drug	Dose	Dosage Forms
Calcium salts (continued)	Orally (carbonate, glubionate, or lactate salts): Neonates: 20–80 mg calcium/kg/day in 4–6 divided doses. Infants and children: 20–40 mg calcium/kg/day in 4–6 divided doses. Adults: 400 mg–1.2 g calcium/day or more.	Syrup: glubionate salt: 1.8 g/5 mL = 115 mg Ca/5 mL Tablets: Acetate salt: 667 mg = 169 mg Ca (PhosLo) Carbonate salt: 650 mg = 250 mg Ca; 1.25 g = 500 mg Ca; 1.5 g = 600 mg Ca Citrate salt: 950 mg = 200 mg Ca (Citracal); 2376 mg = 500 mg Ca (Citracal Liquitab) Gluconate salt: 500 mg = 45 mg Ca; 650 mg = 58.5 mg Ca; 975 mg = 87.75 mg Ca; 1 g = 90 mg Ca Lactate salt: 325 mg = 42.25 mg Ca; 650 mg = 84.5 mg Ca
Calfactant (Infasurf)	Intratracheally: 3 mL/kg divided into 2–4 aliquots. Patients should be ventilated and repositioned between aliquots.	Suspension, intratracheal: 8 mL
Captopril (Capoten)	Orally: Neonates: 0.01–0.05 mg/kg up to t.i.d., initially. Dose may be increased incrementally to a maximum of 0.5 mg/kg administered as frequently as every 6 hours (2 mg/kg/day).	Tablets: 12.5 mg, 25 mg, 50 mg, 100 mg

Carbamazepine (Tegretol)	Infants and children: 0.15–0.3 mg/kg up to t.i.d., initially. Dose may be increased incrementally to a maximum of 6 mg/kg/day in divided doses. Adolescents and adults: 12.5–25 mg every 8–12 hours, initially. May be titrated upward to a maximum of 6 mg/kg/day or 450 mg.	Suspension: 100 mg/5 mL Tablets, chewable: 100 mg Tablets: 200 mg
Carbamide peroxide (Debrox, Gly-Oxide)	Orally: initially 5–10 mg/kg/day in 2–4 divided doses, increasing slowly to a maximum of 30 mg/kg/day (1.6–2.4 g in adults). Suspension formulation should be administered in 3–4 daily doses; tablet formulations may be administered in 2–3 divided doses.	Drops, oral: 10% (Cank-aid, Gly-Oxide, Orajel Brace-aid Rinse) Drops, otic: 6.5% (Auro Ear Drops, Debrox, Murine Ear Drops)
Cefaclor (Ceclor)	Ear: instill up to 5–10 drops in the ear and allow to remain there for several minutes or longer. Orally: apply several drops to the affected area up to q.i.d.	Capsules: 250 mg Suspension: 125 mg/5 mL, 250 mg/5 mL
Cefadroxil (Duricef, Ultracef)	Orally: 20–40 mg/kg/24 hr in 2–3 divided doses to a maximum of 2 g/24 hr.	Capsules: 500 mg Suspension: 125 mg/5 mL, 250 mg/5 mL, 500 mg/5 mL Tablets: 1 g
Cefazolin (Ancef, Kefzol)	Orally: Children: 30 mg/kg/day in 2 divided doses to a maximum of 2 g/day. Adults: 1–2 g/day in a single or 2 divided doses.	Injection: 250-mg, 500-mg, 1-g vials
	IV or IM: 50–100 mg/kg/day in 3 divided doses to a maximum of 6 g/day. Usual adult doses are 500 mg–2 g/dose every 8 hours Dosing adjustment is necessary in renal impairment.	

Continued

TABLE 85.1. Medications (continued)

Drug	Dose	Dosage Forms
Cefdinir (Omnicef)	*Orally:* Age 6 months to 12 years: 14 mg/kg/day in 1 or 2 divided doses. >12 years or 43 kg: 600 mg daily in 1 or 2 divided doses.	Capsules: 300 mg Suspension: 125 mg/5 mL
Cefixime (Suprax)	*Orally:* Children: 8 mg/kg/day in 1 or 2 divided doses to a maximum of 400 mg. Adults: 400 mg/day in 1 or 2 divided doses. *Otitis media:* use suspension formula because higher serum levels are reached at the same dose when the suspension is administered.	Suspension: 100 mg/5 mL Tablets: 200 mg, 400 mg
Cefotaxime (Claforan)	*IV:* *Sepsis:* Infants and children: 100–120 mg/kg/day in 3–4 divided doses. Adults: 1–2 g every 6–8 hours. *Meningitis:* Neonates under age 1 week: 50 mg/kg every 12 hours. Neonates age 1 week or over: 50 mg/kg every 8 hours.	Injection: 1-g, 2-g vials

Continued

	Infants over 4 weeks and children: 200 mg/kg/day in 4 divided doses. A dose of 300 mg/kg/day in 4 divided doses has been used for the treatment of pneumococcal meningitis. Maximum total daily dose is 12 g. Adults: 2 g every 4–6 hours. Dosing adjustment is necessary in renal impairment.	
Cefoxitin (Mefoxin)	*IV:* Neonates: 90–100 mg/kg/day in 3 divided doses. Children: 80–160 mg/kg/day depending on the severity of the infection in 4 divided doses. Adults: 1–2 g every 6–8 hours to a maximum total daily dose of 12 g.	Injection: 1-g, 2-g vials
Cefpodoxime (Vantin)	*Orally* (with food to enhance absorption): Children: 10 mg/kg/day in 2 divided doses to a maximum of 400 mg/day (otitis media) or 200 mg/day (pharyngitis/tonsillitis). Adults: 200 mg/day in 2 divided doses for upper respiratory or uncomplicated urinary tract infection, 400 mg/day in 2 divided doses for lower respiratory tract infection (community-acquired pneumonia), 800 mg/day in 2 divided doses (skin, skin structure infection). Dosage adjustment is necessary in severe renal impairment.	Suspension: 50 mg/5 mL, 100 mg/5 mL Tablets: 100 mg, 200 mg

TABLE 85.1. Medications (continued)

Drug	Dose	Dosage Forms
Cefprozil (Cefzil)	*Orally:* Children: *Otitis media:* 30 mg/kg/day in 2 divided doses to a maximum total daily dose of 1 g. *Pharyngitis, tonsillitis:* 15 mg/kg/day in 2 divided doses to a maximum total daily dose of 500 mg. Adults: *Lower respiratory tract:* 500 mg every 12 hours. *Upper respiratory tract and skin:* 500 mg every 24 hours. Dosage adjustment is necessary in renal impairment.	Suspension: 125 mg/5 mL, 250 mg/5 mL Tablets: 250 mg, 500 mg
Ceftazidime (Fortaz, Tazicef, Tazidime)	*IV:* Neonates: <2,000 g: 60 mg/kg/day in 2 divided doses. ≥2,000 g: 90 mg/kg/day in 3 divided doses. Infants and children: 90–150 mg/kg/day in 3 divided doses to a maximum total daily dose of 6 g. Adults: 3–6 g/day in 3 divided doses. Dosage adjustment is necessary in renal impairment.	Injection: 500 mg, 1 g, 2 g

Continued

Ceftriaxone (Rocephin)

Injection: 250-mg, 500-mg, 1-g, 2-g vials

IV or IM:
PPNG (uncomplicated pharyngeal, urethral, endo-cervical, rectal):
  <45 kg: 125 mg IM as a single dose.
  ≥45 kg: 250 mg IM as a single dose.
PPNG (ophthalmia): >20 kg: 1 g IM as a single dose.
Infants born to a mother infected with PPNG: 50 mg/kg IM to a maximum of 125 mg as a single dose.
Other serious infections (not including meningitis):
Children: 50–75 mg/kg/day in 2 divided doses. Do not exceed 2 g/day.
Adults: usually 1–2 g as a single daily dose or in 2 divided doses.
Otitis media, chancroid: 50 mg/kg as a single dose given IM.
Meningitis:
Children: 100 mg/kg/day in 1–2 divided doses to a maximum total daily dose of 4 g.

Cefuroxime (Ceftin, Kefurox, Zinacef)

Injection: 750-mg, 1.5-g vials
Suspension (axetil): 125 mg/5 mL
Tablets: 125 mg, 250 mg, 500 mg

Orally (administer with food to enhance absorption):
Otitis media (all ages): 30 mg/kg/day in 2 divided doses to a maximum total daily dose of 1 g.
Other infections (all ages): 20 mg/kg/day in 2 divided doses to a maximum total daily dose of 500 mg.
IV:
Children: 50–100 mg/kg/day in 3–4 divided doses. A dose of 150 mg/kg/day in 3 divided doses is recommended for bone and joint infections. Do not exceed adult doses below.

TABLE 85.1. Medications (continued)

Drug	Dose	Dosage Forms
Cefuroxime [Ceftin, Kefurox, Zinacef] (continued)	Adults: 2.25–4.5 g/day in 3 divided doses. Higher dose is necessary for severe infections and bone and joint infections. Dosage adjustment is necessary in renal impairment.	
Cephalexin (Keflet, Keflex)	Orally: Children: 50–100 mg/kg/day in 4 divided doses for otitis media and serious infections. Doses of 25–50 mg/kg/day in 2–4 divided doses may be used for less serious infections. Do not exceed adult doses. Adults: 1–4 g/day in 4 divided doses.	Capsules: 250 mg, 500 mg Drops: 100 mg/mL Suspension: 125 mg/5 mL, 250 mg/5 mL Tablets: 250 mg, 500 mg, 1 g
Cetirizine (Zyrtec)	Orally: Age 2–5 years: 2.5 mg/day. Dose may be increased to 5 mg/day as a single or 2 divided doses. Age 6 years–adults: 5–10 mg/day as a single dose.	Syrup: 1 mg/mL Tablets: 5 mg, 10 mg
Charcoal (Actidose-Aqua, Actidose with Sorbitol, CharcoAid, Liqui-Char)	Orally: usually available as premixed solutions. Solutions containing sorbitol should not be used for multiple doses because diarrhea will occur. Do not administer concomitantly with ipecac because charcoal will adsorb and inactivate the ipecac. Do not administer with milk, ice cream, or sherbet because adsorptive capacity of the charcoal will be decreased.	Liquid: 25 g/120 mL, 30 g/240 mL, 50 g/240 mL Liquid, with sorbitol: 25 g/120 mL, 50 g/240 mL

Single dose:
  Children: 1–2 g/kg up to 15–30 g as soon as possible after the ingestion, preferably after emesis.
  Adults: 30–100 g.
  Dose should be 5 to 10 times the amount of the ingested poison.
Multiple dose (products without sorbitol):
  Infants: 1 g/kg every 4–6 hours.
  Children and adults: 1–2 g/kg (up to 60 g) every 2–6 hours.

Chloral hydrate (Aquachloral, Noctec)

Orally or rectally:
  Sedation before procedures: 60–75 mg/kg 30 minutes to 1 hour before the procedure. May repeat with a half-dose [30–37.5 mg/kg] if the first dose is ineffective. Do not exceed 120 mg/kg or 2 g total.
  Sedation for anxiety: 25 mg/kg/day in divided doses every 6–8 hours to a maximum of the usual adult dose of 750 mg/day. Continuous therapy, especially in infants, is not recommended.

Capsules: 250 mg, 500 mg
Suppositories: 324 mg, 500 mg, 648 mg
Syrup: 500 mg/5 mL

Chloramphenicol (Chloromycetin)

IV or orally:
  Neonates under age 7 days: 25 mg/kg/day in a single daily dose.
  Neonates age 7–21 days: 50 mg/kg/day in 2 divided doses daily.
  Infants and children: 50–75 mg/kg/day in 4 divided doses to a maximum total daily dose of 4 g.

Capsules: 250 mg
Injection: 1-g vial

Continued

TABLE 85.1. Medications (continued)

Drug	Dose	Dosage Forms
Chloramphenicol (Chloromycetin) (continued)	Adults: 50 mg/kg/day in 4 divided doses to a maximum total daily dose of 4 g. Serum levels must be monitored closely, especially in neonates and infants, and patients with renal or hepatic impairment.	Injection: 500 mg Suspension: 250 mg/5 mL Tablets: 250 mg, 500 mg
Chlorothiazide (Diuril)	*Orally:* Infants under age 6 months: 20–40 mg/kg/day in 2 divided doses. Children: 20 mg/kg/day in 2 divided doses. Adults: 0.5–1 g/day in 1 or 2 divided doses. *IV:* Infants under age 6 months: 20–40 mg/kg/day in 2 divided doses, but doses of 2–8 mg/kg/day may be sufficient in some patients. Children: 4–20 mg/kg/day in 2 divided doses. Adults: 0.5–1 g/day.	
Chlorpromazine (Thorazine)	*Nausea and vomiting or psychosis:* Over age 6 months: 0.3–0.5 mg/kg IV every 6–8 hours or 0.5–1 mg/kg PO every 4–6 hours or 1 mg/kg rectally every 6–8 hours as needed. Do not exceed adult doses.	Injection: 25 mg/mL Oral concentrate: 30 mg/mL, 100 mg/mL Suppositories: 25 mg, 100 mg Syrup: 10 mg/5 mL Tablets: 10 mg, 25 mg, 50 mg, 100 mg, 200 mg

Adults: 25–50 mg IV every 6–8 hours or 10–25 mg PO every 4–6 hours or 50–100 mg rectally every 6–8 hours. Doses may be increased in the treatment of psychoses; some adults may require as much as 800 mg/day until control is achieved. Dose should then be decreased to the usual maintenance levels of 200 mg/day for adults.

Cholestyramine resin (Cholybar, Questran, Questran Light)

Orally:
Children: 240 mg/kg/day of the resin administered in 3 divided doses.
Adults: 3–4 g t.i.d. or q.i.d.
Doses should be administered mixed in liquids (4 g in 2–6 oz) or with pulpy fruits (applesauce or pineapple).
Many drugs bind with cholestyramine in the GI tract. Drugs should be administered 1 hour before or 4 hours after cholestyramine. Patients should also be cautioned to ingest plenty of fluids to avoid constipation and fecal impaction.

Bar: 4 g resin/bar (Cholybar)
Powder: 4 g resin/9 g powder (Questran); 4 g resin/5 g powder (Questran Light, contains aspartame)

Cimetidine (Tagamet)

Orally, IV:
Initial dose:
Neonates: 5–10 mg/kg/day in 2–3 divided doses daily.
Infants: 10–20 mg/kg/day in 2–4 divided doses daily.
Children: 20–40 mg/kg/day in 4 divided doses daily.

Injection: 150 mg/mL
Liquid: 300 mg/5 mL
Tablets: 200 mg, 300 mg, 400 mg, 800 mg

Continued

TABLE 85.1. Medications (continued)

Drug	Dose	Dosage Forms
Cimetidine (Tagamet) (continued)	Adults: 300 mg every 6 hours. Orally, doses of 800 mg at bedtime or 400 mg b.i.d. may be used. Doses may be adjusted upward, especially in hypersecretory states, as necessary to maintain the gastric pH of 5 or greater. A maximum total daily dose of 2.4 g should not be exceeded. Dosage must be adjusted in renal impairment.	Injection: 10 mg/mL Solution, ophthalmic: 3.5% Tablets: 250 mg, 500 mg, 750 mg
Ciprofloxacin (Ciloxan, Cipro)	The drug is not approved for use in patients under age 18 due to possible adverse effects; consider risk vs. benefit if for use in patients under age 18. *Orally (on an empty stomach):* Children: 20–30 mg/kg/day in 2 divided doses; up to 40 mg/kg/day may be used for patients with cystic fibrosis. Do not exceed 1.5 g/day. Adults: 500–1,500 mg/day in 2 divided doses. *IV (administer over 1 hour at a concentration of 1–2 mg/mL):* Children: 15–20 mg/kg/day in 2 divided doses; up to 30 mg/kg/day may be used in patients with cystic fibrosis. Do not exceed 800 mg/day. Adults: 400–800 mg/day in 2 divided doses. Dosage must be adjusted in patients with renal dysfunction.	

Continued

		Content per 1 mL*

Citrate and citric acid (Bicitra, Polycitra, Shohl's Solution)

Ophthalmic: administer 1–2 drops every 2 hours while awake for 2 days and then every 4 hours while awake for 5 days.

Orally (dilute in water or juice):
Infants and children: 2–3 mEq/kg/day in 3–4 divided doses.
Adults: 15–30 mL given q.i.d.
Giving doses with meals decreases the saline laxative effect.

Clarithromycin (Biaxin)

Orally:
Children: 15 mg/kg/day in 2 divided doses, not to exceed 1 g/day.
Adults: 500 mg–1 g/day in 2 divided doses.

Suspension: 125 mg/5 mL, 250 mg/5 mL
Tablets: 250 mg, 500 mg

Clindamycin (Cleocin)

IV:
Neonates under age 7 days:
≤2,000 g: 10 mg/kg/day in 2 divided doses.
>2,000 g: 15 mg/kg/day in 3 divided doses.
Neonates over age 7 days:
<1,200 g: 10 mg/kg/day in 2 divided doses.
1,200–2,000 g: 15 mg/kg/day in 3 divided doses.
>2,000 g: 20 mg/kg/day in 3–4 divided doses.
Infants and children: 25–40 mg/kg/day in 3–4 divided doses.
Adults: 1.2–2.7 g/day in 2–4 divided doses.
Maximum total daily dose should not exceed 4.8 g and should be used for life-threatening infections only.

Capsules: 150 mg
Injection: 150 mg/mL
Solution, oral: 75 mg/5 mL
Solution, topical: 1%

TABLE 85.1. Medications (continued)

Drug	Dose	Dosage Forms
Clindamycin (Cleocin) (continued)	*Orally:* Infants and children: 15–25 mg/kg/day in 3–4 divided doses for moderate to severe infections. Adults: 150–450 mg every 6–8 hours to a maximum total daily dose of 1.8 g. *Topically:* apply to the affected area b.i.d. Avoid the eyes, abraded skin, and mucous membranes.	
Clonazepam (Klonopin)	*Orally:* Under age 10 or <30 kg: initially 0.01–0.03 mg/kg/day in 2–3 divided doses. Dose may be increased gradually (every third day) until seizures are controlled or adverse effects are seen. The usual maintenance dose range is 0.1–0.2 mg/kg/day. Adults >30 kg: initially 1.5 mg/day in 3 divided doses. Dose may be increased by 0.5–1 mg every third day to a maximum total daily dose of 20 mg. Usual maintenance dose is 0.05–0.2 mg/kg/day.	Tablets: 0.5 mg, 1 mg, 2 mg
Clonidine (Catapres)	*Orally:* *Hypertension:* 5 to 10 μg/kg/day in 2 to 3 divided doses. In patients who experience sedation, the doses may be divided such that the patient receives a larger dose at bedtime and a smaller dose in the morning. Dose may be incrementally increased	Tablet: 0.1 mg, 0.2 mg, 0.3 mg

if necessary to 25 μg/kg/day to a maximum dose of 0.9 mg/day.

Attention deficit/hyperactivity disorder: 5 μg/kg/day in 4 divided doses has been used in some patients who have failed conventional therapy.

Clorazepate dipotassium (Tranxene)

Orally:
Age 9–12: initially 3.75–7.5 mg b.i.d. Dose may be increased by 3.75 mg at weekly intervals to a maximum total daily dose of 60 mg.
Over age 12 and adults: up to 7.5 mg up to t.i.d. May be increased by 7.5 mg at weekly intervals to a maximum total daily dose of 90 mg.

Capsules or tablets: 3.75 mg, 7.5 mg, 15 mg
Tablets: 11.25 mg, 22.5 mg

Clotrimazole (Lotrimin, Mycelex)

Vaginal cream: 1 full applicator at bedtime for 7–14 days.
Vaginal suppository: 1 suppository intravaginally at bedtime for 7 days or 2 at bedtime for 3 days or 500 mg as a single dose.
Topically: apply to affected areas b.i.d.

Cream, topical: 1% (30-g tube)
Cream, vaginal: 1% (45-g tube)
Solution, topical: 1% (30-mL squeeze bottle)
Suppositories, vaginal: 100 mg, 500 mg

Codeine

Orally:
Analgesic: 0.5–1 mg/kg every 4–6 hours as needed, to a maximum of 60 mg. Usual adult dose is 30 mg.
Antitussive: 0.2–0.25 mg/kg every 4–6 hours as needed, to a maximum of 30 kg.
SC: same doses as above may be used, although the oral route is only two thirds as effective as the SC route. It should not be used IV. (For IV route, use morphine)

Injection (phosphate): 30 mg/mL, 60 mg/mL
Solution, oral (phosphate): 15 mg/5 mL
Tablets (sulfate): 15 mg, 30 mg, 60 mg
Also available in various combinations with acetaminophen:
Elixir, oral: 12 mg codeine with 120 mg acetaminophen
Tablets: 7.5 mg codeine with acetaminophen 300 mg [Tylenol w/Codeine No. 1], 15 mg codeine

Continued

TABLE 85.1. Medications (continued)

Drug	Dose	Dosage Forms
Codeine (continued)		with acetaminophen 300 mg Tylenol w/Codeine No. 2), 300 mg codeine with acetaminophen 300 mg (Tylenol w/Codeine No. 3), 60 mg codeine with acetaminophen 300 mg (Tylenol w/Codeine No. 4)
Colfosceril palmitate (Exosurf Neonatal)	*Intratracheally:* should be used only by physicians familiar with its administration. The usual dose is 5 mL/kg divided equally between the two lungs. Second and third doses may be administered at 12-hour intervals. The infant should be suctioned before administration of colfosceril and ventilator settings should be decreased, depending on the patient's response.	Powder, lyophilized: 108 mg/10 mL
Colistin, neomycin, and hydro-cortisone (Coly-Mycin S Otic)	*Otic* (shake bottle well before administering): *Children:* 3 drops in the affected ear t.i.d. or q.i.d. *Adults:* 4 drops in the affected ear t.i.d. or q.i.d.	Suspension, otic: 5 mL
Cortisone acetate (Cortone Acetate)	Depends on the use of the drug and patient response. *Orally: Physiologic replacement:* 0.5–0.75 mg/kg/day in 3 divided doses. *Antiinflammatory:* 2.5–10 mg/kg/day in 3–4 divided doses.	Injection: 50 mg/mL Tablets: 5 mg, 10 mg, 25 mg

IM:

Physiologic replacement: 0.25–0.35 mg/kg/day as a single dose.

Antiinflammatory: 1–5 mg/kg/day in 1 or 2 divided doses.

In patients requiring physiologic replacement, dosage may need to be increased during periods of stress, including perioperatively and during illness.

Cosyntropin (Cortrosyn)

Injection: 0.25 mg

IV:

Under age 2: 0.125 mg.
Over age 2 and adults: 0.25 mg.

Co-trimoxazole (trimethoprim and sulfamethoxazole; Bactrim, Septra)

Injection: 16 mg trimethoprim and 80 mg sulfamethoxazole per 1 mL
Suspension: 8 mg trimethoprim and 40 mg sulfamethoxazole per 1 mL
Tablets: 80 mg trimethoprim and 400 mg sulfamethoxazole
Tablets, double strength: 160 mg trimethoprim and 800 mg sulfamethoxazole

Orally or IV (based on trimethoprim):
Over age 2 months and adults.
Treatment doses:
Mild to moderate infections (urinary tract or otitis media): 8 mg trimethoprim/kg/day in 2 divided doses. Maximum dose is 320 mg trimethoprim/day.
Pneumocystis carinii pneumonitis: 20 mg trimethoprim/kg/day in 4 divided doses.
Prophylaxis doses:
Urinary tract infection: 2 mg trimethoprim/kg/day as a single dose.

Pneumocystis carinii: 150 mg/m²/day in 1 or 2 divided doses daily on 3 consecutive or alternating days per week.

Continued

TABLE 85.1. Medications (continued)

Drug	Dose	Dosage Form
Co-trimoxazole (trimethoprim and sulfamethoxazole; Bactrim, Septra) (continued)	Dosage adjustment is necessary in patients with renal impairment. IV doses must be administered over 60–90 minutes and should be well diluted (1 mL injection in 25 mL infusate).	
Cromolyn sodium (Crolom, Intal, Nasalcrom, Opticrom)	Children: *Metered-dose inhaler:* 2 inhalations q.i.d. *Spinhaler dry inhalation:* contents of 1 capsule q.i.d. *Nebulizer solution:* 20 mg nebulized q.i.d. *Intranasal spray:* 1 spray in each nostril 3–6 times daily. *Ophthalmic:* 1–2 drops in each eye 4–6 times daily.	Capsules, powder for inhalation: 20 mg Inhalation, metered dose: 800 μg/spray Solution, nasal: 5.2 mg/spray Solution, nebulizer: 20 mg/2 mL Solution, ophthalmic: 4%
Crotamiton (Eurax)	*Topically:* apply a thin layer to all skin surfaces from the neck to the toes and soles of the feet. Be sure to apply to all surfaces, including skin folds. Avoid the face and mucous membranes, including the urethral meatus. A second coat is applied 24 hours later. A cleansing bath should follow 48 hours after the second application. Treatment may be repeated after 7–10 days if the mites reappear. It is safe for use in infants and young children. If signs of irritation or hypersensitivity appear, remove the product immediately by bathing. Contaminated clothing and bed linens should be washed to avoid reinfestations.	Cream: 10% Lotion: 10%

Cyclosporine (Neoral, Sandimmune)

NOTE: The two are *not* bioequivalent. Clinical condition and serum levels must be monitored carefully when a patient's therapy is changed from one to the other, especially in patients receiving large doses (>10 mg/kg/day) of Sandimmune who are changed to Neoral therapy because significant drug toxicity may result.

Orally:
Sandimmune: initially 10–18 mg/kg/day (dose dependent on organ being transplanted) in 2 divided doses, tapering over several weeks with frequent monitoring to a maintenance dose usually in the range of 5–10 mg/kg/day.
Neoral: initially about 10 mg/kg/day in 2 divided doses, tapering over several weeks based on clinical condition and serum levels.
Conversion from Sandimmune to Neoral: Consult with pharmacist
IV (Sandimmune only): 5–6 mg/kg/day in 1 or 2 divided doses. Each dose should be administered over at least 2 hours.

Capsules (Neoral): 25 mg, 100 mg
Capsules (Sandimmune): 25 mg, 50 mg, 100 mg
Injection (Sandimmune): 50 mg/mL
Solution, oral (Neoral and Sandimmune): 100 mg/mL

Dantrolene sodium (Dantrium)

Orally:
Spasticity:
Children >5 years of age: 0.5 mg/kg given b.i.d. initially, but frequency may be increased gradually to t.i.d. or q.i.d. The maximum dose is 100 mg q.i.d.

Capsules: 25 mg, 50 mg, 100 mg
Injection: 20 mg

Continued

TABLE 85.1. Medications (continued)

Drug	Dose	Dosage Forms
Dantrolene sodium (Dantrium) (continued)	Adults: 25 mg daily initially, with increases in frequency and dose to a maximum of 400 mg/day in 4 divided doses. *Malignant hyperthermia prophylaxis:* 4–8 mg/kg/day in 3–4 divided doses daily for 1–2 days prior to surgery. *Intravenously:* *Malignant hyperthermia prophylaxis:* 2.5 mg/kg administered over 1 hour about 1.25 hours before surgery. Repeat doses may be necessary. *Malignant hyperthermia crisis:* 1 mg/kg given rapidly. Repeat doses may be necessary, but it is usually not necessary to exceed 2.5 mg/kg. Maximum dose should not exceed 10 mg/kg.	
Deferoxamine (Desferal)	Children: *Acute iron intoxication:* 15 mg/kg/hr IV continuous infusion; maximum 6 g/24 hr. *Chronic iron overload:* 20–25 mg/kg/day IM or 500 mg–2 g IV with each unit of blood transfused, or 20–40 mg/kg/day SC over 8–12 hours up to 1–2 g/day.	Injection: 500-mg vial

Desmopressin acetate (DDAVP)

Intranasally:
Nocturnal enuresis in patients over age 6: 20 μg at bedtime with half of dose in each nostril. Dose may be increased or decreased depending on the patient's response. Usual range is 10–40 μg/day.
Diabetes insipidus in patients age 7 years–adults: initially 5 μg/day as a single dose or in 2 divided doses. Dosage should be titrated to the patient's response. The usual range is 5–40 μg/day.

Orally:
Diabetes insipidus:
Children: initially, 0.05 mg/dose with careful monitoring to prevent hyponatremia or water intoxication.

Over age 12 and adults: initially, 0.05 mg b.i.d. Dosage may then be adjusted to maintain normal diurnal water turnover. The usual total daily dosage is in the range of 0.1–1.2 mg and may be administered in 2–3 divided doses.

Nocturnal enuresis in children over age 12: 0.2–0.4 mg/day at bedtime.

IV:
To increase factor VIII levels: 0.3 μg/kg over 30 minutes.
Diabetes insipidus: adult doses are 2–4 μg/day in 2 divided doses or approximately one tenth of the intranasal dose necessary to control the patient's symptoms, if that is known.

Injection: 4 μg/mL
Solution, nasal: 100 μg/mL/2.4 mL bottle with calibrated intranasal tube
Spray, intranasal: 10 μg/actuation metered dose
Tablets: 0.1 mg, 0.2 mg

Continued

TABLE 85.1. Medications (continued)

Drug	Dose	Dosage Forms
Dexamethasone (Decadron, Hexadrol, Maxidex)	*IV or orally:* *Bacterial meningitis:* 0.6 mg/kg/day in 4 divided doses for the first 4 days of antibiotic therapy. It must be started at the same time or before the first dose of antibiotic. *Cerebral edema:* 1–1.5 mg/kg/day in 4 divided doses to a maximum total daily dose of 16 mg. *Antiemetic therapy (chemotherapy-induced emesis):* 20 mg/m² /day in 4 divided doses. *Airway edema or extubation:* 0.5–2 mg/kg/day in 4 divided doses beginning 24 hours before and continuing for at least 24 hours after extubation. Doses should be tapered when discontinuing long-term therapy. *Ophthalmic:* instill drops or apply ointment t.i.d. or q.i.d.	Elixir: 0.5 mg/5 mL Injection: 4 mg/mL, 10 mg/mL, 20 mg/mL, 24 mg/mL Ointment, ophthalmic: 0.05% Solution, ophthalmic: 0.05% Solution, oral: 1 mg/mL Tablets: 0.25 mg, 0.5 mg, 0.75 mg, 1 mg, 1.5 mg, 2 mg, 4 mg, 6 mg
Dextroamphetamine sulfate (Dexedrine)	*Orally:* Age 3–5: 2.5 mg/day given in the morning. Dosage may be increased 2.5 mg/day until a response is realized or side effects appear. Usual range is 0.1–0.5 mg/kg/day to a maximum of 40 mg. Age 6 or older: 5 mg/day in the morning or at noon. Dosage may be increased in 5-mg increments at weekly intervals. Usual range is 0.1–0.5 mg/kg/day to a maximum of 40 mg.	Capsules, sustained release: 5 mg, 10 mg, 15 mg Tablets: 5 mg, 10 mg

Diazepam (Diastat Rectal, Valium)	Gel, rectal (in rectal delivery system): 2.5 mg, 5 mg, 10 mg, 15 mg, 20 mg Injection: 5 mg/mL Solution, oral: 5 mg/5 mL Solution, concentrated oral: 5 mg/mL Tablets: 2 mg, 5 mg, 10 mg
	IV: *Status epilepticus:* 0.05–0.3 mg/kg administered over 2–3 minutes and repeated every 15–30 minutes to a total maximum dose of 0.75 mg/kg or 30 mg, whichever is less. May be repeated in 2–4 hours, if necessary. *Sedation:* 0.04–0.2 mg/kg every 2–4 hours to a maximum of 0.6 mg/kg within an 8-hour period. *Orally for sedation or muscle relaxant:* 0.12–0.8 mg/kg/day in 3–4 divided doses to an adult dose of 6–40 mg/day. *Rectally (round dose off to closest dose available from manufacturer):* Children 2–5 years of age: 0.5 mg/kg. Children 6–11 years of age: 0.3 mg/kg Children ≥12 years of age and adults: 0.2 mg/kg. Dose may be repeated every 4–12 hours as necessary.	
Diazoxide (Hyperstat IV, Proglycem)	Capsules: 50 mg Injection: 15 mg/mL Suspension, oral: 50 mg/mL
	IV (hypertensive emergency): 1–3 mg/kg to a maximum of 150 mg. Dose may be repeated in 5–15 minutes. *Orally (hypoglycemia due to hyperinsulinism):* Newborns and infants: initially 8 mg/kg/day in 2 or 3 divided doses. May be increased incrementally if response is inadequate to a maximum of 15 mg/kg/day. Children and adults: 3 mg/kg/day in 2 or 3 divided doses initially. May be increased to a maximum of 8 mg/kg/day.	

Continued

TABLE 85.1. Medications (continued)

Drug	Dose	Dosage Forms
Dicloxacillin (Dycill, Dynapen, Pathocil)	Orally: Children <40 kg: 25–50 mg/kg/day in 4 divided doses. Doses of 50–100 mg/kg/day in 4 divided doses are necessary for follow-up oral therapy of osteomyelitis. Children ≥40 kg and adults: 125–500 mg/dose every 6 hours.	Capsules: 250 mg, 500 mg Suspension, oral: 62.5 mg/5 ml
Didanosine [ddI (dideoxyinisine); Videx]	Orally: doses must be given at 12-hour intervals on an empty stomach, but because the drug is degraded by gastric acids, each formulation contains buffers. Infants and children: 180–300 mg/m²/day in 2 divided doses. If the tablet formulation is used, children over age 1 should receive 2 tablets per dose to assure sufficient buffering. Children under age 1 may receive doses in a single tablet. Adults: <60 kg: 125 mg (tablets) or 167 mg (buffered powder) per dose twice daily. ≥60 kg: 200 mg (tablets) or 250 mg (buffered powder) per dose twice daily.	Powder for oral solution, buffered (single-dose packets): 100 mg, 167 mg, 250 mg, 375 mg Powder for oral solution, pediatric (mixed with an antacid at the time it is dispersed by the pharmacist): 10 mg/mL tablets, buffered, chewable/dispersible: 25 mg, 50 mg, 100 mg, 150 mg
Digoxin (Lanoxicaps, Lanoxin)	Should be based on lean body weight. Dosage adjustment is required in patients with impaired renal function. Total digitalizing dose (TDD) is	Capsules, liquid filled (Lanoxicaps: 0.05 mg, 0.1 mg, 0.2 mg (90–100% bioavailable) Elixir: 0.05 mg/mL (75–87% bioavailable)

administered as follows: half TDD initially, then one fourth TDD 8–12 hours later, then one fourth TDD 8–12 hours after that. Maintenance doses are administered in 2 divided doses beginning 12 hours after the last digitalizing dose. Patients should be under continuous cardiographic monitoring during digitalization. IM doses are the same as oral doses, but that route of administration should be avoided.†

Injection: 0.1 mg/mL, 0.25 mg/mL (100% bioavailable IV)
Tablets: 0.125 mg, 0.25 mg, 0.5 mg (60–80% bioavailable)

Dimercaprol [BAL [British antilewisite]]

Deep IM:
Lead toxicity:
Severe poisoning: 4 mg/kg 6 times a day for 3–5 days.
Arsenic, mercury, or gold toxicity:
Mild:
    Days 1 and 2: 3 mg/kg q.i.d.
    Day 3: 3 mg/kg b.i.d.
    Days 4–14: 3 mg/kg every day.
Severe:
    Days 1 and 2: 3 mg/kg 6 times a day.
    Day 3: 3 mg/kg q.i.d.
    Days 4–14: 3 mg/kg b.i.d.

Injection: 100 mg/mL [3-mL ampul]

Diphenhydramine [Benadryl, Benylin, Nytol, Sleep-Eze 3, Sominex Formula 2]

IV, orally, IM:
Children: 5 mg/kg/day in 3 or 4 divided doses to a maximum of 300 mg/day.
Adults: 10–50 mg repeated as often as every 4 hours, not to exceed 400 mg/day.
The drug may cause paradoxical excitement in children.

Capsules: 25 mg, 50 mg
Elixir (14% alcohol): 12.5 mg/5 mL
Injection: 10 mg/mL, 50 mg/mL
Syrup (5% alcohol): 12.5 mg/5 mL
Tablets: 25 mg, 50 mg

Continued

TABLE 85.1. Medications (continued)

Drug	Dose	Dosage Forms
Dobutamine hydrochloride (Dobutrex)	*IV infusion:* 2–15 μg/kg/min to a maximum of 40 μg/kg/min. Start at the lower end of the range and titrate upward based on the patient's response.	Injection: 12.5 mg/mL
Docusate sodium (dioctyl sodium sulfosuccinate; Colace, D-S-S, Doxinate)	*Orally* (in 1–4 divided doses with a glass of water): Infants and children under age 3: 10–40 mg/day. Age 3–6: 20–60 mg/day. Age >6–12: 40–150 mg/day. Over age 12 and adults: 50–500 mg. Do not administer with mineral oil because absorption of the mineral oil may be increased.	Capsules: 50 mg, 100 mg, 240 mg, 250 mg Liquid: 150 mg/15 mL Solution: 50 mg/mL Syrup: 50 mg/15 mL, 60 mg/15 mL Also available in combination with stimulant laxatives, including senna, phenolphthalein, and casanthranol.
Dopamine hydrochloride (Dopastat, Intropin)	*Continuous IV infusion:* initially 1 μg/kg/min titrated upward based on patient's response to a maximum of 20 μg/kg/min in neonates or 50 μg/kg/min in all other patients. The hemodynamic effects of dopamine occur only at doses >15 μg/kg/min.	Injection in 5% dextrose: 0.8 mg/mL, 1.6 mg/mL, 3.2 mg/mL (premixed infusions) Injection: 40 mg/mL, 80 mg/mL, 160 mg/mL
Dornase alfa (Pulmozyme)	*Inhalation via approved compressor:* Children >5 years of age and adults: 2.5 mg/day.	Solution, inhalation: 2.5 mg/2.5 mL
Doxycycline (Doryx, Doxy-100, Vibramycin)	*Orally or IV:* Children under age 8: should not be used unless there is no alternative. ≥ age 8: 2–5 mg/kg/day to a maximum of 200 mg/day in 1 or 2 divided doses.	Capsules or tablets: 50 mg, 100 mg Injection: 100 mg, 200 mg

Adults: 100–200 mg/day in 1 or 2 divided doses. Inpatient treatment of PID 100 mg IV b.i.d. with cefoxitin 2 g IV every 6 hours for at least 4 days or 2 days after patient improves, whichever is longer. Doxycycline should be continued orally to complete 10–14 days of therapy.

d-Xylose (wood sugar; Xylo-Pfan)

Orally (prepared as a 5–10% aqueous solution): 14.5 g/m² to a maximum dose of 25 g. Alternatively, a dose of 500 mg/kg may be used. Infants should fast for 4–5 hours before the dose and children should fast overnight. Blood xylose levels are then measured to determine extent of intestinal absorption.

Powder for preparing oral solutions: 25 g

Edetate calcium disodium (Calcium Disodium Versenate, Calcium EDTA)

Mild to moderate lead poisoning: 25–50 mg/kg. *Severe lead poisoning:* up to 75 mg/kg/24 hr not to exceed 1.5 g/day.
Usual dosage (children):
Asymptomatic lead toxicity:
Initial: up to 1 g/m²/24 hr in a continuous IV drip if possible or in 2–4 divided doses for 5 days. Subsequent courses: up to 50 mg/kg/24 hr in a continuous IV drip if possible or in 2–4 divided doses for 3–5 days.
Symptomatic lead toxicity or lead encephalopathy:
Initial: up to 1.5 g/m²/24 hr in a continuous IV drip if possible or in 6 divided doses for 5–7 days; give with dimercaprol (BAL).

Injection: 200 mg/mL
For intravenous infusion, dilute to a maximum concentration of 5 mg/mL with D_5W or normal saline.
Infusions should be administered either continuously or over 1–2 hours if intermittent doses are used. Rapid infusion may increase intracranial pressure.

Continued

TABLE 85.1. Medications (continued)

Drug	Dose	Dosage Forms
Edetate calcium disodium (Calcium Disodium Versenate, Calcium EDTA) (continued)	Subsequent courses: as for asymptomatic toxicity above.	
Edrophonium (Enlon, Reversol, Tensilon)	*Myasthenia gravis diagnosis:* Infants: Initially 0.1 mg; if no response, follow with an additional 0.4 mg for a maximum total dose of 0.5 mg. Children: Initial: 0.04 mg/kg followed by 0.16 mg/kg if no response; maximum total dose is 10 mg. Adults: 0.2 mg/kg up to 10 mg. Administer 2 mg initially, then titrate dose. *Titration of therapy:* 0.04 mg/kg one time; if strength improves, an increase in neostigmine or pyridostigmine dose is indicated.	Injection: 10 mg/mL May precipitate cholinergic crisis.
Enalapril, enalaprilat (Vasotec)	*Orally:* initially 0.1 mg/kg/day in 1 or 2 divided doses to the usual adult dose of 2.5–5 mg/kg/day. Dosage may be increased as required to a maximum of 0.5 mg/kg/day or 40 mg. *IV:* 5–10 μg/kg (up to 0.625–1.25 mg) may be administered every 8–24 hours as necessary for control of hypertension.	Injection: 1.25 mg/mL Tablets: 2.5 mg, 5 mg, 10 mg, 20 mg

Dosage must be decreased in patients with compromised renal function and also should be decreased in patients who are hyponatremic or volume depleted, in severe congestive heart failure, or in those who are receiving diuretics.

The oral dosage form (enalapril) is a prodrug that is not stable in aqueous media. The injectable dosage form (enalaprilat) is the active form, but is not absorbed from the GI tract.

Enoxaparin (Lovenox)

Injection: 100 mg/mL

SC:

Prophylaxis:

Infants <2 months of age: 0.75 mg/kg/dose every 12 hours

Infants ≥2 months of age and children: 0.5 mg/kg/dose every 12 hours.

Adults >45 kg: 30 mg every 12 hours

Treatment of DVT or PE:

Infants <2 months of age: 1.5 mg/kg/dose every 12 hours

Infants ≥2 months of age and children: 1 mg/kg/dose every 12 hours

Adults >45 kg: 1 mg/kg/dose every 12 hours. Doses should be adjusted based on anti-factor Xa levels.

Epinephrine (Adrenalin, Sus-Phrine, Vaponefrin)

IV for asystole, or pulseless arrest:

Neonates: 0.01–0.03 mg/kg (0.1–0.3 mL/kg of a 1:10,000 solution) every 3–5 minutes as necessary.

Aerosol: 0.2–0.3 mg/spray, depending on brand (Bronkaid Mist, Primatene Mist, AsthmaHaler Mist)

Injection: 1:10,000 (0.1 mg/mL), 1:1,000 (1 mg/mL)

Continued

TABLE 85.1. Medications (continued)

Drug	Dose	Dosage Forms
Epinephrine (Adrenalin, Sus-Phrine, Vaponefrin) (continued)	Infants to adults: 0.1 mg/kg to a maximum of 1 mg; may be repeated every 3–5 minutes as necessary. A continuous infusion may be started at a dose of 0.1–1 μg/kg/min and titrated to effect. Nebulization: 0.25–0.5 mL of a 2.25% racemic epinephrine solution diluted in 2.5–3 mL of normal saline for inhalation. SC for allergic reactions: 0.01 mg/kg to a maximum dose of 0.5 mg (of the 1:1,000 solution). For a prolonged effect, 0.005 mL/kg/dose of the 1:200 suspension in glycerin (equivalent to 0.025 mg/kg/dose) may be given every 8–12 hours.	Injection pre-filled automatic syringe: 1:200 (EpiPen delivers 0.3 mg IM, EpiPen Jr. delivers 0.15 mg IM) Solution, racemic for inhalation: 2.25% (AsthmaNefrin, S-2, Vaponefrin)
Epoetin alfa (erythropoietin; Epogen, EPO, r-HuEPO)	IV or SC: initially 50–100 U/kg administered 1–3 times weekly until the hematocrit reaches 30–33%. Dosage should be lowered if the hematocrit exceeds that range or increases by more than 4 points in a 2-week period. It may be increased if the hematocrit does not reach the target range or fails to increase by 5–6 points in an 8-week period. The usual maintenance dose is 25 U/kg 3 times weekly. Hematocrit and serum iron levels should be monitored frequently. Blood pressure should also be monitored frequently.	Injection: 2,000 U/mL, 4000 U/mL, 10,000 U/mL

Ergocalciferol (vitamin D$_2$, activated ergosterol; Calciferol, Drisdol)	$1 \mu g = 40$ U. *Orally:* Healthy infants and children: 400 U/day. Infants and children with malabsorption syndromes: 1,000 U/day. Children with liver disease: 4,000–8,000 U/day. Children with vitamin D–dependent rickets: 3,000–5,000 U/day. Nutritional rickets with normal absorption: 1,000–5,000 U/day; with malabsorption: 10,000–25,000 U/day. *IM:* should be retained for patients with rickets due to severe vitamin D deficiency. The dose for vitamin D–resistant rickets ranges from 50,000–500,000 U/day, for hypoparathyroidism from 50,000–200,000 U/day, and for familial hypophosphatemia from 10,000–80,000 U/day. The range between therapeutic and toxic doses is narrow. Patients must be closely monitored.	Capsules: 50,000 U (1.25 mg) Injection (in sesame oil): 500,000 U/mL (12.5 mg/mL) Solution, oral: 8,000 U/mL (200 μg/mL)

Erythromycin (E-Mycin, Ery-Tab, Eryc, Erythrocin, E.E.S., Ilosone, Pediamycin)	*Orally* (do not exceed 2 g/day):
	 Neonates: 20–30 mg/kg/day in 2 or 3 divided doses.
	 Infants and children:
	  Base or ethylsuccinate: 30–50 mg/kg/day in 3 or 4 divided doses.
	  Estolate: 20–50 mg/kg/day in 3 or 4 divided doses.
		Base:
		 Capsules, enteric-coated pellets; 250 mg
		 Ointment, ophthalmic: 0.5%
		 Solution, topical: 1.5%, 2%
		 Tablets, enteric coated: 250 mg, 333 mg, 500 mg
		 Tablets, film coated: 250 mg, 500 mg
		Estolate:
		 Capsules: 250 mg

Continued

TABLE 85.1. Medications (continued)

Drug	Dose	Dosage Forms
Erythromycin (E-Mycin, Ery-Tab, Eryc, Erythrocin, E.E.S., Ilosone, Pediamycin) (continued)	Adults: Base, estolate, or stearate: 250–500 mg every 6–12 hours. Ethylsuccinate: 400–800 mg every 6–12 hours. Endocarditis prophylaxis (penicillin-allergic patients): 20 mg/kg to a maximum of 1 g 2 hours before the procedure and 10 mg/kg to a maximum of 500 mg 6 hours later. Bowel preparation (erythromycin base, only): 20 mg/kg to a maximum of 1 g administered at 1:00, 2:00, and 11:00 P.M. on the day before surgery, usually combined with neomycin and mechanical cleansing of the bowel. IV: 15–20 mg/kg/day to a maximum of 4 g/day administered in 4 divided doses. Ophthalmic ointment for prophylaxis of neonates: apply a 0.5–1 cm ribbon of the ointment to each conjunctival sac. Topically for acne: apply to the affected areas b.i.d. The skin should be washed, rinsed well, and dried before applying the erythromycin. Keep away from the eyes, nose, and mouth.	Suspension: 125 mg/5 mL, 250 mg/5 mL Tablets: 500 mg Ethylsuccinate: Suspension: 200 mg/5 mL, 400 mg/5 mL Tablets, chewable: 200 mg Tablets: 400 mg Stearate: Tablets: 250 mg, 500 mg
Erythromycin and sulfisoxazole (Eryzole, Pediazole)	Orally (based on the erythromycin content): Up to age 2 months: 40–50 mg/kg/day in 3 or 4 divided doses to a maximum of 2 g/day.	Suspension: 200 mg erythromycin and 600 mg sulfisoxazole per 5 mL

	Alternatively, the following patient weights may be used: 8–15 kg: 2.5 mL every 6 hours. 16–23 kg: 5 mL every 6 hours. 24–44 kg: 7.5 mL every 6 hours. ≥45 kg: 10 mL every 6 hours.	
Ethacrynic acid (Edecrin)	*Orally:* 1 mg/kg administered 1–2 times daily. Do not exceed the usual adult dose of 50–100 mg/day. *IV:* 0.4–1 mg/kg up to 50 mg administered 1 or 2 times daily. Serum electrolytes must be closely monitored during ethacrynic acid therapy.	Injection: 50 mg Tablets: 25 mg, 50 mg
Ethambutol (Myambutol)	*Orally* (patient should be old enough to cooperate with an eye exam; optic neuritis is an adverse effect): Children: 15 mg/kg/day in a single dose. Adolescents and adults: 15–25 mg/kg/day in a single dose. Do not exceed 2.5 g/day.	Tablets: 100 mg, 400 mg
Ethosuximide (Zarontin)	*Orally:* Under age 6: 15 mg/kg/day in 2 divided doses to a maximum of 250 mg/dose. ≥ age 6: 250 mg b.i.d. Dose may be increased by 250 mg/day every 4–7 days to a maximum of 1.5 g/day or 40 mg/kg/day.	Capsules: 250 mg Syrup: 250 mg/5 mL
Fentanyl citrate (Sublimaze)	*IV* (slowly over a period of 3–5 minutes to avoid chest wall rigidity and to titrate to effect):	Injection: 50 μg/mL Lozenge, oral transmucosal (Oralet): 100 μg, 200 μg, 300 μg, 400 μg

Continued

TABLE 85.1. Medications (continued)

Drug	Dose	Dosage Forms
Fentanyl citrate (Sublimaze) (continued)	Children: 1–2 μg/kg may be repeated at 30–60-minute intervals. For continuous therapy, after a bolus dose, a dose of 1 μg/kg/hr initially may be increased or decreased as necessary to response. Older children and adults: 0.5–1 μg/kg (25–50 μg) may be repeated at 30–60-minute intervals. The doses listed are analgesic/sedation doses. Doses used for general anesthesia may be higher. Orally (Orally): Children ≥2 years of age who weigh 15–40 kg: 5–15 μg/kg to a maximum of 400 μg. Children ≥40 kg and adults: 5 μg/kg to a maximum of 400 μg.	
Ferrous sulfate (Feosol, Fer-In-Sol)	Orally (doses are expressed as elemental iron; ferrous sulfate contains 20% iron): Iron deficiency anemia: Children: 3–6 mg/kg/day depending on the severity of the deficiency. Higher doses should be administered in 3 divided doses; moderate doses may be administered in 2 divided doses to avoid GI upset. For prophylaxis, 1–2 mg/kg/day in a single dose may be used. Adults: 120–240 mg iron daily in 2–4 divided doses. For prophylaxis, 60 mg iron daily as a single dose.	Capsules: 50 mg Fe Drops: 15 mg Fe/0.6 mL Elixir: 44 mg Fe/5 mL Syrup: 18 mg Fe/5 mL Tablets: 60 mg Fe, 65 mg Fe

Administration between meals increases absorption, but may result in more GI upset. Do not administer with antacids, eggs, or milk because they may decrease absorption of the iron.

Fluconazole (Diflucan)

Orally or IV:
Oropharyngeal or esophageal candidiasis: 6 mg/kg (up to 200 mg) on the first day; then 3 mg/kg/day (up to 100 mg).
Systemic candidiasis or cryptococcal meningitis: 12 mg/kg (up to 400 mg) on the first day; then 6 mg/kg/day (up to 200 mg).
Prevention of candidiasis in bone marrow transplant: 12 mg/kg/day (up to 400 mg) beginning several days before anticipated onset of neutropenia and continued until 7 days after neutrophil count is >1,000/mm^3.
Vaginal candidiasis: 150 mg as a single dose.
Dosage should be adjusted in patients with renal dysfunction.

Injection: 2 mg/mL (ready to administer)
Suspension: 10 mg/mL, 40 mg/mL
Tablets: 50 mg, 100 mg, 150 mg, 200 mg

Flucytosine (Ancobon)

Orally:
Neonates: 50–100 mg/kg/day in 1–2 divided doses.
Children and adults: 50–150 mg/kg/day in 4 divided doses. Dosage must be adjusted in renal impairment.

Capsules: 250 mg, 500 mg

Fludrocortisone (Florinef)

Orally:
Infants and children: 0.05–0.1 mg/day.
Adults: 0.05–0.2 mg/day.

Tablets: 0.1 mg

Continued

TABLE 85.1. Medications (continued)

Drug	Dose	Dosage Forms
Flumazenil (Mazicon, Romazicon)	*IV:* Children (little information is available on dosing in children)—The following are guidelines only: 0.01 mg/kg (to a maximum of 0.2 mg) initially, followed by 0.005 mg/kg (to a maximum of 0.2 mg) every minute until a total cumulative dose of 1 mg has been reached. Adults: *Reversal of sedation:* 0.2 mg over 15 seconds; may repeat 0.2-mg dose every 60 seconds to a maximum of 1 mg. May repeat doses every 20 minutes to a maximum of 3 mg in 1 hour. *Benzodiazepine overdose:* 0.2 mg over 30 seconds, then 0.3 mg over 30 seconds if desired level of consciousness is not reached. Additional 0.5-mg doses may be given every minute until a cumulative dose of 3 mg has been reached. If a partial response is noted, further 0.5-mg doses may be given until a cumulative dose of 5 mg is reached. Resedation may occur in patients who received long-acting benzodiazepines.	Injection: 0.1 mg/mL
Flunisolide (AeroBid, Nasalide)	*Intranasal spray:* Age 6–14: 1 spray in each nostril t.i.d. or 2 sprays in each nostril b.i.d. initially. Maintenance dose is usually 1 spray in each nostril daily.	Oral inhalation: 250 µg/spray Spray, intranasal: 25 µg/metered spray

Continued

Over age 14 and adults: 2 sprays in each nostril b.i.d. or t.i.d. initially. After symptoms are controlled, dosage should be decreased to the lowest dose that will prevent symptoms from recurring. That may be as little as 1 spray in each nostril once daily for perennial rhinitis. The maximum dose is 4 sprays to each nostril daily.

Oral inhalation:
Children 6–15 years of age: 2 inhalations twice a day.
Adults: 2 inhalations twice a day initially, increasing to a maximum of 8 inhalations daily.
Improvement in symptoms may take from several days to several weeks to occur, but therapy should not be continued for more than 3 weeks in the absence of efficacy. Dosage should be decreased to the lowest effective dose when symptoms abate.

Fluocinolone acetonide (Fluonid, Flurosyn, Synalar, Synemol)	*Topically:* apply a thin layer to the affected area b.i.d. to q.i.d. Use the lowest effective potency product. Absorption is greater if the product is covered by anything that is occlusive (plastic pants, tight diapers).	Cream: 0.01%, 0.025%, 0.2% Ointment: 0.025% Shampoo: 0.01% Solution: 0.01%
Fluoride (Fluoritab, Karidium, Luride, Pediaflor)	*Orally:* dosage should be based on the fluoride content of the water supply. Long-term supplementation in areas with fluoridated water may result in dental fluorosis and osseous changes.*	Most multivitamin combinations are available in formulations containing appropriate amounts of fluoride (Poly-Vi-Flor drops or chewable tablets, Tri-Vi-Flo drops, Vi-Daylin/F drops and chewable tablets).

TABLE 85.1. Medications (continued)

Drug	Dose	Dosage Forms
Fluoride (Fluoritab, Karidium, Luride, Pediaflor) (continued)	Fluoride content of drinking water <0.3 ppm: Birth–6 months: do not supplement. >6 months–3 years: 0.25 mg/day. >3–6 years: 0.5 mg/day. >6–16 years: 1 mg/day. Fluoride content of drinking water 0.3–0.6 ppm: Birth–3 years: do not supplement. 3–6 years: 0.25 mg/day. >6–16 years: 0.5 mg/day. Fluoride content of drinking water >0.6 ppm: do not supplement. *Dental gel:* usually applied by a dentist. *Rinses:* over-the-counter rinses may be used for patients over age 6 on a daily basis and contain 0.01–0.02% fluoride.	Products containing only fluoride: Drops: 0.125 mg/drop, 0.25 mg/drop, 0.5 mg/mL Solution: 0.2 mg/mL (may be used orally or as a rinse) Tablets, chewable: 0.5 mg, 1 mg
Fluticasone (Flonase, Flovent)	*Intranasal metered dose spray* Children ≥4 years of age: 1 spray in each nostril daily. Dosage may be increased to 2 sprays in each nostril daily if necessary. Adults: 2 sprays in each nostril daily. *Oral aerosol inhalation:* Children ≥12 years of age and adults: 88 µg twice daily for patients not previously treated with corticosteroids to a maximum of 440 µg twice daily in patients who were previously treated with inhaled corticosteroids.	Powder, oral inhalation: 50 µg (delivers 44 µg), 100 µg (delivers 88 µg), 250 µg (delivers 220 µg) Spray oral inhalation: 44 µg/actuation, 110 µg/actuation, 220 µg/actuation Suspension, nasal: 50 µg/actuation

	Oral powder inhalation: Children 4–12 years of age: 50 µg twice daily to a maximum of 100 µg twice daily. Children >12 years of age and adults: 100 µg twice a day up to 500 µg twice a day based on the patient's previous corticosteroid needs. Patients who previously required oral corticosteroids may require up to 1,000 µg twice a day.	
Folic acid (Folvite)	*Orally, parenterally:* Infants: 50 µg/day. Age 1–10: 1 mg/day initially, then 0.1–0.4 mg/day. Age 11 and over, and adults: 1 mg/day initially, then 0.5 mg/day.	Injection: 5 mg/mL, 10 mg/mL Tablets: 0.1 mg, 0.4 mg, 0.8 mg, 1 mg
Fosphenytoin—See phenytoin		
Furosemide (Lasix)	*Orally, IV, or IM:* Premature neonates (oral absorption may be poor): 1–2 mg/kg every 12–24 hours. Oral doses up to 4 mg/kg may be used. Children: 1–2 mg/kg every 6–12 hours but not to exceed 6 mg/kg/day. Adults: 20–80 mg/day in divided doses to a maximum of 600 mg/day. Serum electrolyte levels should be monitored closely.	Injection: 10 mg/mL Solution: 10 mg/mL, 40 mg/5 mL Tablets: 20 mg, 40 mg, 80 mg
Gabapentin (Neurontin)	*Orally (as add-on therapy):* Patients 3–12 years of age: 10–15 mg/kg/day in 3 divided doses. The maintenance dose for patients 3–4 years of age is usually about 40 mg/kg/day and for patients 5 years and older is 25–35 mg/kg/day.	Capsules: 100 mg, 300 mg, 400 mg Solution: 250 mg/5 mL

Continued

TABLE 85.1. Medications (continued)

Drug	Dose	Dosage Forms
Gabapentin (Neurontin) (continued)	Age >12yr–adults: initially, 300 mg on day 1, followed by rapid titration to 300 mg t.i.d. The usual maintenance dosage range is 900–1,800 mg/day in 3 divided doses to a maximum daily dose of 3,600 mg. It is not necessary to monitor gabapentin levels or the levels of other antiepileptic drugs the patient may be taking because there are no significant drug interactions. Withdrawal of gabapentin therapy should be accomplished over a period of at least 1 week.	
Ganciclovir (Cytovene, DHPG)	IV (as an infusion over 1 hour): Induction: 10 mg/kg/day in 2 divided doses for 2–3 weeks. Maintenance: 5 mg/kg/day as a single dose for 7 days a week to 6 mg/kg/day for 5 days a week. Orally: Maintenance therapy only: in adults, a dose of 1,000 mg t.i.d. with food is used. There are no guidelines for oral use in children. Dosage must be adjusted in patients with renal dysfunction.	Capsules: 250 mg Injection: 500-mg vial

Continued

Gentamicin (Garamycin)

IV or IM (in obese patients it should be based on ideal, rather than actual, body weight):

Neonates under age 7 days:
  <1,000 g: 2.5 mg/kg every 24 hours.
  1,000–1,500 g: 2.5 mg/kg every 18 hours.
  >1,500 g: 2.5 mg/kg every 12 hours.

Neonates over age 7 days:
  1,200–2,000 g: 2.5 mg/kg every 8–12 hours.
  >2,000 g: 2.5 mg/kg every 8 hours.

ECMO patients: 2.5 mg/kg every 18 hours.

Infants and children under age 5: 2.5 mg/kg every 8 hours.

Age 5–10: 2 mg/kg every 8 hours.

Over age 10 and adults: 5 mg/kg/day administered in 3 divided doses.

Ophthalmic solution: 1–2 drops in the affected eye every 2–4 hours. More frequent application (up to every hour) may be used initially in severe infections.

Ophthalmic ointment: apply a ribbon of ointment to the eye b.i.d. or t.i.d.

Intrathecal/intraventricular (use only a preservative-free product):
  Neonates: 1 mg/day as a single dose.
  Children over age 3 months: 1–2 mg/day.
  Older children and adults: 4–8 mg/day.

Dosage must be adjusted in renal dysfunction.

Serum levels should be monitored during therapy in all patients.

Injection: 10 mg/mL, 40 mg/mL
Ointment, ophthalmic: 0.3%
Solution, ophthalmic: 0.3%

TABLE 85.1. Medications (continued)

Drug	Dose	Dosage Forms
Glucagon	*IV, IM, or SC:* *Hypoglycemia* (dose may be repeated in 20 minutes if necessary): Neonates: 0.025 mg/kg/dose. Children: 0.025–0.1 mg/kg/dose to a maximum of 1 mg. Adults: 0.5–1 mg/dose. *Infusion for the treatment of neonatal hyperinsulinemia:* 1–5 ng/kg/min to start and titrate to response. The infusion must be delivered by a pump to maintain a steady rate. Glucose levels must be monitored hourly until they are stable in an acceptable range. Rebound hypoglycemia may occur if the infusion is suddenly discontinued. *Diagnostic aid during radiography:* 0.25–2 mg 10 minutes before the procedure.	Injection: 1 mg-vial, 10 mg-via (1 mg = 1 U)
Glycopyrrolate (Robinul)	*IM:* *Preoperatively:* Under age 2: 4.4–8.8 μg/kg 30–60 minutes before the procedure. ≥ age 2–adults: 4.4 μg/kg 30–60 minutes before the procedure. *Orally:* *To control respiratory secretions* (glycopyrrolate is poorly absorbed from the GI tract): 50 μg/kg administered t.i.d. or q.i.d.	Injection: 0.2 mg/mL Tablets: 1 mg, 2 mg

Continued

Gonadorelin HCl [Factrel, LHRH [luteinizing hormone-release hormone], GnRH [gonadotropin-releasing hormone]]	*Reversal of neuromuscular blockade:* 0.2 mg for each 1 mg neostigmine or 5 mg pyridostigmine administered. IV: 2–5 μg/kg to a maximum of 100 μg.	Injection: 100 μg
Griseofulvin (Microsize products: Fulvicin U/F, Grifulvin V, Grisactin; Ultramicrosize products: Fulvicin P/G, Grisactin Ultra, Gris-PEG)	Absorption of griseofulvin from the GI tract is somewhat dependent on the size of the particles of griseofulvin. The ultramicrosize is absorbed about 1.5 times as well as the microsize. Absorption is also increased by administering the dose with a fatty meal. Duration of therapy is dependent on the site of infection and ranges from 2–4 weeks for tinea corporis, to 4–8 weeks for tinea capitis and tinea pedis, to 3–6 months for tinea unguium. Children: Microsize: 15–20 mg/kg/day in 1 or 2 divided doses. Ultramicrosize: 10–13 mg/kg/day in 1 or 2 divided doses. Older children and adults: Microsize: 500 mg–1 g/day in a single or 2 divided doses. Use higher dose for tinea pedis or tinea unguium. Ultramicrosize: 660–750 mg/day in a single or 2 divided doses. During long-term therapy, renal, hepatic, and hematopoietic function should be monitored. Patients should also be cautioned to avoid sunlight because photosensitivity reactions have occurred.	Microsize: Capsules: 125 mg, 250 mg Suspension: 125 mg/5 mL Tablets: 250 mg, 500 mg Ultramicrosize: Tablets: 125 mg, 165 mg, 250 mg, 330 mg

TABLE 85.1. Medications (continued)

Drug	Dose	Dosage Forms
Haloperidol (Haldol)	*Orally:* Age 3–12: *Agitation or hyperkinesia:* 0.01–0.03 mg/kg/day once daily. *Tourette disorder:* 0.05–0.075 mg/kg/day in 2 or 3 divided doses. *Psychotic disorders:* 0.05–0.15 mg/kg/day in 2 or 3 divided doses. IM: 1–3 mg every 4–8 hours; maximum, 0.1 mg/kg/day. Dose should be individually adjusted to patient. Not recommended for children under age 3. Oral dosage range is 2–100 mg/24 hr.	Injection: 5 mg/mL Solution, concentrated oral: 2 mg/mL Tablets: 1 mg, 2 mg, 5 mg, 1C mg
Heparin sodium	*IV:* *Anticoagulation:* Children and adults: Continuous infusion: 50 U/kg then 15–25 U/kg/hr. Dose may be increased by 2–4 U/kg/hr every 6–8 hours based on the results of the APTT. Intermittent infusion: 50–100 U/kg every 4 hours. This method is less desirable than continuous infusion.	Injection: 1,000 U, 5,000 U, 10 000 U, 20,000 U, 40,000 U/mL Injection, preservative-free: 1,000 U, 5,000 U, 10,000 U/mL Solution, lock flush: 10 U/mL, C0 U/mL (available preserved and preservative-free)

Line flushing:
Central catheters: may be flushed as infrequently as once daily with 2–3 mL of solution containing 10 U/mL for patients under age 1 or 100 U/mL for patients age 1 or older.
Peripheral catheters, locks: usually flushed every 6–8 hours with 10 U/mL concentration with a volume determined by the length of the catheter, but usually about 1 mL.
Lines should be flushed before and after medication or blood administration or if blood is seen in the catheter.
Preservative-free heparin solutions should be used for all line flushes in children under age 2 months.

Hydralazine (Apresoline)

Injection: 20 mg/mL
Tablets: 10 mg, 25 mg, 50 mg, 100 mg

Orally:
Children: 0.75–1 mg/kg/day in 2–4 divided doses, but not to exceed 25 mg/dose initially. May be increased slowly over 3 or 4 weeks to a maximum of 7.5 mg/kg/day (or 200 mg).
Adults: initially 10 mg q.i.d. May be increased by 10–25 mg/dose every 2–5 days to a maximum of 300 mg/day.

IV (ratio of oral to IV dosing is about 4:1):
Children: initially 0.1–0.2 mg/kg (to a maximum of 20 mg) every 4–6 hours. May be increased to a maximum of 1.7–3.5 mg/kg/day.
Adults: initially 10–20 mg every 4–6 hours. May be increased to 40 mg/dose. Dose must be adjusted in renal impairment.

Continued

TABLE 85.1. Medications (continued)

Drug	Dose	Dosage Forms
Hydrochlorothiazide (Esidrix, HydroDIURIL, Oretic)	*Orally* (chlorothiazide, which is available as a suspension, is usually a better choice for children requiring low doses): Children over age 6 months: 2 mg/kg/day in 2 divided doses. Adults: 25–100 mg/day in 1 or 2 doses.	Tablets: 25 mg, 50 mg, 100 mg
Hydrocortisone (Cortef, Cortenema, Cortifoam, Cortril, Hydrocortone, Solu-Cortef)	*Orally:* *Congenital adrenal hyperplasia:* initially 30–36 mg/m²/day divided as one third in the morning and two thirds in the evening or one fourth in the morning, one fourth midday, and half in the evening. *Physiologic replacement:* 0.5–0.75 mg/kg/day. *Antiinflammatory:* 2.5–10 mg/kg/day in 3 or 4 divided doses. *IV:* *Adrenal insufficiency:* Infants and young children: 1–2 mg/kg bolus, then 25–150 mg/day in 3 or 4 divided doses. Older children: 1–2 mg/kg bolus, then 150–250 mg/day in 3 or 4 divided doses. Adults: 15–240 mg/day in 1 or 2 divided doses. *Antiinflammatory:* Infants and children: 1–5 mg/kg/day in 2–4 divided doses. Adults: 15–240 mg every 12 hours.	Cream, topical: 0.5%, 1%, 2.5% Enema: 100 mg/60 mL (Cortenema) Foam, intrarectal: 90 mg/full applicator (Cortifoam), rectal/anal 1% (Proctofoam-HC) Injection (sodium phosphate): 50 mg/mL Injection (sodium succinate): 100-mg, 250-mg, 500-mg, 1-g vials Ointment, topical: 0.5%, 1%, 2.5% Suspension (cypionate): 10 mg/5 mL Tablets: 5 mg, 10 mg, 20 mg

Shock (succinate salt):
  Children: 50 mg/kg then in 4 hours or every
    24 hours as needed.
  Adults: 500 mg–2 g every 2–6 hours.
Rectal retention enemas: 1 enema nightly for 21 days.
  May be continued for a longer period if effective or
  discontinued if no effect is seen.
Intrarectal foam: 1 full applicator rectally nightly or
  b.i.d. for 2 or 3 weeks. Absorption of hydrocortisone
  may be greater from the foam formulation than the
  enema. Discontinue if not effective after 3 weeks.
Topically (low-potency corticosteroid in most
  formulations): apply a thin layer to the affected area
  t.i.d. or q.i.d.

Hydromorphone (Dilaudid)

IV:
  Young children: 0.015–0.03 mg/kg every
    3–4 hours.
  Older children and adults: 1–4 mg every 3–4 hours.
Orally:
  Young children: 0.04–0.07 mg/kg every 3–4 hours.
  Older children and adults: 1–6 mg every 3–4 hours
    depending on size and pain severity.
To convert a patient from oral to IV therapy: start with a
  ratio of 5:1. Ratios of up to 2:1 may be required in
  some patients on long-term chronic therapy.
To convert a patient from IV to oral therapy: in a patient
  who is receiving a stable dose, use an IV to oral ratio
  of 1:3.

Injection: 1 mg/mL, 2 mg/mL, 4 mg/mL, 10 mg/mL
Solution, oral: 1 mg/mL
Suppositories, rectal: 3 mg
Tablets: 2 mg, 4 mg, 8 mg

Continued

TABLE 85.1. Medications (continued)

Drug	Dose	Dosage Forms
Hydromorphone (Dilaudid) (continued)	Equianalgesic doses: Oral: 7.5 mg hydromorphone = 30 mg morphine. Parenteral: 1.5 mg hydromorphone = 10 mg morphine.	
Hydroxyzine (Atarax, Vistaril)	Orally: Children: 2 mg/kg/day in 3 or 4 doses. Adults: 100–400 mg/day in 3 or 4 doses. Use lower doses for pruritus and higher doses for sedation. Parenterally: the use of hydroxyzine parenterally (IM, IV, SC) has been associated with severe adverse effects at the site of the injection. The reactions are characterized by local discomfort, sterile abscess, erythema, and tissue necrosis. Phlebitis and hemolysis have been reported after IV administration. The manufacturers recommend administration by deep IM injection into a well-developed large muscle. SC infiltration of the drug from an IM injection or extravasation of an IV injection must be avoided.	Capsule (pamoate): 25 mg, 50 mg, 100 mg Injection for IM use: 25 mg/mL, 50 mg/mL Solution, oral: 10 mg/5 mL Suspension, oral (pamoate): 25 mg/5 mL Tablets: 10 mg, 25 mg, 50 mg, 100 mg
Ibuprofen (Advil, Motrin, Nuprin)	Orally: Antipyretic: Age 6 months–12 years (repeat doses up to every 6 hours): Temperature <39°C (102.2°F): 5 mg/kg/dose. Temperature ≥39°C (102.2°F): 10 mg/kg/dose.	Suspension, oral: 100 mg/5 mL Tablets: 200 mg, 300 mg, 400 mg, 600 mg, 800 mg

Over age 12 and adults: 200–400 mg/dose to a maximum of 1,200 mg/day.
Juvenile rheumatoid arthritis: 30–70 mg/kg/day in 4 divided doses to a maximum of 2400 mg/day.
Adult antiinflammatory dose: 400–800 mg every 6–8 hours to a maximum of 3200 mg/day.

Imipenem and cilastatin (Primaxin)

IV infusion over 1 hour (expressed as mg of imipenem):
Children: 50–100 mg/kg/day in 4 divided doses to a maximum of 4 g/day.
Adults: 2–4 g/day in 3 or 4 divided doses.
Dosage adjustment is required in renal impairment.

Injection: imipenem 250 mg and cilastatin 50 mg, imipenem 500 mg and cilastatin 500 mg

Imipramine (Tofranil)

Orally:
Enuresis in children under age 6: initially 25 mg 1 hour before bedtime nightly. Dose may be increased to 50 mg in children age 6–12 or 75 mg in children over age 12 if the initial dose is ineffective.
Depression:
Children: 1.5 mg kg/day in 1–4 divided doses initially. May be increased in increments of about 1 mg/kg/day to a maximum of 5 mg/kg/day.
Adolescents: 25–50 mg/day increased gradually to a maximum of 100 mg/day in a single or divided doses.
Adults: 75–100 mg/day increased gradually to a maximum of 300 mg/day in a single or divided doses.

Tablets: 10 mg, 25 mg, 50 mg

Continued

TABLE 85.1. Medications (continued)

Drug	Dose	Dosage Forms
Imipramine (Tofranil) (continued)	Dosage should be decreased to the minimum effective dose after symptom control has been achieved. *Doses used to treat pain:* generally lower than those used in the treatment of depression. A starting dose of 0.2–0.4 mg/kg/day administered at bedtime may be used initially. A gradual increase to 1–3 mg/kg/day may be necessary for some patients. Administration of the total daily dose at bedtime may decrease the daytime sedative effects.	
Immune globulin, intramuscular	IM: *Measles prophylaxis:* 0.25 mL/kg within 6 days of exposure. In immunocompromised patients, use 0.5 mL/kg (15 mL maximum). *Hepatitis A preexposure prophylaxis:* Risk of exposure within 3 months: 0.02 mL/kg. Risk of exposure greater than 3 months: 0.06 mL/kg. *Hepatitis A postexposure:* 0.02 mL/kg given within 2 weeks of exposure. *Immunodeficiency:* IV has largely replaced use of the IM form. An initial dose of 1.2 mL/kg is followed with doses of 0.6 mL/kg at 2–4-week intervals. The usual maximum volumes are 20–30 mL in infants and small children and 30–50 mL in adults.	Injection, IM: 165 ± 15 mg (of protein) per mL (2 mL and 10 mL)

Immune globulin, intravenous (Gamimune N, Gammagard S/D, Gammar-P IV, Iveegam, Polygam S/D, Sandoglobulin, Venoglobulin-I, Venoglobulin-S)	*IV as a slow infusion:* The rate of infusion varies from product to product but should always be initiated at a very slow rate and may be increased every 30 minutes to the manufacturer's maximum recommended rate or less as the patient tolerates. Infusion-related reactions usually abate if the rate of infusion is decreased. Anaphylactic hypersensitivity reactions may occur and are more likely in patients with IgA deficiency. *Immunodeficiency syndromes:* 100–400 mg/kg every 2–4 weeks. *Idiopathic thrombocytopenic purpura:* either 400 mg/kg/day for 2–5 consecutive days or 1 g/kg/day for 1 or 2 consecutive days may be used for induction. Maintenance doses are usually 400 mg/kg/dose every 4–6 weeks but may be increased to 800–1,000 mg/kg if the lower dose is insufficient and are based on platelet counts and clinical response. *Kawasaki disease:* usually 2 g/kg as a single dose. Alternatively, 400 mg/kg/day for 4 days may be used.	Gamimune N: 5% or 10% solution in vials Gammagard S/D: powder with diluent to make 5% solution Gammar-P IV: powder with diluent to make 5% solution Iveegam: powder with diluent to make 5% solution Polygam S/D: powder with diluent to make 5% solution Sandoglobulin: powder with diluent to make 3%, 6%, or 12% solution Venoglobulin-I: powder with diluent to make 5% solution Venoglobulin-S: solution 5%, 10%
Indomethacin IV (Indocin IV)	*IV push:* Further dilution of the reconstituted injection may result in precipitation of insoluble indomethacin. An initial 0.2 mg/kg/dose is followed by 2 doses based on the patient's postnatal age (PNA) *at the time of the first dose:*	Injection (sodium trihydrate): 1 mg

Continued

TABLE 85.1. Medications (continued)

Drug	Dose	Dosage Forms
Indomethacin IV (Indocin IV) (continued)	PNA <48 hours: 0.1 mg/kg at 12–24-hour intervals. PNA 2–7 days: 0.2 mg/kg at 12–24-hour intervals. PNA >7 days: 0.25 mg/kg at 12–24-hour intervals. The patient's renal and hepatic function should be monitored. Oral use in children is generally not recommended.	
Insulin	IV: Treatment of diabetic ketoacidosis: loading dose of 0.1 U/kg followed by a continuous infusion of 0.1 U/kg/hr (usual range 0.05–0.2 U/kg/hr) to maintain steady, but slow, decrease of serum glucose levels of 80–100 mg/dl/hr. Only regular insulin should be used by this route. SC: Maintenance: most patients require 0.5–1 U/kg/day in 2–4 divided doses depending on how well controlled the patient's glucose levels have been. Patients should be warned not to change insulins without prior approval of their physicians. If regular insulin is to be mixed with other types of insulin, the regular insulin should always be measured first.	All insulins below are 100 U/mL. Regular insulin: available in beef and pork; pork; human, recombinant DNA; and human, semisynthetic Isophane (NPH) insulin: available in beef and pork; pork, human, recombinant DNA Lispro (Humalog): human, recombinant DNA Prompt zinc (semilente) insulin: available in beef and pork; pork; and human, recombinant DNA Extended zinc (ultralente) insulin: available in beef and pork; and human, recombinant DNA Fixed combinations: regular insulin 30 U/mL with isophane insulin 70 U/mL; available as pork; human, recombinant DNA; and human, semisynthetic isophane insulin 50 U/mL available as human, recombinant DNA

Continued

Extemporaneously prepared doses of mixed insulins should be used as soon as possible after mixing to minimize the amount of the regular insulin that will be bound by excess protamine or zinc in the other insulin. The activity of regular insulin has a time to onset of 1/2 to 1 hour, peaks at 2–3 hours, and has a duration of 5–7 hours. The activity of isophane (NPH) insulin has a time to onset of about 1–2 hours, peaks at 4–12 hours, and has a duration of 18–24 hours.

Ipecac

Orally (followed by 10–20 mL/kg (up to 300 mL) of water. May be repeated after 20 minutes if vomiting does not occur):
Age 6–12 months: 5–10 mL.
Age >1–12 years: 15 mL.
Over age 12 years: 30 mL.
Do not administer at the same time as activated charcoal, or with milk or carbonated beverages.

Syrup

Ipratropium bromide (Atrovent)

Oral metered dose inhalation:
Children 3–14 years of age: 1–2 inhalations t.i.d.
Children >14 years of age and adults: 2 inhalations q.i.d. Maximum dose should not exceed 12 inhalations in 24 hours.

Nebulization
Children 3–14 years of age: 125–250 μg t.i.d.
Children >14 years of age and adults: 500 μg 3 to 4 times daily.

Aerosol, metered dose: 18 μg/actuation
Solution for nebulization: 0.02%, 2.5 mL

TABLE 85.1. Medications (continued)

Drug	Dose	Dosage Forms

Isoniazid (isonicotinic acid hydrazide, isonicotinyl hydrazide; INH, Nydrazid)	*Orally or IM:*
	Treatment:
	  Children: 20 mg/kg/day in 1 or 2 divided doses (up to 300 mg/day).
	  Adults: 5 mg/kg/day up to 300 mg; 10 mg/kg should be used for disseminated disease.
	Prophylaxis:
	  Children: 10 mg/kg/day in a single dose up to 300 mg/day.
	  Adults: 300 mg/day.
	Liver function should be monitored during therapy because hepatitis may occur at any time. Patients whose diets are low in milk or meat should receive pyridoxine supplements at a dose of about 10–50 mg/day.
		Injection: 100 mg/mL
		Solution, oral: 50 mg/5 mL (with sorbitol 70%)
		Tablets: 100 mg, 300 mg

Isoproterenol (Isuprel)	*IV (by continuous infusion):* 0.05–3 µg/kg/min up to 2–20 µg/min.
	Oral inhalation: 1–2 metered doses up to 6 times daily.
	Nebulization:
	  Age 2–9: 0.25 mL (1:200) in 2.5 mL normal saline solution up to every 4 hours.
	  Over age 9: 0.5 mL (1:200) in 2.5 mL normal saline solution up to every 4 hours.
		Aerosol, metered dose inhaler: 1:400 (0.25%)
		Injection: 1:5,000 (0.2 mg/mL, 1 mg/5 mL)
		Solution for inhalation: 1:200 (0.5%)

Ketoconazole (Nizoral)	*Orally* (acid must be present in the GI tract for the dissolution and absorption of ketoconazole): Children: 3.3–6.6 mg/kg/day in 1 or 2 divided doses to a maximum dose of 400 mg/day. Adults: 200–400 mg/day in a single dose. Do not administer antacids or H_2 antagonists at the same time as ketoconazole. Monitor liver function during therapy. *Topically:* apply to the affected area once or twice daily. *Shampoo for dandruff:* apply shampoo and lather, allow to remain on the scalp for at least 1 minute before rinsing. Reapply shampoo and lather again, allow to remain on the scalp for 3 minutes, and then rinse. Treatments should be done twice weekly with at least 3 days between treatments, for 4 weeks. The frequency of subsequent treatments should be determined individually.	Cream: 2% Shampoo: 2% Tablets: 200 mg
Lamivudine (Epivir)	*Orally:* Age 3 months–12 years: 4 mg/kg b.i.d., to a maximum of 150 mg b.i.d. Adolescents and adults: 150 mg b.i.d. Dosage adjustment may be necessary in patients with renal dysfunction.	Solution: 10 mg/mL Tablets: 150 mg
Leuprolide acetate (Lupron, Lupron Depot)	*SC:* *Anterior pituitary gonadotropic testing:* 10 μg/kg/dose.	Injection for SC use (Lupron): 5 mg/mL Injection, suspension for IM use (Lupron Depot): 3.75 mg, 7.5 mg

Continued

TABLE 85.1. Medications (continued)

Drug	Dose	Dosage Forms
Leuprolide acetate (Lupron, Lupron Depot) (continued)	*Precocious puberty:* 50 μg/kg/day. Dosage may be titrated upward in 10-μg/kg increments if suppression of ovarian or testicular function is incomplete. *IM for precocious puberty* (higher doses may be necessary for younger children. Doses should be based on the patient's weight and age): Girls over age 8 and boys over age 9: 0.3 mg/kg (minimum 7.5 mg) repeated every 4 weeks using the depot product. Dosage may be increased in 3.75-mg increments every 4 weeks until an effective dose is achieved. Therapy should generally be discontinued at age 11 for girls or age 12 for boys.	
Levothyroxine sodium (Levothroid, Synthroid)	*Orally:* Age 0–6 months: 8–10 μg/kg or 25–50 μg/day. Age >6–<12 months: 6–8 μg/kg or 50–75 μg/day. Age 1–5: 5–6 μg/kg or 75–100 μg/day. Age 6–12: 4–5 μg/kg or 100–150 μg/day. Over age 12 and adults: 2–3 μg/kg or >150 μg/day. *IV:* one half to three fourths of the oral dose for children or about half the oral dose for adults. The parenteral form of the drug is very unstable and should be used immediately after reconstitution without admixing with other solutions.	Injection: 200 μg, 500 μg Tablets: 25 μg, 50 μg, 75 μg, 88 μg, 100 μg, 112 μg, 125 μg, 150 μg, 175 μg, 200 μg, 300 μg

Lidocaine hydrochloride (Xylocaine)

IV for cardiac arrhythmias: 1 mg/kg loading dose followed by a continuous infusion of 20–50 μg/kg/min. The loading dose may be repeated twice at 10–15-minute intervals, if necessary.

Infiltration for local anesthesia: dose depends on procedure, degree, and duration of anesthesia required and the vascularity of the site. Maximum recommended dose is 4.5 mg/kg. Doses should not be repeated sooner than 2 hours.

Topical: apply to affected area as needed. Maximum dose should not exceed 3 mg/kg or be repeated within 2 hours. Patients treated with oral lidocaine viscous should be cautioned about the hazards of biting the numbed areas and swallowing difficulties.

Aerosol, metered dose: 10% (for use before endotracheal intubation)

Injection: 0.5%, 1%, 1.5%, 2%, 4%; 0.5% with epinephrine 1:200,000; 1% with epinephrine 1:100,000 or 1:200,000; 1.5% with epinephrine 1:200,000; 2% with epinephrine 1:100,000 or 1:200,000

Jelly: 2%
Liquid, viscous: 2%
Ointment: 2.5%, 5%
Solution, topical: 2%, 4%

Lindane (gamma benzene hexachloride; Kwell)

Topically:
Pediculosis: apply 15–30 mL of shampoo to the scalp and lather for 4–5 minutes, then rinse. The hair should be combed with a fine-toothed comb to remove nits. Treatment may be repeated after 1 week, if necessary.

Scabies: apply a thin layer of the lotion to the skin from the neck to the toes (include the head in infants). The lotion should be removed by bathing after 6 hours for infants, 6–8 hours for children or 8–12 hours for adults. Treatment may be repeated after 1 week, if necessary.

Percutaneous absorption may occur and cause toxicity. Do not apply to inflamed or raw skin.

Lotion: 1%
Shampoo: 1%

Continued

TABLE 85.1. Medications (continued)

Drug	Dose	Dosage Forms
Loperamide (Imodium)	*Orally:* *Acute diarrhea* (dosage is for the initial 24 hours): Age 2 up to age 6 (13–20 kg): 1 mg t.i.d. Age >6–8 (20–30 kg): 2 mg b.i.d. Age >8–12 (>30 kg): 2 mg t.i.d. Adults: 4 mg initially followed by 2 mg after each unformed stool to a maximum of 8 mg in 24 hours (16 mg/24 hr under a physician's care). For subsequent days, use a dose of 0.1 mg/kg for children after each loose stool, but do not exceed dosage guidelines for the first day. *Chronic diarrhea:* Children: 0.08–0.24 mg/kg/day in 2 or 3 doses daily to a maximum of 2 mg/dose. Adults: 4 mg followed by 2 mg after each unformed stool until symptoms are controlled, then decreased to the lowest dose that will control symptoms. Usual maintenance dose is 4–8 mg/day.	Capsules: 2 mg Solution, oral: 1 mg/5 mL Tablets: 2 mg
Loracarbef (Lorabid)	*Orally* (administer doses on an empty stomach): Age 6 months–12 years: *Otitis media:* 30 mg/kg/day in 2 divided doses. Administer only the suspension for otitis because it is absorbed more quickly and results in higher blood levels.	Capsules: 200 mg Suspension, oral: 100 mg/5 mL, 200 mg/5 mL

Continued

Loratadine (Claritin)

Other infections: 15 mg/kg/day in 2 divided doses.
Older children and adults: 200–400 mg/day in 2 divided doses.

Orally:
Age 2–12: 5 mg/day in a single dose.
Adults >30 kg: 10 mg/day in a single dose.

Tablets: 10 mg

Lorazepam (Ativan)

IV:
Status epilepticus:
Neonates: 0.05 mg/kg over 2–5 minutes. Dose may be repeated in 10–15 minutes.
Infants and children: 0.1 mg/kg over 2–5 minutes to a maximum of 4 mg/dose. A second dose of 0.05 mg/kg may be given.
Adolescents: 0.07 mg/kg over 2–5 minutes to a maximum of 4 mg. Dose may be repeated in 10–15 minutes.
Adults: 4 mg over 2–5 minutes. Dose may be repeated in 10–15 minutes.
Adjunct to antiemetic therapy: 0.02–0.04 mg/kg up to every 6 hours. Do not exceed a maximum of 2 mg/dose.
Orally or IV:
Anxiety and sedation:
Infants and children: 0.03–0.04 mg/kg/day, in 3–4 divided doses.
Adults: 2–6 mg/day, usually orally, in 2 or 3 divided doses.

Injection: 2 mg/mL, 4 mg/mL
Solution, oral: 2 mg/mL
Tablets: 0.5 mg, 1 mg, 2 mg

TABLE 85.1. Medications (continued)

Drug	Dose	Dosage Forms
Magnesium citrate (Citrate of Magnesia, Evac-Q-Mag)	*Orally* (chill for better palatability): Under age 6: 2–4 mL/kg. Age 6–12: 100–150 mL. Over age 12: 150–300 mL.	Solution: 300 mL (carbonated contains 3.85–4.71 mEq Mg/5 mL)
Magnesium gluconate (Almora, Magonate, Magtrate)	*Orally* (expressed in terms of mEq of magnesium): Children: 0.5–0.75 mEq/kg/day in 3 or 4 divided doses. Adults: 2.2–4.4 mEq administered b.i.d. or t.i.d.	Liquid: 1,000 mg/5 mL (54 mg Mg = 4.4 mEq Mg) Tablets: 500 mg (27 mg Mg = 2.2 mEq Mg)
Magnesium hydroxide (Milk of Magnesia)	*Orally:* Under age 2: 0.5 mL/kg/dose. Age 2–5: 5–15 mL/day. Age 6–12: 15–30 mL/day. Over age 12: 30–60 mL/day.	Suspension: contains about 13.7 mEq Mg/5 mL
Magnesium sulfate (Epsom Salts)	*IV* [expressed in terms of magnesium sulfate (and mEq Mg)]: *Hypomagnesemia* (monitor serum magnesium levels closely): Neonates: 25–50 mg/kg (0.2–0.4 mEq/kg) every 8–12 hours for 2–3 doses. Infants and children: 25–50 mg/kg (0.2–0.4 mEq/kg) every 4–6 hours for 3 or 4 doses with a maximum single dose of 2,000 mg (16 mEq). Doses up to 100 mg/kg have been used in severe hypomagnesemia.	Injection: 500 mg/mL (4 mEq magnesium = 49 mg Mg)

Continued

Adults: 1 g (8 mEq) every 6 hours for 4 doses. Doses of 2–3 g (16–24 mEq) have been used for severe hypomagnesemia.

Maintenance dose: 30–60 mg/kg/day (0.25–0.5 mEq/kg/day) in 3 or 4 divided doses.

Management of seizures or hypertension in children: 25–100 mg/kg (0.2–0.8 mEq/kg) every 4–6 hours as needed. Administer the drug slowly (over 1–2 hours) in a concentration not greater than 10 mg/mL. Blood pressure should be monitored frequently during infusions because hypotension has been reported with too-fast administration.

Mannitol (Osmitrol)

Injection: 5%, 10%, 15%, 20%, 25%

IV: initial dose of 2 g/kg followed by doses of 0.25–0.5 g/kg every 4–6 hours.

A test dose of 0.2 g/kg (to a maximum of 12.5 g) over 3–5 minutes should produce a urine flow of about 1 mL/kg/hr for 2 or 3 hours. It should be used for patients with marked oliguria or inadequate renal function.

Mebendazole (Vermox)

Tablets, chewable: 100 mg

Orally:
Over age 2 and adults:
Enterobiasis (pinworm): 100 mg as a single dose. May be repeated at 2 weeks.
Ascariasis (roundworm), trichuriasis (whipworm), hookworm, or mixed infections: 200 mg/day in 2 divided doses for 3 days. A second course may be administered 3–4 weeks later.

TABLE 85.1. Medications (continued)

Drug	Dose	Dosage Forms
Meperidine hydrochloride (Demerol)	Oral doses are about half as effective as IV doses but are generally used for less severe pain; therefore, the doses listed are for all routes of administration, but that should be kept in mind if a patient is being switched from parenteral to oral therapy. Children: 1–1.5 mg/kg every 3–4 hours. A single dose of 3 mg/kg (to a maximum of 100 mg) may be used preoperatively. Adults: 50–150 mg every 3–4 hours. Dosage adjustment is necessary in renal impairment. Long-term or high-dose therapy may result in accumulation of normeperidine, an active metabolite that is a CNS stimulant, especially in patients with renal failure.	Injection: 25 mg/mL, 50 mg/mL, 75 mg/mL, 100 mg/mL Solution, oral: 50 mg/5 mL Tablets: 50 mg, 100 mg
Meropenem (Merrem IV)	*IV:* *Intraabdominal infections:* Age 3 months–adults: 60 mg/kg/day in 3 divided doses to a maximum total daily dose of 3 g. *Meningitis:* Age 3 months–adults: 120 mg/kg/day in 3 divided doses to a maximum total daily dose of 6 g.	Injection: 500 mg, 1 g
Mesalamine (Asacol, Pentasa, Rowasa)	*Orally:* Adults: 1 g (capsules) q.i.d. or 800 mg (tablets) t.i.d.	Capsules (Pentasa): 250 mg Suspension, rectal: 4 g/60 mL

	Rectally: 4 g enema administered at bedtime daily. The enema should be retained overnight (8 hours) for best results. The oral forms of the drug are formulated with an enteric coating to slowly release the drug.	Tablets (Asacol): 400 mg
Metaproterenol (Alupent, Metaprel)	*Orally:* Under age 6: 1.3–2.6 mg/kg/day in 3 or 4 divided doses. Age 6–9 (<27 kg): 10 mg/dose t.i.d. or q.i.d. Over age 9 (>27 kg) and adults: 20 mg/dose t.i.d. or q.i.d. *Oral inhalation:* Over age 12 and adults: 2–3 inhalations every 3–4 hours, up to 12 inhalations daily. *Nebulizer:* Age 6–12: 0.1 mL of a 5% solution diluted in 0.9% sodium chloride solution to 3 mL, repeated up to every 4 hours. Over age 12 and adults: 0.2–0.3 mL of 5% solution (or 2.5 mL of 0.4% or 0.6% commercially available diluted solution) administered t.i.d. or q.i.d.	Inhalation: Aerosol: 0.65 mg/inhalation spray Solution: 5%, 0.4% in normal saline solution, 0.6% in normal saline solution Solution, oral: 10 mg/5 mL Tablets: 10 mg, 20 mg
Methylene blue (Urolene Blue)	*IV for methemoglobinemia:* 1–2 mg/kg injected slowly over a period of several minutes. The dose may be repeated in 1 hour, if necessary. *Orally for adults with chronic methemoglobinemia:* 100–300 mg/day.	Injection: 10 mg/mL Tablets: 65 mg

Continued

TABLE 85.1. Medications (continued)

Drug	Dose	Dosage Forms
Methylphenidate (Ritalin)	*Orally:* Over age 6: initially 0.3 mg/kg/day (2.5–5 mg/dose) before breakfast and lunch. That may be increased to the usual dosage range of 0.5–1 mg/kg/day or a maximum of 2 mg/kg/day or 60 mg. The sustained-release form may be given as a single dose at breakfast.	Tablets: 5 mg, 10 mg, 20 mg Tablets, extended release: 20 mg
Methylprednisolone (A-methaPred, Depo-Medrol, Medrol, Solu-Medrol)	*IV:* *Status asthmaticus:* 1 mg/kg every 6 hours. *Acute spinal cord injury:* 30 mg/kg over 15 minutes followed in 45 minutes by an infusion of 5.4 mg/kg/hr for 23 hours. *Shock:* 30 mg/kg and may be repeated every 4–12 hours, but not to continue for longer than 48–72 hours. *"Pulse" therapy for lupus nephritis in older children and adults:* 1 g/day for 3 days. A dose of 30 mg/kg every other day for 6 doses has been used for children. *Orally:* Children: 0.117–1.6 mg/kg/day in 4 divided doses. Adults: 2–60 mg/day in 4 divided doses. *Intraarticular, intralesional doses (acetate):* 4–40 mg or up to 80 mg for large joints every 1–5 weeks.	Injection (acetate; Depo-Medrol) 20 mg/mL, 40 mg/mL, 80 mg/mL Injection (sodium succinate): 40-mg, 125-mg, 500-mg, 1-g, 2-g vials Tablets: 2 mg, 4 mg, 8 mg, 16 mg, 24 mg, 32 mg

Metoclopramide (Maxolon, Octamide, Reglan)	*Orally or IV:* *Gastroesophageal reflux:* Children: initially 0.1–0.5 mg/kg/day in 4 divided doses before meals. Dosage may be increased to a maximum of 0.8 mg/kg/day. Adults: 10–15 mg 30 minutes before meals and at bedtime. *IV:* *Intubation of GI tract or radiographic exam:* Under age 6: 0.1 mg/kg. Age 6–14: 2.5–5 mg. Adults: 10 mg. *Antiemetic in chemotherapy-induced nausea:* 1–2 mg/kg administered 30 minutes before the chemotherapy and every 2–4 hours as necessary thereafter to a maximum of 3 doses. Extrapyramidal reactions are common at this dose and may be treated with diphenhydramine IV (1 mg/kg up to 50 mg) every 6 hours.	Injection: 5 mg/mL Solution, oral: 5 mg/5 mL, 10 mg/5 mL Tablets: 5 mg, 10 mg
Metolazone (Zaroxolyn)	*Orally:* Infants and children: 0.2–0.4 mg/kg/day in 1–2 divided doses. Adults: 2.5–5 mg/day for the treatment of hypertension. Edema due to cardiac or renal disease may require doses of 5–20 mg/day.	Tablets: 2.5 mg, 5 mg, 10 mg
Metronidazole (Flagyl, Protostat)	*Orally or IV:* *Anaerobic bacterial infections* (IV initially, then orally): Infants other than neonates to adults: 30 mg/kg/day in 4 divided doses, not to exceed 4 g/day.	Injection: available 5 mg/mL ready to infuse solution or 500-mg vial Tablets: 250 mg, 500 mg

Continued

TABLE 85.1. Medications (continued)

Drug	Dose	Dosage Forms

Metronidazole (Flagyl, Protostat) (continued)	*Amebiasis (usually orally):*
	  Infants and children: 35–50 mg/kg/day in 3 divided doses.
	  Adults: 500–750 mg every 8 hours.
	Other parasitic infections (usually orally):
	  Infants and children: 15–30 mg/kg/day in 3 divided doses.
	  Adults: 250 mg every 8 hours or a single 2-g dose.
	Pelvic inflammatory disease:
	  Adults: 500 mg every 12 hours.
	Antibiotic-associated pseudomembranous colitis:
	  Infants and children: 20 mg/kg/day in 4 divided doses.
	  Adults: 250–500 mg t.i.d. or q.i.d.
	Oral doses may be taken with food to minimize stomach upset.	

Midazolam (Versed)	IV (titrate dose slowly to avoid excessive dosing):
	Conscious sedation:
	  Children: 0.05 mg/kg just before the procedure to a maximum dose of 2 mg. Dose may be repeated every 3 or 4 minutes up to 4 times.
	  Adults: 0.5–2 mg over 2 minutes. Titrate to effect by repeating doses every 2–3 minutes to a usual dose of 2.5–5 mg.
		Injection: 1 mg/mL, 5 mg/mL

	Infusion for sedation during mechanical ventilation: administer a loading dose of 0.05–0.2 mg/kg followed by a continuous infusion of 1–2 μg/kg/min and titrate to effect. *Orally:* 0.5 mg/kg to a maximum dose of 15 mg. *Intranasally:* 0.2–0.3 mg/kg/dose. The oral and intranasal routes of administration are not FDA approved.	
Mineral oil	*Orally* (do not administer concomitantly with docusate): Children: 5–20 mL/day. Adults: 15–45 mL/day. *Rectally* (as a retention enema): Children: 30–60 mL. Adults: 60–150 mL.	Enema: 133 mL Liquid
Mometasone Elocon	*Topically:* Apply a thin film to the affected area once daily. The cream and ointment have been used twice daily.	Cream: 0.1% Lotion: 0.1% Ointment: 0.1%
Montelukast (Singulair)	*Orally:* Children 2–6 years of age: 4 mg once daily. Children >6–14 years of age: 5 mg once daily. Children >14 years of age and adults: 10 mg once daily.	Tablets, chewable: 4 mg, 5 mg Tablets: 10 mg
Morphine sulfate (Astramorph PF, Duramorph, MSIR, MS Contin, Roxanol)	*IV or IM:* Neonates and infants under age 6 months: these patients are particularly sensitive to the respiratory depressant effects of opiates; therefore, the doses recommended are lower: 0.03 mg/kg every 3 or	Injection: 0.5 mg/mL, 1 mg/mL, 2 mg/mL, 3 mg/mL, 4 mg/mL, 5 mg/mL, 8 mg/mL, 10 mg/mL, 15 mg/mL Solution: 10 mg/5 mL, 20 mg/5 mL, 20 mg/mL Suppositories: 5 mg, 10 mg, 20 mg, 30 mg *Continued*

TABLE 85.1. Medications (continued)

Drug	Dose	Dosage Forms
Morphine sulfate (Astramorph PF, Duramorph, MSIR, MS Contin, Roxanol) (continued)	4 hours. Infusions have been used in neonatal patients at a dose of 0.01 mg/kg/hr. The dose may be increased if necessary but should not exceed 0.015–0.02 mg/kg/hr. Infants over 6 months and children: 0.025–0.1 mg/kg every 3 to 6 hours. Doses of up to 2.5 mg/kg have been used in severe pain such as sickle cell or cancer pain. The usual maximum dose is 10 mg. Adults: 2.5–10 mg every 2–6 hours. *Epidurally:* 0.5–5 mg in the lumbar region. Dose may be repeated every 24 hours. Maximum dose is 10 mg/24 hr. *Intrathecally:* one tenth of epidural dose or about 0.2–1 mg/dose. Repeat doses are not recommended. *Orally:* prompt-release preparations are administered every 3 or 4 hours; controlled-release preparations are administered every 8–12 hours. Oral doses are about one third as effective as IV doses. Infants over 6 months and children: 0.3 mg/kg every 3 or 4 hours (prompt release) or 0.3–0.6 mg/kg every 8–12 hours (extended release). Adults: 10–30 mg every 3–4 hours (prompt release) or 15–30 mg every 8–12 hours (extended release).	Tablets: 15 mg, 30 mg Tablets, controlled release: 15 mg, 30 mg, 60 mg, 100 mg

Continued

Mumps virus vaccine (Mumpsvax)	*SC into the outer aspect of the upper arm:* 0.5 mL at age 15 months or older. Trivalent MMR vaccine is preferred for most vaccinations. Federal law requires that the date of administration, manufacturer, lot number, and expiration date of the vaccine, and the name, title, and address of the person administering the dose be entered into the patient's permanent medical record. It also requires providers to distribute information on vaccines before each vaccination.	Injection: ≥20,000 TCID$_{50}$/0.5 mL
Mupirocin (pseudomonic acid A; Bactroban)	*Topically:* *Impetigo:* apply ointment to affected area t.i.d. for 3–5 days. *Lacerations, minor suture infections or abrasions:* apply cream to the affected area t.i.d. for 10 days. *Intranasal Staphylococcus aureus infection:* apply 1/2 of the contents of a unit-dose tube of intranasal cream into each nostril 2–4 times daily for 5–14 days.	Cream (as mupirocin calcium): 2% mupirocin Cream, intranasal (as mupirocin calcium): 2% Ointment: 2%
Nafcillin (See oxacillin)	*Neonates:* 60 mg/kg/24 hr in 4–6 divided doses. *Children:* 100–200 mg/kg/24 hr in 4–6 divided doses.	Injection: 500 mg, 1 g, 2 g
Nalbuphine (Nubain)	*Parenterally:* *Reversal of morphine infusion side effects:* 0.025–0.05 mg/kg repeated every 6 hours as necessary. *Analgesia:* Children over age 10 months: 0.1–0.14 mg/kg every 3–6 hours as necessary to a maximum dose of 10 mg.	Injection: 10 mg/mL, 20 mg/mL

TABLE 85.1. Medications (continued)

Drug	Dose	Dosage Forms
Nalbuphine (Nubain) (continued)	Adults: 10–20 mg every 3–6 hours. Its use in narcotic-dependent patients may cause symptoms of withdrawal.	
Naloxone (Narcan)	IV (preferred), IM, or SC: Neonatal opiate depression: 0.01 mg/kg every 2 or 3 minutes until the desired response is obtained. Additional doses may be necessary at 1–2-hour intervals. Opiate overdosage: 0.1 mg/kg to a dose of 2 mg administered every 2 or 3 minutes until 5 doses (up to 10 mg) have been given. If the depressive condition is not reversed, causes other than opiate ingestion should be considered. Additional doses may be necessary because the duration of effect of the opiate is generally longer than that of naloxone. The drug may also be administered via continuous infusion, especially if higher doses are necessary. Postoperative narcotic reversal (partial reversal): 0.005–0.01 mg/kg every 2–3 minutes until the desired degree of reversal is achieved. Care should be taken to avoid excessive dosage because that might result in a decrease in analgesia and an increase in blood pressure.	Injection (neonatal): 0.02 mg/mL Injection: 0.4 mg/mL, 1 mg/mL
Naproxen (Aleve, Naprosyn)	Orally: 5–10 mg/kg every 8–12 hours to a maximum daily dose of 1 g.	Suspension: 125 mg/5 mL Tablets: 250 mg, 375 mg, 500 mg

Nelfinavir (Viracept)	*Orally* (to be used in combination with nucleoside analogs): Age 2–13: 60–90 mg/kg/day in 3 divided doses with food. Adolescents and adults: 750 mg/dose t.i.d.	Powder: 50 mg/g (1 g scoop provided to measure doses) Tablets: 250 mg
Neomycin, polymyxin B, and hydrocortisone (Cortisporin)	*Ophthalmic:* Solution: 1–2 drops to the affected eye every 4–6 hours; apply finger pressure to the lacrimal sac for 1 minute after instillation. Ointment: apply about 1/2-inch ribbon of ointment to the eye t.i.d. or q.i.d. *Otic* (both a suspension and a solution formulation are available. The solution form may sting when instilled, but allows the ear canal to be examined easily): instill 3–4 drops into the affected ear t.i.d. or q.i.d.	Ointment, ophthalmic: neomycin 0.35%, bacitracin 400 U, polymyxin B 10,000 U, and hydrocortisone 1% Solution or suspension, otic: neomycin 5 mg/mL, polymyxin B 10,000 U/mL, and hydrocortisone 1% Suspension, ophthalmic: neomycin 0.35%, polymyxin B 10,000 U, and hydrocortisone 1%
Neomycin sulfate (Mycifradin)	*Orally:* *Bowel preparation:* 15 mg/kg (up to 1 g) at 1 P.M., 2 P.M., and 11 P.M. on the day before surgery (with erythromycin, cleansing enemas). *Hepatic coma:* 50–100 mg/kg/day in 3 or 4 divided doses up to 12 g/day.	Solution, oral: 125 mg/5 mL Tablets: 500 mg
Neostigmine (Prostigmin)	*IM:* *Myasthenia gravis test:* 0.04 mg/kg single dose *IV:* Reversal of nondepolarizing neuromuscular blockade after surgery in conjunction with atropine or glycopyrrolate: Infants: 0.025–0.1 mg/kg/dose.	Injection: 0.25 mg/mL, 0.5 mg/mL, 1 mg/mL

Continued

TABLE 85.1. Medications (continued)

Drug	Dose	Dosage Forms
Neostigmine (Prostigmin) (continued)	Children: 0.025–0.08 mg/kg/dose. Adults: 0.5–2.5 mg, total dose not to exceed 5 mg.	
Nitrofurantoin (Furadantin, Macrodantin)	Orally: Active infection: Children: 5–7 mg/kg/day in 4 divided doses to a maximum of 400 mg/day. Adults: 200–400 mg/day in 4 divided doses. Chronic suppression therapy: Children: 1–2 mg/kg/day in 1 or 2 divided doses. Adults: 50–100 mg at bedtime daily. Administer with food or milk to decrease rate of absorption because high peak levels are associated with increased GI upset.	Capsules (macrocrystals): 25 mg, 50 mg, 100 mg Suspension: 25 mg/5 mL
Nitroprusside sodium (Nipride, Nitropress)	IV as a continuous infusion: 0.3–0.5 µg/kg/min initially, then titrate to effect. Usual dose is 3 µg/kg/min. The maximum dose is 10 µg/kg/min. Cyanide toxicity may occur during prolonged therapy or in patients with hepatic dysfunction. Administration of sodium thiosulfate may decrease blood cyanide levels. Thiocyanate may accumulate in patients with renal impairment.	Injection: 50 mg Protect solutions from light. Do not use if highly colored (blue, green, or red).
Norepinephrine (Levarterenol, Levophed, Noradrenalin)	IV as a continuous infusion: initially 0.05–0.1 µg/kg/min, titrated to response. Maximum dose: 1–2 µg/kg/min.	Injection: 1 mg/mL

Nystatin (Mycostatin, Nilstat)	*Orally:* Neonates: 100,000 U administered q.i.d. Infants: 200,000 U administered q.i.d. Children and adults: 400,000–1 million U administered q.i.d. *Topically:* apply ointment or cream to the affected area t.i.d. or q.i.d.	Cream: 100,000 U/g [also available with triamcinolone, a topical steroid (Mycolog)] Ointment: 100,000 U/g [also available with triamcinolone, a topical steroid (Mycolog)] Suspension: 100,000 U/mL Tablets: 500,000 U (intestinal infections only) Troches: 200,000 U
Octreotide (somatostatin analog; Sandostatin)	*IV or SC:* the subcutaneous route is generally preferred because absorption is not immediate and the activity is somewhat prolonged. The drug may also be administered as a continuous infusion. Pediatric experience is limited, but initial doses of 1–10 µg/kg with total daily doses of 2–50 µg/kg in 2–4 divided doses. Usual adult doses are 50 µg 1 or 2 times daily initially, then titrate dose to the patient's response. The long-term effects of octreotide on growth hormone release have not been determined.	Injection: 50 µg/mL, 100 µg/mL, 200 µg/mL, 500 µg/mL, 1,000 µg/mL
Ofloxacin (Floxin Otic, Ocuflox)	*Ophthalmic infections:* *Bacterial conjunctivitis:* 1–2 drops in the affected eye every 2–4 hours while awake for 2 days, then 4 times a day for up to 5 more days. *Bacterial keratitis:* 1–2 drops in the affected eye every 30 minutes while awake and 4–6 hours after retiring for 2 days, then every hour while awake for up to 4–6 more days, then 4 times a day until cure is affected.	Solution, ophthalmic: 0.3% Solution, otic: 0.3%

Continued

TABLE 85.1. Medications (continued)

Drug	Dose	Dosage Forms
Ofloxacin (Floxin Otic, Ocuflox) (continued)	*Otic infections:* *Otitis externa:* Children 1–12 years of age: 5 drops in the affected ear canal twice a day for 10 days. Children >12 years of age and adults: 10 drops in the affected ear canal twice a day for 10 days. *Suppurative otitis media in patients with perforated tympanic membranes:* 10 drops in the affected ear twice a day for 14 days. The tragus of the ear should be pumped several times to make sure the solution is in the ear canal and the patient should remain in a position with the ear up for 5 minutes. *Otitis media in patients with tympanostomy tubes:* 5 drops in the affected ear twice a day for 10 days. The tragus of the ear should be pumped as above and the patient should remain in a position with the ear up for 5 minutes.	
Olopatadine (Patanol)	*Ophthalmic:* Children ≥3 years of age to adults: 1–2 drops in each eye daily at 6–8 hours intervals.	Solution, ophthalmic: 0.1%
Omeprazole (Prilosec)	*Orally with food or a meal:* Children: while safety and efficacy in children has not been established, a dose of 0.6–0.7 mg/kg/day as a single dose in the morning has been used. If necessary, a second dose may be given	Capsules: 10 mg, 20 mg, 40 mg The capsules contain enteric coated spheres. If the patient is unable to swallow capsules, the spheres may be put into an acidic juice, such as apple juice, for administration. Do not crush the spheres. The

12 hours later. The usual range of doses used is 0.3–3.3 mg/kg/day.

Adults: 20 mg daily. Higher doses may be used for pathologic hypersecretory conditions. The usual starting dose is 60 mg daily, but doses of up to 360 mg daily have been used. Doses >80 mg/day should be given in 2–3 divided doses.

Capsules: 10 mg, 20 mg, 40 mg. The capsules contain enteric coated spheres. If the patient is unable to swallow capsules, the spheres may be put into an acidic juice, such as apple juice, for administration. Do not crush the spheres. The spheres may be crushed for administration through a jejunostomy tube if a 650-mg tablet of sodium bicarbonate is added.

spheres may be crushed for administration through a tube if a 650 mg tablet of sodium bicarbonate is added to the diluent.

Oseltamivir (Tamiflu)

Orally (within 2 days of onset of symptoms):
≥13 years of age: 75 mg twice a day for 5 days.

Capsules: 75 mg

Oxacillin (Bactocill)

IV:
Neonates under age 7 days:
  <2,000 g: 50 mg/kg/day in 2 divided doses.
  ≥2,000 g: 100 mg/kg/day in 2 divided doses.
Neonates over age 7 days:
  <1,200 g: 50 mg/kg/day in 2 divided doses.
  1,200–2,000 g: 75 mg/kg/day in 3 divided doses.
  >2,000 g: 100 mg/kg/day in 4 divided doses.
Infants and children (depends on severity and site of infection):
  Mild to moderate infections: 50 mg/kg/day in 4 divided doses.

Capsules: 250 mg, 500 mg
Injection: 250 mg, 500 mg, 1 g, 2 g, 4 g, 10 g
Solution, oral: 250 mg/5 mL

Continued

TABLE 85.1. Medications (continued)

Drug	Dose	Dosage Forms
Oxacillin (Bactocill) (continued)	*Severe infections, including osteomyelitis:* 100–200 mg/kg/day in 4–6 divided doses. Total maximum dose is 12 g/day. Adults: *Mild to moderate infections:* 250–500 mg every 6 hours. *Severe infections:* 1–2 g every 4–6 hours. *Orally:* Infants and children: 50–100 mg/kg/day in 4 divided doses. Adults: 500 mg–1 g every 4–6 hours.	
Oxybutynin (Ditropan)	*Orally:* Children ≤age 5: 0.2 mg/kg/dose given 2–3 times daily. Children over age 5: 5 mg administered b.i.d. or t.i.d. Adults: 5 mg b.i.d. or t.i.d., to a maximum of q.i.d.	Solution, oral: 5 mg/5 mL Tablets: 5 mg
Pancrelipase (Cotazym, Cotazym-S, Creon, Pancrease MT, Ultrase, Zymase)	*Orally:* depends on the condition being treated and the dietary content of the patient. Dosage is usually determined by the fat content of the diet. The usual starting dose is 4,000–8,000 U of lipase activity before or with each meal or snack for children age 1–7, 4,000–12,000 U for children age >7–12, or 4,000–33,000 U for adults. Further dosage adjustments may be made based on the patient's	Capsules, delayed release, containing enteric-coated spheres, microspheres, or microtablets‡

	symptoms. The newer, enteric-coated products are designed to release the enzymes at pH >6 and are therefore more resistant to destruction by gastric acids.	
Paregoric	*Analgesic:* 0.25-0.5 mL/kg from once daily to q.i.d. *Antidiarrheal:* 0.1 mL/kg after each loose stool up to q.i.d. Contains 0.4 mg/mL morphine.	Tincture: 16-oz bottle
Penicillamine (Cuprimine, Depen)	Do not exceed a dose of 30 mg/kg/day. *Rheumatoid arthritis:* Children: Initial: 3 mg/kg/day (≤250 mg/day) for 3 months, then 6 mg/kg/day (≤500 mg/day) in divided doses b.i.d. for 3 months. Maximum: 10 mg/kg/day in 3 or 4 divided doses. *Wilson disease:* Children: 20 mg/kg/day in 4 divided doses.	Capsules: 125 mg, 250 mg Tablets: 250 mg
Penicillin G, aqueous (potassium and sodium salts)	*IV:* Neonates under age 7 days: <2,000 g: 25,000 U/kg every 12 hours. For meningitis, use 50,000 U/kg every 12 hours. >2,000 g: 20,000 U/kg every 8 hours. For meningitis, 50,000 U/kg every 8 hours. Neonates over age 7 days: <2,000 g: 25,000 U/kg every 8 hours. For meningitis, 50,000 U/kg every 8 hours. >2,000 g: 25,000 U/kg every 6 hours. For meningitis, 50,000 U/kg every 6 hours.	Injection, potassium salt: 1 million U, 5 million U, 10 million U Injection, sodium salt: 5 million U

Continued

TABLE 85.1. Medications (continued)

Drug	Dose	Dosage Forms
Penicillin G, aqueous (potassium and sodium salts) (continued)	Infants and children: 100,000–250,000 U/kg/day in 6 divided doses. Up to 500,000 U/kg/day may be used for severe infections to a maximum of 20 million U/day. Adults: 2–20 million U/day in 6 divided doses. The potassium salt contains 1.7 mEq of potassium and 0.3 mEq of sodium per 1 million U. The sodium salt contains 2 mEq of sodium per 1 million U. The potassium salt must be administered slowly at high doses due to the effect of the potassium.	
Penicillin G procaine, benzathine	*Deep IM:* results in low but prolonged serum levels. May be given as a single daily dose. A dose of penicillin G benzathine will result in low serum levels for up to 4 weeks. Newborns: avoid use in these patients because sterile abscess and procaine toxicity are of greater concern. Infants: 50,000 U/kg up to 600,000 U. Children and adults: 600,000–1.2 million U/day. Maximum dose is 4.8 million U.	Injection, benzathine: 600,000 U/mL Injection, benzathine and procaine combined equal parts of each in 300,000 U, 600,000 U, 1.2 million U, 2.4 million U; 900,000/300 (900,000 U benzathine, 300,000 U procaine) Injection, procaine: 600,000 U/mL
Penicillin V potassium (phenoxymethylpenicillin; Pen Vee K, V-Cillin K, Veetids)	*Orally:* Children: 25–50 mg/kg/day in 4 divided doses. Adults: 125–500 mg/dose every 6 hours.	Liquid, oral: 250 mg/5 mL Tablets: 125 mg, 250 mg, 500 mg

Pentobarbital (Nembutal)

Prophylaxis:
Under age 5: 125 mg b.i.d.
Over age 5 and adults: 250 mg b.i.d.

Orally, IM:
Sedation before surgery:
Children: 2–6 mg/kg/day to a maximum of 100 mg.
IV:
For sedation before procedures: dose should be
administered slowly and incrementally to avoid
oversedation. Patients must be closely observed.
Dosing is very patient-specific. The rate of injection
should not exceed 1 mg/kg/min (50 mg/min in
adults). Allow at least 1 minute to reach full effect.
Children: initially 2 mg/kg to a maximum of 100 mg.
Incremental doses of 1–2 mg/kg may be used to a
maximum total dose of 200 mg.
Adults: initially 100 mg. Incremental doses of
100–200 mg may be given to a maximum dose of
500 mg for healthy adults.
Barbiturate coma: 10–15 mg/kg administered over
1–2 hours, followed by a maintenance infusion of
1 mg/kg/hr. Dosage may be increased to 2–3 mg/
kg/hr to maintain burst suppression on EEG.
Hypothermia may necessitate a decrease in dosage.
Rectally (do not divide suppositories):
4.5–9 kg: 30 mg.
>9–18 kg: 30–60 mg.
19–36 kg: 60 mg.
>36–50 kg: 60–120 mg.
>50 kg: 120–200 mg.

Capsules: 50 mg, 100 mg
Elixir: 20 mg/5 mL
Injection: 50 mg/mL
Suppositories: 30 mg, 60 mg, 120 mg, 200 mg

Continued

TABLE 85.1. Medications (continued)

Drug	Dose	Dosage Form
Permethrin (Elimite Cream, Nix Cream Rinse)	*Scabies:* Children >2 months of age and adults: apply cream from head to toe. Wash cream off after 8–14 hours. May be reapplied after 1 week if live mites appear. *Head lice:* apply cream rinse to hair that has been thoroughly washed, rinsed and towel dried. Saturate hair and scalp with cream rinse. Also apply to the ears and hairline at the nape of the neck. Rinse off after 10 minutes and remove remaining nits with the comb provided. May be repeated after 1 week if necessary.	Cream, topical 5% Cream rinse: 1%
Phenobarbital	*IV or orally:* *Loading doses (usually IV for status epilepticus):* Neonates: 20 mg/kg in a single or 2 divided doses. Infants, children and adults: 15–18 mg/kg a single or 2 divided doses. Allow 15–30 minutes for the drug to distribute into the CNS and for the seizures to stop. *Maintenance doses:* Neonates: 5 mg/kg/day in 2 divided doses. Infants: 5–6 mg/kg/day in 2 divided doses. Age 1–5: 6 mg/kg/day in 2 divided doses. Age >5–12: 4 mg/kg/day in 1 or 2 divided doses. Over age 12 and adults: 1–2 mg/kg/day in 1 or 2 divided doses.	Elixir: 15 mg/5 mL, 20 mg/5 mL Injection (sodium): 30 mg/mL, 60 mg/mL, 65 mg/mL, 130 mg/mL Tablets: 15 mg, 30 mg, 60 mg, 100 mg

Phentolamine mesylate	Test dose (pheochromocytoma): 1 mg IM or IV.	Injection: 5-mg ampul
Phenylephrine (Neo-Synephrine, Mydfrin ophthalmic)	Intranasally (do not use for longer than 3–5 days): Under age 6: 0.125% solution 2–3 drops every 4 hours as needed. Age 6–12: 0.25% solution 2–3 drops or 1–2 sprays every 4 hours as needed. Over age 12 and adults: 0.5% solution 2–3 drops or 1–2 sprays every 4 hours as needed. 1% solution may be used in adults with extreme congestion. Ophthalmic: Infants: 1 drop of 2.5% solution 15–30 minutes before procedure. Children and adults: 1 drop of 2.5% or 10% solution; may repeat in 15–30 minutes. IV for severe hypotension or shock: a bolus dose of 5–20 μg/kg (2–5 mg in adults) may be repeated every 10–15 minutes. For infusion, initial doses of 0.1–0.5 μg/kg/min are titrated to effect.	Drops only: 0.125% Injection: 10 mg/mL Solution, nasal drops or spray: 0.25%, 0.5%, 1% Solution, ophthalmic: 2.5%, 10%
Phenytoin (Dilantin) and fosphenytoin (Cerebyx)	Care must be taken when changing from one dosage form of the drug to another because some contain phenytoin sodium and some contain the free acid form of the drug. The free acid form is used for the Infatabs and the suspension. Phenytoin sodium is used for the injection and capsules. Phenytoin sodium contains 92% phenytoin. Injection labeled as 50 mg/mL phenytoin sodium contains 46 mg of phenytoin and capsules labeled 100 mg contain 92 mg phenytoin. Fosphenytoin should be ordered in terms of phenytoin equivalents.	Capsule, phenytoin sodium, extended: 30 mg, 100 mg Injection, for phenytoin: 75 mg/1 mL (equivalent to 50 mg phenytoin sodium) Injection, phenytoin sodium: 50 mg/mL Suspension, phenytoin: 125 mg/5 mL Tablet, chewable, phenytoin: 50 mg

Continued

TABLE 85.1. Medications (continued)

Drug	Dose	Dosage Forms
Phenytoin (Dilantin) and fosphenytoin (Cerebyx) (continued)	The patient's serum levels should be monitored whenever the dosage form is changed. In addition, the different brands of phenytoin capsules have different dissolution characteristics. Dilantin capsules are considered extended and may be dosed in adults as a single daily dose. The serum level range usually associated with clinical effectiveness is 10–20 μg/mL; that associated with mild to moderate toxicity may be as low as 25–30 μg/mL. *Loading dose (IV or PO):* 15–20 mg/kg in a single or divided doses. *Maintenance dose (IV or PO):* 5 mg/kg/day in 2 or 3 divided doses initially and then adjusted to response and serum levels. Usual ranges based on age (divided into 2 or 3 doses daily): Neonates: 5–8 mg/kg/day. Age 6 months–3 years: 8–10 mg/kg/day. Age 4–6: 7.5–9 mg/kg/day. Age 7–9: 7–8 mg/kg/day. Age 10–16: 6–7 mg/kg/day. Adults: 5–6 mg/kg/day may be given as a single dose if extended-capsule preparation is used. Higher doses are required in infants and young children due to lower absorption of the drug from the GI tract.	

	IV doses of phenytoin should be administered at a maximum rate of about 1 mg/kg/min (50 mg/min in adults) to avoid cardiovascular side effects. The injection is not compatible with many solutions or medications. The line must be flushed well with saline before administration to avoid precipitation of phenytoin in the line. Extravasation of the drug must also be avoided because it is very alkaline and may cause severe tissue necrosis. Thorough flushing of the vessel after phenytoin administration will also decrease the incidence of local tissue inflammation that may occur even in the absence of extravasation. Fosphenytoin injection should be diluted with either 5% dextrose or normal saline to a concentration of 1.5–25 mg of phenytoin equivalents (2.3–37.5 mg fosphenytoin) per mL of diluent and may be administered at a rate of 2–3 mg phenytoin equivalents/kg/min (100–150 mg phenytoin equivalents/min in adults).
Phosphate (potassium and/or sodium)	Should be guided by the patient's serum phosphorus and potassium levels. Severe deficits should be replaced by the IV route because the oral route may result in diarrhea and oral absorption is unreliable. In general, the deficit should be made up by incorporating it into the patient's maintenance fluids. Intermittent infusions should follow the guidelines outlined below for potassium infusions because the IV form is potassium phosphate and each 3 mmol of phosphate will also deliver 4.4 mEq of potassium. The guidelines below are meant for use in patients with severe hypophosphatemia (<1 mg/dL in adults):	Injection (potassium phosphate): 3 mmol (94 mg) phosphorus and 4.4 mEq potassium per milliliter Packets or capsules (Neutra-Phos): 250 mg (8 mmol) phosphorus, 7 mEq potassium, and 7 mEq sodium Packets or capsules (Neutra-Phos K): 250 mg (8 mmol) phosphorus, 14.25 mEq potassium Tablets (K-Phos Neutral): 250 mg (8 mmol) phosphorus, 1.1 mEq potassium, and 13 mEq sodium Tablets (Uro-KP-Neutral): 250 mg (8 mmol) phosphorus, 1.27 mEq potassium, and 10.9 mEq sodium

Continued

TABLE 85.1. Medications (continued)

Drug	Dose	Dosage Forms

Phosphate (potassium and/or sodium) (continued)	Neonates: 0.5 mmol/kg up to 1–2 mmol/kg/day.
	Children: 0.15–0.3 mmol/kg with subsequent doses only after serum levels are checked and if the patient is symptomatic.
	Adults: 0.08 mmol/kg (uncomplicated hypophosphatemia) or 0.16 mmol/kg for prolonged deficits. Do not exceed 0.24 mmol/kg/day (serum phosphorus ≥0.5 mg/dl) or 0.5 mmol/kg/day (serum phosphorus <0.5 mg/dl).
	IV doses should be administered over a 6-hour period.
	Maintenance doses:
	  Children: 0.5–1.5 mmol/kg/day.
	  Adults: 15–30 mmol/day.
	Orally: should be taken with food to increase GI tolerance. Each packet or capsule should be mixed in 75 mL of water. Tablets should be taken with a full glass of water.
	Maintenance doses:
	  Children: 2–3 mmol/kg/day in 4 divided doses.
	  Adults: 32–64 mmol/day (4–8 packets) in 4 divided doses.
	Do not administer at the same time as aluminum- and/or magnesium-containing antacids, sucralfate, or calcium because they may act to bind phosphorus.	

Continued

Phytonadione (vitamin K;
AquaMEPHYTON, Konakion,
Mephyton)

IM or SC:
Hemorrhagic disease of the newborn, prophylaxis:
0.5–1 mg within 1 hour of birth and again 6–8
hours later, if needed.
Treatment: 1–2 mg/day.
Treatment of deficiency caused by malabsorption or
decreased synthesis or due to drugs (administer IV
cautiously and slowly):
Children: 1–2 mg/day.
Adults: 10 mg/day
Treatment of oral anticoagulant overdose:
Infants: 1–2 mg repeated every 4–8 hours.
Children and adults: 2.5–10 mg repeated in
6–8 hours.
Orally:
Prevention of deficiency in malabsorption:
Children: 2.5–5 mg every other day or daily.
Adults: 5–25 mg/day.

Injection: 2 mg/mL, 10 mg/mL
Tablets: 5 mg

Piperacillin (Piperacil)

IV:
Neonates: 150 mg/kg/day in 3 divided doses.
Infants and children: 300 mg/kg/day in 4–6
divided doses. Doses of 300–500 mg/kg/day in
6 divided doses have been used in the treatment of
children with cystic fibrosis.
Adults: 2–4 g every 4–8 hours. Do not exceed
18 g/day.

Injection: 2-g, 3-g, 4-g, 40-g bulk package

TABLE 85.1. Medications (continued)

Drug	Dose	Dosage Forms
Piroxicam (Feldene)	*Orally:* Children: 0.2–0.3 mg/kg/day in a single daily dose to a maximum of 15 mg/day. Adults: 10–20 mg/day in a single dose.	Capsules: 10 mg, 20 mg
Polyethylene glycolelectrolyte solution (Colovage, Colyte, GoLYTELY, OCL)	*Orally after a 3–4-hour fast:* Children: 25–40 mL/kg/hr. Adults: 240 mL every 10 minutes. The patient should continue to drink the solution until the rectal effluent is clear. Rapid drinking of each portion is more effective than slow consumption. The first bowel movement should occur about an hour after starting. The solution is more palatable if chilled, but must not be poured over ice. Nothing, including other flavorings, should be added to the solution. *Nasogastric tube administration:* Adults: 240 mL every 10 minutes.	Powder for oral solution to make 4 L: PEG3350 236 g, sodium sulfate 22.74 g, sodium bicarbonate 6.74 g, sodium chloride 5.86 g, and potassium chloride 2.97 g
Potassium chloride	*Orally:* liquid doses must be well diluted before administration to avoid GI adverse effects. Capsules or tablets should be taken with a full glass of water. Capsules may be opened and emptied onto a soft food, but the beads should not be crushed or chewed. Total daily dose may be given in 1 or 2 divided doses if tolerated, or may be given in	Capsules, controlled release: 8 mEq (600 mg), 10 mEq (750 mg). Injection, concentrated: 2 mEq/mL, 3 mEq/mL Liquids: 20 mEq/15 mL (10%), 30 mEq/15 mL (15%), 40 mEq/15 mL (20%) Powders, effervescent packets: 15 mEq, 20 mEq, 25 mEq

3 or 4 divided doses to decrease GI upset. Dose is usually based on each patient's requirements and may depend on concurrent medications or medical conditions that result in potassium losses. The following may be used as general guidelines:

Normal daily requirement for either PO or IV replacement:
  Newborn: 2–6 mEq/kg/day.
  Children: 2–3 mEq/kg/day.
  Adults: 40–80 mEq/day.

During diuretic therapy:
  Children: 1–2 mEq/kg/day.
  Adults: 20–40 mEq/day.

For treatment of hypokalemia:
  Children: 2–5 mEq/kg/day.
  Adults: 40–100 mEq/day.

IV: doses should be well diluted. Usually they are incorporated into the patient's daily fluid requirement. The maximum desirable concentration is 80 mEq/L. Greater concentrations should be used cautiously and only in patients with documented hypokalemia with a serum potassium level <2.5 mEq/L.

In the case of a patient in whom a shorter infusion of potassium is necessary, the following guidelines may be used: Maximum concentration of the solution must not exceed 30 mEq/100 mL (1 mEq/3 mL) and rate of infusion should not exceed 1 mEq/kg/hr in children or 40 mEq/hr in adults. The solutions should be infused using a pump to control the infusion rate.

Tablets, effervescent: 20 mEq, 25 mEq, 50 mEq
Tablets, extended release: 6.7 mEq (500 mg), 8 mEq (600 mg), 10 mEq (750 mg)
Other potassium salts are also available and may be desirable in patients who are acidotic. They include bicarbonate, citrate, acetate, and gluconate salts.

Continued

TABLE 85.1. Medications (continued)

Drug	Dose	Dosage Forms
Potassium chloride (continued)	Infusion over 2–3 hours (0.3–0.5 mEq/kg/hr) is more desirable. Administration of doses greater than 0.3 mEq/kg/hr should be done only if the patient has an ECG monitor in place. Solutions should be mixed well to prevent layering of the potassium chloride, which may result in inadvertent rapid administration.	
Prednisolone and prednisone	*Orally:* depends on the condition being treated and the patient's response. The lowest dose possible should be used. Withdrawal of long-term therapy must be accomplished slowly by gradually tapering the dose. The guidelines below may be used for initial dosing. Children: *Antiinflammatory or immunosuppressive:* 0.1–2 mg/kg/day in 1–4 divided doses. *Acute asthma:* 1–2 mg/kg/day in 1 or 2 divided doses for up to 5 days. *Inflammatory bowel disease:* 1–3 mg/kg/day in 1–2 divided doses. *Nephrotic syndrome:* 2 mg/kg/day in 3 or 4 divided doses. *Organ transplants:* 1 mg/kg/day in 2 divided doses, tapering gradually to 0.15 mg/kg/day or lowest effective dose.	Prednisolone: Liquid, as sodium phosphate: 5 mg/5 mL (Pediapred), 15 mg/5 mL (OraPred) Syrup (Prelone): 15 mg/5 mL Tablets: 5 mg Prednisone: Solution: 5 mg/5 mL Syrup (Liquid Pred): 5 mg/5 mL Tablets: 1 mg, 2.5 mg, 5 mg, 10 mg, 20 mg, 50 mg

Primidone (Mysoline)	*Orally:* Under age 8: initially 50–125 mg/day at bedtime or in 2 divided doses. Increase dose by 50–125 mg/day at weekly intervals in the normal range of 125–250 mg t.i.d. or 10–25 mg/kg/day. Over age 8 and adults: initially 125–250 mg/day at bedtime or in 2 divided doses. Increase dose by 125–250 mg/day at weekly intervals to the usual maintenance dose of 250 mg t.i.d. or q.i.d. Do not exceed 500 mg q.i.d. (2 g). Primidone is metabolized to phenobarbital and phenylethylmalonamide (PEMA). Phenobarbital levels should be monitored in addition to primidone levels.	Suspension: 250 mg/5 mL Tablets: 50 mg, 250 mg
Probenecid (Benemid)	*Uricosuric:* Children under age 2: not recommended. Age 2–14: *Initial:* 25 mg/kg for 1 dose. *Maintenance:* 40 mg/kg/24 hr in 4 divided doses.	Tablets: 500 mg
Procainamide (Procanbid, Pronestyl)	*IV:* Children: loading dose of 3–6 mg/kg to a maximum of 100 mg over 5 minutes. This may be repeated every 5–10 minutes to a maximum of 15 mg/kg. Follow with a maintenance infusion at a dose of 20–80 µg/kg/min. Adults: loading dose of 50–100 mg, repeated every 5–10 minutes to maximum of 15–18 mg/kg or 1–1.5 g. Follow with a maintenance infusion at a usual dose of 3–4 mg/min (range 1–6 mg/min).	Capsules, immediate release: 250 mg, 375 mg, 500 mg Injection: 100 mg/mL, 500 mg/mL Tablets, immediate release: 250 mg, 375 mg, 500 mg Tablets, sustained release: 250 mg, 500 mg, 750 mg, 1,000 mg Tablets, sustained release, 12-hour duration (Procanbid): 500 mg, 1,000 mg

Continued

TABLE 85.1. Medications (continued)

Drug	Dose	Dosage Forms
Procainamide (Procanbid, Pronestyl) (continued)	Orally (immediate-release products must be administered every 3 hours; controlled-release products must be administered every 6 hours or every 12 hours depending on the formulation used): Children: 15–50 mg/kg/day to a maximum dose of 4 g/day. Adults: usual range is 1–4 g/day in divided doses as above.	
Prochlorperazine (Compazine)	Orally or rectally as an antiemetic: 0.4 mg/kg/day in 3 or 4 divided doses or alternatively by the patient's weight: 9–14 kg: 2.5 mg every 12–24 hours as needed, to a maximum of 7.5 mg/day. >14–18 kg: 2.5 mg every 8–12 hours as needed, to a maximum of 10 mg/day. >18–39 kg: 2.5 mg every 8 hours or 5 mg every 12 hours as needed, to a maximum of 15 mg/day. >40 kg: Rectally: 25 mg every 12 hours. Orally: 5–10 mg t.i.d. or q.i.d. IM (IV is not recommended in children): 0.13 mg/kg; may be repeated if necessary up to t.i.d. or q.i.d. Usual adult dose is 5–10 mg every 4 hours to a maximum of 40 mg/day.	Capsules, sustained release: 10 mg, 15 mg, 30 mg Injection: 5 mg/mL Suppositories: 2.5 mg, 5 mg, 25 mg Syrup: 5 mg/5 mL Tablets: 5 mg, 10 mg, 25 mg

Promethazine (Phenergan)

Antihistamine (usually orally):
 Children: 0.1 mg/kg every 6 hours during the day.
  A dose of 0.5 mg/kg may be used at bedtime.
 Adults: 12.5 mg every 6 hours during the day with a
  25-mg dose at bedtime.
Antiemetic (orally, IV, IM, or rectally):
 Children: 0.5 mg/kg up to every 4 hours.
 Adults: 12.5–25 mg every 4 hours as needed.
Motion sickness (orally):
 Children: 0.5 mg/kg 30 minutes to 1 hour before
  traveling; then every 12 hours as needed.
 Adults: 25 mg 30 minutes to 1 hour before traveling;
  then every 12 hours as needed.
Sedation (all routes):
 Children: 0.5–1 mg/kg every 6 hours as needed.
 Adults: 25–50 mg every 6 hours as needed.

Injection: 25 mg/mL, 50 mg/mL
Suppositories: 12.5 mg, 25 mg, 50 mg
Syrup: 6.25 mg/5 mL, 25 mg/5 mL
Tablets: 12.5 mg, 25 mg, 50 mg

Propranolol (Inderal)

Orally:
Arrhythmias:
 Children: 0.5–1 mg/kg/day in 3 or 4 divided
  doses. Dosage may be titrated upward at 3–7-day
  intervals to the usual range of 2–4 mg/kg/day. If
  higher doses are necessary, up to 16 mg/kg/day
  [up to 640 mg] may be used.
 Adults: usually 10–30 mg every 6–8 hours.
Hypertension:
 Children: 0.5–1 mg/kg/day in 2–4 divided doses,
  increasing at 3–7-day intervals to the usual range
  of 1–5 mg/kg/day.

Capsules, sustained release: 60 mg, 80 mg,
 120 mg, 160 mg
Injection: 1 mg/mL
Solution: 4 mg/mL, 8 mg/mL
Tablets: 10 mg, 20 mg, 40 mg, 60 mg, 80 mg,
 90 mg

Continued

TABLE 85.1. Medications (continued)

Drug	Dose	Dosage Forms
Propranolol (Inderal) (continued)	Adults: 40 mg b.i.d., increasing at 3–7-day intervals to a maximum dose of 640 mg/day. *Migraine prophylaxis:* Children: 0.6–1.5 mg/kg/day in 3 divided doses. Adults: 80 mg/day in 3 or 4 divided doses. Dose may be increased to a maximum of 240 mg/day in divided doses. *Tetralogy spells:* Children: 1–2 mg/kg every 6 hours. *Thyrotoxicosis:* Neonates: 2 mg/kg/day in 2–4 divided doses. Children: 1 mg/kg/day q.i.d. Adolescents and adults: 10–40 mg every 6 hours. *IV:* reserve for life-threatening arrhythmias. To be administered as an IV bolus *slowly* under ECG monitoring. The IV dose is much smaller than the oral dose. Children: 0.01–0.1 mg/kg to a maximum of 1 mg for arrhythmias. For tetralogy spells, 0.15–0.25 mg/kg, which may be repeated once after 15 minutes. Adults: 1–3 mg. A second dose may be given, if necessary, after 2 minutes.	

Continued

Propylthiouracil

Orally: Initially:
Neonates: 5–10 mg/kg/day in 3 divided doses.
Under age 10: 5–7 mg/kg/day in 3 divided doses.
≥ age 10: 150–300 mg/day in 3 divided doses.
Adults: 300 mg/day in 3 divided doses.
After control of symptoms has been achieved, the dose may be decreased to the lowest dose possible, usually one third to two thirds of the initial dose, administered in 3 doses daily.

Tablets: 50 mg

Protamine sulfate

IV: 1 mg of protamine sulfate neutralizes 90 mg of lung-derived heparin or 115 U of intestinal mucosa-derived heparin. Because heparin disappears rapidly from the circulation, the dose of protamine decreases rapidly with time elapsed since the heparin infusion. The dose of protamine necessary after 30 minutes is half the dose above and that necessary after 2 hours is one fourth the dose above. Because protamine itself is an anticoagulant, avoid overdosing. Protamine should be administered slowly, over a 1-minute period, and the dose should not exceed 50 mg.

Injection: 10 mg/mL

Protirelin (Thyrel TRH)

IV (as a bolus over 15–30 seconds with the patient remaining supine for an additional 15 minutes):
Children: 7 μg/kg to a maximum of 500 μg.
Adults: 500 μg.

Injection: 500 μg/mL

TABLE 85.1. Medications (continued)

Drug	Dose	Dosage Forms
Psyllium (Fiberall, Hydrocil, Konsyl, Metamucil, Perdiem Fiber, Serutan).	*Orally* (each dose should be accompanied by a full glass of water or other liquid): Children: half the adult dose (1/2 to 1 packet or 1.7–3.4 g of psyllium) once daily to t.i.d. Adults: 1–2 packets or 3.4–6.8 g of psyllium once daily to t.i.d.	Powder: ~3.4 g/dose Powder, effervescent
Pyrantel pamoate (Antiminth)	*Orally* (may be taken with juice or milk and without regard to the ingestion of food): 11 mg/kg to a maximum of 1 g.	Suspension: 50 mg/mL
Ranitidine (Zantac)	*Orally:* Children: 2–4 mg/kg/day in 2 divided doses initially. Dose may be higher in hypersecretory conditions. Adults: 150 mg b.i.d. or 300 mg at bedtime. Dose may be higher or more frequently administered. Up to 6 g/day has been used. *IV:* Children: 1–2 mg/kg/day in 3 or 4 divided doses. Do not exceed 6 mg/kg/day or 300 mg/day. Adults: 50 mg every 6–8 hours. Do not exceed 400 mg/day.	Injection: 25 mg/mL Syrup: 15 mg/mL Tablets: 75 mg, 150 mg, 300 mg
Ribavirin (Virazole)	Aerosol administered via the manufacturer's small particle aerosol generator (SPAG). 6 g of the drug are solubilized in sterile water and aerosolized over	Powder for reconstitution for aerosol: 6 g

12–18 hours daily for 3–7 days. Therapy must be started within the first 3 days of lower respiratory tract infection due to RSV. The manufacturer recommends against using the drug for patients who require assisted ventilation. Precipitation of the drug in respiratory equipment has occurred, as has accumulation of fluid in tubing. Either condition may compromise the patient.

Rifampin (Rifadin, Rimactane)	*Orally* (on an empty stomach):

Tuberculosis:
Children: 10–20 mg/kg/day as a single daily dose to a maximum of 600 mg.
Adults: 600 mg/day.
Meningococcal carriers:
Under age 1 month: 10 mg/kg/day in 2 divided doses for 2 days.
Infants and children: 20 mg/kg/day in 2 divided doses for 2 days, to a maximum dose of 1,200 mg/day.
Adults: 600 mg/dose b.i.d. for 2 days.
Haemophilus influenzae type b prophylaxis:
Under age 1 month: 10 mg/kg/day as a single dose for 4 days.
Over age 1 month and children: 20 mg/kg/day as a single dose for 4 days.
Adults: 600 mg/day for 4 days.
IV (over 30 minutes to 3 hours): same doses as for the oral route. Rifampin may cause a red-orange discoloration of the sweat, urine, tears, and other body fluids; soft contact lenses may be permanently stained.

Capsules 150 mg, 300 mg
Injection: 600 mg
Suspension: not commercially available, but may be made by mixing the powder from the capsules with simple syrup to form a 10 mg/mL suspension. Such suspensions are stable for 4 weeks at room temperature or refrigerated.

Continued

TABLE 85.1. Medications (continued)

Drug	Dose	Dosage Forms
Rimantadine (Flumadine)	*Orally:* Under age 10: 5 mg/kg once daily to a maximum dose of 150 mg. Over age 10 and adults: 100 mg b.i.d. Therapy may be continued for up to 6 weeks. Rimantadine does not completely prevent an immune response to influenza vaccine; therefore, vaccination is not contraindicated. Rimantadine should be continued for 2–4 weeks after vaccination to allow for antibody production.	Syrup: 50 mg/5 mL Tablets: 100 mg
Ritonavir (Norvir)	*Orally with food to increase absorption:* Children 2–12 years of age: 250 mg/m²/dose given twice a day initially to decrease the nausea that usually occurs. The dose is gradually increased by 50 mg/m²/dose every 2–3 days as tolerated to a maximum of 400 mg/m²/dose (or 600 mg/dose). Children >12 years of age and adults: 300 mg/dose twice daily initially, increasing by 100 mg/dose over 3–5 days to a maximum dose of 600 mg twice a day.	Capsule, liquid filled, oral: 100 mg Solution, oral: 80 mg/mL
Salmeterol (Serevent, Serevent Diskus)	*Powder (Diskus) for oral inhalation:* Children ≥4 years of age to adults: 1 inhalation	Inhalation, metered dose: 21 μg/actuation Inhalation, powder: 50 μg/foil blister

(50 μg) twice daily about 12 hours apart is used for chronic asthma.

Metered dose inhalation:

Children ≥12 years of age and adults: 2 inhalations (42 μg) twice daily about 12 hours apart. For exercise-induced asthma, 1 puff should be inhaled 30–60 minutes prior to exercise and may be repeated 12 hours later. Patients on regular twice a day doses should not add a third dose prior to exercise.

Scopolamine (hyoscine; Isopto Hyoscine)

IM, SC, or IV:

Children: 0.006 mg/kg to a maximum dose of 0.3 mg.

Adults: 0.3–0.65 mg.

Ophthalmic:

Children: 1 drop (up to q.i.d. for uveitis).

Adults: 1–2 drops (up to q.i.d. for uveitis).

Injection: 0.3 mg/mL, 0.4 mg/mL, 0.86 mg/mL, 1 mg/mL

Solution, ophthalmic: 0.25%

Sermorelin acetate (growth hormone-releasing hormone; Geref)

IV (in the morning after an overnight fast):

1 μg/kg IV push followed by a 3-mL saline flush.

Injection: 50-μg vials

Silver sulfadiazine (Silvadene, SSD, Thermazene)

Topically: applied to a thickness of 1/16-inch under sterile conditions (using a sterile glove) once or b.i.d. to a clean, debrided wound. Wound should always be covered with cream; reapply if it rubs off.

Cream: 10 mg/g

Continued

TABLE 85.1. Medications (continued)

Drug	Dose	Dosage Forms
Sodium bicarbonate (baking soda, $NaHCO_3$)	*IV:* *Cardiac arrest* (only after adequate ventilation has been established): 1 mEq/kg IV push initially; may repeat with a dose of 0.5 mEq/kg. Further doses should not be given until the patient's acid-base status has been determined. In infants, the concentration should not exceed 4.2% (0.5 mEq/mL). *Metabolic acidosis* (after measurement of blood gases and pH): Children: mEq HCO_3 = 0.3 × weight (kg) × base deficit (mEq/L) OR mEq HCO_3 = 0.5 × weight (kg) × [24-serum HCO_3 (mEq/L)]. Adults: mEq HCO_3 = 0.2 × weight (kg) × base deficit (mEq/L) OR mEq HCO_3 = 0.5 × weight (kg) × [24-serum HCO_3 (mEq/L)]. Doses should be administered slowly with frequent monitoring of acid-base balance. *Orally:* *Urine alkalinization* (titrate dose to desired pH): Children: 1–10 mEq/kg/day in divided doses. Adults: 48 mEq initially followed by 12–24 mEq every 4 hours. Doses up to 192 mEq/day have been used.	Injection: 4.2% (0.5 mEq/mL), 7.5% (0.9 mEq/mL), 8.4% (1 mEq/mL) Tablets: 325 mg, 650 mg
Sodium polystyrene sulfonate (Kayexalate)	*Orally:* Children: base the dose on the exchange rate of 1 mEq K^+/g of resin in smaller children.	Powder Suspension: 15 g/60 mL (with sorbitol)

Alternatively, a dose of 1 g/kg every 6 hours may be used.
Adults: 15 g administered once daily to q.i.d.
Rectally as a retention enema:
Children: 1 g/kg every 2–6 hours.
Adults: 30–50 g every 6 hours.
Enemas should be retained for as long as possible to increase ion exchange. Evacuation of the enema should be followed by a non-sodium-containing cleansing enema. Sorbitol is frequently used for making solutions because it helps to prevent constipation.
Administer cautiously to patients who may be at risk of serum sodium level increases. It is not totally selective for potassium; small amounts of calcium and magnesium may also be lost.

Sodium sulfacetamide (Ak-Sulf, Bleph-10, Cetamide, Sodium Sulamyd)

Topically to the eye:
Solutions: apply 1–2 drops in the affected eye up to every 2 or 3 hours while awake.
Ointment: apply to the eye once daily to q.i.d. Drops will cause burning or stinging sensation.
Ointment will cause blurred vision.

Ointment, ophthalmic: 10%
Ointment, ophthalmic: 10% with prednisolone 0.2%, 0.25%, or 0.5%
Suspension, ophthalmic: 10%, 15%, 30%
Suspension, ophthalmic: 15% with phenylephrine 0.125% (Vasosulf)
Suspension, ophthalmic: 10% with prednisolone 0.2%, 0.25%, or 0.5%

Spironolactone (Aldactone)

Orally:
Edema (response may not be evident for up to 5 days):

Tablets: 25 mg, 50 mg, 100 mg (a stable suspension may be made by crushing tablets and suspending the powder in simple syrup or cherry syrup.)
Continued

TABLE 85.1. Medications (continued)

Drug	Dose	Dosage Forms
Spironolactone (Aldactone) (continued)	Children: 1–3 mg/kg/day in 1 or 2 divided doses. Adults: 100 mg/day with a range of 25–200 mg/day. *Primary aldosteronism:* Children: 125–375 mg/m²/day in divided doses. Adults: 400 mg/day in 1 or 2 divided doses.	
Stavudine (Zerit)	*Orally:* Age 6 months–15 years: dose has not been established, but doses of 1–2 mg/kg/day have been well tolerated. Adults: <60 kg: 30 mg b.i.d. ≥60 kg: 40 mg b.i.d. Dosage must be adjusted in patients with renal dysfunction.	Capsules: 15 mg, 20 mg, 30 mg, 40 mg
Streptomycin	*IM:* Newborn: 20–30 mg/kg/24 hr in 2 divided doses for 10 days. Children: 20–40 mg/kg/24 hr in 2 divided doses for 10 days. Adults: 1–2 g in 1 or 2 doses daily. Maximum dose 2 g/24 hr.	Injection: 400 mg/mL
Sucralfate (Carafate)	Sucralfate is not absorbed from the GI tract. It may bind with other drugs administered at the same time,	Suspension: 1 g/10 mL Tablets: 1 g

Continued

lowering their effectiveness; therefore, it should be administered at least 2 hours before or after other drugs.

Orally:

Children: dosage has not been established, but 40–80 mg/kg/day in 4 divided doses has been used.

Adults: 1 g q.i.d.

The dose for stomatitis or mucositis is about 500 mg–1 g of suspension swished around the mouth and then spit out or swallowed, repeated q.i.d.

Sulfasalazine (Azulfidine)

Orally:

Over age 2: initially 40–60 mg/kg/day in 3–6 divided doses (not to exceed 6 g/day) then decreasing to a maintenance dose of 20–40 mg/kg/day in 4 divided doses to a maximum dose of 2 g/day.

Adults: initially 3–4 g/day in equally divided doses. Although doses as high as 12 g/day have been used, they are generally accompanied by an increased incidence of adverse effects.

Maintenance doses are usually 2 g/day in 4 divided doses.

The drug may cause a yellow discoloration of urine and skin.

Tablets: 500 mg

Tablets, enteric coated: 500 mg

TABLE 85.1. Medications (continued)

Drug	Dose	Dosage Forms
Sulfisoxazole (Gantrisin)	*Orally:* Over age 2 months: 150 mg/kg/day in 4 or 6 divided doses to a maximum daily dose of 6 g. An initial dose of 75 mg/kg may be given. Adults: 2–4 g initially followed by 4–8 g/day in 4–6 divided doses.	Solution or suspension: 500 mg/5 mL Tablets: 500 mg
Sumatriptan (Imitrex)	*SC:* Children ≥6 years of age and ≤30 kg: 0.06 mg/kg or 3 mg. Children >30 kg and adults: 6 mg. A second dose may be given at least 1 hour after the first dose if necessary. Do not exceed 2 doses in 24 hours.	Injection: 12 mg/ml
Tacrolimus (FK-506, Prograf)	Patients are usually treated concurrently with an adrenal corticosteroid. *Orally:* Children: 0.1–0.5 mg/kg/day in 2 divided doses. Adults: 0.15–0.3 mg/kg/day in 2 divided doses. Doses may be decreased to a lower maintenance dose. *IV (as a continuous infusion):* Children: 0.1 mg/kg/day. Adults: 0.05–0.1 mg/kg/day. Conversion to oral therapy should take place as soon as the patient is able to tolerate oral medication.	Capsules: 1 mg, 5 mg Injection: 5 mg/mL

Terbinafine (Lamisil AF)	*Topically:* ≥12 years of age: apply to affected area and surrounding skin for at least 1 week, but not more than 4 weeks.	Cream: 1%
Terbutaline (Brethine, Bricanyl)	*Orally:* Under age 12: initially 0.05 mg/kg t.i.d., increased gradually as required to a maximum of 0.15 mg/ kg t.i.d. or total of 5 mg/24 hr. Over age 12: initially 2.5 mg t.i.d. Maintenance: usually 5 mg or 0.075 mg/kg t.i.d. *Parenteral, SC:* Under age 12: 0.01 mg/kg to a maximum of 0.3 mg every 15–20 minutes for 3 doses. Over age 12: 0.25 mg, repeated in 15–30 minutes if needed once only; a total dose of 0.5 mg should not be exceeded within a 4-hour period. *Inhalation:* 2 puffs every 4–6 hours.	Aerosol, oral: 0.2 mg/activation Injection: 1 mg/mL (1-mL ampul) Tablets: 2.5 mg, 5 mg
Tetracycline (Achromycin V, Panmycin, Robitet, Sumycin)	*Orally* (should be given on an empty stomach): Over age 8: 25–50 mg/kg/day in 4 divided doses. Adults: 1–2 g/day in 2–4 divided doses.	Capsules: 250 mg, 500 mg Suspension: 125 mg/5 mL Tablets: 250 mg, 500 mg
Theophylline	*IV or orally for apnea in infants:* Premature neonates (postconceptional age under 40 weeks): 2 mg/kg/day in 2 divided doses. Term neonates under age 4 weeks: 5 mg/kg loading dose followed by 2–4 mg/kg/day in 2 or 3 divided doses.	*Immediate release:* Capsules: 100 mg, 200 mg Injection in D_5W: 0.4 mg/mL, 0.8 mg/mL, 1.6 mg/mL, 2 mg/mL, 3.2 mg/mL, 4 mg/mL Solution: 27 mg/5 mL, 50 mg/5 mL, 90 mg/5 mL (provided by 105 mg/5 mL of aminophylline) *Continued*

TABLE 85.1. Medications (continued)

Drug	Dose	Dosage Forms
Theophylline (continued)	Term neonates over age 4 weeks: 5–7.5 mg/kg loading dose followed by 3–6 mg/kg/day in 3 divided doses. Acute bronchospasm (all dosing should be based on lean body weight): Loading dose: 1 mg/kg will increase serum theophylline concentration by 2 μg/mL. Patients who have received no theophylline in the previous 24 hours may be given 6 mg/kg. Patients who have received theophylline within the previous 24 hours may receive 3 mg/kg. Serum theophylline level should be monitored 30 minutes after the end of a bolus infusion. Loading dose should be administered IV over 30 minutes or PO using an immediate-release product. For patients requiring a continuous IV infusion of theophylline, it should be started at the completion of the bolus dose at the following rate for children: Age 6 months–1 year: 0.5 mg/kg/hr. Age >1–9: 0.9 mg/kg/hr. Age >9–12 and adolescent smokers: 0.8 mg/kg/hr. Age >12–16 (nonsmokers): 0.7 mg/kg/hr. Theophylline levels should be monitored 12–24 hours after beginning the infusion and daily while therapy continues.	Tablets: 100 mg, 125 mg, 200 mg, 250 mg, 300 mg Controlled release: Capsules and tablets of various strengths and release properties: Frequency of dosing must be based on the characteristics of the product chosen. Immediate-release products must be administered every 6 hour. Extended-release products may be administered every 8–12 hours or even every 24 hours in adolescents using products designed for daily administration. Serum levels should be monitored frequently during early therapy to maintain serum levels between 10–20 μg/mL. After a stable dose is achieved, monitoring should be done at least every 6–12 months.

Oral therapy for chronic bronchospasm:
Age 6 months–1 year: 12–18 mg/kg/day.
Age >1–9: 20–24 mg/kg/day.
Age >9–12 and adolescent smokers: 20 mg/kg/day.
Age >12–16 (nonsmokers): 18 mg/kg/day.
Over age 16 (nonsmokers): 13 mg/kg/day (not to exceed 900 mg/day).

Ticarcillin (Ticar)

IV (for the treatment of severe infections):
Neonates under age 1 week:
<2 kg: 75 mg/kg every 12 hours.
≥2 kg: 75 mg/kg every 8 hours.
Neonates from age 1–4 weeks:
<2 kg: 75 mg/kg every 8 hours.
≥2 kg: 100 mg/kg every 8 hours.
Infants over age 4 weeks and children:
200–300 mg/kg/day in 4–6 divided doses.
Children weighing over 40 kg and adults:
200–300 mg/kg/day in 4–6 divided doses to a maximum daily dose of 24 g.
Dosage must be adjusted in patients with renal or hepatic dysfunction.

Injection: 1 g, 3 g, 6 g (20-g and 30-g pharmacy bulk packages)

Ticarcillin and clavulanate potassium (Timentin)

IV (may be expressed in terms of ticarcillin content alone or in terms of the fixed ratio (30:1) of the commercially available combination product):
Children:
<60 kg: 200–300 mg/kg/day of ticarcillin (207–310 mg of ticarcillin/clavulanic acid) in 4–6 divided doses.

Injection: 3 g ticarcillin + 0.1 g clavulanic acid labeled as a combined total potency of 3.1 g (pharmacy bulk package containing 30 g ticarcillin + 1 g clavulanic acid)

Continued

TABLE 85.1. Medications (continued)

Drug	Dose	Dosage Forms
Ticarcillin and clavulanate potassium (Timentin) (continued)	≥60 kg: 3 g ticarcillin + 0.1 g clavulanic acid (3.1 g of combination) every 4–6 hours to a maximum of 24 g of ticarcillin daily. Dosage must be adjusted in patients with renal or hepatic dysfunction.	
Tobramycin (Nebcin, TobraDex, Tobrex)	*IV:* Infants and children: 7.5 mg/kg/day in 3 divided doses. Older children and adults: 5 mg/kg/day in 3 divided doses. Patients with cystic fibrosis usually require higher doses (10 mg/kg/day in 3 divided doses). Dosage may be increased based on the results of serum level monitoring. Dosage must be adjusted in patients with renal dysfunction. *Ophthalmic:* Ointment: apply a 1-cm ribbon of ointment to the eye b.i.d. or t.i.d. Solution: apply 1–2 drops into the eye up to every 30–60 minutes in severe infections or every 3–4 hours for moderate infections.	Injection: 10 mg/mL, 40 mg/mL Ointment, ophthalmic: 0.3% Ointment, ophthalmic: 0.3% with dexamethasone 0.1% Solution, ophthalmic: 0.3% Solution, ophthalmic: 0.3% with dexamethasone 0.1%
Tolmetin (Tolectin)	*Orally for rheumatoid arthritis:* Over age 2: initially 20 mg/kg/day in 3 or 4 divided doses, adjusted to the patient's response.	Capsules: 400 mg Tablets: 200 mg, 600 mg

Topiramate (Topamax)	Usual maintenance dosage range is 15–30 mg/kg/day. Adults: 600 mg–1.8 g/day in 3 divided doses.	
	Orally Children 2–16 years of age: initially, 1–3 mg/kg/day (or 25 mg) given daily at bedtime for 1 week. Gradually increase dose by 1–3 mg/kg/day and increase frequency to twice daily to the usual maintenance dosage range of 5–9 mg/kg/day. Children >16 years of age and adults: initially, 50 mg daily in two divided doses, then increase at weekly intervals by 50 mg/day to a usual adult dose range of 200–400 mg daily in 2 divided doses.	Capsule, sprinkle: 15 mg, 25 mg Tablet: 25 mg, 100 mg, 200 mg. Tablets should not be crushed since the drug has a very bitter taste. Broken tablets should be used immediately as the drug is not stable.
Tretinoin (retinoic acid; Retin-A)	*Topically:* apply to the affected area once daily after cleaning, generally at bedtime. Avoid application to areas not being treated. Use should be discontinued if severe reddening, swelling, or peeling occurs. After healing, therapy may be restarted with the same or a different formulation administered less frequently.	Cream: 0.025%, 0.05%, 0.1% Gel: 0.01%, 0.025% Solution: 0.05%
Trifluridine (Viroptic)	*Topically to the eye:* apply 1 drop every 2 hours while awake until re-epithelialization has occurred. Maximum daily dose of 9 drops should not be exceeded. After re-epithelialization has occurred, dosage should be reduced to 1 drop every 4 hours for an additional 7 days to prevent recurrence, but the total length of therapy should not exceed 21 days.	Solution, ophthalmic: 1%

Continued

TABLE 85.1. Medications (continued)

Drug	Dose	Dosage Forms

Trimethobenzamide (Tigan)	*IM* (not for infants or young children): 200 mg t.i.d. or q.i.d.
	Rectally (not for neonates or infants):
	  <13.6 kg: 100 mg t.i.d. or q.i.d.
	  13.6–45 kg: 100–200 mg t.i.d. or q.i.d.
	  >45 kg: 200 mg t.i.d. or q.i.d.
	Orally:
	  13.6–45 kg: 100–200 mg t.i.d. or q.i.d.
	  >45 kg: 250 mg t.i.d. or q.i.d.
	Alternatively, a dose of 5 mg/kg administered t.i.d. or q.i.d. rectally or orally may be used.
		Capsules: 100 mg, 250 mg
		Injection: 100 mg/mL
		Suppositories: 100 mg, 200 mg

Trimethoprim (Primsol, Proloprim, Trimpex)	*Orally:* *UTI:* Infants and children <12 years of age: 4–6 mg/kg/day in 2 divided doses for 10 days. Children ≥12 years of age and adults: 100 mg twice daily or 200 mg once daily for 10 days *Pneumocystis carinii pneumonia treatment (given with dapsone):* 15–20 mg/kg/day in 4 divided doses.	Solution: 50 mg/5 mL Tablet: 100 mg, 200 mg
Tropicamide (Mydriacyl, Ocu-Tropic, Tropicacyl)	*Topically to the eye:* 1 to 2 drops into the eye(s) 15–20 minutes before exam. 0.5% solution is usually sufficient for exam. If cycloplegia for refraction is necessary, 1% solution must be used and repeated in 5 minutes. Exam must take place within 30 minutes because its effect is short.	Solution, ophthalmic: 0.5%, 1%

Valproic acid, valproate sodium, and divalproex sodium (Depacon, Depakene, Depakote)	*Orally* (expressed in terms of valproic acid): initially 15 mg/kg/day increasing by 5–10 mg/kg/day at weekly intervals until seizures are controlled or side effects occur. Usual maximum total daily dose is 60 mg/kg. Frequency of administration in part depends on dosage form, but dosage is usually divided. To prevent adverse GI effects, capsules (valproic acid) and solution are usually administered in 2 or 3 divided doses. Divalproex usually may be administered in 2 divided doses. The usual therapeutic serum concentration range is 50–100 μg/mL. The oral solution has been administered rectally in patients who are NPO by diluting it 1:1 with tap water and administering it as a retention enema. *IV (over 1 hour):* for patients who are not on valproic acid therapy, use the dosing and frequency of administration guidelines outlined above for oral dosing. For patients already on valproic acid therapy, use the patient's total oral daily dose and frequency of dosing for the IV route. The use of the injectable form for periods of more than 14 days has not been studied.	Capsules (divalproex sodium): 125 mg valproic acid Capsules (valproic acid): 250 mg Injection: 100 mg/mL Solution (valproate sodium): 250 mg valproic acid/ 5 mL Tablets (divalproex sodium): 125 mg, 250 mg, 500 mg valproic acid

Vancomycin (Lyphocin, Vancocin, Vancoled)	*IV (over at least 1 hour):*
	Neonates under age 7 days:
	  <1,000 g: 10 mg/kg every 24 hours.
	  1,000–2,000 g: 10 mg/kg every 18 hours.
	  >2,000 g: 10 mg/kg every 12 hours.
		Capsules: 125 mg, 250 mg
		Injection: 500 mg, 1 g, (5-g, 10-g pharmacy bulk packages)
		Solution, oral: 1 g, 10 g

Continued

TABLE 85.1. Medications (continued)

Drug	Dose	Dosage Forms
Vancomycin (Lyphocin, Vancocin, Vancoled) (continued)	Neonates age 7–30 days: <1,000 g: 10 mg/kg every 18 hours. 1,000–2,000 g: 10 mg/kg every 12 hours. >2,000 g: 10 mg/kg every 8 hours. Infants age 31–60 days: 10 mg/kg every 8 hours. Infants over age 2 months and children: 40 mg/kg/day in 4 divided doses to a maximum dose of 2 g/day. Adults: 0.5 g every 6 hours or 1 g every 12 hours. Dosage adjustment is necessary in renal impairment. Higher doses, up to 60 mg/kg/day, may be required in children with staphylococcal central nervous system infections. *Intrathecal:* Neonates: 5–10 mg/day. Children: 5–20 mg/day. Adults: 20 mg/day. *Orally* (not absorbed; do not use for systemic infections): Children: 40 mg/kg/day in 4 divided doses to a maximum daily dose of 2 g. Adults: 0.5–2 g/day in 3 or 4 divided doses.	
Verapamil (Calan, Isoptin, Verelan)	*IV* (push over 2 to 3 minutes): Under age 1: 0.1–0.2 mg/kg (usually 0.75–2 mg).	Capsules, extended release: 120 mg, 180 mg, 240 mg

Age 1–16: 0.1–0.3 mg/kg to a maximum of 10 mg.
   May be repeated once in 30 minutes if not
   effective.
Over age 16: 0.075–0.15 mg/kg (5–10 mg) with a
   repeat dose in 30 minutes if necessary.
Orally (not well established in children):
   Age 1–5: 4–8 mg/kg/day in 3 divided doses or
      about 40–80 mg every 8 hours.
   Over age 5: 80 mg every 6–8 hours.
   Adults: 240–480 mg/day in 3 or 4 divided doses
      (1–2 doses daily using extended-release products
      for the treatment of hypertension).

Injection: 2.5 mg/mL
Tablets: 40 mg, 80 mg, 120 mg
Tablets, extended release: 120 mg, 180 mg, 240 mg

Vitamin A (Aquasol A)

Orally:
For malabsorption syndromes (water miscible product):
   Under age 8: 5,000–15,000 U/day.
   Over age 8 and adults: 10,000–50,000 U/day.
For severe deficiency with xerophthalmia:
   Age 1–8: 5,000 U/kg/day for 5 days or until
      recovery.
   Over age 8 and adults: 500,000 U/day for 3 days,
      then 50,000 U/day for 14 days, then 10,000–
      20,000 U/day for 2 months.
Deficiency (without corneal change):
   Under age 1: 10,000 U/kg/day for 5 days, then
      7,500–15,000 U/day for 10 days.
   Age 1–8: 5,000–10,000 U/kg/day for 5 days, then
      17,000–35,000 U/day for 10 days.
   Over age 8 and adults: 100,000 U/day for 3 days,
      then 50,000 U/day for 14 days.

Capsules: 10,000 U, 25,000 U, 50,000 U

Continued

TABLE 85.1. Medications (continued)

Drug	Dose	Dosage Forms
Vitamin A (Aquasol A) *(continued)*	*Dietary supplementation:* Infants up to age 6 months: 1,500 U/day. Age >6 months–3 years: 1,500–2,000 U/day. Age 4–6: 2,500 U/day. Age 7–10: 3,300–3,500 U/day. Over age 10 and adults: 4,000–5,000 U/day.	
Vitamin E [alpha tocopherol, alpha tocopheryl acetate, tocopherol polyethylene glycol succinate (TPGS), Aquasol E]	*Orally* (water miscible or water soluble TPGS products are recommended, especially for patients with malabsorption): *Deficiency:* Infants: 25–50 U/day. *Children with malabsorption:* 15–25 U/kg/day to raise and maintain plasma tocopherol levels. Patients with cystic fibrosis, thalassemia, or sickle-cell disease may require larger daily doses (400–800 U/day). Adults: 60–75 U/day.	Capsules: 100 U, 200 U, 400 U, 600 U, 1,000 U, 1,000 U Capsules, water miscible: 100 U, 200 U, 400 U Solution, water miscible: 50 U/mL Solution (TPGS): 400 U/15 mL
Warfarin sodium (Coumadin)	*Orally:* Infants and children: 0.1 mg/kg/day with a range of 0.05–0.34 mg/kg/day adjusted to achieve the desired PT. Adults: 5–15 mg/day initially for 2–5 days until desired PT is reached. Usual maintenance dosage range is 2–10 mg/day.	Tablets: 1 mg, 2 mg, 2.5 mg, 4 mg, 5 mg, 7.5 mg, 10 mg

Continued

Zafirlukast (Accolate)	*Orally on an empty stomach:* Children 7–12 years of age: 10 mg twice daily. Children >12 years of age and adults: 20 mg twice daily.	Tablet: 10 mg, 20 mg
Zalcitabine (ddC, Hivid)	*Orally:* Under age 13: 0.01 mg/kg/dose given every 8 hours. Adolescents age 13–adults: 0.75 mg every 8 hours on an empty stomach. Adjust dose in patients with renal dysfunction.	Tablets: 0.375 mg, 0.75 mg
Zanamivir (Relenza)	*Oral inhalation:* Children ≥12 years of age and adults: 2 inhalations twice a day for 5 days beginning within 2 days of the onset of symptoms.	Powder for inhalation with device: 5 mg/actuation
Zidovudine (Retrovir)	*Orally:* Age 3 months–12 years: 180 mg/m^2 every 6 hours to a maximum of 200 mg every 6 hours. Dosage may be decreased in patients who develop anemia and/or granulocytopenia. Adults: *Asymptomatic:* 100 mg every 4 hours while awake (500 mg/day). *Symptomatic:* 100 mg every 4 hours (600 mg/day). *IV:* Age 3 months–13 years: 0.5–1.8 mg/kg/hr as a continuous infusion or 100 mg/m^2 by infusion over 1 hour every 6 hours. Adults: 1–2 mg/kg every 4 hours 6 times daily.	Capsules: 100 mg Injection: 10 mg/mL Solution: 50 mg/5 mL

TABLE 85.1. Medications (continued)

Drug	Dose	Dosage Forms
Zidovudine (Retrovir) (continued)	*Maternal–fetal HIV transmission prevention:* Maternal (> 14 weeks of pregnancy): 100 mg every 4 hours while awake (500 mg/day) until the onset of labor. During labor and delivery, 2 mg/kg over 1 hour followed by a continuous IV infusion of 1 mg/kg/hr until the umbilical cord is clamped. Infant: 2 mg/kg orally every 6 hours starting within 12 hours of birth and continuing for 6 weeks. For infants unable to tolerate oral drugs, 6 mg/kg/day IV in 4 evenly divided doses may be used. Dosage adjustment is necessary in severe renal impairment.	
Zinc	Response may not occur for 6–8 weeks. *Orally:* Infants and children: 0.5–1 mg/kg/day of elemental zinc in 1–3 divided doses. Adults: 25–50 mg elemental zinc t.i.d. *Acrodermatitis enteropathica:* 10–45 mg/day elemental zinc. Zinc sulfate 4.4 mg = 1 mg elemental zinc (220 mg = 50 mg).	Zinc sulfate (23% zinc): Capsules: 220 mg (50 mg zinc) Injection: 1 mg/mL, 5 mg/mL (zinc) Tablets: 66 mg (15 mg zinc), 110 mg (25 mg zinc), 220 mg (45 mg zinc) Zinc gluconate (14.3% zinc): Tablets: 10 mg (1.4 mg zinc), 15 mg (2 mg zinc), 50 mg (7 mg zinc), 78 mg (11 mg zinc)

* See Table 83.2 for a discussion of the content of each milliliter of these products.

† See Table 83.3 for dosage recommendations.

‡ See Table 83.4 for the lipase, amylase, and protease content of each form of pancrelipase.

TABLE 85.2. Citric Acid and Citrate Dosage Forms (Content per 1 mL)

Product	Sodium Citrate	Potassium Citrate	Citric Acid	Bicarbonate Equivalent
Bicitra solution	100 mg (1 mEq Na)	. . .	66.8 mg	1 mEq
Oracit solution	98 mg (1 mEq Na)	. . .	128 mg	1 mEq
Polycitra K solution	. . .	220 mg (2 mEq K)	66.8 mg	2 mEq
Polycitra-LC solution	100 mg (1 mEq Na)	110 mg (1 mEq K)	66.8 mg	2 mEq

TABLE 85.3. Digoxin Dosing

Age	Total Digitalizing Dose (µg/kg)		Daily Maintenance Dose (µg/kg divided in 2 doses)	
	PO	IV	PO	IV
Preterm infant	20–30	15–25	5–7.5	4–6
Full-term infant	25–40	20–30	6–10	5–8
1 month to 2 years	35–60	30–50	10–15	7.5–12
2 years to adult	30–40	25–35	7.5–15	6–9
Maximum dose	0.75–1.5 mg	0.5–1 mg	0.125–0.5 mg	0.1–0.4 mg

IV, intravenously; PO, orally.

TABLE 85.4. Pancrelipase Dosage Forms

	Lipase (USP Units)	Amylase (USP Units)	Protease (USP Units)
Capsules (enteric-coated or delayed-release microspheres)			
Cotazym-S	5,000	20,000	20,000
Creon	8,000	30,000	13,000
Creon-10	10,000	33,200	37,500
Creon-20	20,000	66,400	75,000
Pancrease	4,500	20,000	25,000
Pancrease MT-4	4,500	12,000	12,000
Pancrease MT-10	10,000	30,000	30,000
Pancrease MT-16	16,000	48,000	48,000
Pancrease MT-20	20,000	56,000	44,000
Ultrase MT-12	12,000	39,000	39,000
Ultrase MT-20	20,000	65,000	65,000
Zymase	12,000	24,000	24,000
Capsules (filled with non–enteric coated powder)			
Cotazym, Ku-Zyme HP	8,000	30,000	30,000
Powder (not enteric-coated)			
Viokase (per 0.7 g)	16,800	70,000	70,000
Tablets (not enteric-coated)			
Ilozyme	11,000	30,000	30,000
Viokase	8,000	30,000	30,000

Laboratory Values

HENRY R. DROTT

TABLE 86.1. Normal Laboratory Values

% Saturation	20%–40%
Absolute B_1 count	76–462/μL
Absolute lymphocyte count (ALC)	1266–3022/μL
Absolute T3	919–2419/μL
Absolute T4	614–1447/μL
Absolute T8	267–1133/μL
Absolute T11	1025–2587/μL
Acetaminophen	10–20 μg/ml
Acid phosphatase total	2–10 U/L
Alanine aminotransferase (ALT)	5–45 U/L
Albumin	3.7–5.6 g/dl
Aldolase	< 6 U/L
Alkaline phosphatase (AP)	130–560 U/L
Alpha$_1$-antitrypsin	210–500 mg/dl
Alpha-fetoprotein (AFP)	0.6–5.6 ng/ml
Amikacin	
Peak	20–30 μg/ml
Trough	0–10 μg/ml
Ammonia	9–33 μmol/L
Amylase	30–100 U/L
Anion gap	7–20 mmol/L
Antithrombin III	91%–128%
Apolipoprotein A–I	102–215 mg/dl
Apolipoprotein B	45–125 mg/dl
Aspartate aminotransferase	
Newborn	35–140 U/L
Child	10–60 U/L
B_1 (Total B cells)	4%–21%
Bands	0%–4%
Bicarbonate	20–26 mEq/L
Bilirubin	
δ	0.3–0.6 mg/dl
Neonatal	2.0–12.0 mg/dl
Total	0.6–1.4 mg/dl
Unconjugated	0.2–1.0 mg/dl
Blasts	0%
Caffeine	5–20 μg/ml
Calcium	8.9–10.7 mg/dl
Ionized	1.12–1.30 mmol/L
Stool	0–640 mg/24 h.
Carbon dioxide	20–26 mmol/L
Carboxyhemoglobin	0%–2%
CD3+ and CD8+	17.4%–34.2%
CD14+	0%–10%
CD45+ and CD14–	90%–100%
Ceruloplasmin	23–48 mg/dl
CH_{50}	104–356 U/ml
Chloramphenicol	5–20 μg/ml

TABLE 86.1. Normal Laboratory Values (continued)

Chloride	96–106 mmol/L
Sweat	0–40 mmol/L
Cholesterol	111–220 mg/dl
High-density lipoprotein (HDL)	35–82 mg/dl
Low-density lipoprotein (LDL)	59–137 mg/dl
Complement	
C3	
Newborn	67–161 mg/dl
Child	90–187 mg/dl
C4	16–45 mg/dl
Copper	67–147 μg/dl
Cortisol	
AM	10–25 μg/dl
PM	2–10 μg/dl
C-reactive protein (CRP), quantitative	0–1.2 mg/dl
Creatine kinase	
< age 1 year	60–305 U/L
> age 1 year	60–365 U/L
Creatinine	0.6–1.2 mg/dl
Cryoglobulin	
C3	0.0–0.028 mg/dl
IgA	0.0–0.026 mg/dl
IgG	0.0–0.157 mg/dl
IgM	0.0–0.224 mg/dl
Cyclosporin A	150–400 μg/L
Digoxin	0.5–2.0 ng/ml
DNA binding	0–149 IU/ml
D-Xylose, post-test	36–63 mg/dl (25-g dose)
Erythrocyte sedimentation rate (ESR)	0–20 mm/h
Ethosuximide	25–100 μg/ml
Factor II assay	27%–108%
Factor V assay	50%–200%
Factor VII assay	50%–200%
Factor VIII assay	50%–200%
Factor IX assay	
Newborn	14.5%–58.0%
Child	50%–200%
Factor X assay	50%–200%
Factor XI assay	50%–200%
Ferritin	23–70 ng/ml
Fibrin split products	0–10 μg/ml
Fibrinogen	180–431 mg/dl
G6PD assay, quantitative	4.6–13.5 U/g Hb
γ-Glutamyltransferase (GGT)	14–26 U/L
Gentamicin	
Peak	4–10 μg/ml
Trough	0–2 μg/ml
Glucose	75–110 mg/dl
CSF	32–82 mg/dl
Whole blood	60–115 mg/dl
Ham test	
Acidified	0%–1%
Unacidified	0%–1%
Haptoglobin	13–163 mg/dl

Continued

TABLE 86.1. Normal Laboratory Values (continued)	
Hematocrit	36%–46%
Spun	36%–41%
Hemoglobin	13.5–17.0 g/dl
A_1C	3.8%–5.9%
Total	
Newborn	10–18 g/dl
Child	12–16.0 g/dl
HbA_2, quantitative	1.8%–3.6%
HbF, quantitative	0%–1.9%
Immunoglobulin A	
Newborn	0–5 mg/dl
Infant	27–169 mg/dl
Child	70–486 mg/dl
Immunoglobulin E	
Newborn	0–15 IU/ml
Child	0–200 IU/ml
Immunoglobulin G	
CSF	0.5–6 mg/dl
Child	635–1775 mg/dl
Immunoglobulin M	
Child	71–237 mg/dl
Iron	50–180 µg/dl
Urine	0–2.0 mg/24 h.
Iron-binding capacity	250–420 µg/dl
Lactate	
CSF	0–3.3 mmol/L
Plasma	0.6–2.0 mmol/L
Lactate dehydrogenase (LDH)	340–670 U/L
Latex IgE	0–20 U
Lead, blood	0–10.0 µg/dl
Lipase	25–110 U/L
Lyme antibodies (IgG/IgM)	0.00–0.79
Magnesium	1.5–2.5 mg/dl
Mean corpuscular hemoglobin (MCH)	26.0–34.0 pg
Mean corpuscular volume (MCV)	80.0–100.0 μm^3
Mean platelet volume	7.4–10.4 fl
Methemoglobin	0.0%–1.9%
Netilmicin	
Peak	5–10 µg/ml
Trough	0–2 µg/ml
Osmolality	
Urine	
Newborn	50–645 mOsm/kg
Child	50–1500 mOsm/kg
Whole blood	275–296 mOsm/kg
Partial thromboplastin time	25.0–38.0 seconds
Peroxide hemolysis	0%–20%
Phenobarbital	15–40 µg/ml
Phenytoin	10–20 µg/ml
Phosphorus	2.7–4.7 mg/dl
Platelet aggregation, 10 µm	> 60.1%
Platelet count	150–400 $10^3/\mu L$
Potassium	3.8–5.4 mmol/L
Prealbumin	22.0–45.0 mg/dl
Primidone	5–12 µg/ml
Procainamide	4–10 µg/ml
Prolactin	2.7–15.2 ng/ml

TABLE 86.1. Normal Laboratory Values (continued)

Protein, 24-hour total	0–150 mg/24 h.
Protein C	
Immunological	50%–122%
Functional	59%–116%
Protein S, free	40%–111%
Protein, total	6.3–8.6 g/dl
Prothrombin time	10–12 seconds
Protoporphyrin, free RBC	30–80 μmol/mol Hb
Pyruvate kinase assay	1.8–2.3 IU/ml RBC
RBC distribution width	11.5%–14.5%
Reptilase	18–22 seconds
Reticulocyte count	0.5%–1.5%
Ristocetin cofactor	48%–220%
Salicylate	< 35 mg/dl
Sodium	136–145 mmol/L
Sucrose hemolysis	0%–5%
T3 (total T cells)	69%–86%
T4 (helper T cells)	39%–57%
T4–T8 ratio	0.7–2.5
T8 (suppressor T cells)	18%–45%
T11 (SRBC receptor)	75%–93%
Theophylline	10–20 μg/ml
Thrombin time	11.3–16.3 seconds
Thyroxine binding globulin	1.8–4.2 mg/dl
Thyroid stimulating hormone (thyrotropin)	0.5–5.0 μIU/ml
Thyroxine	
Newborn	3.0–14.4 μg/dl
Infant	4.6–13.4 μg/dl
Child	4.5–10.3 μg/dl
Tobramycin	
Peak	4–10 μg/ml
Trough	0–2 μg/ml
Total cell count	100
Total eosinophil count	100–300 mm^3
Total protein	
CSF	
Newborn	40–120 mg/dl
Child	15–40 mg/dl
Urine	0–20 mg/dl
Triglycerides	34–165 mg/dl
Triiodothyronine	0.9–2.25 ng/ml
Trypsin, stool	80–740 μg/g
Urea nitrogen	2–19 mg/dl
Uric acid	2.1–5.0 mg/dl
Urine specific gravity: TS meter	1.003–1.035
Urine pH	4.8–7.8
Valproic acid	50–100 μg/ml
Vancomycin	
Peak	20–30 μg/ml
Trough	0–12 μg/ml
White blood cell count	
Newborn	9–30 10^3/μL
Child	4.5–11.0 10^3/μL
Zinc	68–94 μg/dl

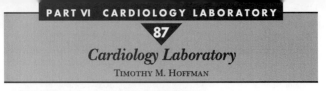

87

Cardiology Laboratory

TIMOTHY M. HOFFMAN

▼ BLOOD PRESSURE MEASUREMENT

Accurate measurement of the blood pressure depends on **selection of an appropriate cuff size.** The recommended width of the cuff is **40%–50% of the circumference of the measured extremity.** If the cuff size is too small, then the blood pressure will be overestimated, whereas if it is too large, the blood pressure will be underestimated.

Auscultation of the diastolic component of the blood pressure exhibits **two endpoints, Korotkoff phases IV and V,** respectively. **In children, phase IV** (i.e., the point of diminution or muffling of the Korotkoff sound) is generally considered a **more accurate representation** of the diastolic pressure. Phase V (i.e., the disappearance of the Korotkoff sounds) should be **considered the diastolic endpoint if it falls within 6 mm Hg of phase IV.** Standard blood pressure measurements for children from birth to 18 years of age are shown in Figure 87.1.

Pulsus Paradoxus

Pulsus paradoxus, a **decrease of more than 10 mm Hg in the systolic blood pressure during inspiration,** may be associated with **cardiac tamponade** (e.g., as a result of pericardial effusion), **constrictive pericarditis, or severe respiratory compromise** (e.g., asthma exacerbation).

▨ HINT Pulsus paradoxus must not be confused with pulsus alternans (i.e., a decrease in the systolic pressure on alternate contractions that indicates left ventricular failure).

Using a sphygmomanometer, the clinician **inflates the cuff until the pressure is 20 mm Hg above the systolic pressure.** She then **slowly deflates** the bladder **until the first Korotkoff sound is heard** independent of the respiratory cycle—this is the first data point. She **continues to slowly deflate** the bladder **until the Korotkoff phase I sound is noted in all respiratory cycles** (in inspiration and expiration)—the second data point. The difference between the points is considered the reduction in systolic pressure during inspiration and is abnormal if it is greater than 10 mm Hg.

Figure 87.2 schematically depicts pulsus paradoxus.

▼ HYPEROXITEST

The hyperoxitest can be useful for **differentiating cardiac and pulmonary causes of cyanosis,** and is **one of the first evaluations** performed when confronted **with a cyanotic newborn.** Cyanosis usually becomes apparent at a mean capillary concentration of 3–4 g/dl of reduced hemoglobin, a concentration that corresponds to an oxygen saturation of 70%–80%.

In infants with **cyanosis and hypoxemia,** the **arterial oxygen tension** (Pao_2) can range from **10–60 mm Hg.** In an infant with a **pulmonary cause** for the cyanosis, administration of **100% oxygen increases the Pao_2** to a level significantly **greater than 150 mm Hg.** In an infant with **cardiac cyanosis,** the Pao_2 **does not increase beyond 150 mm Hg** in response to the administration of 100% oxygen. In patients with **congenital heart disease,** this phenomenon is

A. Girls

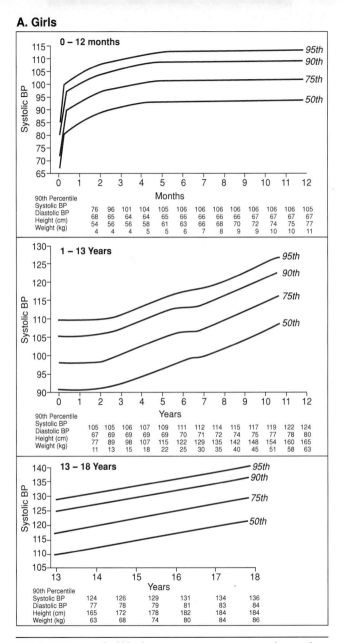

FIGURE 87.1. Standard blood pressure measurements in accordance with age and gender.
(A) Girls. (B) Boys. BP = blood pressure. (Reproduced with permission from Horan MJ: Report of the Second Task Force on Blood Pressure Control in Children—1987. *Pediatrics* 79:1–25, 1987.)

B. Boys

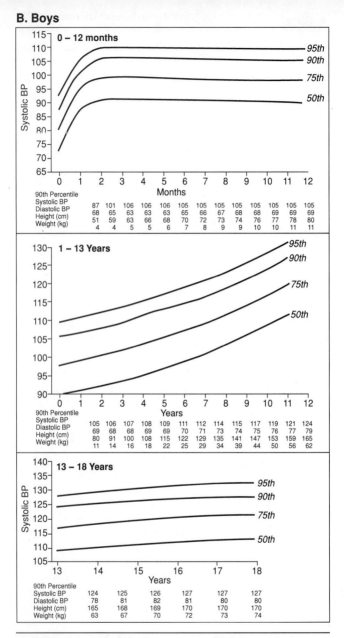

FIGURE 87.1. Standard blood pressure measurements in accordance with age and gender. (continued)

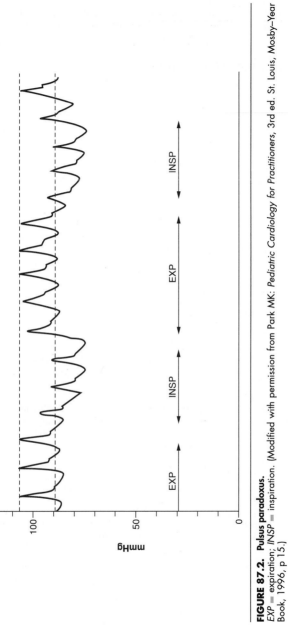

FIGURE 87.2. Pulsus paradoxus.
EXP = expiration; *INSP* = inspiration. (Modified with permission from Park MK: *Pediatric Cardiology for Practitioners*, 3rd ed. St. Louis, Mosby–Year Book, 1996, p 15.)

attributable to **right-to-left shunting** (i.e., the mixing of unoxygenated blood and oxygenated blood within the circulatory system). Right-to-left shunting may be either **intracardiac or extracardiac** in nature.

▼ ELECTROCARDIOGRAPHY

The EKG provides data concerning the following:

▼ Rhythm
▼ Rate
▼ Intervals
▼ Axis
▼ Hypertrophy
▼ Wave changes (Q waves and ST/T waves)

Rhythm

Rhythm diagnosis is beyond the scope of this chapter.

Rate

The heart rate is determined accurately by **dividing 60 by the RR interval** (measured in seconds). For example, if the RR interval is 0.4 second (10 small boxes), the heart rate is 60 divided by 0.4, or 150 beats/min.

Intervals (Figure 87.3)

Interval standards include the **PR, QRS, and QT intervals.** The **normal heart rate, PR interval, and QRS duration vary with age** (Table 87.1).

PR Interval

First-degree atrioventricular block is characterized by a **PR interval that is greater than the standard** range for age. A short PR interval associated with a **delta wave** is indicative of **Wolff-Parkinson-White syndrome.**

QRS Interval

The QRS duration represents the **intraventricular conduction time** and is normally **less than 0.09 second** (in children **younger than 4 years**) or **0.1 second** (in children **older than 4 years**). A QRS duration **greater than normal is identified as a bundle branch block:**

▼ **Left bundle branch block** is diagnosed when there is a monophasic R wave in lead I and no Q wave in lead V_6.
▼ **Right bundle branch block** is diagnosed when there is a wide S wave in leads I and V_6, right axis deviation, and an M-shaped (RSR' pattern) QRS complex in lead V_1.
▼ **Left anterior hemiblock** can be diagnosed in the setting of left axis deviation associated with right bundle branch block.

QT Interval

The QT measurement is **corrected for heart rate** using the following formula:

$$QTc = \frac{\text{measured QT (seconds)}}{\sqrt{\text{RR interval (seconds)}}}$$

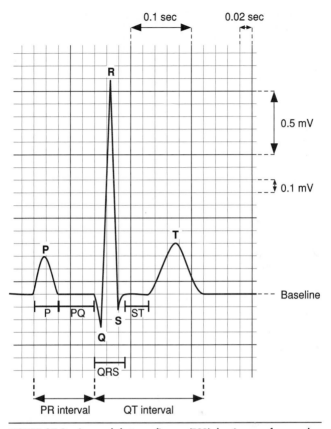

FIGURE 87.3. A normal electrocardiogram (ECG) showing waveforms and intervals.
The standard paper speed is 25 mm/sec; therefore, a single 1-mm box equals 0.04 seconds, and a large (5-mm) box equals 0.20 seconds.

The QTc interval is **less than 0.45 second for infants younger than 6 months,** and **less than 0.44 second for children.**

Axis

The frontal axis should be determined for the **P, QRS, and T waves from the limb leads** (I, II, III, aVR, aVL, aVF). The **hexaxial reference system** (Figure 87.4) is usually used. The **normal** axis falls **between 0 and 90 degrees.**

The axis is **equal to the direction of the largest positive force on depolarization.** A cursory way to determine the frontal axis is to **note the complex that is isoelectric** and **locate the two planes perpendicular to it.** The **perpendicular plane with the greatest positive deflection** is indicative of the axis.

TABLE 87.1. Normal Heart Rate, PR Interval, and QRS Duration for Age

Age	Heart Rate (beats/min) Mean	Heart Rate (beats/min) Range	PR Interval in Lead II (seconds) Mean	PR Interval in Lead II (seconds) Range	QRS Duration (seconds) Mean	QRS Duration (seconds) Range
<1 day	126	95–155	0.106	0.082–0.138	0.05	0.025–0.069
1–7 days	135	100–180	0.107	0.079–0.130	0.05	0.025–0.068
8–30 days	160	120–190	0.100	0.075–0.128	0.053	0.026–0.075
1–3 months	147	95–200	0.098	0.075–0.126	0.052	0.027–0.069
3–6 months	139	114–170	0.105	0.078–0.137	0.053	0.028–0.075
6–12 months	130	95–170	0.105	0.077–0.138	0.055	0.03–0.070
1–3 years	121	95–150	0.113	0.090–0.140	0.056	0.032–0.070
3–5 years	98	70–130	0.119	0.092–0.150	0.058	0.03–0.069
5–8 years	86	65–120	0.124	0.094–0.155	0.059	0.035–0.075
8–12 years	86	65–120	0.129	0.093–0.165	0.062	0.038–0.079
12–16 years	86	65–120	0.135	0.098–0.169	0.065	0.040–0.081

Adapted with permission from Liebman J, Plonsey R, Gillette PC: *Pediatric Electrocardiography*. Baltimore, Williams & Wilkins, 1982, pp 96–97 and Cassels DE, Ziegler RF: *Electrocardiography in Infants and Children*. Philadelphia, WB Saunders, 1966, p 100.

P-Wave Axis

The location of the P-wave axis **determines the origin of an atrial-derived rhythm:**

▼ 0 to 90 degrees = a high right atrial rhythm (normal sinus rhythm)
▼ 90 to 180 degrees = a high left atrial rhythm

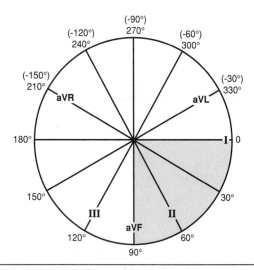

FIGURE 87.4. Hexaxial reference system (frontal axis). The *shaded area* represents the normal axis.

▼ 180 to 270 degrees = a low left atrial rhythm
▼ 270 to 0 degrees = a low right atrial rhythm

✄ HINT Classic "mirror image" dextrocardia is associated with a P-wave axis of 90–180 degrees in conjunction with high amplitude forces in the right chest leads and low voltage in the left chest leads (i.e., lead V_{4R} has a greater amplitude than does lead V_4).

QRS Axis

The QRS axis value is **age-specific** (Table 87.2), but **may correlate with congenital heart disease** in certain clinical settings. For example, a **northwest axis or left axis deviation** (−30 to −120 degrees) may correlate with an **endocardial cushion defect or tricuspid atresia. Left axis deviation is always abnormal in a newborn.**

T-Wave Axis

The T-wave axis helps **determine strain associated with ventricular hypertrophy.** A T-wave axis that is **90 degrees different from the QRS** axis suggests strain.

Hypertrophy

Right Atrial Hypertrophy

Diagnostic findings on EKG include a **peaked P wave that exceeds 2.5 mm in any lead** (often best seen in lead II).

Left Atrial Hypertrophy

A **P wave with a notched contour** and a duration of **more than 0.08 second in lead II** is diagnostic. Alternatively, a **biphasic P wave in lead V_1 or V_{3R} with a terminal inverted portion** that measures 1×1 **mm** will suffice to make the diagnosis.

TABLE 87.2.   Age-Specific QRS Axis Values

Age	Mean (Degrees)	Range (Degrees)
< 1 day	135	60–180
1–7 days	125	60–180
8–30 days	110	0–180
1–3 months	80	20–120
3–6 months	65	20–100
6–12 months	65	0–120
1–3 years	55	0–100
3–5 years	60	0–80
5–8 years	65	340–100
8–12 years	65	0–120
12–16 years	65	340–100

Adapted with permission from Liebman J, Plonsey R, Gillette PC: *Pediatric Electrocardiography.* Baltimore, Williams & Wilkins, 1982, p 90.

TABLE 87.3. Normal Range of Values (5th–95th Percentile) for R and S Waves in Leads V$_1$ and V$_6$

Age	Lead V$_1$		Lead V$_6$	
	R Wave (mm)	S Wave (mm)	R Wave (mm)	S Wave (mm)
<1 day	7.0–20.0	2.5–27.0	2.3–7.0	1.6–10.3
1–7 days	9.0–27.4	4.6–10.0	2.2–13.1	0.8–9.9
8–30 days	4.2–19.8	2.5–12.8	1.7–20.5	0.6–9.0
1–3 months	3.6–17.9	2.0–17.4	3.6–12.9	0.8–5.8
3–6 months	6.1–16.7	2.1–11.8	5.0–15.8	0.6–4.9
6–12 months	4.0–16.0	1.9–14.4	5.5–17.6	0.7–3.3
1–3 years	3.6–15.0	2.2–20.5	5.0–17.5	0.6–3.4
3–5 years	2.6–15.6	5.0–24.8	5.4–20.6	0.6–2.4
5–8 years	2.6–13.5	5.3–21.0	7.9–20.5	0.6–2.9
8–12 years	3.6–11.3	4.8–22.3	8.4–19.2	0.6–2.8
12–16 years	2.1–11.1	5.5–22.3	7.9–17.4	0.7–3.1

Adapted with permission from Liebman J, Plonsey R, Gillette PC: *Pediatric Electro-cardiography.* Baltimore, Williams & Wilkins, 1982, pp 84–85.

Right Ventricular Hypertrophy

Table 87.3 summarizes the normal measurements of R and S waves in leads V$_1$ and V$_6$ by age. Right ventricular hypertrophy can be diagnosed if any one of the following is seen:

▼ An R wave in lead V$_1$ that is greater than the ninety-eighth percentile for age
▼ An S wave in lead V$_6$ that is greater than the ninety-eighth percentile for age
▼ An upright T wave in lead V$_1$ in a patient older than 4 days
▼ Pure qR in leads V$_{3R}$ or V$_1$
▼ An RSR' pattern in leads V$_{3R}$ or V$_1$, in which the R' portion is 15 mm greater than the R wave (in a child younger than 1 year) or 10 mm greater than the R wave (in a child older than 1 year)

Left Ventricular Hypertrophy

Left ventricular hypertrophy can be diagnosed if any one of the following is seen:

▼ An R wave in lead V$_6$ that is greater than the ninety-eighth percentile for age
▼ A Q wave in lead V$_5$ or V$_6$ that is greater than 4 mm
▼ An R wave in lead V$_1$ that is below the fifth percentile for age
▼ An S wave in lead V$_1$ that is greater than the ninety-eighth percentile for age

Wave Changes

▼ **ST segment elevation** of greater than 2 mm in the precordial leads may indicate pericarditis, myocardial injury, ischemia, infarction, or digitalis effect.
▼ **Tall, peaked T waves** may be seen in patients with hyperkalemia.
▼ **Flat T waves** can occur in children with myocarditis, hypokalemia, or hypothyroidism.

▼ CHEST ROENTGENOGRAPHY

When examining a chest radiograph, one must comment on the **cardiac size, organ situs, and the pulmonary vascular markings** (normal, increased, or decreased).

Cardiac Size

Cardiac size is determined by **estimating the cardiothoracic ratio.** The ratio is calculated by **dividing the largest diameter of the heart by the largest internal diameter of the thorax.** If the result is **greater than 0.5, cardiomegaly is** present.

Organ Situs

The normal cardiac silhouette in the anterior–posterior and lateral views is depicted in Figure 87.5.

Pulmonary Vascular Markings

Pulmonary vascular markings **reflect the appearance of the pulmonary arteries and veins** on a chest radiograph **over the lung fields.**

These markings can be **increased in states of excessive pulmonary arterial flow** [e.g., ventricular septal defect, atrial septal defect, patent ductus arteriosus (PDA)], as well as in states characterized by **excessive pulmonary venous flow** (e.g., congestive heart failure, conditions characterized by pulmonary edema or pulmonary venous obstruction). On the radiograph, **increased pulmonary vasculature is noted when cephalization occurs and the vascular shadows extend more than two-thirds across the lung field.**

Decreased pulmonary vasculature markings are manifested radiographically as **hyperlucency of the lung field** and a **paucity of pulmonary vasculature,** as seen in patients with **tetralogy of Fallot.**

⚡ HINT The following signs, seen on the anterior–posterior projection, offer clues to the diagnosis:

▼ A **"boot-shaped" heart** is often seen in newborns with tetralogy of Fallot.
▼ An **"egg on a string"** is noted in newborns with a narrow mediastinum owing to absence of a large thymus, and is associated with transposition of the great arteries.
▼ A **"snowman sign"** is associated with supracardiac total anomalous pulmonary venous return. The left vertical vein, innominate vein, and the superior vena cava form the superior aspect of the "snowman."

▼ ECHOCARDIOGRAPHY

In pediatric patients, echocardiography is **performed in a stepwise fashion** to obtain **subcostal views, apical four-chamber views, parasternal views, and suprasternal views** (Figure 87.6).

M-Mode Echocardiography

A parasternal short axis view using M-mode echocardiography reveals a **cross-section of the left ventricle** and, therefore, can be used to **estimate cardiac dimensions.** Most commonly, it is used to obtain a **shortening fraction** (SF),

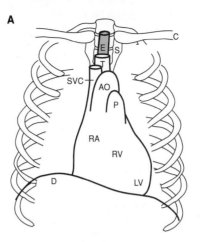

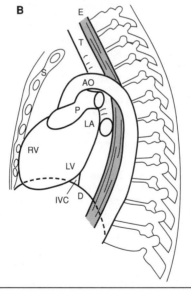

FIGURE 87.5. Normal cardiac silhouette.
(A) Anterior-posterior view. (B) Lateral view. AO = aorta; C = clavicle; D = diaphragm; E = esophagus; IVC = inferior vena cava; LA = left atrium; LV = left ventricle; P = pulmonary outflow tract; RA = right atrium; RV = right ventricle; S = sternum; SVC = superior vena cava; T = trachea. (Modified with permission from Sapire DW: *Understanding and Diagnosing Pediatric Heart Disease*. East Norwalk, CT, Appleton & Lange, 1991, p 64.)

A. Subcostal views

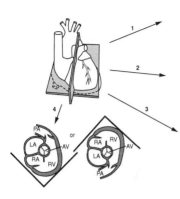

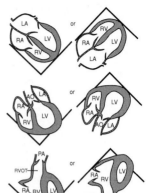

B. Apical views

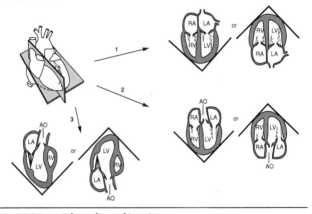

FIGURE 87.6.   Echocardiographic series.
The *numbers* represent different planes along a sweep of the echocardiographic beam. (*A*) Subcostal views. (*B*) Apical views. (*C*) Parasternal views. (*D*) Suprasternal views. *AO* = aorta; *AV* = aortic valve; *IA* = innominate artery; *LA* = left atrium; *LCA* = left coronary artery; *LPA* = left pulmonary artery; *LSA* = left subclavian artery; *LV* = left ventricle; *MPA* = middle pulmonary artery; *MV* = mitral valve; *PA* = pulmonary artery; *PM* = papillary muscle; *PV* = pulmonary valve; *RA* = right atrium; *RCA* = right coronary artery; *RPA* = right pulmonary artery; *RV* = right ventricle; *RVOT* = right ventricular outflow tract; *SVC* = superior vena cava. (Modified with permission from Park MK: *Pediatric Cardiology for Practitioners*, 3rd ed. St. Louis, Mosby–Year Book, 1996, pp 70–73.)

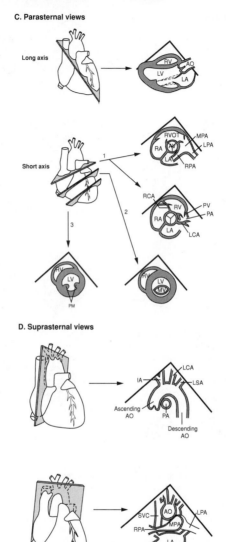

FIGURE 87.6. Echocardiographic series. (continued)

calculated in the following manner:

$$SF = \frac{\text{LV end-diastolic dimension} - \text{LV end-systolic dimension}}{\text{LV end-diastolic dimension}} \times 100$$

The **normal value** for the SF is generally considered to be **28%–32%,** independent of age.

Doppler Echocardiography

Doppler echocardiography detects a **frequency shift** that reflects the **direction and velocity of blood flow.** Doppler echocardiography is used to detect **valvular insufficiency or stenosis and abnormal vasculature flow patterns.**

▼ CARDIAC CATHETERIZATION

Cardiac catheterization allows **sampling of oximetric and hemodynamic data.** The normal pressures and oxygen saturations for children are depicted in Figure 87.7. Cardiac catheterization, an **invasive procedure,** is often used in **conjunction with angiography** to confirm the **diagnosis and physiology** of certain **acquired and congenital heart diseases.** The technique also has **therapeutic applications,** such as PDA coil embolization, coil embolization of aortopulmonary collaterals, pulmonary artery angioplasty and stent placement, and balloon valvuloplasty of semilunar valvular stenosis.

Shunts

Data obtained from cardiac catheterization can be used to calculate the **degree and direction of an intracardiac or extracardiac shunt.** The calculation is based on the **Fick principle,** using oxygen as the indicator.

The **oxygen content equals the dissolved oxygen** (which is usually negligible) **plus the oxygen capacity** [hemoglobin (g/dl) $\times$ 1.36 ml O_2/dl $\times$ 10] **multiplied by the oxygen saturation** (as a percentage).

Flow (Q) is the **oxygen consumption divided by the arteriovenous oxygen content difference:**

$$Qp = \frac{\dot{V}o_2}{PV - PA} \quad Qs = \frac{\dot{V}o_2}{AO - MV}, \text{ where}$$

Qp = pulmonary flow
Qs = systemic flow
$\dot{V}o_2$ = oxygen consumption per unit time
PV = pulmonary venous oxygen content
PA = pulmonary arterial oxygen content
MV = mixed venous oxygen content
AO = aortic oxygen content

To calculate the **amount of a shunt,** one needs to **calculate the effective pulmonary blood flow** ($Qp\ eff$):

$$Qp\ eff = \frac{\dot{V}o_2}{PV - MV}$$

$$Rs = \frac{AO - RA}{Qs}$$

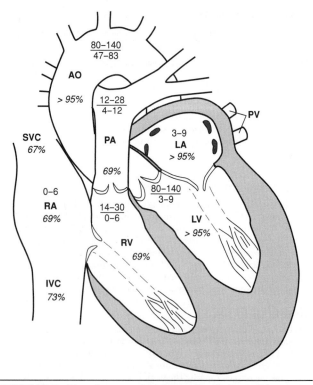

FIGURE 87.7. Normal pressures (systolic over diastolic, in mm Hg), mean pressures, and oxygen saturations for children.
The data are based on information compiled from healthy patients between the ages of 2 months and 20 years. *AO* = aorta; *IVC* = inferior vena cava; *LA* = left atrium; *LV* = left ventricle; *PA* = pulmonary artery; *PV* = pulmonary vein; *RA* = right atrium; *RV* = right ventricle; *SVC* = superior vena cava.

A **left-to-right shunt** is the **pulmonary flow less the effective pulmonary flow** (Qp − Qp eff), and a **right-to-left shunt** is the **systemic flow less the effective pulmonary flow** (Qs − Qp eff).

Resistance

Systemic and pulmonary vascular resistance can also be calculated using the **catheterization data.** This calculation is based on the **Ohm law** (essentially, the pressure change across the vascular bed divided by flow equals resistance):

$$Rp = \frac{PA - LA}{Qp}, \text{ where}$$

Rs = systemic resistance
Rp = pulmonary resistance

AO = mean aortic pressure
RA = mean right atrial pressure
PA = mean pulmonary artery pressure
LA = mean left atrial pressure

A pulmonary resistance (Rp) of **2.5 Wood units or less** is considered within the **normal** range; however, no vascular bed is rigid and **variations in flow can affect the result** obtained.

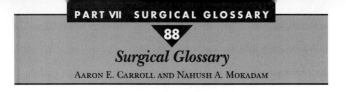

88

Surgical Glossary

AARON E. CARROLL AND NAHUSH A. MOKADAM

aortopexy—a procedure in which the aorta is approximated to the anterior thoracic wall; for the treatment of tracheomalacia.

Bishop-Koop procedure—resection of a dilated loop of bowel proximal to meconium obstruction, with end-to-side anastomosis between the proximal bowel and obstructed loop, combined with end ileostomy; for the treatment of meconium ileus.

bladder augmentation—a procedure in which a portion of the intraabdominal gastrointestinal tract is used to increase the volume of the bladder.

Blalock-Taussig shunt—a procedure in which the subclavian artery is anastomosed to the pulmonary artery; for the temporary treatment of tetralogy of Fallot.

Boix-Ochoa procedure—restoration of the intraabdominal esophageal length, repair of the esophageal hiatus, fixation of the esophagus to the hiatus, and restoration of the angle of His; for the treatment of incompetent lower esophageal sphincter.

chordee correction—a procedure in which the corpus spongiosum is moved ventrally and the corpus cavernosa are approximated dorsally; for the treatment of chordee (abnormal penile curvature associated with epispadias or hypospadias).

Clatworthy mesocaval shunt—division of the common iliac veins and side-to-end anastomosis of the inferior mesenteric vein to the left renal vein; for the treatment of portal hypertension.

Cohen procedure—trigonal reimplantation of the ureter; for the treatment of vesicoureteral reflux.

colonic conduit diversion—a procedure involving two stages: (1) a loop diversion using a colonic segment, and (2) an end-to-side anastomosis of the colonic segment to the gastrointestinal tract.

colonic interposition—replacement of the esophagus with a colonic segment; for treatment of esophageal atresia or stricture when gastric mobilization is not feasible.

diaphragmatic plication—surgical shortening of the diaphragm (abdominal, transthoracic, or bilateral); for the treatment of diaphragmatic eventration.

distal splenorenal shunt—see **Warren shunt**.

Drapanas mesocaval shunt—prosthetic graft implantation from the inferior mesenteric vein to the inferior vena cava; for the treatment of portal hypertension.

Duckett transverse preputial island flap—technique in which a flap of foreskin is used to elongate the urethra; for the treatment of hypospadias.

Duhamel procedure—resection of the aganglionic colon above the dentate line with stable anastomosis to the rectal stump, normally performed in children 6 to 12 months of age for the treatment of Hirschsprung disease (see **Martin modification**).

end-to-side portocaval shunt—procedure in which the portal vein is divided and anastomosed to the inferior vena cava; for the treatment of portal hypertension.

esophagectomy—resection of the esophagus, with gastric pull-up and anastomosis with the cervical esophagus; for the treatment of esophageal atresia or stricture.

Fontan procedure—a procedure in which a graft is created to connect the pulmonary artery to the right atrium; for the treatment of hyperplastic right heart syndrome.

Glenn shunt—a shunt from the superior vena cava to the pulmonary artery; for the treatment of tricuspid atresia or stenosis.

gridiron incision—see **McBurney incision**.

Hegman procedure—surgical release of the tarsal, metatarsal, and intertarsal ligaments; for the treatment of metatarsus adductus.

Heller myotomy—myotomy of the anterior lower esophagus (always accompanied by a Thal fundoplication); for the treatment of achalasia.

ileal loop diversion—resection and implantation of ureters into an isolated ileal segment, with an ileal stoma and primary anastomosis of ileum to cecum.

ileal ureter—ileal interposition between the renal pelvis and bladder when the ureteral length is insufficient for anastomosis; for the treatment of urinary obstruction.

ileocecal conduit diversion—bilateral ureteral diversion and anastomosis to an isolated ileocecal segment and cecostomy with primary anastomosis of ileum to the right colon.

J-pouch—creation of an ileal reservoir in the distal ileum using a J-shaped configuration; used following colectomy.

Jateene procedure—arterial retransposition; for the treatment of transposition of the great vessels.

Kasai procedure—resection of atretic extrahepatic bile ducts and gallbladder with Roux-en-Y anastomosis of the jejunum to the remaining common hepatic duct; for the treatment of biliary atresia or other extrahepatic obstruction.

Kimura procedure (parasitized cecal patch)—a multistep operation in which (1) a side-to-side anastomosis is made with a portion of the distal ileum and the right colon, and (2) an ileoanal pull-through is performed; for the treatment of Hirschsprung disease.

King operation—resection of the knee with placement of a Küntscher rod to fix the femur to the tibia, followed by a Syme amputation for the treatment of proximal focal femoral deficiency (PFFD).

Koch pouch diversion—a procedure involving bilateral ureteral diversion with anastomosis to a neobladder formed from an isolated ileal segment, combined with an ileal stoma and primary anastomosis of ileum to ileum.

Ladd operation—restoration of intestinal anatomy from a malrotated state; for the treatment of intestinal malrotation.

Lanz incision—an abdominal incision made in the left iliac fossa; for colostomy formation.

left hepatectomy—resection of the left hepatic lobe (medial and lateral segments).

Magpi procedure—distal advancement of the urethral meatus and granuloplasty; for the treatment of hypospadias.

Mainz pouch diversion—a procedure involving bilateral ureteral division with anastomosis to a neobladder formed from isolated cecum and terminal ileum; combined with an ileal stoma and primary anastomosis of the ileum to the right colon.

Martin modification (of Duhamel procedure)—right and transverse colectomy with ileoanal pull-through and side-to-side anastomosis of the remaining left colon to the ileum; procedure preserves some absorptive capacity of the large bowel; for the treatment of total colonic Hirschsprung disease.

McBurney (gridiron) incision—abdominal incision from the anterior superior iliac spine to the umbilicus; used for appendectomy.

Mikulicz procedure—a diverting enterostomy performed proximal to the meconium obstruction without resection; for the treatment of meconium ileus.

mini-Pena procedure—anterior sagittal anorectoplasty; for the treatment of anterior rectoperianal fistula (boys) or rectal-fourchette fistula (girls).

Mitrofanoff technique—a modification of neobladder diversion procedures, in which vascularized appendix is used to create the stoma.

Mustard technique—redirection of blood through an atrial septal defect (ASD) using a pericardial pathway; for the treatment of transposition of the great vessels; because of associated increased turbulence, this technique is not widely used today.

Mustarde procedure—correction, using simple mattress sutures, of a prominent ear with normal or absent antihelical folds.

Nissen fundoplication—a technique involving a 360-degree wrap of the gastric fundus around the gastroesophageal junction; for the treatment of incompetent lower esophageal sphincter; patient is rendered unable to vomit or belch.

Norwood procedure—a three-stage palliative procedure including (1) atrial septectomy, transection, and ligation of the pulmonary artery, "neoaorta" formation using the proximal pulmonary artery, and creation of a synthetic porto-aortal shunt; (2) creation of a Glenn shunt; and (3) performance of a modified Fontan procedure; for the treatment of hypoplastic left heart syndrome.

onlay island flap—a technique in which a flap of foreskin is used to elongate the urethra; for the treatment of hypospadias.

orchidopexy—testicular pull-down and attachment; for the treatment of undescended testis.

orthoplasty—surgical correction of excessive penile curvature.

parasitized cecal patch—see **Kimura procedure**.

Pena procedure—posterior sagittal anorectoplasty performed in children 1 to 6 months of age; for the treatment of imperforate anus.

Pfannenstiel incision—an abdominal incision used to gain access to the lower abdomen and bring pelvic organs within reach without dividing muscular tissue.

pharyngoplasty—elevation of the posterior pharyngeal wall following a primary cleft palate repair (to narrow the pharyngeal space); for the treatment of velopharyngeal incompetence.

Potts shunt—anastomosis of the descending aorta to the pulmonary artery for the permanent treatment of tetralogy of Fallot.

proximal splenorenal shunt—end-to-side anastomosis of the splenic vein to the left renal vein with splenectomy; for the treatment of portal hypertension.

pyeloplasty—resection of an atretic ureter with primary anastomosis to the renal pelvis; for the treatment of ureteropelvic junction obstruction.

Ramstedt operation—relaxation of the pyloric sphincter; for the treatment of pyloric stenosis.

Rashkind procedure—balloon atrial septostomy; for the treatment of palliation of the great vessels.

Rastelli repair—a technique involving the closure of a ventricular septal defect (VSD) with a patch and the creation of a conduit from the distal pulmonary artery to the right ventricle; for the treatment of transposition of the great vessels.

Ravitch procedure—a procedure involving (1) creation of osteotomies between the manubrium and costal cartilages, (2) a greenstick fracture of the manubrium, and (3) the temporary insertion (for 6 to 12 months) of a stabilizing bar; for the treatment of pectus excavatum or pectus carinatum.

right colon pouch—a procedure involving bilateral ureteral division with anastomosis to a neobladder (formed from an isolated segment of the right colon), combined with an ileal stoma and primary anastomosis of the ileum to the transverse colon.

right hepatectomy—resection of the right hepatic lobes (anterior and posterior segments).

rooftop (bilateral subcostal) incision—an abdominal incision used to access the liver and portal structures.

Roux-en-Y anastomosis—division of the jejunum distal to the ligament of Treitz with end-to-side anastomosis of the duodenum to the distal jejunum and anastomosis of the proximal jejunum (typically) to the bile duct.

S-pouch—the creation of an ileal reservoir in the distal ileum using an S-shaped configuration following colectomy.

Santulli-Blanc enterostomy—a modification of the Bishop-Koop procedure that involves the resection of a distal dilated bowel segment with side-to-end anastomosis to the proximal enterostomy; for the treatment of meconium ileus.

Senning procedure (venous switch)—technique involving intraatrial redirection of venous return so that systemic caval return is shunted through the mitral valve to the left ventricle, and pulmonary return is brought through the tricuspid valve to the right ventricle; for the treatment of transposition of the great vessels.

side-to-side portocaval shunt—a procedure in which the portal vein is anastomosed to the inferior vena cava; for the treatment of portal hypertension.

side-to-side splenorenal shunt—side-to-side anastomosis of the splenic vein to the left renal vein; for the treatment of portal hypertension.

Sistrunk operation—complete excision of a thyroglossal duct cyst.

Soave procedure—a technique involving endorectal pull-through; for the correction of rectal resection.

Stamm gastrostomy—placement of an open gastrostomy tube; the opening is designed to close spontaneously on removal of the tube.

Sting procedure—subureteric Teflon injection; for the endoscopic correction of vesicoureteral reflux.

Sugiura procedure—a technique that involves lower esophageal transection and primary anastomosis, devascularization of the lower esophagus and stomach, and splenectomy; for the treatment of esophageal varices.

Swenson procedure—resection of the posterior rectal wall to the dentate line (aganglionic region); for the treatment of Hirschsprung disease; technically difficult and rarely performed.

Syme amputation—amputation of the foot, calculated to bring the end of the stump above the opposite knee at maturity; for the treatment of proximal focal femoral deficiency (PFFD).

Thal procedure—a procedure involving a 180-degree anterior wrap of the gastric fundus around the gastroesophageal junction, preserving the patient's ability to vomit and belch; for the treatment of incompetent lower esophageal sphincter.

Thiersch operation—a procedure in which a distal rectal segment that has prolapsed is approximated to the external sphincter muscle; for the treatment of rectal prolapse.

trisegmentectomy—resection of the right hepatic lobe and the quadrate lobe of the liver (right posterior segment, right anterior segment, and medial segment).

ureteropyelostomy—partial resection and side-to-side anastomosis of a partially duplicated ureter.

uretocalycostomy—a technique for the treatment of urinary obstruction involving division of the ureter (distal to the obstruction) and intrarenal anastomosis to the most dependent renal calyx; when the renal pelvis is insufficient for anastomosis, the lower pole of the kidney is resected.

vaginal switch operation—a procedure in which the vagina is separated from the urinary tract; for treatment of duplicated vagina.

Van Ness procedure—rotational 180-degree osteotomy of the femur in which the foot and ankle are brought to the level of the opposite knee; for prosthetic attachment for the treatment of femoral deficiency.

venous switch—see **Senning procedure.**

ventricular shunt procedure—a procedure in which a Silastic catheter is positioned in a lateral ventricle and tunneled subcutaneously to drain into the central venous system or peritoneal cavity; for the treatment of hydrocephalus

Warren (distal splenorenal) shunt—a procedure in which the splenic vein is anastomosed to the left renal vein; for the treatment of portal hypertension.

Waterston aortopulmonary anastomosis—a procedure involving anastomosis of the ascending aorta and the right pulmonary artery; for the temporary treatment of tetralogy of Fallot.

Whipple procedure—resection of the pancreatic head, duodenum, and gallbladder with gastrojejunostomy, hepatojejunostomy, and pancreaticojejunostomy.

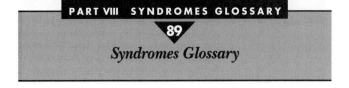

4p syndrome—characterized by a round face, prominent nasal tip, polydactyly, and scoliosis.

5p syndrome—characterized by macrocephaly; small mandible; long, thin fingers; short, big toes; and anorectal and renal anomalies.

13q syndrome—typically involves malformations of the brain, heart, kidneys, and digits; usually lethal.

Aagene syndrome—hereditary (autosomal-recessive transmission); characterized by recurrent intrahepatic cholestasis, with lymphedema.

Aarskog syndrome—an x-linked recessive disorder characterized by short stature, and musculoskeletal and genital anomalies of unknown etiology. Physical features include short stature (90%), hypertelorism, small nose with anteverted nares, broad philtrum and nasal bridge, abnormal auricles and widow's peak, brachyclinodactyly (80%), broad feet with bulbous toes (75%), simian crease (70%), ptosis (50%), syndactyly (60%), "shawl" scrotum (80%), cryptorchidism (75%), inguinal hernia (60%), hyperopic astigmatism, large corneas, ophthalmoplegia, strabismus, delayed puberty, mild pectus excavatum, prominent umbilicus. Radiographs show delayed bone age.

abetalipoproteinemia—recessive transmission; characterized by progressive cerebellar ataxia and pigmentary degeneration of the retina (starts with malabsorption of fat and progresses to ataxia); absent or reduced lipoproteins and low carotene, vitamin A, and cholesterol levels; and acanthocytosis [spiny projections on red blood cells (RBCs)].

acanthosis nigricans (Lawrence-Seip syndrome)—characterized by hyperpigmented lichenoid plaques in the neck and axilla; may be associated with insulin resistance.

acrodermatitis enteropathica—autosomal-recessive transmission; characterized by zinc deficiency, vesicobullous and eczematous skin lesions in the perioral and perineal areas, cheeks, knees, and elbows; photophobia, conjunctivitis and corneal dystrophy; chronic diarrhea; glossitis; nail dystrophy; growth retardation; and superinfections and *Candida* infections.

Adie syndrome—characterized by a large pupil with little or no reaction to light; pupil may react to accommodation; patients have hyperreflexia.

agenesis of corpus callosum—cause unknown (rarely, X-linked recessive); absence of the major tracts connecting the right and left hemispheres is usually associated with hydrocephalus, seizures, developmental delay, abnormal head size, and hypertelorism.

Alagille syndrome (arteriohepatic dysplasia)—characterized by paucity or absence of intrahepatic bile ducts with progressive destruction of bile ducts; patients have a broad forehead, deep-set eyes that are widely spaced and underdeveloped, a small, pointed mandible, cardiac lesions, vertebral arch defects, and changes in the renal tubules and interstitium.

Albers-Schönberg disease (osteopetrosis tarda, marble bone disease)—most cases are autosomal dominant, a few are autosomal recessive; patients are prone to fractures and have mild anemia and craniofacial disproportion; radiologic changes include increased cortical bone density, longitudinal and transverse dense striations at the ends of the long bones, lucent and dense bands in the vertebrae, and thickening at the base of the skull.

Albright syndrome—see **McCune-Albright syndrome.**

Alexander disease—unknown pathogenesis; characterized by megaloencephaly in infants, dementia, spasticity and ataxia; may cause seizures in younger children; patients become mute, immobile, and dependent; hyaline eosinophilic inclusions occur in the footplates of astrocytes in subpial and subependymal regions.

Alport syndrome—several forms are hereditary male-to-male autosomal dominant, and an X-linked form also exists; characterized by neurosensory deafness and progressive renal failure.

Anderson disease (glycogen storage disease, type IV)—caused by a defect in the glycogen branching enzyme 1, 4-α-glucan branching enzyme; characterized by hepatomegaly and failure to thrive in the first few months, progressing to liver cirrhosis and splenomegaly.

Apert syndrome (acrocephalosyndactyly)—autosomal dominant; characterized by high and flat frontal bones, underdevelopment of the middle third of the face, hypertelorism and proptosis; a narrow, high, arched palate; a short, beaked nose; and syndactyly of the toes and digits.

arthrogryposis multiplex congenita—characterized by fixed contractures of the middle joints; present at birth.

Asperger syndrome—a developmental disorder on the higher-functioning end of the autism spectrum. These patients, often viewed as brilliant, eccentric, and physically awkward, fail to develop relationships with peers, have repetitive and stereotyped behaviors, usually with hand movements. See *www.aspergersyndrome.org.*

Bart syndrome—autosomal dominant; congenital aplasia of the skin; characterized by nail defects and recurrent blistering of the skin and mucous membranes.

Bartter syndrome—hypertrophy of the juxtaglomerular apparatus; characterized by hypokalemic alkalosis, hypochloremia, and hyperaldosteronism; patients have normal blood pressure but the renin level is elevated; may lead to mental retardation and small stature.

Beckwith-Wiedemann syndrome—characterized by hypoglycemia, macrosomia, and visceromegaly; patients have umbilical anomalies and renal medullary dysplasia.

Behçet syndrome—unknown cause; involves relapsing iridocyclitis and recurrent oral and genital ulcerations; 50% of patients have arthritis.

blind loop syndrome—stasis of small intestine, usually secondary to incomplete bowel obstruction or a problem of intestinal motility.

Bloch-Sulzberger syndrome (incontinentia pigmenti)—characterized by mental retardation; one third of patients have seizures and ocular malformations.

Bloom syndrome—autosomal recessive; characterized by erythema and telangiectasia in a butterfly distribution, photosensitivity, and dwarfism.

Blount disease (tibia vara)—characterized by irregularity of the medial aspect of the tibial metaphysis adjacent to the epiphysis; bowing starts as angulation at the metaphysis.

blue diaper syndrome—defective tryptophan absorption; characterized by bluish stains on the diapers, digestive disturbances, fever, and visual difficulties.

Brill disease (Brill-Zinsser disease)—repeat episode of typhus; caused by a *Rickettsia* infection.

bronchiolitis obliterans—begins with necrotizing pneumonia secondary to viral infection (e.g., adenovirus, influenza, measles); tuberculosis (TB); or inhalation of fumes, talcum powder, or zinc; and involves the obstruction of small bronchi and bronchioles by fibrous tissue.

Byler disease—autosomal-recessive familial cholestasis; characterized by hepatomegaly, pruritus, splenomegaly, elevated bile acids, and gallstones.

Caroli disease—autosomal recessive; cystic dilatation of the intrahepatic bile ducts; characterized by recurrent bouts of cholangitis and biliary abscesses secondary to bile stasis and gallstones.

cat's eye syndrome—autosomal dominant; characterized by ocular coloboma, down-slanting eyes, congenital heart disease, and anal atresia.

Charcot-Marie-Tooth disease (peroneal muscular atrophy)—most common cause of chronic peripheral neuropathy; characterized by foot drop, high-arch foot; patients may have stocking-glove sensory loss.

Chèdiak-Higashi syndrome—autosomal-recessive disorder; involves partial oculocutaneous albinism, increased susceptibility to infection, lack of natural killer cells, and large, lysosome-like granules in many tissues; patients have splenomegaly, hypersplenism, hepatomegaly, lymphadenopathy, nystagmus photophobia, and peripheral neuropathy.

Coat disease—telangiectasia of retinal vessels, with subretinal exudate.

Cobb syndrome—intraspinous vascular anomaly and port-wine stains.

Cockayne syndrome—autosomal recessive; characterized by dwarfism, mental retardation, bird-like facies, premature senility, and photosensitivity.

Cornelia de Lange syndrome—prenatal growth retardation; characterized by microcephaly, hirsutism, anteverted nares, down-turned mouth, mental retardation, and congenital heart defects.

cri du chat syndrome—characterized by growth retardation, mental deficiency, hypotonia, microcephaly, round "moon face," hypertelorism, epicanthal folds, and down-slanting palpebral fissures.

Crigler-Najjar syndrome (congenital nonhemolytic unconjugated hyperbilirubinemia)—type 1 is recessive; a deficiency of uridine diphosphate (UDP) glucuronyl transferase causes a rapid increase in the unconjugated bilirubin level on the first day of life; no hemolysis occurs and patients have no conjugation activity; type 2 is autosomal dominant and is characterized by variable penetrance and partial activity of UDP glucuronyl transferase.

Cronkhite-Canada syndrome—diffuse intestinal polyps involving large and small intestine; characterized by alopecia, brown skin lesions, and onychatrophia; patients have diarrhea and protein-losing enteropathy (PLE).

Crouzon syndrome (craniofacial dysostosis)—autosomal dominant with a range of expressivity; characterized by exophthalmos, hypertelorism, and hypoplasia of maxilla; patients have oral cavity anomalies and premature closure of the external auditory meatus.

cyclic neutropenia—syndrome involving lack of granulocyte macrophage colony-stimulating factor (GM-CSF); characterized by fever, mouth lesions, cervical adenitis, and gastroenteritis occurring every 3 to 6 weeks; neutrophil count may be zero.

de Toni-Fanconi-Debré acute syndrome—fatal; infantile myopathy with renal dysfunction; involves abnormal mitochondria and lipid and glycogen accumulation; patient has weak cry, poor muscle tone, poor suck, and lactic acidosis.

De Sanctis-Cacchione syndrome—autosomal recessive; characterized by xeroderma pigmentosum with mental retardation, dwarfism, and hypogonadism; skin is unable to repair itself after exposure to ultraviolet light; patients may have erythema, scaling bullae, crusting telangiectasia keratoses, photophobia, corneal opacities, and tumors of the eyelids.

Diamond-Blackfan syndrome (congenital hypoplastic anemia)—failure of erythropoiesis; characterized by macrocytic anemia; patients have anemia, pallor, and weakness, no hepatomegaly, elevated fetal hemoglobin, and defect in abduction with retraction of the eye on adduction.

DiGeorge syndrome—thymic hypoplasia with hypocalcemia; patients have tetany, abnormal facies, congenital heart disease, and increased incidence of infection.

Dubin-Johnson syndrome—autosomal recessive; characterized by elevated conjugated bilirubin, large amounts of coproporphyrin I in urine, and deposits of melanin-like pigment in hepatocellular lysosomes.

Dubowitz syndrome—Children with this syndrome nearly always have a history of intrauterine growth retardation involving both low birth weight and reduced length. Primary microcephaly. Facial characteristics include triangular face; small, receding chin; and broad and sometimes flat nasal bridge. As the child matures, the nasal bridge appears less wide and often becomes prominent, producing a continuous line with the forehead when viewed in profile. Tip of nose is frequently wide, rounded, or prominent, hypertelorism, shortened palpebral fissure that may be slanted, ptosis, sloping and high forehead, scanty hair and eyebrows, ear abnormalities.

Eagle-Barrett syndrome (prune-belly syndrome)—characterized by deficiency of the abdominal musculature, dilatation and dysplasia of the urinary tract, cryptorchidism, dilatation of the posterior urethra, and a hypoplastic or absent prostate.

ectodermal dysplasia—characterized by the poor development, or absence, of teeth, nails, hair, and sweat glands; patients have hyperextensible skin, hypermobile joints, and easy bruisability.

Eisenmenger syndrome—characterized by ventricular septal defect (VSD) with pulmonary hypertension.

Fabry disease—X-linked, lipid storage disease; involves a defect of the ceramide trihexoside α-galactosidase; characterized by tingling and burning in the hands and feet; small, red maculopapular lesions on the buttocks, inguinal area, fingernails, and lips; and an inability to perspire; patients have proteinuria, progressing to renal failure.

Farber syndrome—autosomal recessive; involves a deficiency of acid ceramidase; characterized by hoarseness; painful, swollen joints; and palpable nodules over affected joints and pressure points.

fetal alcohol syndrome—characterized by a small body, head, and maxillary bone; abnormal palpebral fissures; epicanthal folds; cardiac septal defect; delayed development; and mental deficiency.

fetal hydantoin syndrome—characterized by hypoplasia of the midface, low nasal bridge, ocular hypertelorism, cupid bow upper lip; patients experience slow growth, may have mental retardation, cleft lip, and cardiac malformation.

Friedreich ataxia—mostly autosomal recessive; appears in late childhood or in adolescence; involves progressive cerebellar and spinal cord dysfunction; patients have high-arched foot, hammer toes, and cardiac failure.

fructose intolerance, hereditary—autosomal recessive; involves deficiency of fructose-1-phosphate aldolase or fructose 1,6-diphosphatase; characterized by vomiting, diarrhea, hypoglycemic seizures, and jaundice.

Gardner syndrome—characterized by multiple gastrointestinal polyps with malignant transformation, skin cysts, and multiple osteoma.

Gaucher disease—abnormal storage of glucosylceramide in the reticuloendothelial system; three types: (1) adult, or chronic, (2) acute neuropathic, or infantile, (3) subacute neuropathic, or juvenile; characterized by splenomegaly, hepatomegaly, delayed development, strabismus, swallowing difficulties, laryngeal spasm, opisthotonos, and bone pain.

Gianotti-Crosti syndrome—papular acrodermatitis and hepatitis B virus (HBV) infection; usually benign and self-limited.

Gilles de la Tourette syndrome—dominant trait with partial penetrance; characterized by multiple tics (e.g., blinking, twitching, grimacing) and involvement of muscles of swallowing and respiration; patient may exhibit swearing behavior and may have learning disabilities.

Glanzmann disease—autosomal recessive; involves defective primary platelet aggregation (size and survival of platelets is normal).

Goldenhar syndrome—characterized by oculoauriculovertebral dysplasia and mandibular hypoplasia; patients have a hypoplastic zygomatic arch; malformed, displaced pinnae, and hearing loss.

Goltz syndrome—focal dermal hypoplasia; herniations of fat through thinned dermis produce tan papillomas associated with other skin defects and skeletal anomalies (e.g., syndactyly, polydactyly, spinal defects); patients also have colobomas, strabismus, and nystagmus.

Gradenigo syndrome—acquired palsy of the abducens nerve and pain in the trigeminal nerve distribution, usually occurs after otitis media; produces diplopia, ocular and facial pain, photophobia, and lacrimation.

Hand-Schüller-Christian disease—see **histiocytosis X.**

Hartnup disease—autosomal recessive defect in transport of monoamine monocarboxylic amino acids by intestinal mucosa and renal tubules; characterized by photosensitivity and a pellagra-like skin rash; patients may have cerebellar ataxia.

histiocytosis X—(reticuloendotheliosis) formerly called eosinophilic granuloma, Hand-Schüller-Christian disease, or Letterer-Siwe disease; patients may have a few solitary bone lesions or seborrheic dermatitis of scalp, lymphadenopathy, hepatosplenomegaly, tooth loss, exophthalmos, or pulmonary infiltrates.

Hunter syndrome (mucopolysaccharidosis II)—X-linked recessive; characterized by an accumulation of heparan sulfate and dermatan sulfate and enzyme deficiency of L-iduronate sulfatase.

Hurler syndrome (mucopolysaccharidosis IH)—autosomal recessive; characterized by an accumulation of heparan sulfate and dermatan sulfate, and enzyme deficiency of α-L-iduronidase.

hyper-IgE—characterized by recurrent deep tissue and skin staphylococcal infections; patients have eosinophilia and IgE levels that are 10 times greater than normal.

incontinentia pigmenti—see **Bloch-Sulzberger syndrome.**

Jeune thoracic dystrophy—characterized by respiratory distress, short limbs, and polydactyly; may progress to renal insufficiency.

Job syndrome—characterized by severe staphylococcal infections, chronic skin disease, and cold abscesses; patients may have elevated IgE.

Kallmann syndrome—familial; characterized by isolated gonadotropin deficiency and anosmia.

Kartagener syndrome—characterized by sinusitis, bronchiectasis, and immotile cilia.

Kasabach-Merritt syndrome—characterized by hemangioma and consumption coagulopathy, platelet trapping, and microangiopathic hemolytic anemia.

Kleine-Levin syndrome—characterized by unusual hunger, somnolence, and motor restlessness.

Klinefelter syndrome—XXY karyotype; characterized by seminiferous tubule dysgenesis, testicular atrophy, eunuchoid habitus, and gynecomastia.

Klippel-Feil syndrome—characterized by a short neck, limited neck motion, and low occipital hairline.

Krabbe leukodystrophy—autosomal recessive; characterized by cerebroside lipidosis and lack of myelin in white matter; usually presents by age 1 year; patients have hyperreflexia, rigidity, swallowing difficulties, lack of development.

Larsen syndrome—usually autosomal dominant; characterized by hyperlaxity, multiple dislocations, and skin hyperplexity.

Laurence-Moon-Biedl syndrome—characterized by retinitis pigmentosa, polydactyly, obesity, and hypogonadism.

Lennox-Gastaut syndrome (childhood epileptic encephalopathy)—characterized by severe seizures, mental retardation, and characteristic electroencephalography (EEG) pattern (i.e., generalized bilaterally synchronous sharp wave and slow wave complexes); patients have seizures starting in infancy; condition is difficult to treat; mental retardation is common.

Lesch-Nyhan syndrome—X-linked recessive disorder; characterized by a defect in purine metabolism; patients have hyperuricemia as a result of diminished or absent hypoxanthine guanine phosphoribosyl transferase (HG-PRT) activity, choreoathetosis, compulsive self-mutilation, mental retardation, and growth failure.

Letterer-Siwe disease—component of histiocytosis X; characterized by acute disseminated histiocytosis; patients have seborrheic-looking skin lesions, bone lesions, gingival lesions, and liver and lung infiltrates.

Lowe syndrome (oculocerebral dystrophy)—X-linked recessive; patients have congenital cataracts, glaucoma, hypotonia, hyperreflexia, severe mental retardation, rickets, osteopenia, pathologic fractures, aminoaciduria, and organic aciduria.

Maffucci syndrome—multiple enchondromata and hemangioma of the bone and overlying skin; patients have short stature, skeletal deformities, scoliosis, and limb disproportion.

Marfan syndrome—connective tissue disorder characterized by ectopia lentis; dilatation of the aorta; long, thin extremities; pectus excavatum or carinatum; scoliosis; and pneumothorax.

McCune-Albright syndrome—polyostotic fibrous dysplasia; found more commonly in girls and in patients living on the coast of Maine; characterized by prominent skin discoloration with ragged edges; patients may have precocious puberty, hyperthyroidism, gigantism headaches, epilepsy, and mental deficiency.

MELAS syndrome—*mi*tochondrial *e*ncephalopathy, *la*ctic *a*cidosis, and *s*troke-like episodes; causes seizures, alternating hemiparesis, hemianopsia, or cortical blindness; patients have lactic acidosis, spongy degeneration of the brain, sensorineural hearing loss, and short stature.

Menkes syndrome—X-linked recessive; patients have short scalp hair, hypopigmentation, hypothermia, growth failure, skeletal defects, arterial aneurysms, seizures, and progressive central nervous system (CNS) failure.

Möbius syndrome—characterized by cranial nerve defects and a hypoplastic tongue or digits.

Morquio syndrome (mucopolysaccharidosis)—characterized by severe skeletal deformities, pectus carinatum, kyphoscoliosis, short neck, hypoplasia of the odontoid processes, C1 and C2 dislocation, neurosensory deafness, and aortic insufficiency.

multiple cartilaginous exostosis—characterized by bony projections near the ends of the tubular bones and ribs, scapula, vertebral bodies, and iliac crest; the exostoses become calcified and cause skeletal deformities; appears after the age of 3 years.

nail-patella syndrome—autosomal dominant; characterized by dystrophic and hypoplastic nails, hypoplastic patellae and iliac horns, and malformed radial heads; may lead to nephrotic syndrome and renal failure.

Niemann-Pick disease—four types; storage of sphingomyelin and cholesterol causes hepatomegaly; patients are normal at birth but experience delayed development; 50% have a macular cherry red spot.

Noonan syndrome—normal karyotype; syndrome is characterized by cardiac lesions [atrial septal defect (ASD) or pulmonic stenosis]; facial changes (palpebral slant, broad flat nose); webbed neck; short stature; a high, arched palate; and malformed ears.

Osler-Weber-Rendu syndrome—hereditary hemorrhagic telangiectasia; patients have telangiectasia in the skin, respiratory tract mucosa, lips, nails, conjunctiva, and nasal and oral mucosae.

Parinaud syndrome—characterized by weakness of upward gaze, poor convergence and accommodation, refractive nystagmus with upward gaze, and pupillary changes.

Patau syndrome—see **trisomy 13**.

Pelizaeus-Merzbacher disease—characterized by dancing eye movements, delayed motor development and spasticity, small head, poor head control, and possible optic atrophy and seizures.

Peutz-Jeghers syndrome—autosomal dominant; patients have bluish-black macules around the mouth and intestinal polyposis in the small bowel.

Pickwickian syndrome—characterized by obesity and hypoventilation syndrome; patients may have respiratory arrest, restless sleep.

Pierre Robin syndrome—characterized by severe micrognathia, glossoptosis, and cleft palate.

Poland syndrome—characterized by a unilateral hypoplastic pectoral muscle with ipsilateral upper limb deficiency, syndactyly, and a defect of the subclavian artery.

Prader-Willi syndrome—characterized by hypotonia, hypomentia, hypogonadism, obesity, narrow bifrontal diameter, and hypotonia; patients may have a deletion in chromosome 15.

progeria—characterized by premature aging, severe growth failure, atherosclerosis, alopecia, and dystrophic nails.

prune-belly syndrome—see **Eagle-Barrett syndrome**.

Rieger syndrome—sporadic autosomal dominant; characterized by microcornea with opacity, iris hypoplasia, anterior synechiae, hypodontia, and maxillary hypoplasia.

Riley-Day syndrome—familial dysautonomia; affects sensory and autonomic functions; patients have poor feeding, aspiration, no tears, high threshold to pain, markedly decreased reflexes, smooth tongue and impaired taste, and erratic blood pressure and temperature.

Rotor syndrome—autosomal recessive; characterized by elevated conjugated bilirubin, elevated coproporphyrin I and coproporphyrin in urine, and normal liver biopsies.

Rubinstein-Taybi syndrome—characterized by broad thumbs and toes, short stature, mental retardation, beaked nose, hypoplastic mandible, and congenital heart defect.

Russell-Silver dwarf syndrome—characterized by intrauterine growth retardation (IUGR), subnormal growth velocity, triangular facies, clinodactyly, simian creases, and genitourinary malformations.

Sandhoff GM$_2$-gangliosidosis type II—characterized by deficient hexosaminidase activity leading to cherry red spot in macula, failure to develop motor skills, blindness, weakness, and seizures.

Sanfilippo type A syndrome (mucopolysaccharidosis IIIA)—autosomal recessive; characterized by accumulation of heparan sulfate, dermatan sulfate, and sulfatidase.

Sanfilippo type B syndrome (mucopolysaccharidosis IIIA)—autosomal recessive; characterized by accumulation of heparan sulfate, dermatan sulfate, and α-*N*-acetylglucosaminidase.

Scheie syndrome (mucopolysaccharidosis IS)—autosomal recessive; characterized by accumulation of heparan sulfate and dermatan sulfate, and an enzyme defect affecting α-L-iduronidase.

scimitar syndrome—characterized by hypoplasia of the right lung with systemic arterial supply, anomalous right pulmonary vein, and dextroposition of heart.

Seckel syndrome—characterized by intrauterine growth retardation (IUGR), microcephaly, sharp facial features with underdeveloped chin, and mental retardation.

Shwachman syndrome—characterized by pancreatic dysfunction, short stature, bone marrow dysfunction, and skeletal abnormalities.

silo filler disease—acute pneumonitis caused by inhalation of nitrogen dioxide; patients have chills, fever, cough, dyspnea, and cyanosis; associated with a high mortality rate.

Smith-Lemli-Opitz syndrome—characterized by short stature, microcephaly, ptosis, anteverted nares, micrognathia, syndactyly, cryptorchidism, and mental retardation.

Sotos syndrome—characterized by cerebral gigantism, large head and ears, prominent mandible, mental retardation, and poor coordination.

Stickler syndrome—autosomal dominant; characterized by high myopia, cataract formation, and retinal detachment.

Sturge-Weber syndrome—characterized by a port-wine stain on the face at the first branch of the trigeminal nerve; patients have seizures and mental retardation.

Swyer-James syndrome—characterized by unilateral hyperlucent lung following bronchiolitis obliterans.

Tourette syndrome—see **Gilles de la Tourette syndrome.**

Treacher Collins syndrome—autosomal dominant with incomplete penetration; characterized by mandibulofacial dysostosis; patients have hypoplastic mandible; hypoplastic zygomatic arches; antimongoloid slant to eyes; deformities of the pinna; and a high, arched palate with or without cleft palate.

trisomy 9—characterized by deep-set eyes, bulbous nasal tip, an anxious facial expression, and cleft lip.

trisomy 13 (Patau syndrome)—characterized by cleft lip, microphthalmia, postaxial polydactyly, and cardiovascular anomalies.

trisomy 18—characterized by a small face, high nasal bridge, short palpebral fissures, micrognathia, small mouth, overriding fingers, and hypoplastic nails; patients have mental retardation and intrauterine growth retardation (IUGR).

tuberous sclerosis—characterized by epiloia; patients have seizures, mental deficiency, adenoma sebaceum foci of intracranial calcification, hypopigmented macules, ash leaf spots, connective tissue nevi (shagreen spots), adenoma sebaceum, and angiofibroma.

Turcot syndrome—characterized by adenomatous colonic polyposis associated with malignant brain tumors, especially glioblastomas.

Turner syndrome—characterized by gonadal dysplasia (streak gonads stem from XO karyotype), short stature, sexual infantilism, atypical facies, low hairline, webbed neck, congenital lymphedema of the extremities, coarctation of the aorta, and increased carrying angle.

Usher syndrome—autosomal recessive; characterized by retinitis pigmentosa, cataracts, and sensorineural deafness.

vanishing testes syndrome—characterized by bilateral gonadal failure with normal external male genitalia, normal 46,XY karyotype, absent testes, and no male puberty.

VATER syndrome—syndrome involving *v*ertebral defects, *a*nal atresia, *t*racheo*e*sophageal atresia, *r*adial dysplasia, *r*enal dysplasia, and congenital heart defect.

Vogt-Koyanagi-Harada syndrome—characterized by vitiligo, uveitis, dysacousia, and aseptic meningitis.

von Gierke disease (type 1 glycogenosis)—glucose-6-phosphate dehydrogenase (G6PD) is absent in the liver, kidney, and intestinal mucosa; characterized by hypoglycemia under stress (e.g., fasting), hepatomegaly, and seizures.

von Hippel–Landau disease—autosomal dominant (linked to chromosome 3); characterized by hemangioblastoma of the cerebellum and retina; patients have cystic cerebellar neoplasm with increased intracranial pressure (ICP).

Waardenburg syndrome—autosomal dominant; characterized by white forelock, heterochromic irides, displacement of the inner canthi, broad nasal root, and confluent eyebrows.

Wegener granulomatosis—necrotizing granulomatous vasculitis of the arteries and veins; involves airways, lungs, and kidneys with resultant rhinorrhea, nasal ulceration, hemoptysis, and cough; patients have hematuria caused by necrotizing vasculitis.

Werner syndrome—autosomal recessive; characterized by short stature, juvenile cataracts, hypogonadism, gray hair in second decade.

Williams syndrome—characterized by mental retardation, hypoplastic nails, periorbital fullness, supravalvular aortic stenosis, growth delay, and stellate iris.

Wilson-Mikity syndrome—characterized by pulmonary immaturity; occurs in premature infants; patients have slow onset of respiratory distress, retractions, and apnea; may clear in several weeks.

Wiskott-Aldrich syndrome—characterized by thrombocytopenia, severe eczema, and recurrent skin infections.

Wolff-Parkinson-White syndrome—characterized by a short PR interval and slow upstroke of the QRS-delta wave; usually occurs in patients with a normal heart but also may occur in patients with Ebstein anomaly and cardiomyopathy.

Wolman disease—fatal condition characterized by primary xanthomatosis, adrenal insufficiency, vomiting, failure to thrive, steatorrhea, hepatomegaly, and adrenal calcification.

Zellweger syndrome—cerebrohepatorenal syndrome; characterized by hepatic fibrosis and cirrhosis; patients have seizures, mental retardation, hypotonia, glaucoma, congenital stippled epiphyses, and cysts of the renal cortex.

Zollinger-Ellison syndrome—characterized by islet cell tumors that produce duodenal and jejunal ulcers; patients have high gastrin levels and excessive acid secretion.

Page numbers in *italics* indicate figures. Page numbers followed by "t" indicate tables.